SKIN DEEP

SKIN DEEP

Third Edition

Carol Turkington
Jeffrey S. Dover, M.D.

Medical Illustrations
Birck Cox

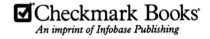
Checkmark Books®
An imprint of Infobase Publishing

To the memory of Dottie Kennedy,
for her unfailing support

Skin Deep, Third Edition

Copyright © 1996, 2002, 2007 by Carol Turkington

Checkmark Books
An imprint of Infobase Publishing
132 West 31st Street
New York NY 10001

Library of Congress Cataloging-in-Publication Data

Turkington, Carol.
Skin deep / Carol Turkington, Jeffrey S. Dover ; medical illustrations, Birck Cox.— 3rd ed.
p. cm.
Includes index.
ISBN 0-8160-6403-2 (hc: alk. paper) — ISBN 0-8160-6404-0 (pbk. : alk. paper)
1. Dermatology—Encyclopedias. 2. Skin—Diseases—Encyclopedias. 3. Skin—Encyclopedias.
I. Dover, Jeffrey S. II. Title.
RL41.T87 2006
616.5003—dc22   2005057402

Text design by Cathy Rincon
Cover design by Salvatore Luongo

Printed in the United States of America

VB FOF 10 9 8 7 6 5 4 3 2 1

This book is printed on acid-free paper.

CONTENTS

FOREWORD

The future of skin disease prevention and treatment is bright. Better understanding of the genetics of disease will help researchers to discover the causes of many common ailments, and continued technological developments will ensure even better treatments. The major advances in dermatology over the last decade include revolutionary anti-acne medication and drugs that combat immune diseases; advances in skin cancer awareness; new lasers and light sources engineered to improve skin appearance, texture, and tone; and the development of Botulinum Exotoxin A and fillers to decrease facial lines and creases.

The single most notable event in the field of acne treatment was the crucial discovery of isotretinoin in 1979 for the treatment of severe acne. This drug's approval in 1982 revolutionized therapy; today the drug remains the treatment of choice for resistant severe nodular cystic acne, although it is under increasing regulatory scrutiny because of uncommon but potentially significant side effects of birth defects and depression. Isotretinoin belongs to a class of compounds called retinoids, which are vitamin A derivatives. It is the only truly effective treatment against severe cystic acne and has been shown to prevent scarring, a disastrous result of acne. Isotretinoin affects the sebaceous gland, suppressing sebum production to preteen levels and causes a decrease in the levels of bacteria responsible for acne. It also promotes shedding of skin cells. Isotretinoin can reduce acne by 90 percent or more within three months. Its effects are prolonged, lasting months to years after a 20-week course, a result unable to be achieved by any other acne medication. Some side effects from isotretinoin are seen in most of its users, but usually resolve one to three weeks after treatment. These include dryness of the skin, mouth, and membranes, as well as chapped lips and patches of eczema. Fragile skin and susceptibility to sunburn are frequently reported. Dry eyes, nosebleeds, hair shedding, muscle and joint pains are common. Bone and blood lipid abnormalities can also occur. Recently, depression and suicide have been reported among patients taking isotretinoin, although in the past some studies had shown an improvement in emotional well-being. Whether isotretinoin plays a role in depression is unclear. A recent large study failed to show an increased risk of depression in isotretinoin users compared with other acne patients.

One of the most significant problems with isotretinoin is its risk of the development of serious birth defects in the infants of women who conceive while on treatment. This requires that no woman being put on the drug become pregnant under any circumstances. To prevent pregnancy in women undergoing isotretinoin treatment, contraceptive counseling prior to starting treatment is essential, and strict monitoring of women of childbearing age during the treatment course is performed. Two negative pregnancy tests are required prior to the start of therapy, and monthly testing is compulsory for sexually active females during treatment. Guidelines suggest that pregnancy is safe one month after stopping the drug.

Immunologic Drugs

IFN-a Interferon alpha is an agent that can modulate the immune system used in the treatment of cancers of the blood, immune diseases, and in the treatment of genital warts. A large number of new clinical uses of interferon are being developed. The recent introduction of interferon alpha into current therapies for malignant melanoma is notable. As immune control mechanisms seem to be important in the behavior of melanoma, biological agents have been the subject of many studies involving treatment. Results suggest that interferon alpha may be beneficial, most clearly in preventing recurrence but also perhaps in overall survival. Further studies are needed in order to determine its benefit, and it cannot yet be recommended as a standard therapy in high-risk malignant melanoma, although it remains a promising mode of treatment.

Topical Immunomodulators Imiquimod cream induces the release of interferons and has been approved in the United States for the treatment of genital warts, as well as actinic keratoses (pre–skin cancers). Research also shows that it is effective in the treatment of superficial spreading basal cell carcinoma, a slowly growing local type of skin cancer; studies are currently under way that examine its effectiveness in the treatment of precancerous skin growths due to the sun, nongenital warts, molluscum, and alopecia areata.

Tacrolimus ointment (Protopic) and pimecrolimus cream (Elidel) are powerful topical anti-inflammatory agents approved for the treatment of eczema. The greatest development in the treatment of eczema since the discovery of steroids in the 1950s, its major advantage over topical corticosteroids, the mainstay of treatment of atopic dermatitis treatment, is that it is not associated with the development of the side effects such as thinning of the skin and the formation of prominent blood vessels and stretch marks. These new agents are particularly useful at sites where the skin is more delicate, such as the face, groin, and underarms. They should be used only on the affected area until it clears and then treatment should be discontinued until the next outbreak in an effort to reduce the risk of overuse of these highly effective treatments.

Systemic Biologics

Recent advances in technology have led to a proliferation of new strategies for treating diseases with agents that can be designed to act specifically on the immune system and may prove to be safer than traditional therapies. Biologic agents are proteins that can be extracted from animal tissue or synthesized in the laboratory. These medications are divided into two categories: monoclonal antibodies and fusion receptor proteins. Monoclonal antibodies are usually derived from mouse antibodies and engineered to be better tolerated by human beings. Fusion receptor proteins are human antibodies that are constructed in the laboratory from components that are not normally combined by the human body.

Over the last decade, immune mediated diseases such as Crohn's disease and rheumatoid arthritis have been successfully treated with biologic agents. In 2003 the Food and Drug Administration (FDA) approved alefacept, a fusion receptor protein, for the treatment of moderate to severe psoriasis. This drug reduces the number and function of specific white blood cells important in inflammatory reactions of the skin. Efulizumab, an example of a monoclonal antibody, similarly decreases the ability of white blood cells to participate in inflammation. Etanercept, a fusion receptor protein, binds the inflammatory molecule tumor necrosis factor-alpha (TNF-a). The reduction of TNF-a leads to the improvement of many inflammatory disorders of the skin.

These three drugs have been approved for the treatment of moderate to severe psoriasis. Other biologics, such as adalimumab and infliximab, have been used to successfully treat psoriasis, though they are not approved by the FDA for this use. Many of these biologics have demonstrated the ability to improve other inflammatory diseases of the skin such as hidradenitis suppurativa and pyoderma gangrenosum. These agents and their effectiveness in treating other diseases will remain an area of intense investigation in the future.

Systemic biologics are an exciting new option in the management of some skin diseases. These drugs are significantly more expensive than traditional systemic medications such as methotrexate and acitretin, though they may prove to be safer for chronic use. Long-term evaluation of the cost effectiveness and safety of these new medications will determine their ultimate role in dermatology.

Antifungals

Today most cases of nail fungus can be cured using new oral antifungal agents terbinafine or itraconazole. Terbinafine was discovered in 1974 and was first approved internationally for the management of nail fungus in the United Kingdom in 1990. It was introduced into the United States in 1991, and is now available worldwide. The preferred mode of treatment for nail fungus and fungal skin infection is continuous therapy, although there are some reports where an intermittent treatment regimen with terbinafine has been used. Terbinafine inhibits a fungal enzyme causing buildup of squalene, which leads to disruption and destruction of the fungal cell wall, ultimately killing the fungus. It is taken up into already formed nail through the entire nail bed, and spreads through the whole nail as treatment continues. It is able to reach infected sites rapidly, is detected in nail clippings at three weeks, and has been found to remain in the nail for 10 months, well after drug administration has ended.

Itraconazole was discovered in 1980 and was first approved for treatment of nail fungus in 1987. Since then, there has been a change to a pulsed form of treatment—a seven-day course given four weeks apart, which is now preferred. Itraconazole has been detected in skin within hours of administration, and in the far ends of the fingernails and toenails within one and two weeks of starting treatment. Following two pulses of itraconazole for fingernail fungus, the drug has been detected in the far end of the nail nine months from the start of treatment, and at the far end of toenails after three pulses, 12 months from the start of treatment. In contrast, in the blood the drug concentration decreases to almost undetectable levels within 10–14 days of stopping a course of pulse therapy.

Advantages of pulse therapy include effectiveness with a similar or decreased frequency of side effects, economy, and convenience.

UVB narrow band

Among the most effective therapies for psoriasis is ultraviolet light phototherapy at 290–320 nm wavelength, and more recently narrowband UVB at 311 nanometers wavelength, which has been shown to be more effective than broadband UVB. Using phototherapy, the optimal wavelength for clearing psoriasis is 313 nanometers. In narrowband UVB phototherapy, conventional bulbs emitting primarily at 311–312nm are used. UVB phototherapy typically requires 30 sessions to produce clearing. However, the development of skin cancer in response to UVB phototherapy is a real concern.

Excimer laser

The excimer laser emits laser light at 308 nanometers, within the ultraviolet B range and holds promise for the treatment of localized psoriasis and vitiligo. It is thought that the light tissue interaction may be different for ultraviolet light in the form of laser light as opposed to conventional light. Also, because laser light is emitted from a hand piece only, psoriatic plaques are exposed while uninvolved skin is spared exposure, unlike conventional ultraviolet light treatments. Preliminary studies have indicated that excimer laser has great potential in the treatment of psoriasis and vitiligo.

Surgical Updates

Mohs Surgery   In the 1930s Frederick Mohs pioneered the unique concept of using a zinc chloride paste for the treatment of skin cancers. In 1970 Tromovitch and Stegman developed a technique of using the Mohs approach without zinc chloride, with frozen sections. This method, called the "fresh tissue technique," allowed similar cure rates. The chief advantage of this approach was that the defects created could be repaired immediately. Initially the tumor is debulked, tissue is excised by a beveled (saucer-shaped) excision just beyond the debulked area, the excised specimen is subdivided, mapped, and unfolded (flattened) to allow the entire margins to be examined. Instant slides of the specimen are prepared using a frozen technique in the lab for examination under the microscope, enabling the dermatologist to determine whether the entire cancer has been removed. The cancer is removed layer by layer until a negative margin is obtained. Today dermatologists perform these repairs in a day surgery setting, with tremendous cost savings over traditional hospital surgery.

The introduction of Mohs surgery also encouraged dermatologic interest in the science of wound healing. Dermatologists have been leaders in research on the biology of healing wounded skin and have also been instrumental in developing new biological dressings based on wound healing research.

Sentinel node biopsy Sentinel lymph node biopsy has recently gained acceptance in the surgical management of high-risk melanoma. The technique is becoming routine in many medical centers. Its use enables the identification of movement of microscopic cancer cells to lymph nodes, may reduce the number of unnecessary lymph node removals, and may lead to a survival benefit.

Skin cancer awareness, early detection, and sunscreens

Malignant melanoma continues to present a significant public health problem as its incidence is rising faster than that of any other cancer in the United States. At current rates, one in 74 Americans will develop melanoma. In the United States, primary prevention of melanoma and non-melanoma skin cancer has focused on encouraging sensible sun-exposure behaviors through public education. One of the most effective measures of protection is minimization of ultraviolet exposure from sunlight, by the use of sunscreens containing relatively new physical sun block agents such as micronized titanium dioxide and zinc oxide, or Parsol 1789. Other effective sun protective measures include the use of hats and protective clothing and avoidance of greatest sun exposure at peak times during the day.

Secondary prevention consists of a national campaign that promotes greater public awareness about the significance of risk factors, early warning signs of evolving tumors, and skin awareness, as well as self-examination and free examinations to detect evolving tumors, sponsored by the American Academy of Dermatology and the American Cancer Society. Melanoma and non-melanoma skin cancer have a high chance for cure if detected and treated in an early phase of development. Most melanoma deaths are related to patient delay in seeking medical care, attributed mostly to lack of knowledge. More attention is needed to encourage timely consultation for changing tumors and predisposing risk factors and to focus screening and surveillance efforts of those people at greatest risk.

It is hoped that increased public and professional awareness and education in all areas relating to the prevention, detection, and treatment of malignant melanoma will contribute to decreasing trends in the incidence and mortality from this cancer in the future.

Cosmetic Treatment of the Aging Face

Fillers Over the past two decades, dermatologists have been at the forefront of development and experience with various filling agents and techniques. These have become increasingly popular for patients in whom age-related changes develop as contour defects or who desire volume enhancement for various areas of the face. A variety of agents and techniques are currently available that, when used appropriately, can improve or correct wrinkles and facial volume loss.

The ideal filler agent should be safe and effective, easy to maintain and administer, have a minimal risk for infection, extrusion, or migration, produce no allergy, and last for an acceptable degree of time. It should also be cost effective, show consistency and reproducibility, and ultimately yield highly acceptable positive aesthetic results with no clumping or puffiness.

Collagen With formal approval by the U.S. Food and Drug Administration, collagen became the preferred filling agent for superficial wrinkles or skin depressions that do not originate with movement. Until recently, bovine collagen was the collagen type most readily available. More recently, human-derived collagen has replaced bovine collagen as the collagen of choice. It is used to fill fine lines around the mouth, skin folds between the nose, mouth, and chin area, and for lip enhancement, currently a much sought after procedure, which returns the lip to its fuller, more youthful state. Skin testing to determine whether the patient is allergic to collagen, something that had to be done twice with bovine collagen, is unnecessary with human collagen because of the low risk of allergic reaction. As collagen resorts over a period of months, enhancement is temporary with touch-ups required approximately every three months.

Fat Deep cosmetic defects, such as age-related changes of the face with loss of volume, are best addressed by replacing the substance that has been depleted—fat. Fat injections are most often administered at the time of fat harvesting, a procedure in which excess fat below the skin is taken from the patient's abdomen, buttocks, or outer thigh. Fat is then processed into a less viscous form, which can be injected below the skin.

Fat transplantation was repopularized with the development of liposuction in the 1980s. Klein's development of the tumescent technique has profoundly altered the way liposuction and fat transplantation are performed. The new procedure of microlipoinjection was introduced in May 1986. Fat could be aspirated and reinjected without major incisions or scars. Dermatologists in the United States have played an important role in the refinements and development of fat transplantation. These procedures continue to be increasingly popular today.

Dermalogen Recently, injectable human collagen has become available. Dermalogen is a suspension of collagen fibers and human collagen tissue matrix from skin donors from approved tissue banks accredited by the American Association of Tissue Banks. Skin tests are presently recommended before treatment to ensure the absence

of local allergic reaction. A positive skin test has not occurred in any recipient to date. Autologen is a dispersion of intact collagen fibers and collagen tissue matrix made from a patient's own skin, obtained during a cosmetic surgical procedure. Excised skin is placed in sterile containers and sent to laboratories on ice by express mail. "Custom collagen" is then created and sent back to the physician's office to be used for the same patient. Collagen can then be made at any time in the future by request.

Hyaluronic acid Injectable hyaluronic acid, a natural component of the skin, has recently emerged. This agent is derived from rooster combs or produced through bacterial fermentation and stabilized. It is used for the correction of contour defects of the skin, particularly in cases of aging or to increase the lips. Twenty years of experience with hyaluronan from rooster combs confirm its reliability. It is used extensively in Canada and in Europe and so far it has been used in study sites in the United States. Approval by the USFDA is pending.

Cymetra Cymetra is particulated tissue bank–quality skin. It has been available since 2005 and is injected into the lower part of the skin for filling in one to two sessions. However, long-term results are not yet available. Studies so far on at least 200 patients have revealed no allergic reactions, but side effects related to the injection of Cymetra have not yet been fully evaluated.

Others A number of other modern filler agents have recently become popular. These include particulate human fascia lata from tissue banks, expanded polytetrafluoroethylene (a suture-like material that can be implanted below the skin), micro droplet injectable liquid silicone, and collagen–wrapped polymethylmethacrylate microspheres.

Lifts Until recently, face-lifting and eyelid lifting were the only treatments available for the aging face. While there have been many important recent developments that have revolutionized the treatment of the aging face, lifting remains an important aspect of facial rejuvenation. Refined and simplified face-lift techniques including endoscopic procedures are improving outcomes.

Relaxers

Botox Botulinum neurotoxin is a paralyzing agent that prevents the release of a molecule called acetycholine from nerve junctions. Botox has been used throughout the 1990s to treat muscular neck disorders. More recently, cosmetic uses of botulinum A toxin for reduction of wrinkles caused by facial expressions in the aging face and neck have become popular. By relaxing the muscles involved, it can dramatically reduce frown lines of the forehead, between the eyebrows, and crow's-feet. Dermatologic surgeons also pioneered its use for sweat reduction of the palms and underarms. However, an important potential side effect of Botox is drooping of the upper eyelid. The effects of Botox are temporary necessitating touch-ups at four to five monthly intervals.

The development and launch of Myobloc, a commercially available Botox neurotoxin-B complex, will add to the two currently available Botox neurotoxin-A products. It has been studied widely in clinical trials, and as it has a different site of action it is believed that exotoxin B will be effective in individuals who have no response to exotoxin A.

Smoothers

Laser Skin Renewal R. Anderson and J. Parrish developed the theory of selective photothermolysis and the pulsed dye laser at Harvard Medical School in the early 1980s. The concept that selective tissue injury can be produced by using appropriate laser wavelengths and pulse duration has revolutionized treatment of a variety of skin disorders. Through the 1980s and 1990s into the new century, many useful laser applications have been developed, including treatments for pigmented lesions, tattoos and blood vessels, excessive hair, and sun-damaged skin.

The carbon dioxide laser is the best treatment for severe sun damage and emits an infrared beam, which heats and destroys thin layers of the skin and promotes new collagen formation, resulting in an improvement in wrinkles and appearance of the skin. The erbium laser emits laser energy in the near-infrared invisible light spectrum and leads to superficial skin removal and new collagen formation with less heat injury than the carbon dioxide laser and hence a faster healing time with less risk of side effects. Both these resurfacing lasers create wounds in the skin, resulting in downtime and can be associated with complications such as redness, delayed healing, pigment changes, and scarring.

Subsurface remodeling, also termed photo-rejuvenation, represents the newest approach to improving damaged skin. High rates of undesirable side effects associated with traditional techniques have led to the development of new non-ablative laser technologies. The non-ablative technique is meant for those individuals who do not wish to take time away from their daily activities in order to laser improve the quality of their sun-damaged skin. These systems improve wrinkles without the creation of a wound. Selective heating below the skin surface leading to formation of collagen without surface damage is produced using cooling techniques such as cryogen sprays to protect the skin surface. Non-ablative lasers hold potential for skin tightening, as well as the treatment of stretch marks, scars, and a variety of other conditions. In the future lasers may be created that can cause the same degree of improvement as that seen with ablative systems without the potential complications and downtime from such systems.

Erasers Intense pulsed light sources emit light in the 500–1,200 nm range and is a safe new technology effective in hair removal, treatment of vascular lesions, and removal of lesions such as sunspots and freckles. Intense pulsed light selectively targets and destroys pigment of hair follicle, allowing hair removal. Pigment irregularities due to sun damage are one of the newest uses of intense pulsed light.

Chemical peels have been performed to enhance the tone of skin since the time of Cleopatra. Widespread use of more superficial peeling agents such as alpha-hydroxy acids started in the 1980s and 1990s to the point where they have become standard treatment to maintain skin glow and tone.

Aluminum oxide crystal microdermabrasion, a technique developed in Italy in 1985, has become extremely popular within the last few years in the offices of plastic surgeons, dermatologists, and lay spas for the management of fine wrinkles, sun damage, mild surgical scars, acne, skin discoloration and irregularities. It is a nonsurgical procedure being used to rejuvenate the skin. The device gently pulls the skin into a hand piece by mild suction, which initiates the flow of crystals. Surface debris and dead skin cells are removed by the impact of the particle on the skin's surface. The treatment is typically performed in a series of weekly visits. After the procedure the subject can return to normal daily activities with no interrup-

tion. There has been an overwhelming perceived benefit in the skin's appearance and texture from patients undergoing a course of therapy.

Retinoids, derived from vitamin A, are highly effective in treatment of moderate sun damage. An increase in collagen in the skin has been observed with use of topical tretinoin (Retin A®). Patients who are not candidates for tretinoin therapy may benefit from other newer retinoids, such as adapalene and tazarotene, which were developed in the 1990s.

—Jeffrey S. Dover, M.D., FRPCP

INTRODUCTION

Skin Deep, Third Edition has been designed as a reference guide to a wide range of terms related to skin and skin disorders. It also includes extensive appendixes with information and addresses for organizations that deal with skin problems. It is not a substitute for prompt assessment and treatment by experts trained in the diagnosis of dermatological problems.

In this new, revised edition, we have tried to present the latest developments, based on the newest information in the field, the latest research, and current FDA approvals of new treatments. In this revision, readers will find a number of completely new topics, including entries on:

- autologous fat transplants
- biological implants
- dermal stimulator
- dihydroxyacetone (DHA)
- elephantiasis
- infantile acropustulosis
- laser hair removal
- Louis-Bar syndrome
- Merkel cell cancer
- microdermabrasion
- nevi entries
- pemphigoid
- post-inflammatory pigmentation
- prohibited cosmetic ingredients
- skin fillers
- spider bites
- syringomas

In addition, almost every entry has been revised and updated to include the latest information on cause and treatments of certain diseases and conditions, such as Addison's disease, basal cell carcinoma, Behcet's syndrome, bites and infestations, Bowen's disease, Bloom's syndrome, burns, *Candida paronychia*, canker sore, chicke pox, chloasma, Cockayne-Touraine syndrome, contact urticaria, collodion baby, cradle cap, cutaneous diphtheria, dermatitis artefacta, dermatofibrosarcoma protuberans, drug-induced acne, ecthyma, EPS, erythema multiforme, fifth disease, folliculitis, gangrene, granuloma faciale, Homer's syndrome, HPV, hyperhydrosis, Kawasaki disease, latex allergies, Lawrence-Seip syndrome, lentigines, leptospirosis, leukoplakia, Lyme disease, measles, neurocutaneous syndromes, panniculitis, pressure sores, psoriasis, scabies, scleroderma, scorpions, seaweed dermatitis, strawberry birthmarks, strep infections, ulerythema, and vitiligo.

The newest updates on terrorist-related poisoning with effects on the skin include revisions on entries about smallpox, bubonic plague, dioxin, and anthrax. The latest genetic updates include the newest information on alopecia, congenital Lawrence-Seip, Darier's disease, erythropoietic protoporphyria, Louis-Bar syndrome, neurofibromatosis, porphyria, psoriasis, rosacea, scleroderma,

Sturge-Weber disease, tuberous sclerosis, and Urbach-Wiethe disease.

Skin-related medications and product updates include the newest revisions in entries about AHA peels, Accutane, benzoyl peroxide, Drysol, lindane, NSAIDs, and retinoids. Techniques also continue to advance at a dizzying pace, and this encyclopedia updates the latest information on cosmetic acupuncture, dermabrasion, interferon, lasers, laser resurfacing, prohibited cosmetic ingredients, pulsed dye laser, and silicone implants.

Vaccines are always being developed, discarded, or improved upon, and this revision includes the latest information on new shingles prevention vaccines related to the chicken pox shot, the Lyme vaccine recall, and new skin cancer vaccines now being developed. At the same time, skin-related medications and products are also continually changing; revised updates include entries on AHA peels, Accutane, benzoyl peroxide, Drysol, lindane, and thalidomide. Techniques also continue to advance at a dizzying pace, and this encyclopedia updates the latest information on cosmetic acupuncture, dermabrasion, interferon, lasers, laser resurfacing, prohibited cosmetic ingredients, pulsed dye laser, and silicone implants.

In addition, aging-related issues are a big part of dermatology, and we have revised many entries related to the effects of age on the skin and related structures along with the newest methods to improve aging skin. Revised entries related to these subjects include topics such as aging and the skin, alopecia, alpha hydroxy acids, anthralin, Artecoll, Autologen, biological implants, bovine collagen, collagen injections, composite cultured skin, CosmoDerm, Cymetra, human-derived collagen, hyaluronic acid gel, liposuction, and soft tissue fillers.

As researchers uncover more and more problems with sun exposure, the revision has included information on a variety of solar-related entries, such as sun protective clothing, hats and the sun, skin cancer, malignant melanoma, Melanotan, tanning beds, tanning pills, sunscreen, SPR regulations, and solar urticaria.

In addition, the appendixes have been completely updated; many new organizations have been added, and the latest addresses, phone numbers, and Web sites added and checked for accuracy.

Information in this book comes from the most up-to-date sources available and includes some of the most recent research in dermatology. Readers should keep in mind, however, that changes occur very rapidly in this field. References have been provided for readers who seek additional sources of information. All entries are cross-referenced, and appendixes provide additional information.

—Carol Turkington
Cumru, Pennsylvania

ACKNOWLEDGMENTS

Thanks to Birck Cox, for providing terrific drawings; to my editors, James Chambers and Vanessa Nittoli, for patient editing; and to my agents, Ed Claflin, Gene Brissie, and Bert Holtjer, for their tireless efforts.

Thanks also to the staffs of the American Academy of Dermatology, the American Dermatological Association, the American College of Allergy and Immunology, Jeff Bender at the American Academy of Allergy and Immunology, the American Hair Loss Council, Susan Kastner at the American Leprosy Missions, the American Society for Dermatologic Surgery, the American Society of Plastic and Reconstructive Surgeons, the Dystrophic Epidermolysis Bullosa Research Association of America, the Foundation for Ichthyosis and Related Skin Types, the National Tuberous Sclerosis Association, the National Institutes of Health, Maggie Bartlett and Donna at the National Cancer Institute, the National Institute of Arthritis, Musculoskeletal and Skin Diseases, the Society for Pediatric Dermatology, the Psoriasis Research Institute, the National Vitiligo Foundation, the Skin Cancer Foundation, Suzanne Corr at the National Rosacea Society.

Thanks also to the librarians of Hershey Medical Center medical library, the National Library of Medicine, the Reading Public Library, the Reading Hospital Medical Library, the Chester County Library, and the Pennsylvania State Library/Berks Campus.

Finally, thanks to Kara and Michael for unfailing support.

ENTRIES A–Z

abdominoplasty A surgical technique used to tighten up a sagging abdominal wall that has become flaccid due to pregnancy or weight loss. The most common of these techniques involves a long incision in the lower abdomen or directly above the pubic hairline. The skin and subcutaneous tissues of the abdominal wall are lifted off the muscle, where they are redraped and the excess skin removed. After the wounds are closed, a new opening is made for the navel, which is sutured into place.

Risks/Complications
Risks include scars, numbness in the lower abdominal wall, and blood clots in the veins of the lower legs.

Outlook and Lifestyle Modifications
This operation is considered major surgery and requires general anesthesia and post-surgical recovery of up to a week in a hospital and several weeks more rest at home. LIPOSUCTION can be used as an alternative to abdominoplasty in some patients.

abrasion A graze that involves a superficial loss of epithelium, the tissue that covers the external surface of the body that results in oozing and crusting. No treatment is necessary.

abscess An inflammatory nodule containing a collection of PUS, usually caused by a bacterial infection. The pus is made up of dead and live microorganisms and destroyed tissue from white blood cells carried to the area to fight the infection. An abscess may become larger or smaller depending on whether the white blood cells or the bacteria win the fight.

Abscesses may be found in the soft tissues beneath the skin, such as the armpit and the groin—two areas with a large number of lymph glands responsible for fighting infections.

Bacteria (such as staphylococci) are the most common cause of abscesses. Fungal infections sometimes cause abscesses as well.

Symptoms and Diagnostic Path
Most larger abscesses cause body-wide symptoms such as fever and chills. Abscesses close to the skin usually cause inflammation with redness, increased skin temperature, and tenderness.

Abscesses usually can be diagnosed visually, although an imaging technique (CAT scan, MRI or radionuclide scans) also may be used to confirm the extent of the wound.

Treatment Options and Outlook
Antibiotics are usually prescribed to treat a bacterial infection, and antifungal agents are used to treat fungi. However, the lining of the abscess tends to cut down on the amount of drug that can get into the source of the infection from the blood. Therefore, the abscess cavity itself needs to be drained by cutting into the lining, and allowing the pus to escape either through a drainage tube or by leaving the cavity open to the outside of the skin.

Many abscesses heal after drainage alone; others require both drainage and medication.

acantholysis Disruption of intercellular connections between KERATIN-producing cells in the outer skin layer. It is caused when the cementing substance between cells dissolves, and is associated with a form of blisters in diseases such as PEMPHIGUS.

acanthosis Increased thickness of the surface layer of the skin (EPIDERMIS), found in a wide variety of skin disorders.

See ACANTHOSIS NIGRICANS.

acanthosis nigricans A rare untreatable condition characterized by thick velvety dark gray or brown patches of skin on the groin, armpits, neck, and other skin folds.

It can either be an inherited genetic disorder appearing during childhood or adolescence, as a result of an endocrine or metabolic disorder (such as Cushing's syndrome) or a symptom of malignant tumors. In addition, at least one drug (nicotinic acid) may cause acanthosis nigricans.

When caused by obesity or heredity, the condition progresses very slowly; however, acanthosis nigricans associated with cancer appears and develops more rapidly.

Symptoms and Diagnostic Path

"Pseudoacanthosis" nigricans is a far more common condition found in overweight patients with dark complexions. Skin in the fold areas (groin, armpits, or neck) is both thicker and darker than the surrounding skin. There also may be excessive sweating in this area.

Treatment Options and Outlook

Treatment for patients with acanthosis nigricans is aimed at recognizing and treating the underlying disorder. With treatment of the malignancy, the condition should improve.

acarophobia See DELUSIONS OF PARASITOSIS.

Accutane See ISOTRETINOIN.

acid mantle A fluid made up of an oily substance called SEBUM, sweat, and dissolved cells that bathes the top layer of the skin and protects against infection. Care of this acidic fluid mantle is very important, especially in people with oily skin prone to infection or ACNE lesions.

acne A very common inflammatory reaction in oil-producing follicles. While most common in adolescence, the problem may affect people of any age, including infants and the middle-aged.

Acne is the most common skin disease in the United States, and accounts for 25 percent of all visits to dermatologists. Because it most commonly affects the face and can lead to permanent scarring, acne can have profound and long-lasting psychological effects.

In boys, acne usually begins in early adolescence; it tends to be more severe than in girls and improves in the early to mid-twenties. In girls, acne usually begins slightly later (mid-teens), and is often less severe. In some individuals, acne can last into the 30s. Patients with severe acne often have a family history of severe acne.

Normally, oil is produced in the oil glands in the skin, travels up to the hair follicles, and flows out onto the surface of the skin. When oil glands within the hair follicles are stimulated and begin to enlarge (usually as a result of the hormonal change at puberty), they produce more oil. Acne bacteria inside the follicles multiply and produce fatty acids, which irritate the lining of the pores. Simultaneously, there is an increased number of thicker cells in the lining of the pores, which tend to clump together, narrowing and clogging the pore openings with a backup of oil, skin cells, and debris inside the pores.

As the pressure builds within these clogged pores, the constant production of oil together with irritation from bacterial action ruptures the pore walls. When the oil pathway gets blocked and the plug pushes up to the surface, it causes a blackhead (open COMEDO). When the opening is very tightly closed, the material behind it causes a whitehead (closed comedo).

While there are many factors behind the inflammatory changes in acne, one of the most important is the different levels of bacteria found on the skin. While acne is *not* a bacterial infection, it is believed that inflammation results from the byproducts released by the bacterium PROPIONIBACTERIUM ACNES, found deep in the hair follicle.

Emotional stress, cosmetics, and certain drugs (such as the birth control pills that have higher amounts of progesterone and lower amounts of estrogen) may worsen the condition. Estrogen, however, will improve acne; women who use an estrogen-dominant birth control pill usually notice their acne improves.

Acne is hereditary, and the tendency to develop the condition runs in families. If both parents have acne, then three out of four of their children also will have acne.

Oil in cosmetics can contribute to acne. Cosmetic products that contain lanolin, sodium lauryl sulfate, isopropyl myristate, laureth-4, and D&C red dyes should be avoided, since all of these ingredients can promote acne. Makeup should be washed off each night with a mild soap; patients should be sure to rinse six or seven times with fresh water.

(To find out how oily a cosmetic is, patients should rub a thick blob of makeup on a piece of typing paper; within 24 hours, the oil will make a ring on the paper; the bigger the ring, the more oil in the makeup.)

Acne is *not* caused by diet, dirt, or surface oil. Oily foods have nothing to do with the oil on the skin; oil on the skin is manufactured locally in the oil glands, no matter *what* a person eats.

Symptoms and Diagnostic Path

Acne is characterized by lesions on the face, neck, chest, back, shoulders, and upper arms, including several types: pimples, cysts, pustules, whiteheads and blackheads.

Treatment Options and Outlook

There are excellent types of therapy for all kinds of acne, including topical treatment, systemic antibiotics and other medications, and hormonal manipulation. A properly-structured regimen is required for all those with acne, but most people benefit from a combination of skin peeling, bacterial destruction, and comedo-affecting products.

Patients should wash with soap and water every night, eat well, and exercise regularly. For milder cases of acne, medications containing BENZOYL PEROXIDE (beginning with a 5 percent solution) or those containing SULFUR, or a combination of sulfur and RESORCINOL or SALICYLIC ACID are effective.

Since oil accumulation attracts bacteria, and the bacteria's enzymes produce fatty acids that irritate the skin and cause inflammation, one of the best ways to fight acne is to kill the bacteria. Those products that are effective in treating acne actually cut down the oil production of the glands slightly, and destroy (or decrease) bacteria in the follicles. The most popular antibiotics in the treatment of acne are tetracycline, minocycline, and erythromycin. For mild cases of acne, antibiotics are used directly on the skin. For more advanced disease, they are taken by mouth.

Retin-A, a drug made with TRETINOIN (an acid related to vitamin A) is an effective treatment for comedones, inflammatory papules, and pustules. It is also effective in reversing sun-induced skin aging. Retin-A is often used in combination with benzoyl peroxide or antibiotics.

Those with the most severe types of acne may be given a stronger vitamin-A related drug called Accutane (ISOTRETINOIN). This drug has more serious side effects, including birth defects, and requires strict medical supervision. *No woman should become pregnant when taking Accutane.* It is not safe to become pregnant until two months after the course of medication is finished.

TYPES OF ACNE

Acne conglobata Severe hereditary acne that generally causes scarring on face and back

Acne detergens Acne caused by overuse of abrasive cleansers

Acne excoriée A psychosomatic disease involving neurotic picking of the face

Acne mallorca Acne caused by sunbathing

Acne mechanica Acne caused by mechanical irritation (such as under the chin straps in football players)

Acne medicamentosa Acne caused by medications

Acne neonatorum Infant acne caused by hormones from the mother to the newborn that usually disappears without treatment

Chloracne Acne induced by constant exposure to hydrocarbons in motor oil or insecticides

Imaginary acne Imagining acne where none exists

Pitch acne Lesions caused by coal tars or dandruff tar shampoos

Premenstrual acne Acne breakouts induced by hormonal change that flare each month prior to starting a period

Steroid acne An inflammation of hair follicles caused by internal steroids or from topical corticosteroids on the face

Tropical acne Acne first described in World War II by soldiers in the Tropics who developed severe acne with terrible scars.

It is possible that some cases of acne can be controlled by regulating the androgen/estrogen hormone balance in those women who have an increased activity of the enzyme that converts testosterone (a male androgen) into a more potent form that affects the oil glands. Since androgen has been implicated in the increased secretion of sebum that starts an acne blemish, androgen blockers that reduce the size of oil glands may help women whose acne is associated with other changes, such as excessive hair growth or balding. These drugs could be in the form of high-estrogen birth control pills. However, this benefit should be balanced against the health risks associated with taking estrogen, including heart problems and breast cancer.

Steroids (cortisone) are very effective for inflammatory or cystic acne when injected into a lesion; it can heal the cyst in about 24 hours. The injection is relatively painless, clears the skin rapidly and prevents scarring.

See also ACNE, ADULT; ACNE, COSMETIC; ACNE, CYSTIC; ACNE, DRUG-INDUCED; ACNE, INFANT; ACNE, OIL; ACNE, TREATMENT FOR; ACNE DETERGENS; ACNE FULMINANS; ACNE KELOIDALIS; ACNE MECHANICA; ACNE MYTHS; ACNE VULGARIS.

acne, adult Pimples, pustules, and papules may be the bane of the teenage years, but they can also crop up in adulthood—even in people who were never troubled with breakouts during their adolescence. In fact, some estimates suggest that acne affects 70 to 80 percent of all individuals in their 20s and 30s.

Why these skin blemishes suddenly occur in older patients is a mystery. The hormonal upheaval that triggers acne in teenagers is not usually a factor in adult acne, and while stress, dirt, and pollution are prime suspects, there is no direct evidence that either is the cause. In 30- to 40-year-old women, the cause is clearly related to hormones.

Treatment Options and Outlook

Treatment is the same as for teenage ACNE.

See also ACNE, COSMETIC; ACNE, CYSTIC; ACNE, DRUG-INDUCED; ACNE, INFANT; ACNE, OIL; ACNE, TREATMENT OF, ACNE; ACNE DETERGENS; ACNE FUL-

MINANS; ACNE KELOIDALIS; ACNE MECHANICA; ACNE MYTHS; ACNE VULGARIS.

acne, cosmetic True cosmetic ACNE is probably quite rare. While it is commonly believed that most acne seen in adult women is related to their use of cosmetics containing comedogenic material, this is probably inaccurate. There are three main groups of ingredients that may aggravate acne. These are lanolins, isopropyl myristate, and some pigments.

LANOLIN (sheep skin oil) is an extremely common ingredient in cosmetics, but the fatty acids in lanolin tend to aggravate acne in some people. Many lanolin derivatives in cosmetics, such as etoxylated lanolins and acetylated lanolins, are harmful to acne-prone individuals. The partially synthetic lanolins are able to penetrate skin PORES even better than natural lanolin. Lanolin oil itself is acceptable.

Another problem ingredient in cosmetics is a penetrating oil called isopropyl myristate, which is used to give cosmetics a slicker, sheer feel. There are many chemicals similar to isopropyl myristate in cosmetics, including isopropyl palmitate, isopropyl isothermal, putty sterate, isostearyl neopentonate, myristyl myristate, decyl oleate, octyl sterate, octyl palmitate and isocetyl stearate, and PPG myristyl propionate. All can worsen acne.

Another ingredient in cosmetics that may trigger acne are the red tints used in blushes. Some of the red dyes are comedogenic. The easiest way to avoid these agents is to check the label for ingredients and to be sure to use only noncomedogenic products that do not worsen or cause acne.

See also ACNE, ADULT; ACNE, CYSTIC; ACNE, DRUG-INDUCED; ACNE, INFANT; ACNE, OIL; ACNE DETERGENS; ACNE FULMINANS; ACNE KELOIDALIS; ACNE MECHANICA; ACNE MYTHS; ACNE VULGARIS.

acne, cystic A type of severe ACNE in which the SEBUM (together with dead cells and bacterial products) ruptures through the follicle wall, causing an inflammatory reaction that may end in scarring.

See also ACNE, ADULT; ACNE, COSMETIC; ACNE, DRUG-INDUCED; ACNE, INFANT; ACNE, OIL; ACNE

DETERGENS; ACNE FULMINANS; ACNE KELOIDALIS; ACNE MECHANICA; ACNE MYTHS; ACNE VULGARIS.

acne, drug-induced Many drugs can cause ACNE when administered systemically. The most common are phenytoin (Dilantin), isoniazid, lithium, bromides, iodides, androgens, and corticosteroids. Of these, topical and systemic corticosteroids are the most common acne inducers. In drug-induced acne there may not be any blackheads; instead, patients experience uniform papules and pustules.

Lithium worsens ACNE VULGARIS, and can cause a severe case of acne in patients who never before had a skin problem. Oral contraceptives containing agents such as norgestrel or norethindrone can induce or worsen acne vulgaris; this may improve when pill prescriptions are switched. Medications containing potassium iodide, bromide (especially cold remedies) and chlorine (chloral hydrate) may cause acne with very small pustules.

Steroids may cause acne several days to weeks after treatment begins with either oral or topical steroids. Steroid-induced acne is distinctive, with tiny red papules and pustules limited to the area where the steroid was applied, or on the chest, back and shoulders in people on systemic therapy. Steroids thin the outer skin layer, making follicles more susceptible to rupture. Because inflammation is controlled by steroids, the lesions are usually small or they may appear after the drug is stopped. Acne fades after the medicine is stopped, but it may take some time to completely clear.

Other substances associated with acne are dioxin, actinomycin D, cod liver oil, halothane, thiouracil, thiourea, trimethadione and vitamin B_{12}.

The chemical dioxin also can cause a type of severe acne called CHLORACNE. In 2004 dioxin was used by his enemies to poison Ukrainian president Viktor Yushchenko during his presidential campaign. The strikingly handsome Yushchenko was terribly disfigured by the dioxin, with swollen, distorted facial features and a severe case of chloracne that pitted and scarred his face. Experts say it is impossible for Yushchenko to have naturally acquired levels of dioxin more than 6,000 times higher than normal—the second highest ever recorded in human history. What constitutes a lethal dose of dioxin has never been established because no one has ever been known to die from it. However, dioxin poisoning at such lethal levels is linked to the development of chloracne, cancer, and system-wide organ failure. Scientists confirm he was poisoned by TCDD, the most harmful dioxin, a key ingredient of Agent Orange, an herbicide defoliant used as a weapon during the Vietnam War, and blamed for myriad health problems in U.S. Vietnam veterans.

See also ACNE, ADULT; ACNE, COSMETIC; ACNE, CYSTIC; ACNE, INFANT; ACNE, OIL; ACNE DETERGENS; ACNE FULMINANS; ACNE KELOIDALIS; ACNE MECHANICA; ACNE MYTHS.

acne, infant ACNE is not unusual among newborns; it is triggered by hormones passed from the mother to the child before birth. The hormones cause the SEBACEOUS GLANDS in the skin to produce oil; if these glands become blocked and inflamed, WHITEHEADS and pimples may develop on the baby's face. Newborn acne usually clears up on its own in three or four months. If it is troublesome or persistent a pediatrician may prescribe a topical medication.

Contrary to popular belief, infant acne is not associated with the development of acne in adolescence or later in life. However, on rare occasions infantile acne becomes severe and persists for months to a few years. This is associated with a family history of acne, usually in the father, and often is followed by severe acne at adolescence.

See also ACNE, ADULT; ACNE, COSMETIC; ACNE, CYSTIC; ACNE, DRUG-INDUCED; ACNE, OIL; ACNE DETERGENS; ACNE FULMINANS; ACNE KELOIDALIS; ACNE MECHANICA; ACNE MYTHS; ACNE VULGARIS.

acne, oil A form of ACNE caused by heavy petroleum lubricating oils and greases that irritate the follicles, resulting in plugging of comedones or pustular folliculitis.

Symptoms and Diagnostic Path

The lesions usually occur on the hands and forearms, but they may be severe on covered areas of the body if clothing is saturated with oil. The appearance of lesions in places other than outside the bridge of nose, chin, forehead, back, and chest, plus a history of exposure to oils, is a good way to distinguish oil acne from ACNE VULGARIS or bacterial FOLLICULITIS.

Treatment Options and Outlook

This condition responds immediately when the exposure to the irritating oil is stopped. Eliminating skin and clothing contact with the offending oil and grease is the best way to avoid oil acne. Applications of BENZOYL PEROXIDE may also help.

See also ACNE, ADULT; ACNE, COSMETIC; ACNE CYSTIC; ACNE, DRUG-INDUCED; ACNE, INFANT; ACNE DETERGENS; ACNE FULMINANS; ACNE KELOIDALIS; ACNE MECHANICA; ACNE MYTHS.

acne, pomade A type of ACNE that occurs primarily in African-American patients who use pomades or thick oils daily on their hair to eliminate the curl. The pomade gets transferred to the skin from the fingers and hair, and blocks the skin's oil glands, causing acnelike lesions. In this condition, which was first described in 1970, many closed comedones and sometimes inflamed lesions are packed close together on the head and temples near the hairline.

Risk Factors and Preventive Measures

Patients should wash hands after applying the oil, keep hands away from the face and avoid hairstyles where the hair constantly touches the skin of the face.

acne, treatment for There are a range of therapies for all kinds of acne, including topical treatment, systemic antibiotics, hormonal manipulation, or ISOTRETINOIN (Accutane), a synthetic derivative of vitamin A.

For milder cases, some people find relief with over-the-counter medications containing BENZOYL PEROXIDE or SULFUR, a combination of sulfur and RESORCINOL, or SALICYLIC ACID. These medications are sold as liquids, gels, lotions, or creams; the water-based gels are least likely to irritate the skin.

Probably the most popular of these over-the-counter products is benzoyl peroxide, an extremely effective topical antibacterial agent. When applied to the skin it markedly suppresses the bacterium *Propionibacterium acnes*. The benzoyl in the product draws the peroxide into the pore where it releases oxygen, killing the bacteria that can aggravate acne. Benzoyl peroxide also suppresses fatty acid cells that irritate pores, and it helps to open up BLACKHEADS and WHITEHEADS. Benzoyl peroxide is most effective for patients with inflammatory acne; by inhibiting bacteria growth, it decreases the inflammatory components in the skin.

Benzoyl peroxide is sold in strengths ranging between 2.5 percent to 10 percent, but dermatologists usually advise patients to start with a 2.5 or 5 percent product, since the lower concentration is usually just as effective and less likely to cause irritation. Most over-the-counter products contain benzoyl peroxide in a lotion base or in treated pads; the prescription items contain the chemical in a gel base. Some irritation, redness, and swelling may follow use of benzoyl peroxide, and allergic sensitization has occasionally occurred.

For more severe cases, dermatologists may prescribe Retin-A, a drug made with TRETINOIN (an acid related to vitamin A), or topical or oral antibiotics. Tretinoin is the principal drug for topical use in acne with comedones (open whiteheads), and is available as a gel, cream, or lotion. (The lotion is potentially more irritating and the creams are less irritating.) Less irritation develops if tretinoin is applied at least 30 minutes *after* washing. Tretinoin, like benzoyl peroxide, should be started in the lowest concentration available and be applied only every other day. Patients should protect their skin from exposure to the sun, since tretinoin increases the skin's sensitivity to ultraviolet radiation.

While tretinoin is best used for acne with open whiteheads, it may also help patients with inflammatory acne since it helps to prevent inflammation.

Topical antibiotics (including TETRACYCLINE, ERYTHROMYCIN, CLINDAMYCIN, and meclocycline) have been used topically as an antibacterial approach to treating acne. Experts believe antibiotics are not as effective as benzoyl peroxide except in mild inflammatory acne. A preparation combining 3 percent erythromycin with 5 percent benzoyl peroxide in a gel base may be more effective than either component by itself.

Systemic Therapy

About 10 percent of all tetracycline sold in the United States is used to treat acne, although the condition is not a bacterial disease. The effectiveness of oral antibiotics is probably related to the fact that the drugs interfere with inflammatory byproducts of some types of bacteria, which prevents the development of new inflammatory lesions. It does take some time, however, before the antibiotic approach works. Erythromycin and minocycline are probably as effective as tetracycline, but minocycline is much more expensive.

Preparations that interfere with the production of sebum (an oily substance produced by sebaceous glands) may also be effective, including corticosteroids and estrogens. (Estrogens should only be used for women whose acne has not responded to other types of treatment). In addition, a medication called cyproterone acetate has been used in Europe to successfully treat acne.

Those with the most severe types of acne may be given an even stronger vitamin-A related drug called Accutane (isotretinoin). Accutane is the only treatment that can potentially cure acne. Sixty percent of those with severe scarring acne who receive Accutane never again need treatment. Accutane is very effective against the most stubborn cases of acne, and has produced remarkable clearing in those with severe cystic acne. The drug has also resulted in remissions that have persisted for years in most patients.

Unfortunately, Accutane has serious side effects and requires strict medical supervision. Side effects include those found in excess levels of vitamin A (dry mouth, itching, small red spots on the skin and eye irritation). Its most serious side effect is that it can cause serious birth defects. Acutane *must not* be given during pregnancy.

Research suggests it may also trigger serious depression, and in rare cases, suicidal thoughts.

This seems to affect those with an existing tendency toward depression. It is important for patients to discuss all these potential side effects with their doctor before starting Accutane.

Acne medications may cause reactions if the skin is exposed to the sun; experts recommend staying away from sunlight, infrared heat lamps, and sunscreens until patients understand how the product works.

Surgical Techniques

Acne surgery removes open and closed comedones and sometimes very small pustules; removal of the closed comedones is important, since they can lead to inflammatory lesions. Open comedones are removed only for cosmetic reasons, since they do not usually become inflamed.

The direct injection of corticosteroids into a lesion can reduce inflammation in larger cysts in order to avoid a depressed scar. This technique is not used for papules and pustules.

Topical Applications

The directions on most topical acne medications say to "apply to the affected area" after washing. This does *not* mean apply to pimples only, since these medications do not really fight pimples that already exist. However, there is the possibility that benzoyl peroxide applied to a pimple may cause it to go away a bit faster.

It's not a good idea to mix acne medications. If a patient is using a nonprescription acne product, it should be stopped if a prescription product is used.

What Not to Do

Picking or squeezing blemishes can inhibit healing and lead to scarring. For this reason, patients should never squeeze pimples or whiteheads. Because regular pimples are the result of inflammation, squeezing can simply worsen the inflammation and cause an infection. However, pimples with a little yellow PUS head in the middle *can* be gently squeezed, which will pop the pimple and allow it to heal more quickly. Unfortunately, nothing can make a pimple go away faster—the life of a pimple lasts between one and four weeks.

Whiteheads, which do not involve inflammation, should never be squeezed. If a whitehead is squeezed, the wall of the plugged pore can break and the contents can leak out into the skin, causing a pimple. (A pimple forms from the rupture of a whitehead pore.)

Blackheads may be squeezed, since they will not result in a pimple. Blackheads are simply open comedones or open whiteheads. The black color is from melanin and from oxidation of the pore contents.

Risk Factors and Preventive Measures

Acne sufferers should try to avoid excess stress if prone to breaking out. Patients taking birth control pills that cause acne (especially Ovral, Loestrin, Norlestrin, and Norinyl) may be able to switch to a different pill or use an alternative birth control method.

acne detergens This form of ACNE occurs in some patients who are compulsive face washers. There is some evidence that this may be a variety of ACNE MECHANICA.

See also ACNE, ADULT; ACNE, COSMETIC; ACNE, CYSTIC; ACNE, DRUG-INDUCED; ACNE, INFANT; ACNE, OIL; ACNE FULMINANS; ACNE KELOIDALIS; ACNE MECHANICA; ACNE MYTHS; ACNE VULGARIS.

acne excoriée One of a group of disorders in which a patient, because of an exaggerated sense of abnormal conditions, causes a skin rash by constantly picking or squeezing facial blemishes. In these cases, one or a few small blemishes are so upsetting that the individual constantly picks or washes them, actually making the lesions worse. People with this problem may refuse to believe their actions are making the lesions worse by constant irritation, and may seek plastic surgery to correct the problem. However, in these cases they are quite often dissatisfied with the results of surgery. Severely distraught patients may even attempt suicide.

See also ACNE, ADULT; ACNE, COSMETIC; ACNE, CYSTIC; ACNE, DRUG-INDUCED; ACNE, INFANT; ACNE DETERGENS; ACNE OIL; ACNE KELOIDALIS; ACNE MECHANICA; ACNE MYTHS; ACNE VULGARIS.

acne fulminans This is an acute, severe necrotic variety of ACNE that is accompanied by systemic symptoms such as fever and joint pain.

Acne fulminans may be triggered by high levels of testosterone, either legally prescribed or illegally taken to enhance muscle growth.

Symptoms and Diagnostic Path

The condition, which almost always affects males, includes the following symptoms:

- abrupt onset
- inflammatory and ulcerated nodular acne on chest and back
- severe acne scarring
- fluctuating fever
- painful joints
- malaise
- loss of appetite and weight loss
- high white blood cell count

Treatment Options and Outlook

Management can be difficult, and several medications are usually required, including high doses of oral antibiotics such as ERYTHROMYCIN or anti-inflammatory medications such as aspirin. Most cases require Accutane and oral corticosteroids such as prednisone, DAPSONE, or ISOTRETINOIN. Acne medications applied directly to the skin are not helpful.

See also ACNE, ADULT; ACNE, COSMETIC; ACNE, CYSTIC; ACNE, DRUG-INDUCED; ACNE, INFANT; ACNE, OIL; ACNE DETERGENS; ACNE KELOIDALIS; ACNE MECHANICA; ACNE MYTHS; ACNE VULGARIS.

acne keloidalis Also called *dermatitis papillaris capillitii,* this disorder affects hair follicles in people of African descent.

Symptoms and Diagnostic Path

It creates firm papules and pustules on the nape of the neck. In severe cases, large lesions may result in significant scarring and permanent hair loss. Complications may include infection, scarring resulting in limited range of neck movement; squamous cell cancer may rarely develop.

Treatment Options and Outlook

While no single treatment is effective for all patients, therapies include corticosteroid injections and topical corticosteroid preparations, which may limit the formation of scars. A variety of surgical techniques also may be attempted, including removal of individual papules with scissors, a scalpel, or lasers. In more severe cases, the entire affected area is removed and the wound is stitched closed.

See also ACNE, ADULT; ACNE, COSMETIC; ACNE, CYSTIC; ACNE, DRUG-INDUCED; ACNE, INFANT; ACNE, OIL; ACNE DETERGENS; ACNE FULMINANS; ACNE MECHANICA; ACNE MYTHS; ACNE VULGARIS.

acne mechanica Acne caused by physical trauma such as rubbing, tight clothes, or underneath chin straps of helmets worn by athletes. Heat and sweat also contribute to this condition.

Treatment Options and Outlook

Topical treatments such as a solution of salicylic acid, Retin-A, or benzoyl peroxide can be applied directly to the affected area.

Risk Factors and Preventive Measures

Acne mechanica can be prevented by wearing clean clothes made of cotton or another material that wicks moisture away from the skin, and washing the area after exercise.

See also ACNE, ADULT; ACNE, COSMETIC; ACNE, CYSTIC; ACNE, DRUG-INDUCED; ACNE, INFANT; ACNE, OIL; ACNE DETERGENS; ACNE KELOIDALIS; ACNE FULMINANS; ACNE MYTHS; ACNE VULGARIS.

acne medicamentosa See ACNE, DRUG-INDUCED.

acne myths A wide range of ACNE taboos are groundless, such as the idea that acne is worsened by chocolate, nuts, fatty foods, and shellfish.

See also ACNE, ADULT; ACNE, COSMETIC; ACNE, CYSTIC; ACNE, DRUG-INDUCED; ACNE, INFANT; ACNE, OIL;

ACNE DETERGENS; ACNE FULMINANS; ACNE KELOIDALIS; ACNE MECHANICA; ACNE VULGARIS.

acne neonatorum See ACNE, INFANT.

acne products, over-the-counter There are a number of ingredients found in non-prescription products that are considered safe and effective in the treatment of ACNE by the U.S. Food and Drug Administration. They include BENZOYL PEROXIDE 2.5 to 10 percent, RESORCINOL 2 percent (in certain combinations), resorcinol monacetate 3 percent (in certain combinations), SALICYLIC ACID 0.5 to 2 percent, and SULFUR 3 to 10 percent (in certain combinations).

All of these products dry and peel the skin to some degree. However, used together they may increase skin dryness and cause irritation.

acne rosacea See ROSACEA.

acne vulgaris Another name for common ACNE.

acrochordon See SKIN TAG.

acrocyanosis A condition induced by abnormal cold sensitivity, which causes spasms in small blood vessels. These spasms result in a loss of oxygen in the blood, which makes hands and feet blue, cold and sweaty. The problem is usually worsened by cold weather, and young women are particularly susceptible. Acrocyanosis is distantly related to RAYNAUD'S DISEASE, a more serious circulatory disorder in which the skin of the fingers and toes may be damaged by chronically reduced blood flow.

Treatment Options and Outlook

Treatment is often unnecessary. Drugs to dilate the blood vessels are not usually prescribed.

Risk Factors and Preventive Measures

The condition can be prevented by avoiding cold and tobacco.

acrodermatitis enteropathica A rare inherited disease in which the skin of the fingers, toes, mouth, anus, mouth, and scalp of infants is reddened, ulcerated and covered with pustules. In rare instances, the disorder can lead to blood poisoning and death if unrecognized and untreated.

The disease is caused by low levels of zinc in the skin as a result of problems in zinc metabolism. The problem occurs after weaning because human breast milk contains a substance (believed to be picolinic acid) that permits zinc absorption even when the intestinal factor normally controlling the absorption of zinc is deficient or absent. After weaning from breast milk, symptoms in affected babies occur in both boys and girls.

Symptoms and Diagnostic Path

Symptoms appear about four to 10 weeks after birth in bottle-fed babies, or after weaning in breastfed babies. They include failure to thrive, diarrhea, hair loss, nail problems, conjunctivitis and photophobia (hypersensitivity to light), emotional instability, decreased appetite, and skin problems.

Treatment Options and Outlook

Zinc dietary supplements reverse all symptoms. The supplements should not be taken with food (especially bread); nausea is a common side effect.

While the disease is lifelong, proper treatment leads to remission and a normal life span. The disease usually improves during adolescence, but it may persist into adulthood when it begins to resemble PSORIASIS.

acrodermatitis, papular See GIANOTTI-CROSTI SYNDROME.

acroparesthesia A medical term for the feeling of tingling in the fingers or toes.

See also PINS AND NEEDLES SYNDROME.

actinic Pertaining to changes caused by the ultraviolet rays of the Sun.

actinic conditions Conditions caused by overexposure to the sun. These include actinic dermatitis (inflammation of the skin), ACTINIC KERATOSIS (a sun-induced premalignant condition characterized by redness and swelling), BASAL CELL CARCINOMA, and SQUAMOUS CELL CARCINOMA. All these conditions can be prevented by avoiding the sun and using sunscreens from an early age.

See also DERMATITIS, ACTINIC.

actinic dermatitis See DERMATITIS, ACTINIC.

actinic keratosis Also known as solar keratosis, this lesion is a dry, scaly, rough pink-to-tan thickening of the skin caused by long-standing overexposure to the sun. This common skin lesion affects one out of six people; it is a precancerous condition that can lead to malignant skin tumors (SQUAMOUS CELL CARCINOMA).

Symptoms and Diagnostic Path

The condition is usually found in older patients; however, with increased exposure to the sun it is being seen in younger and younger patients.

Lesions occur most often on the face, back of the hands and forearms, neck, and exposed scalp. The lesions develop slowly, eventually growing to the size of a quarter inch, sometimes fading and reappearing. There are usually several keratoses at one time on areas of the body exposed to sunlight. The skin surrounding the lesion often shows evidence of chronic sun damage, including scaling, pigment variation, wrinkling, and atrophy.

Actinic damage of the lips is called "actinic cheilitis," if it proceeds to squamous cell carcinoma, about one-fifth of these lesions will spread.

Untreated, this type of cancer can invade the surrounding tissues or internal organs. The presence of this skin lesion indicates that the sun has damaged the skin, and any type of skin cancer can develop.

Since more than half a person's lifetime sun exposure usually occurs before age 20, keratoses *can* appear in a person's 20s if that person has not been sufficiently protected from sun damage.

Treatment Options and Outlook

While not all keratoses need to be removed, there are a number of treatments for those that do. The most common treatment is cryotherapy with LIQUID NITROGEN. With cryosurgery, the physician freezes the lesions by applying liquid nitrogen with a special spray or a cotton-tipped applicator and removes the lesions. This method does not require anesthesia and produces no bleeding. White spots may sometimes appear afterward on the skin's surface, but if done properly this is relatively uncommon.

In another method, CURETTAGE AND ELECTRO-DESICCATION, the physician scrapes the lesion and takes a biopsy to test for malignancy. During the procedure, bleeding is controlled by electrocautery (heat produced by an electric needle).

Alternatively, a physician could shave the keratosis by a process called "shave removal" to obtain a specimen for testing; the base of the lesion is destroyed and the bleeding is stopped by cauterization (heat).

DERMABRASION removes the upper layers of the skin by sanding or using a fine wire brush; redness and pain usually disappear after a few days.

Chemical peeling causes the top layers of the skin to slough off by applying glycolic acid, trichloroacetic acid or phenol while the patient is sedated; the skin is usually replaced within seven days by a new growth of skin.

LASER SURGERY may be used to treat actinic cheilitis by focusing a beam of light from a carbon dioxide laser; the damaged skin can be vaporized.

Two medicated creams—5-FLUOROURACIL or masoprocol are also effective in removing keratoses (especially when there are many lesions). A solution or cream of 1 to 5 percent fluorouracil is applied by the patient twice a day from two days a week to daily for four to nine weeks. Treatments cause the skin to become intensely red, causing some pain and skin breakdown. After treatment, the skin may be treated with a topical steroid (such as hydrocortisone 1 percent) to alleviate the inflammation.

Masoprocol cream (10 percent) is applied for four weeks and is now available by prescription. Redness and flaking are common side effects.

Risk Factors and Preventive Measures

Those at greatest risk for these lesions have fair skin, blond or red hair, and blue, green or gray eyes because their skin has less protective pigment. However, even those with dark skin can develop keratoses if they are exposed to the sun without protection, although those with black skin rarely have these lesions. Individuals with compromised immune systems as a result of chemotherapy, AIDS, or organ transplants are at higher risk.

Actinic keratoses are more likely to appear in older people because of the cumulative effects of the sun; one recent survey of individuals who had been exposed to large amounts of sunlight found keratoses in more than half of the men and a third of the women aged 65 to 74. Some experts believe that most people who live to be 80 or older have actinic keratoses.

actinic lentigo   See LENTIGO SIMPLEX.

actinomycosis   A deep bacterial infection of the skin caused by *Actinomyces israelii* or *Arachnia propionica*, normal bacteria always present in the mouth and tonsils that can cause infection when introduced into broken tissue. It is also possible to transmit this bacteria via a human bite.

Symptoms and Diagnostic Path

The most common form of the disease affects the mouth and jaw, causing a painful swelling. Small openings later develop on the skin of the face around the mouth, discharging PUS and characteristic yellow granules. Poor oral hygiene may contribute to this form of the infection.

A diagnosis is usually confirmed by presence of the granules.

Treatment Options and Outlook

Adequate surgical drainage is important, together with bed rest and good diet. Treatment with large doses of penicillin injections is usually successful, although medication may be needed for several months in severe infections.

acyclovir (Trade name: Zovirax) An antiviral drug introduced in 1982 used in treating the virus causing HERPES SIMPLEX INFECTION, SHINGLES, and CHICKEN POX. Acyclovir is available in topical or oral form. Severe cases may be treated with intravenous (IV) acyclovir.

Oral Acyclovir

Acyclovir is effective in managing both the initial infection and recurrent infections of herpes (including ECZEMA HERPETICUM) and in the treatment of shingles. It is effective in preventing subsequent viral attacks if taken continuously soon after infection. In patients with recurrent genital herpes, acyclovir therapy reduces the duration of viral shedding, and makes the lesions heal quicker, providing symptom relief.

In addition, acyclovir has been helpful to patients receiving bone marrow transplants to prevent the subsequent development of herpes simplex infection.

Topical Acyclovir

The topical form does not prevent new lesions from forming during the course of the disease, nor does it prevent the development of latency. When applied to an existing blister, however, it may relieve symptoms, speed healing, and shorten the duration of the infection and the contagious period.

Adverse Effects

Adverse effects are rare. The ointment may cause skin irritation or rash. Taken by mouth, the drug may cause headache, dizziness, or nausea/vomiting, confusion, or hallucinations. Rarely, acyclovir injections may cause kidney damage.

See also VALACYCLOVIR; FAMCICLOVIR.

Addison's disease A rare endocrine or hormonal disorder characterized by a deficiency of the hormones hydrocortisone and aldosterone. The disease, which affects about one in 100,000 people, occurs in all age groups and afflicts men and women equally. It was invariably fatal before hormone treatment became available in the 1950s.

The disease was named for the English physician Thomas Addison (1793–1860), who first diagnosed the disorder. It is likely that the late president John F. Kennedy suffered from this disease.

Addison's disease occurs when the adrenal glands do not produce enough of the hormone cortisol and in some cases, the hormone aldosterone. For this reason, the disease is sometimes called chronic adrenal insufficiency, or hypocortisolism.

Failure to produce enough cortisol can occur for different reasons. The problem may be due to a disorder of the adrenal glands themselves (primary adrenal insufficiency) or to inadequate secretion of acrinocorticotropic hormone (ACTH) by the pituitary gland (secondary adrenal insufficiency). Most cases of Addison's disease are caused by the gradual destruction of the adrenal cortex, the outer layer of the adrenal glands, by the body's own immune system. About 70 percent of reported cases of Addison's disease are due to autoimmune disorders, in which the immune system makes antibodies that attack the body's own tissues or organs and slowly destroys them. Adrenal insufficiency occurs when at least 90 percent of the adrenal cortex has been destroyed. As a result, often both glucocorticoid and mineralocorticoid hormones are lacking. Sometimes only the adrenal gland is affected; sometimes other glands also are affected.

Less common causes of primary adrenal insufficiency are chronic infections, mainly fungal infections; cancer cells spreading from other parts of the body to the adrenal glands; amyloidosis; and surgical removal of the adrenal glands.

Symptoms and Diagnostic Path

The disease begins with a feeling of malaise and is characterized by weight loss, muscle weakness, and fatigue. The symptoms of adrenal insufficiency usually begin gradually. Nausea, vomiting, and diarrhea occur in about 50 percent of cases. Blood pressure is low and falls further when standing, causing dizziness or fainting. Skin changes also are common in Addison's disease, with areas of dark tanning covering exposed and nonexposed parts of the body. This darkening of the skin is most visible on scars; skin folds; pressure points, such as the elbows, knees, knuckles, and toes; lips; and mucous membranes.

Addison's disease also can cause irritability and depression. Because of salt loss, craving of salty foods is common. Low blood sugar is more severe in children than in adults. In women, menstrual periods may become irregular or stop.

Because the symptoms progress slowly, they are usually ignored until a stressful event like an illness or an accident causes them to become worse.

In its early stages, adrenal insufficiency can be difficult to diagnose. A review of a patient's medical history based on the symptoms, especially the dark tanning of the skin, will lead a doctor to suspect Addison's disease. A diagnosis is made by biochemical laboratory tests to determine whether there are low levels of cortisol. X-ray exams of the adrenal and pituitary glands also are useful in helping to establish the cause, as are the ACTH stimulation and insulin-induced hypoglycemia tests.

Treatment Options and Outlook

The pigmentation disappears slowly when the patient receives glucocorticosteroid replacement therapy. Still, most patients retain a slight tan color for the rest of their lives.

adenoma sebaceum   See ANGIOFIBROMA.

adenosine monophosphate (AMP)   A metabolism byproduct that may help ease the pain of SHINGLES. The treatment has no side effects, and works best within the first few months of pain when the nerve endings have experienced minimal damage.

Otherwise, the pain following a shingles outbreak (POSTHERPETIC NEURALGIA) is treated with the painkillers Tylenol and codeine, if necessary. In addition, ZOSTRIX (CAPSAICIN) has been found to be effective.

adenovirus   One of a group of viruses that cause infections of the upper respiratory tract, producing measleslike eruptions and symptoms of the common cold. Adenoviruses are often diagnosed in the winter and spring.

Most infections are mild and require no therapy or only symptomatic treatment. Because there is no virus-specific therapy, serious adenovirus illness can be managed only by treating symptoms and complications of the infection.

adipose nevi   A rare type of connective tissue BIRTHMARK characterized by grouped yellowish nodules that form plaques, usually appearing on the lower torso and upper thighs. The condition, also known as *nevus lipomatosus superficialis Hoffmann and Zurhelle*, does not require treatment.

adipose tissue   A layer of fat beneath the skin and around internal organs. After puberty, the distribution of this superficial adipose tissue changes in males and females; women have a greater proportion of total body weight in adipose tissue accumulated on breasts, hips, and thighs. In adult males, adipose tissue accumulates around the shoulders, waist, and abdomen.

Adipose tissue is constructed from fat deposits left by excess food intake and serves as an energy store; too much adipose tissue causes obesity. The tissue is an insulator and keeps the body warm, especially in babies, and it also helps absorb shock in areas subject to sudden or frequent pressure (such as the buttocks and feet).

adnexa of skin   The cutaneous structures that make up the hair, nails and sebaceous, eccrine, and APOCRINE GLANDS.

See also SEBACEOUS GLANDS.

age spots   Blemishes that appear on the skin as a person ages. The most common of these spots are SEBORRHEIC KERATOSES—brown or yellow-brown raised spots that may occur anywhere on the body. Other common age spots in the elderly are LIVER SPOTS (lentigines), ACTINIC KERATOSES, and Campbell De Morgan's spots (cherry ANGIOMAS)—red, pinpoint blemishes.

Treatment is usually not necessary except for actinic keratoses, which may become malignant. Freezing the keratoses with liquid nitrogen and removing them is the usual treatment, although they may be removed surgically with a local anesthetic.

While most age spots are harmless, any inexplicable blemish (or one that bleeds or grows rapidly) may represent skin cancer and should be examined by a physician. Brown spots that have irregularities of brown color or irregular borders also should be shown to a physician.

See also KERATOSIS.

aging and skin Loss of elastic tissue and COLLAGEN causes the skin to sag and wrinkle; weakened blood capillaries cause skin to bruise more easily. This damage is accelerated by exposure to the sun or by smoking. In fact, there are really two types of skin aging—chronological aging and photoaging.

Chronological aging is just what it sounds like—the inherited tendency to age. Photoaging (or solar-induced aging) is caused by damage from exposure to the sun, and this type of skin problem is more common today than skin problems due to chronological aging.

As a person ages, the skin produces fewer cells and repairs damaged cells more slowly, while cells in the horny layer of the skin become dryer and rougher. At the same time, the number of melanin-producing cells (MELANOCYTES) drops, leading to patchy skin color. Wound healing is also slowed down, and there is usually a decreased ability to clear foreign material and fluid. Increasing rigidity, inelasticity, and a decrease of dermal collagen and elastin fibers make the skin begin to wrinkle and sag.

Fat distribution in the skin also changes with age, redistributing itself to the waist in men and the thighs in women. At the same time, the SUBCUTIS begins to thin in certain areas such as the face, hands, feet, and shins.

In addition, aging glands produce less oil and smaller amounts of perspiration, and so there is less oil to trap moisture on the skin's surface and less perspiration to moisturize skin. Heat, air conditioning, and wind can further dehydrate the skin.

Age also affects hair color, graying or whitening it because of a decrease in the number of melanin-producing cells. Most people also notice thinning and slower hair regrowth rate, while on the other hand, hair begins to appear in unwanted places (ears, nose, and eyebrows in men and upper lip and chin in women).

Treatment Options and Outlook

There are literally hundreds of products on the market that claim to reverse the consequences of aging. Lotions containing ALPHA HYDROXY ACID and Retin-A have been shown to reverse some features of skin aging; no other skin products have ever been shown to improve or slow the aging process.

Alternatively, it is possible not to reverse aging but to erase it with injectable soft tissue fillers, which are designed to produce a smoother, more youthful appearance with minimal recovery time and maximum safety. In the past, doctors have used bovine (cow) collagen and the patient's own body fat to safely diminish creases and give the face a more youthful appearance.

While these methods are effective, the fillers (especially collagen) were not a long-term solution; they required frequent office visits to maintain the youthful look.

However, in early 2003 the U.S. Food and Drug Administration (FDA) approved two injectable products containing human collagen that plump up the skin. Later in the year and in 2004, they approved two hyaluronic acid fillers that lasted longer than collagen injections. Injectable soft tissue fillers are used to improve the appearance of fine lines and wrinkles, fill out hollow cheeks, lighten scars, lessen deep folds, and repair other facial flaws. Results are, or close to, immediate; however, it may take more than one treatment to achieve the desired effect. The length of time that you can expect the results to last varies.

Bovine collagen The oldest and best-known filler is purified bovine collagen, which dermatologists use to fill in fine lines around the eyes and deep lines from the nose to the corners of the lips, as well as enlarge lips and erase acne scars. Typically, a series of injections will help fill out the imperfections and give almost immediate results, each session lasting about 10 to 30 minutes.

While this method is certainly effective, the procedure must be done again within three to four months, depending on the size of the area treated, how much collagen was injected, and how healthy the filled skin was. The procedure often causes some redness, swelling, or bruising around the injection site, which usually disappeared in a few days. Patients with a history of allergic reactions or cold sores risk further possible outbreaks.

Patient's body fat For years dermatologists also have been successfully injecting the patient's own body fat. Since the patient's own body fat is used to fill in the creases, potential allergic reactions are not an issue and allergy testing is not required.

In this procedure, the dermatologist transfers the patient's own fat from a part of the patient's body with excess fat to an area that has lost fat as a result of aging. Typically, the fat is used to plump up deep creases around the nose and mouth, to fill scars, or to replace fat pads in the cheeks. This technique may require follow-up visits to achieve the desired effects. Results last longer than with bovine collagen—typically between one to three years. Treatment of scars with this method tends to last longer.

Potential side effects with this method are similar to other fillers; swelling and bruising and sometimes lumps can develop around the lips or the eyes where body fat does not naturally occur.

Human-based collagen Two products containing human-based collagen (COSMODERM and COSMOPLAST) received FDA approval in March 2003 for the correction of facial wrinkles, acne scars, restoration of the lip border, and other soft-tissue contour problems. Allergy testing is not required with these fillers, which makes same-day treatment possible. Side effects are usually limited to temporary redness and swelling around the injection site. As with bovine collagen, results are noticeable almost right away, and last about three to four months. Repeated treatments may be needed to achieve the desired effects.

Although human collagen was an improvement over bovine collagen because it did not trigger allergies, dermatologists still needed a filler that could safely and effectively fill folds but last longer than three to four months. Finally, two new fillers have been approved by the FDA that can replace the skin's hyaluronic acid lost during aging. These fillers work by pulling water into the skin, plumping up the skin and adding volume.

Hyaluronic acid gel For years, dermatologists have known that wrinkles result from the loss of three crucial skin components—collagen, elastin, and hyaluronic acid. Today, doctors can replace two of these components (collagen and hyaluronic acid).

Hyaluronic acid holds together collagen and elastin, providing a framework for the skin. When injected into the skin in gel form, hyaluronic acid binds to water and adds volume to easily fill in larger folds of skin around the mouth and cheeks. Patients notice an immediate plumping of the skin in the treated areas.

HYALURONIC ACID GEL (Restylane) and hylan-Bgel (Hylaform), both approved in 2005 by the FDA, are injected into facial tissue to smooth wrinkles and folds, especially in the folds around the nose and mouth. Hyaluronic acid is a protective, lubricating and binding gel substance that is produced naturally by the body. These two fillers work by temporarily adding volume to facial tissue and restoring a smoother appearance to the face for an effect that lasts for about six months.

The hyaluronic fillers are injected by a doctor into areas of facial tissue where moderate to severe facial wrinkles and folds occur. The gel temporarily adds volume to the skin and can give the appearance of a smoother surface. Restylane and Hylaform will help smooth moderate to severe facial wrinkles and folds. In one study, most patients needed just one injection to smooth out the wrinkles; about one-third of patients needed more than one injection to get a satisfactory result.

One of the main advantages of hyaluronic acid gel is that it rarely triggers allergic reactions, nor is there a risk of transmitting animal diseases by injection as there is with bovine collagen. Since a skin check for allergies is not required with hyaluronic acid gel, patients can be treated on their first visit to the dermatologist. In addition, hyaluronic acid treatments last about four to six months or longer and require less volume to fill wrinkles and hard-to-treat skin folds compared to collagen.

Hyaluronic acid fillers have side effects, and pain is a problem. Since hyaluronic acid gel does not contain the anesthetic lidocaine, injections are painful. In addition, there is usually temporary inflammation that produces swelling and redness following injection with hyaluronic acid gel—especially in the lip area.

Some dermatologists combine hyaluronic acid and collagen. Injecting collagen first numbs and supports the area, stabilizing the skin to prevent bruising. Then hyaluronic acid gel is injected painlessly. Using these fillers together replaces two of the skin components that are lost with skin aging.

Silicone Until it was banned by the FDA in 1992, injectable silicone was used in the United States for many years to successfully treat wrinkles and ACNE scars as well as enhance lips, cheekbones, and the chin. However, problems emerged when medical-grade silicone was diluted with foreign substances, such as mineral oil, when non-medical grade silicone was injected and when it was injected in large volumes.

What makes silicone unique is that the results are permanent. Studies are showing that once the desired results are achieved, there is no need for future treatments unless it becomes necessary as the patient ages or disease processes continue.

Unfortunately, side effects may include delayed reactions that trigger redness and lumpiness as the body rejects the silicone. In the past, more problems were reported with silicone breast implants. However, side effects are rare when silicone is injected by a dermatologic surgeon skilled in the microdroplet technique, in which tiny amounts of silicone are injected at four- to eight-week intervals until the desired effect is achieved. Using silicone as a filler is not approved by the FDA, but it is used by some physicians as a filler in the United States in an off-label manner.

Fibroblasts Harvesting the patient's own collagen-producing cells (FIBROBLASTS) holds promise for filling fine facial lines, enhancing lips and correcting scars. Results reportedly last a bit longer than bovine collagen, and side effects are minimal. However, the procedure is time-consuming and it is not FDA-approved. First, a dermatologist must remove a small amount of the patients skin tissue and close the area with adhesive or sutures. The tissue is shipped to a company that cultures the fibroblasts, using its patented process. In six weeks, the harvested cells are delivered to the dermatologist's office, and the patient must return for skin testing because the substance in which the cells are grown can cause an allergic reaction. If no allergic reaction occurs within two weeks, treatment can begin.

Risk Factors and Preventive Measures

Obviously, prevention offers the best chance to avoid excess age-related damage to the skin. Those who have stayed away from the sun's rays for most or all of their lives will have much healthier skin than the senior citizen who has been a sun-worshipper for decades.

Health habits also play a role—getting enough sleep, fresh air, exercise, and good food. Cutting down or eliminating smoking will also improve the condition of the skin. Research suggests that smokers (whether young or old, male or female, smiling or unsmiling) tend to look five or more years older than their chronological age.

AIDS and skin disorders The skin symptoms of AIDS can range from a severe form of normally mild eruptions to unusual lesions such as the pink-purple spots of KAPOSI'S SARCOMA, and oral hairy LEUKOPLAKIA. In fact, skin symptoms may be the very first sign of a suppressed immune system.

Viral Infections

A wide range of viral infections may plague the patient with AIDS, including HERPES SIMPLEX (1 and 2), SHINGLES, MOLLUSCUM CONTAGIOSUM, WARTS, and oral hairy leukoplakia. Herpes attacks are far more common in patients with AIDS than in the general population, and they are more likely to be deep, painful, and slow to heal (especially in the perianal area). Occasionally, herpes simplex infections in patients with AIDS are resistant to ACYCLOVIR, the primary drug treatment for herpes simplex.

The appearance of shingles in an individual is highly suggestive of HIV infection, and the likelihood that the patient will go on to develop full-blown AIDS is high. In addition, recurrent shingles may also occur in patients with AIDS.

Both common WARTS and CONDYLOMATA ACUMINATA are common and can be very difficult to treat in this patient population. Warts in the anal area may become large and require surgical removal.

The lesions of oral hairy leukoplakia which are fairly specific to patients with AIDS, appear on the side of the tongue as white linear lesions.

Bacterial Infections

Treatment of SYPHILIS may be difficult in patients with AIDS, and one dose of penicillin may not cure the disease. Other bacterial infections that may be seen include CAT SCRATCH FEVER, mycobacterial infections, ECTHYMA, CELLULITIS, ABSCESSES, IMPETIGO, and FOLLICULITIS.

Fungal Infections

Oral CANDIDIASIS is very common. Fungal infections are frequent, including ATHLETE'S FOOT, JOCK ITCH and nail infection. CRYPTOCOCOCCIS as either a single skin lesion or as herpeslike ulcers or histoplasmosis are also common.

Parasitic Infections

AMEBIASIS or SCABIES may occur among patients with AIDS.

Skin Tumors

In addition to Kaposi's sarcoma, patients with AIDS have a high incidence of lymphoma.

Miscellaneous Skin Lesions

Patients with AIDS are much more likely than other patients to experience drug reactions. Explosive PSORIASIS may occur in these patients. Often, patients with AIDS develop seborrheic DERMATITIS of the scalp, face (especially center of the face), armpits, chest, groin, and genitals.

In addition, these patients may experience itchy papular eruptions over the body, acquired ICHTHYOSIS and very dry skin. An atopic-like dermatitis has developed in about half of all children with AIDS.

Hair Problems

As the disease progresses, patients report their hair becomes softer, lighter, thinner, and silkier.

Nail Problems

Yellow colored nails have been reported; others notice bluish bands that occur during administration of zidovudine (AZT).

air travel and the skin Frequent airplane travel can have a negative effect on skin and hair, especially for those with dry skin. The low humidity and lack of fresh air on board can greatly increase flaky skin, dryness, and irritation. Even those with oily skin complain that they develop dry patches of skin on cheeks and chin during plane travel, followed by a "rebound effect" of excess oiliness.

If possible, women should not wear makeup during air travel, but apply a moisturizer and eye cream the morning of the flight, reapplying it during any trip longer than two hours. For those who *must* wear makeup during air travel, use a water-based foundation and undermakeup primer or moisturizer.

Travelers should refrain from drinking alcohol or caffeinated beverages on a plane, since alcohol and caffeine are natural diuretics, minimizing the amount of moisture available to skin cells. Some travelers carry a mineral water spritzer to refresh and moisturize complexions. Travelers should always wear a lip balm or moisturized lip color on board, to prevent lips from drying and cracking, and reapply hand cream several times during the trip (especially if hands are washed during the flight).

For irritated eyes (especially for those who wear contact lenses), cotton pads soaked in distilled water or milk should be applied to closed lids for several minutes. Contact lens wearers might consider abandoning the lenses altogether for the duration of the flight.

A few minutes before landing, the face should be cleansed and moisturizer should be applied; women can then apply water-based foundation, mascara, blusher, and lip gloss.

albinism A rare congenital inherited condition characterized by a partial or total lack of the pigment MELANIN that gives color to skin, eyes, and hair. Found in people of all races, albinos often suffer visual problems, skin inflammations, severe sunburn, and a tendency toward SKIN CANCER.

The most common type of albinism is inherited in an autosomal recessive pattern. Usually parents have normal skin coloring, but they carry the gene defect in a hidden form. If parents with normal pigmentation have an albino child, there is a one in four chance that future children will be affected.

Less than five per 100,000 people in the United States and Europe are affected, although the prevalence is much higher in some parts of the world (about 20 per 100,000 in southern Nigeria, for instance).

The most serious complication of the disease is the lack of melanin, which protects the skin against the harmful radiation in sunlight. Because the skin cannot tan, it ages prematurely and is prone to skin cancers. Visual problems common in albinos can also cause problems.

Symptoms and Diagnostic Path

The most common type of albinism is called oculocutaneous albinism, in which the hair, skin, and eyes are all affected. In the more severe form, the skin and hair are snowy white throughout life. Less severely affected individuals may be born with white skin and hair, but both darken slightly with age and numerous FRECKLES develop on sun-exposed parts of the body. In both forms, the eyes cannot tolerate bright lights and are often affected with abnormal flickering movements, squinty eyes, and nearsightedness. More rare types of albinism affect either only skin, hair, or the eyes.

Albright's syndrome   The popular term for fibrous dysplasia, a condition characterized by a few large dark flat spots with very irregular borders (often compared to the coast of Maine). There are also developmental abnormalities, such as bony lesions and endocrine problems, such as precocious sexual development.

The syndrome is not genetic, although it is more common in girls.

Symptoms and Diagnostic Path

Symptoms include bone pain, fractures, and skin pigment changes. Other related symptoms include mental deficiency, epilepsy, and headaches.

Treatment Options and Outlook

There is no specific treatment for this disorder other than observation and treatment of bone fractures or deformities, together with screening for the development of endocrine disorders. There is an increased incidence of sudden death caused by heart rhythm problems.

alcohol   An organic compound with strong grease-cutting properties used in many cosmetics as an antiseptic astringent. Alcohol cools the skin as it evaporates. It is very drying, however, and people with dry skin should avoid products containing alcohol. Alcohol can be found in some soaps, deodorants, skin fresheners, colognes, acne products, mousses, gels, and setting lotions.

alcohol and skin cancer   Research suggests that alcohol use can contribute to malignant melanoma (the most deadly form of skin cancer). Several studies appear to have uncovered a link between alcohol and melanoma. Experts recommend women limit themselves to one drink a day, and men to no more than two drinks a day.

See also MELANOMA, MALIGNANT.

alkaptonuria   See OCHRONOSIS.

allergens   Foreign substances that induce allergic reactions that include skin rashes. Some common examples are certain foods, dust, plants, and so on.

allergies and the skin   The skin is one of the first sites where the symptoms of allergy may appear. A rash occurs when the immune system tries to fight off a foreign substance (called an ALLERGEN) that comes in contact with the skin. Some of the most common skin allergens include poison ivy (more than 50 percent of people are allergic to these plants), fragrances, preservatives, hair dyes, formaldehyde, nickel, cement, shoe leather, and rubber.

Chromium/Chromates

Contact with these substances is the most common cause of rash in men, usually occurring on the job. Chromium is typically found in the environment, and therefore is not easy to avoid. A primary source of chromium is in cement, widely used in machining and construction. Shoes made from leather tanned with chromates can cause ECZEMA on the feet of sensitive people.

Collagen (Injectable)

About 3 percent of healthy people are allergic to injectable collagen, used to smooth out facial wrinkles and creases; about half of them experience the allergy after the actual treatment has begun. Once an allergy develops, further treatments are not advisable.

Cosmetics

Allergic reactions to cosmetics are usually caused by fragrances such as cinnamic alcohol, cinnamic aldehyde, hydroxycitronnella, musk ambrette, isoeugenol, and geraniol.

Drugs

Almost any medication can cause an allergic reaction in a sensitive individual, although allergic reactions to most drugs are uncommon. A reaction is caused by a hypersensitive immune system triggering a misdirected response against a substance that does not affect most people. The body becomes sensitized by the first exposure to the medication, and subsequent exposure will then trigger an immune response. Reactions can range from a mild rash or hives to life-threatening anaphylaxis. Serum sickness is a delayed type of drug allergy that occurs a week or more after exposure to a medication or vaccine.

Penicillin and other antibiotics in that family are the most common cause of drug allergies. Other allergy-causing drugs include sulfa medications, barbiturates, anticonvulsants, insulin preparations (especially from animal sources), local anesthetics, and iodine (found in many X-ray contrast dyes).

Common symptoms include hives, skin rash, and itchy skin or eyes. Other symptoms include wheezing and facial swelling. Anaphylaxis may trigger nasal congestion, difficulty breathing, cough, blue skin, fainting, light-headed dizziness, anxiety, confusion, slurred speech, rapid pulse, palpitations, nausea, vomiting, diarrhea, abdominal pain, or cramping.

Skin testing may confirm allergy to penicillin, but it may be ineffective for other medications.

Antihistamines usually ease common symptoms; prednisone or topical steroids may also be prescribed. Epinephrine treats anaphylaxis.

Foods

A range of common foods may bring on allergic reactions on the skin, including citrus fruits, eggs, fish, artificial coloring, sugar alcohols, or milk. Acute hives usually result from an allergic reaction to foods such as shellfish, nuts, berries, tomatoes, eggs, citrus fruits, chicken, and pork. Less commonly, individuals develop hives from contact of food with skin (chicken, fish, and certain vegetables). Allergy prick or scratch skin testing to determine food allergies is often ineffective, sometimes producing a false positive (showing an allergy when no symptoms actually appear when the food is eaten) or a false negative (showing no reaction when tested on the skin but having strong reactions when the food is eaten).

Footwear

It is possible to develop a contact allergy to footwear chemicals, especially rubber or rubber cements, leather-tanning products, or dyes. They cause itching, redness, swelling, and small blisters. These symptoms appear most readily on the thin sensitive skin of the tops and sides of the feet. Avoiding such an allergy may mean buying special shoes and keeping the feet dry, since potential allergens can be leached out of footwear by sweat.

Fragrances

A wide variety of products contain fragrances that may trigger an allergic reaction in some people, including soaps, tissues, creams, and deodorants. Since manufacturers closely guard the specific ingredients in scented products (the products usually simply list "fragrance" on their label), sensitive consumers may find the "fragrance free" products to be their best choice. Those marked "hypoallergenic," while good for sensitive people, may still contain some scent that may cause a reaction in very sensitive individuals. "Unscented" products are not a good choice because they contain some fragrance traces that have been included to mask unpleasant odors naturally found in the product.

Some eaux de cologne, which contain oil of bergamot, can cause a berloque DERMATITIS (dark color when exposed to the sun on neck and cleavage of women) in the area of skin where the cologne is applied. Those sensitive to some types of perfume could try spraying the product on hair or clothing instead of skin.

Genital Deodorants

These products can produce a contact dermatitis, including swelling and itching.

Hair Dye

Permanent dyes contain *paraphenylenediamine,* which can cause an oozing red rash in allergic patients. This is the reason why patch tests are recommended before dyeing hair. For sensitive people, temporary or vegetable hair dyes are a good alternative.

Lanolin

This type of animal fat derived from sheep oil glands is commonly included in moisturizers. Many people with sensitive skin are allergic to lanolin.

Nail Products

Allergic reactions can occur from a wide variety of nail products, including nail polishes, nail hardeners, and artificial nails. Most nail products contain toluenesulfonamide formaldehyde resin, which can set off an allergic response when it comes in contact with eyelids, the neck, or other sensitive areas. If nail products contain this chemical, women should be sure the nails have dried for an hour before touching the skin.

Nickel

This shiny stainless metal is often used in surface plating of metal objects such as buttons, costume jewelry, and kitchen equipment. It is also an element in many alloys, and is widely used in dentistry. Allergy to nickel occurs 10 times more often in women then men, and is often triggered by ear piercing. Having the ears pierced and using earrings with nickel posts causes subsequent rashes

to appear in other areas of the body whenever the person touches objects containing nickel. In allergic individuals, necklaces, bracelets, belt buckles, and other jewelry that have never before caused a problem may suddenly cause a rash after the ears are pierced. Those at high risk for developing an occupational nickel allergy include hairdressers, nurses, cashiers, and metal industry employees.

People with newly pierced ears should wear only steel posts until earlobes heal (about three weeks). Surgical steel is the best choice and is available most often in earrings specifically designed for sensitive skin. Individuals should avoid the heat when wearing this type of jewelry, and buy only high-quality jewelry that is at least 14-karat gold; the higher the karat, the lower the percentage of nickel. A few dermatologists warn highly sensitive patients to avoid foods that may contain traces of nickel, such as coffee, beer, tea, apricots, chocolate, and nuts.

Parabens

A group of often-used preservatives, parabens can be found in a variety of products (especially cosmetics).

Plastics

Plastics such as epoxy resin can affect workers; finished plastic products rarely cause sensitivity.

Preservatives

A wide variety of cosmetics, shampoos, creams, and lotions contain preservatives to extend their shelf life and prevent bacteria buildup. The most toxic of these are quaternium 15, imidazolidinyl urea and dialozolidinyl urea.

Rubber (Latex)

The stretchy material used in many types of surgical gloves and condoms, bras, waistbands, and sneakers cause two types of allergic reactions. Most common is a red, oozing, blistering eruption. Less common are hives. About a third of those who develop hives from contact with latex also develop other symptoms, including hay fever, asthma and even anaphylactic shock. This type of reaction is often seem among medical workers because of the extensive use of latex gloves. Those sensitive to rubber should avoid clothes with exposed rubber, since rubber covered by cloth usually does not cause a problem. Women who are allergic to rubber condoms should have their partner wear a lambskin condom over a latex one (a lambskin condom alone won't protect against HIV). Men allergic to rubber should wear a lambskin condom under a latex condom.

Sun

While most people think of the sun as the source of a so-called "healthy" tan, it can also cause allergies in some people, who develop bumps, blotches, hives, or blisters. Some people are allergic to the sun alone, others to a combination of cosmetics, soaps, detergents, perfumes, or topical or systemic medications, that react with the sun.

Topical Agents

Many people are sensitive to the active or inactive ingredients in topical drugs or cosmetics, including lanolin, bacitracin, neomycin, local anesthetics, formaldehyde, and preservatives.

See also FORMALDEHYDE, SENSITIVITY TO; SOLAR URTICARIA; OIL OF BERGAMOT; POLYMORPHIC LIGHT ERUPTION.

allergy tests See PATCH TESTS.

AlloDerm A soft SKIN FILLER made of human tissue donated in much the same way as other transplantable organs and approved by the U.S. Food and Drug Administration (FDA) for cosmetic use. AlloDerm may be used to enhance the lips or to fill in lines and creases that develop with aging.

AlloDerm is processed from donated human cadaver tissue prepared in such a way that it retains its underlying structure. It has been used for a variety of surgical reconstructive procedures to replace lost, damaged, or diseased tissues, and is now used to fill in facial wrinkles, where it is considered stable and may last from one to two years.

A micronized form of AlloDerm, called CYMETRA, is also available. This material is rehydrated with lidocaine in the physician's office before injection so the procedure is much less painful.

Because it is human derived, no skin test is required by the manufacturer. Studies so far have found no evidence of allergic reactions, although temporary bruising, redness, and swelling occur in a few patients.

AlloDerm is obtained from tissue banks, which surgically remove a thin layer of skin from deceased donors, using sterile operating room techniques. The skin is placed into an antibiotic solution and processed to remove the top layer of skin cells and all of the cells in the deepest layer. The remaining material—the AlloDerm—is a COLLAGEN framework that provides strength to the skin, but without any components left to cause rejection or inflammation. Therefore, when transplanted to a patient, the AlloDerm graft gradually becomes a natural part of the patient's own tissue. Before any processing of the skin takes place, the tissue donors are rigorously screened by the tissue bank and extensively tested for infectious diseases. The donor must be found free of hepatitis B and C, HIV and AIDS, and SYPHILIS. In any case, human viruses including HIV need cells to live and reproduce; the AlloDerm process removes all cells, getting rid of the components necessary for the survival and transmission of these viruses.

AlloDerm was first used in 1992 to treat burn patients and in 1994 for periodontal and plastic surgery. Currently, more than 50,000 patients have received AlloDerm grafts.

AlloDerm is the only available product capable of regenerating normal soft tissue. Since it is human tissue, it does not trigger an inflammatory or allergic reaction, and the pretreatment skin testing required with bovine collagen is not needed. In addition, patients report that the graft does not feel hard the way other synthetic materials do. When AlloDerm is used as an implant, it completely eliminates any need to take donor fat or skin from one part of the body to transplant to another area.

Although AlloDerm appears to be long lasting, there have been reports of a small number of patients completely absorbing the AlloDerm within six months. AlloDerm lip enhancement is irreversible after a period of seven to eight weeks. Given the increasing number of safe and effective fillers available in the United States, the use of AlloDerm has declined dramatically by the early 2000s.

See also BIOLOGICAL IMPLANT.

allograft A type of tissue or organ graft (also known as homograft) between two members of the same species.

See also AUTOGRAFT; PINCH GRAFT; SKIN GRAFT.

aloe vera A wild succulent (*Aloe barbadensis* Miller) of the lily family used for centuries as a healing agent and beauty aid. Aloe vera juice (obtained from slicing the tip of leaf and squeezing out the gel) appears to be effective in relieving the pain and inflammation of sunburn. The aloe vera gel contains vitamins B_1, B_2 and B_6, calcium, potassium, chlorine, enzymes, and other ingredients that have not yet been identified.

alopecia, androgenetic The most common type of hair loss that includes hereditary HAIR LOSS and male pattern baldness. Normal genes and male hormones (especially testosterone) cause progressive shrinking of certain scalp follicles over time. The shrinking follicle produces a smaller, finer hair with each growth cycle. In addition to a smaller follicle, androgenetic alopecia is characterized by a shortened growth phase, which results in shorter hair.

The balding process is a gradual conversion of active, large hair follicles to less active, smaller follicles, resulting in short, thin hairs that are barely visible and that eventually disappear completely. In men, hereditary baldness is characterized by a receding hairline above the forehead and loss of hair at the crown. If male pattern baldness progresses to its final stage, the person is left with hair only around the sides and back of the head.

In women, hereditary hair loss is a general or diffuse thinning of the hair over the top of the head; half of all women have a notable thinning by age 50, but rarely lose all their hair. The hairline in front is almost always maintained.

Treatment Options and Outlook

A topical solution of MINOXIDIL (Rogaine) 2 percent applied twice daily to the scalp lessens falling hair and stimulates new hair growth; one third of patients using this product report moderate hair growth after one year. Treatment with minoxidil is most effective if begun early; patients who have been balding for less than five years or who have smaller bald patches report the best results. It may take several months for hair growth to begin, and if the treatment is stopped, the newly regrown hair will fall out. Minoxidil is effective for both men and women. It was developed to treat high blood pressure, and it increases the diameter of blood vessels.

Alternatively, HAIR TRANSPLANTS or scalp reduction (removal of the bald area of the scalp) are effective treatments for men with male pattern baldness.

See also ALOPECIA, FRICTION; ALOPECIA, TRACTION; ALOPECIA AREATA.

alopecia, friction The loss of hair caused by constantly wearing snug-fitting wigs or hats.

See also ALOPECIA, ANDROGENETIC; ALOPECIA, TRACTION; ALOPECIA AREATA; HAIR LOSS.

alopecia, traction Loss of hair caused by ponytails, braids, or cornrows that are pulled too tight, pulling the hair out by its roots.

See also ALOPECIA, ANDROGENETIC; ALOPECIA, FRICTION; ALOPECIA AREATA; HAIR LOSS.

alopecia areata A common form of hair loss that usually begins with a small, round bare spot on the scalp; in extreme cases it progresses to total hair loss on the entire body. It can affect people of all ages, although it most often occurs in children and young adults.

The condition is generally believed to be an autoimmune disorder in which the body produces antibodies that cause hair follicles to stop hair production. It may run in families, especially those with a history of asthma, ECZEMA, or autoimmune disorders such as rheumatoid arthritis or LUPUS ERYTHEMATOSUS. Alopecia areata affects about 4 million Americans of both sexes and all ages and ethnic backgrounds. It often begins in childhood. Patients with a close family member with the disease have a slightly higher risk of developing the condition. If the family member lost the first patch of hair before age 30, the risk to other family members is greater.

Overall, one in five people with the disease have a family member who has it as well. In those who are genetically predisposed, some type of trigger—perhaps a virus or something in the person's environment—brings on the attack against the hair follicles.

Alopecia areata often occurs in people whose family members have other autoimmune diseases, such as diabetes, rheumatoid arthritis, thyroid disease, VITILIGO, systemic lupus erythematosus, pernicious anemia, or ADDISON'S DISEASE. People who have alopecia areata do not usually have other autoimmune diseases, but they do have a higher occurrence of thyroid disease, atopic eczema, nasal allergies, and asthma.

Symptoms and Diagnostic Path

In *alopecia totalis*, hair suddenly falls out in a generalized pattern, ending in complete baldness of the scalp but body hair is preserved. In *alopecia areata universalis* all body hair is lost, including head, pubic, underarm, eyebrow, and eyelid hair. The most common form of alopecia areata (also known as localized alopecia) is characterized by a complete loss of hair on the head in one circular patch from one to 10 cm in diameter; the nails also may be affected by pitting, ridging, or splitting.

Treatment Options and Outlook

While there is no cure, in the localized form hair frequently regrows without treatment.

CORTICOSTEROIDS are powerful anti-inflammatory drugs that suppress the immune system, and are often used to treat various autoimmune diseases, including alopecia areata. Corticosteroids may be administered in three ways for alopecia areata—by injection, orally, or topically.

Local injections Injections of steroids directly into hairless patches on the scalp can boost hair growth in most people within a month. Injections deliver small amounts of CORTISONE to affected areas, avoiding the more serious side effects encountered with long-term oral use. The main side effects of injections are temporary pain, mild swelling, and sometimes changes in pigmentation, as well as small indentations in the skin that go away when injections are stopped. Because injections can be painful, they may not be the preferred treatment for children. After a month or two, new hair growth becomes visible; the injections usually have to be repeated monthly. Large areas cannot be treated, however, because the discomfort and the amount of medicine involved is too large and affects the entire body.

Oral corticosteroids Corticosteroids taken by mouth may be used in more severe cases of alopecia areata. However, because of the risk of side effects (such as high blood pressure and cataracts), they are used only occasionally for alopecia areata and for shorter periods of time.

Topical ointments Ointments or creams containing steroids rubbed directly onto the affected area are less painful than injections and are sometimes preferred for children. However, corticosteroid ointments and creams alone are less effective than injections; they work best when combined with other topical treatments, such as MINOXIDIL or ANTHRALIN, a skin irritant.

Minoxidil (5%) (Rogaine) Topical minoxidil solution promotes hair growth in several conditions in which the hair follicle is small and not growing to its full potential. As well as in pattern thinning or genetic baldness, Minoxidil is approved for nonprescription use in treating male and female pattern hair loss, and may also be useful in promoting hair growth in alopecia areata. The solution, applied twice a day, has been shown to promote hair growth in both adults and children, and may be used on the scalp, brow, and beard areas. With regular and proper use of the solution, new hair growth appears in about 12 weeks.

Anthralin (Psoriatec) This synthetic tarlike substance alters immune function in the affected skin, and is an approved treatment for PSORIASIS. It is also commonly used to treat alopecia areata, where it is applied for 20 to 60 minutes. When it works, new hair growth is usually visible in eight to 12 weeks. Anthralin is often used in combination with other treatments, such as corticosteroid injections or minoxidil, for improved results.

Topical sensitizers These drugs provoke an allergic reaction when applied to the scalp that leads to itching, scaling, and eventually hair growth. If the medication works, new hair growth is usually established in three to 12 months. Two topical sensitizers are used in alopecia areata: squaric acid dibutyl ester (SADBE) and diphenylcyclopropenone (DPCP).

Oral cyclosporine Originally developed to keep people's immune systems from rejecting transplanted organs, oral cyclosporine is sometimes used to suppress the immune system response in psoriasis and other immune-mediated skin conditions. However, suppressing the immune system can lead to a higher risk of serious infection, kidney problems, and possibly skin cancer and lymphoma. Although oral cyclosporine may regrow hair in alopecia areata, it does not turn the disease off, and most experts believe the dangers of the drug outweigh its benefits for alopecia areata.

Photochemotherapy In this treatment used only for extensive disease, a person is given a light-sensitive drug (a PSORALEN) and then exposed to an ultraviolet light—a combination treatment called PUVA. Used primarily to treat psoriasis, it also triggers cosmetically acceptable hair growth in alopecia areata using photochemotherapy. However, the relapse rate is high, and patients must go to a treatment center where the equipment is available at least two to three times per week. Furthermore, the treatment carries the long-term risk of developing skin cancer.

See also ALOPECIA, ANDROGENETIC; ALOPECIA, FRICTION; ALOPECIA, TRACTION; HAIR LOSS.

alpha hydroxy acids (AHA) A generic term that refers to any one of several organic chemicals that serve as mild chemical peels, working to loosen and slough off dead skin cells to expose newer, fresher skin. In six to eight weeks, skin treated with alpha hydroxy acids appears softer and smoother; AGE SPOTS and FRECKLES also appear to fade.

Also called "fruit acids," these products are derived from sugar cane, apples, grapes, and citrus. The popular GLYCOLIC ACID derived from sugar cane is one of the alpha hydroxy acids, all of which are applied as an ointment, cream or lotion directly to the skin.

Alpha hydroxy acids are available over the counter in mild strengths of 10 percent; in beauty shops in concentrations of up to 40 percent, and in the dermatologist's office in concentrations of up to 70 percent.

Precisely how the acids interact with the skin is not entirely understood, but the products do improve the appearance of the skin by accelerating the natural process of shedding dead skin cells. Used properly, the acids work gently, producing only a slight tingling or stinging sensation in some users. AHA peels are much quicker and milder way to freshen the skin than a deeper peel or LASER RESURFACING. An AHA peel takes about 15 to 20 minutes, and is usually repeated every two to four weeks. The face is cleansed thoroughly and then the peel solution is applied for three to four minutes. The solution is then neutralized and washed off. Treated skin may be a little pink immediately after treatment, and less often, a little peeling may occur over the next few days. It can be disguised with moisturizer or normal makeup.

With repeated use, the acids can clear up ACNE-prone skin, soften tiny lines around the eyes and mouth, smooth dry skin, and fade dark spots caused by sun or hormonal changes (such as those caused by pregnancy). Fastest results occur in the physician's office, since dermatologists can prescribe the strongest products.

Legally, these acid products are considered COSMETICS, not drugs, and therefore are not regulated by the Food and Drug Administration. However, alpha hydroxy acids can be dangerous; the availability of "bootleg" formulations in high concentrations have caused irritations and even burns in some people. Due to an increasing number of lawsuits by injured consumers, the U.S. Food and Drug Administration is reviewing the products to see whether strength thresholds should be established by law.

Over-the-counter products manufactured by reputable companies are safe and generally quite mild, containing less than 10 percent AHA. Responsible firms do not sell products with stronger concentrations over the counter because of the danger to consumers and the resulting liability threat. Because these acids have caused problems for people with sensitive skin (being acids, they can sting), the newest products are formulated to work effectively without irritating.

Some of these products contain only 4 percent glycolic acid. Many company experts state that most women can safely switch to the new 8 percent formula once their skin adjusts to this acid. Other companies have introduced a four-step program that gradually accustoms skin to increasing levels of AHAs. However, some experts believe these nonprescription products are not really strong enough to do anything more than soften the skin.

While the acids are less powerful than Retin-A for wrinkle removal, AHA formulations, according to some dermatologists, may prove useful in preventing and treating fine wrinkles.

See also BETA HYDROXY ACIDS.

aluminum acetate   See BUROW'S SOLUTION.

amebiasis   Infection with the protozoa *Entamoeba histolytica,* which is found throughout the world (primarily in tropical countries), may produce painful skin ulcers, although skin symptoms with this infection are not common.

The amoeba is transmitted by ingesting contaminated food and beverages.

The skin also may be infected following surgical procedures, by spread of amoebic liver abscess, or by direct inoculation by the protozoa.

Symptoms and Diagnostic Path

Infections with *E. histolytica* occur primarily in people who show no symptoms. The skin ulcer is a painful lesion that can last from 10 days to two years. Rapid skin destruction occurs more often among children.

Treatment Options and Outlook

Combinations of medication may be required; in those with skin symptoms, metronidazole is probably the safest drug and is most effective when given in single daily doses.

amino acids   The basic building blocks of protein that make up the skin and hair. The process by which amino acids build skin is extremely com-

plex, and slathering on products containing amino acids will not necessarily help the skin utilize these chemicals to produce new skin. However, shampoos and hair conditioners that contain amino acids do help fill in cracks in the hair shaft caused by harsh soaps and processing; these new proteins do not *rebuild* the hair shaft, but they do lend support.

ammoniated mercury   A bleaching agent that reduces skin color by stopping the formation of MELANIN. It was once used to treat IMPETIGO, PSORIASIS, and other skin conditions. Because it is not very effective and has toxic effects in humans, ammoniated mercury in cosmetics has been banned by the U.S. Food and Drug Administration.

amphotericin B   An intravenous drug used to treat fungal infections of the skin. Fungus infections may include anything from a minor problem such as ATHLETE'S FOOT or vaginal yeast infections to more serious problems if these infections invade the blood or internal organs when the immune system is not working well. Amphotericin B is only used for life-threatening systemic fungal infections.

The incidence of serious fungus infections has risen dramatically in this country, mostly because profoundly ill patients are living longer than in the past. Those most susceptible to serious fungal infections include chemotherapy patients, AIDS and burn patients, and transplant recipients.

Side Effects

Vomiting, fever, headache, or seizures are among the drug's adverse effects. Amphotericin B is administered in a hospital setting because side effects may be severe.

See also ANTIFUNGAL AGENTS; FLUCYTOSINE; FUNGAL INFECTIONS; KETOCONAZOLE.

amyloidosis   The general term for a group of fairly uncommon conditions in which amyloid (a substance that contains protein and starch) builds up in tissues and organs.

Symptoms and Diagnostic Path

Primary amyloidosis is often characterized by deposits of amyloid in the skin, causing raised, waxy spots clustered around the armpits, groin, face, and neck. Male Caucasians between age 50 and 60 are most commonly affected. Skin manifestations occur in 40 percent of patients. The most common sign is a "pinch purpura" (development of a purple lesion after pinching or stroking the skin). Lesions may appear to be translucent, waxy, or amber-colored papules or nodules; less often the skin may look yellow, red, or with heightened pigment. There may be a thickening of the palms and enlargement of ears, lips, and eyelids, and the scalp may develop deep folds; there may be hair loss and some patients develop blisters. The nails may be brittle, crumbling, or streaked, and on some fingers there may be no nails. About 40 percent of deaths related to this condition occur because of heart problems; 30 percent of deaths may result from kidney failure caused by deposits of amyloid. Diagnosis depends on microscopic examination of a biopsy of tissue from the affected organ.

Secondary amyloidosis (or reactive systemic amyloidosis) often occurs as a result of an infectious process such as tuberculosis or osteomyelitis, or a chronic noninfectious inflammatory disease such as rheumatoid arthritis. It also may occur in association with certain nonlymphoid tumors and some lymphomas (the two most common are renal cell carcinoma and Hodgkin's disease).

There are no skin symptoms in secondary amyloidosis.

Treatment Options and Outlook

Primary amyloidosis can be treated with anti-cancer drugs; secondary amyloidosis may be stopped or even reversed when the underlying disorder is treated.

anaphylaxis A severe, life-threatening, allergic reaction that may occur in individuals who have an extreme sensitivity to a particular substance (ALLERGEN).

Symptoms and Diagnostic Path

The reaction, which often includes an itchy red rash or HIVES, is most common after an insect sting or as a reaction to an injected or ingested drug, such as penicillin or tetanus serum. As the allergen enters the bloodstream, it provokes the release of massive amounts of histamine and other chemicals that affect the body by widening blood vessels and lowering blood pressure.

Treatment Options and Outlook

A person who experiences such a reaction following a sting or injection should lie down with legs raised to improve blood flow to the heart and brain, while emergency medical care is obtained. An injection of epinephrine must be given as soon as possible to save the person's life.

Ancobon   See FLUCYTOSINE.

androgens and acne   In some women, ACNE can be caused by excess androgens (male hormones). Women and teenage girls with acne may have excess levels of testosterone and other male hormones. Some estimates suggest that one-third of female patients in the general community have an elevated level of androgen.

Androgens stimulate oil glands in the skin and are known to play a role in acne development. Genes and hormone changes throughout the menstrual cycle also contribute to the skin condition.

Individuals with acne should follow a dermatologist's recommendations for topical and systemic treatment. If the acne only gets worse despite treatment, patients may need to have their hormone levels evaluated.

Excess androgen can be due to a more serious disease such as polycystic ovarian syndrome, which can cause infertility. Elevated androgen also may signal a genetic disorder of the adrenal gland. Different treatment may be indicated if acne is being triggered by excess male hormones than by other more common causes. Topical solutions, for example, may not work for hormone-related acne. Instead, birth control pills may be a more effective treatment because they suppress the production of androgen and help balance a woman's hormone levels.

anergy Inability to react to common skin test ALLERGENS (foreign substances that produce allergic reactions), which represents a deficit in a part of the immune system.

angioedema An allergic reaction characterized by large, well-defined swellings that appear suddenly in the skin and larynx. The swellings may last several hours (or days, if untreated). Angioedema is primarily found in young people in their 20s and those who tend to have allergies.

The most common cause of angioedema is a sudden allergic response to food (especially strawberries, eggs, or seafood). Less often, it occurs in response to drug injections or ingestion (especially penicillin), insect stings, snake bite, infection, emotional stress, and exposure to animals, molds, pollens, or cold.

Symptoms and Diagnostic Path
Angioedema may cause sudden breathing problems, difficulty swallowing, and obvious swelling of the lips, face, and neck. The swelling it produces in the throat may lead to suffocation by blocking the victim's airway.

Treatment Options and Outlook
Severe cases respond to injections of epinephrine, but use of a breathing tube or even tracheotomy may be necessary to prevent suffocation. In less severe cases, antihistamine drugs often relieve symptoms.

angioedema, hereditary A form of acquired ANGIOEDEMA (an allergic reaction characterized by itching and swelling) that is passed on from parents to child. Attacks, which are characterized by diffuse nonitching swelling, are not usually accompanied by HIVES. The condition may be set off by trauma or may appear to occur spontaneously.

Symptoms and Diagnostic Path
In addition to the swelling of the skin, symptoms may include swelling of the gastrointestinal tract that may cause abdominal pain severe enough to suggest the need for surgery.

Swelling of the upper respiratory tract may cause marked swelling of the uvula and larynx. Acute laryngeal swelling is the most serious manifestation of this disorder and can be fatal (due to asphyxiation) in nearly 20 percent of patients.

Attacks usually fade within three to four days, but during this time the individual must be observed carefully for signs of laryngeal obstruction.

Treatment Options and Outlook
Epinephrine, antihistamines, and CORTICOSTEROIDS are usually prescribed, but the success of these agents is limited. If the larynx becomes obstructed, tracheostomy (a surgical hole in the trachea to relieve obstruction) may be required.

angiofibroma Several different types of benign lesions (also called adenoma sebaceum) that may appear as a solitary lesion or in groups. It may be an important skin symptom of TUBEROUS SCLEROSIS.

Symptoms and Diagnostic Path
The condition may include a fibrous papule of the nose—a single lesion on the nose that sometimes looks like a red or flesh-colored mole; this is not related to tuberous sclerosis.

Lesions on the face that show a great deal of fibrous tissue around hair follicles are called perifollicular fibromas. Smaller, similar lesions around the penis are called pearly penile papules.

Treatment Options and Outlook
Because these lesions are benign, treatment is not necessary. Single lesions may be removed; groups of lesions related to tuberous sclerosis may be removed with a CARBON DIOXIDE LASER or DERMABRASION to improve the appearance. Pearly papules on the penis are not usually treated.

angiokeratoma A condition resembling KERATOSIS, characterized by benign lesions that are usually soft and pink to red-purple, often found over bony prominences of the body (especially in children and young adults). Sometimes they may occur on the scrotum or in groups on the legs and feet. Occasionally the lesions appear singly.

Angiokeratomas may occur as part of the rare fatal disease known as *angiokeratoma corporis diffusum of Fabry* (FABRY'S DISEASE); other symptoms include heart and kidney disease and high blood pressure. Patients with this variation usually die from heart or kidney failure.

Treatment Options and Outlook

Angiokeratomas may be surgically removed.

angiokeratoma corporis diffusum See FABRY'S DISEASE.

angioma A small collection of blood vessels overlying and compressing the brain; when associated with a PORT-WINE STAIN, this is known as STURGE-WEBER SYNDROME.

See also CHERRY ANGIOMA; HEMANGIOMA.

angiosarcoma See SARCOMA.

anhidrosis The absence of the ability to SWEAT. This problem may be caused by processes that control the sweating response, or it may appear as a symptom in certain skin diseases (PSORIASIS, atopic DERMATITIS), as a side effect of certain drugs (anticholinergics, quinacrine). Many patients who cannot sweat in some areas have a compensatory sweating response in other sweat glands.

ANHIDROTIC ECTODERMAL DYSPLASIA causes a decrease or absence of sweating that is most commonly inherited in an X-linked pattern (primarily affecting males). In this case, hair may be sparse, light, coarse, or strawlike, with sparse eyelashes and eyebrows and dental abnormalities.

Since the body relies on sweating to cool itself, the inability to sweat can lead to excessively high internal body temperatures.

Treatment Options and Outlook

Treatment is aimed at controlling the underlying cause. Those with untreatable anhidrosis should be careful when exposed to excessive heat, work, or physical activity that would normally provoke intense sweating.

anhidrotic ectodermal dysplasia See ECTODERMAL DYSPLASIA.

animal bites Each year 5 million Americans are bitten by animals; in most cases the animal involved is a dog. Less common but more dangerous are bites from skunks, raccoons, bats, and other wild animals.

Treatment Options and Outlook

If the skin has been broken by a bite, treatment depends on its depth and location and on what is known about the animal.

The area is first cleaned using an antiseptic, followed by an antibiotic (the best one is amoxicillin). Stitches may be required, but it is usually best for these wounds to heal without being sewn to prevent any dangerous organism from getting trapped in the body. (Exception: Bites on the face probably will need to be stitched to avoid disfigurement).

ANSI sunglass standard A voluntary labeling program by the American National Sunglass Institute (ANSI) and the Sunglass Association of America, groups working with the U.S. Food and Drug Administration to provide consumers with uniform and useful labeling for nonprescription sunglasses. The ANSI standard is found on a label attached to sunglasses, describing how much and what types of ULTRAVIOLET RADIATION is blocked out. According to ANSI, the minimum requirement for a pair of sunglasses would filter out 99 percent of UVB rays and 60 percent of UVA rays.

anthralin preparations A topical prescription compound used to treat PSORIASIS (a skin disease caused by excess skin cell production) and other skin conditions. Available as a cream or ointment, anthralin works by slowing the skin cell multiplication rate; its effects may be improved by using ultraviolet light treatments at the same time. Anthralin is applied to the skin and left on for a short period of time or overnight (depending on doctor's orders).

Anthralin should not be applied to raw or blistered areas of the skin; even so, anthralin commonly causes redness and irritation. The healthy skin around patches of psoriasis can be protected from inflammation by applying PETROLEUM JELLY or ZINC OXIDE paste before using the anthralin. The higher-strength compounds may cause irritation and skin staining; lower strength compounds have been developed that make this therapy more tolerable. Because anthralin can stain skin, hair, and clothing, users should wear gloves and old clothes when applying.

Short contact treatment   After applying anthralin, the medicine is allowed to remain on the affected area for 10 to 30 minutes. It is then removed by bathing with soap (if applied to the skin) or by shampooing (if applied to the scalp).

Cream form for overnight treatment   If anthralin cream is applied to the skin, any medicine remaining on the affected areas the next morning should be removed by bathing. If anthralin cream is applied to the scalp, shampoo will remove the scales and any medicine remaining on the affected areas from the previous application. The hair should be dried, and after parting, the cream should be rubbed into the affected areas. The physician will recommend when the cream should be removed.

Ointment form for overnight treatment: If anthralin ointment is applied to the skin at night, any ointment remaining on the affected areas the next morning should be removed with warm liquid petrolatum followed by bathing. If anthralin ointment is applied to the scalp at night, it should be shampooed away the next morning to clean the scalp.

anthrax, cutaneous   A serious and sometimes fatal bacterial skin infection that in the past primarily affected livestock, although it had occasionally spread to humans. Following the September 11, 2001 terrorist attacks on the World Trade Center in New York City and the Pentagon in Washington, D.C., a series of envelopes containing anthrax spores were mailed to a variety of news and media organizations and government offices. Anyone who touched or inhaled the spores were at risk for infection with the skin form of the infection (via touch) or the far deadlier respiratory form of anthrax (by inhalation).

For both livestock and humans, anthrax is a notifiable disease in the United States.

Cutaneous anthrax is caused by the bacterium *Bacillus anthracis*, which produces spores that can remain dormant for years in soil and animal products. Once reactivated, the spores can cause a skin infection if they enter an open wound or abrasion. The only way cutaneous anthrax can be transmitted from one person to another is by direct contact with the spores. Anthrax is not spread from person to person by casual contact, sharing space, or by coughing or sneezing.

It can also be contracted by touching objects contaminated by the spores, such as in the anthrax-contaminated mail. Cross-contamination of the mail could occur during the processing, sorting, and delivery of mail when an envelope comes in contact with another envelope, piece of equipment (such as an electronic sorting machine), or other surface that is contaminated with *Bacillus anthracis* spores. In addition, airborne spores in contaminated postal facilities might play a role.

Symptoms and Diagnostic Path

Symptoms usually begin to appear in less than seven days; in most cases, symptoms occur within 48 hours of exposure. The most common symptom is a raised, itchy area at the site of entry that resembles a boil; this progresses to a large blister and then a black scab with swelling of surrounding tissue. Nearby lymph glands may swell, in addition to flu-like symptoms such as fatigue, fever, and nausea. If symptoms do not develop within seven days of exposure, there is only a very remote chance of developing the disease.

Anthrax is diagnosed by isolating *B. anthracis* from the blood, skin lesions, or respiratory secretions, or by measuring specific antibodies in the blood of someone with suspected infection.

Treatment Options and Outlook

Cutaneous anthrax is curable in the early stages if treatment is begun promptly with antibiotics such as ciprofloxin or penicillin. However, even the skin form of this infection can be fatal if untreated. If they are not treated, 20 percent of patients with cutaneous anthrax will die.

Risk Factors and Preventive Measures

Individuals who have been exposed to anthrax but have no signs and symptoms of the disease can take preventive antibiotics, such as CIPROFLOXACIN, penicillin, or doxycycline, depending on the particular strain of anthrax.

There is no known case of transmission of cutaneous anthrax from person to person. Therefore, household contacts of individuals with anthrax do not need antibiotics unless they have also been exposed to the same source of anthrax.

Preventive antibiotics are not recommended for persons who routinely open or handle mail, either at home or at the workplace. Antimicrobial prevention is recommended only in certain specific situations, such as for persons exposed to an air space known to be contaminated with aerosolized *Bacillus anthracis* or for persons in a postal sorting facility in which an envelope containing *B. anthracis* spores was processed.

If there is a risk for inhalational anthrax associated with exposure to cross-contaminated mail, it is very low. For example, about 85 million pieces of mail were processed on the few days in 2001 after envelopes containing *Bacillus anthracis* (addressed to two U.S. senators) passed through the New Jersey and District of Columbia sorting facilities until they were closed. Despite the fact that both of these facilities had evidence of widespread environmental contamination with *B. anthracis* spores and the fact that public health officials had been aggressively looking for anthrax cases, no new cases of anthrax were identified during that time.

There are no scientifically proven recommendations for preventing exposure via contaminated mail, according to the U.S. Centers for Disease Control and Prevention. Nevertheless, there are some commonsense steps people can take. Individuals should:

- not open suspicious mail
- hold mail away from the face as it is opened
- not blow or sniff mail or mail contents
- avoid vigorous handling of mail, such as tearing or shredding
- wash hands after handling the mail
- discard envelopes after opening mail.

If an individual receives a suspicious package or envelope, the CDC recommends:

- The person should not shake or empty the contents of any suspicious package or envelope.
- The person should not carry the package or envelope, show it to others, or allow others to examine it.
- The person should put the package or envelope down on a stable surface without sniffing, touching, tasting, or looking closely at it or at any contents that may have spilled.
- The person should alert others in the area about the suspicious package or envelope.
- The person should leave the area, close any doors, and prevent others from entering the area. If possible, the ventilation system should be shut down.
- The person should wash hands with soap and water to prevent spreading potentially infectious material to face or skin.
- The person should notify a supervisor, a security officer, or a law enforcement official if the package or envelope arrives at work. If at home, the person should contact the local law enforcement agency.
- The person should, if possible, create a list of people who were in the room or area when the suspicious letter or package was recognized and a list of people who also may have handled this package or letter. This list should be given to both the local public health authorities and law enforcement officials.

Cutaneous anthrax also can be prevented by the anthrax vaccine (Anthrax Vaccine Adsorbed, or AVA), the only anthrax vaccine licensed in the United States. The six-dose vaccine is only recommended for individuals who may come in contact with animal products that may be contaminated with anthrax spores and for anyone who may come in contact with the spores. Vaccination is recommended for persons at high risk, such as veterinarians and those working at certain high risk post offices.

Because of biological warfare threats, the vaccine is mandated for all military personnel. It is currently not available or recommended for use in the general public.

The vaccine contains no dead or live bacteria. The immunization consists of three subcutaneous injections given two weeks apart followed by three more subcutaneous injections given at six, 12, and 18 months. Annual booster injections of the vaccine are recommended thereafter. Slight tenderness and redness at the injection site occur in 30 percent of recipients.

Severe local reactions are infrequent and consist of extensive swelling of the forearm in addition to the local reaction. Systemic reactions occur in fewer than .2 percent of recipients.

antibacterial drugs   A group of drugs used to treat infections caused by bacteria. These drugs act in the same way as ANTIBIOTIC DRUGS, but unlike antibiotics they always have been produced synthetically. The largest group of antibacterial agents is the sulfonamides.

Antibacterial ointments contain combinations of the "nonabsorbable" antibiotics (bacitracin, neomycin, polymyxin B, and gramicidin). While these may help for mild skin wounds, more extensive bacterial skin infections require systemic antibiotics.

Bacitracin is effective against organisms including *Streptococcus, Staphylococcus,* and pneumococcus. Neomycin is effective against most gram-negative organisms (gram staining is a way of identifying bacterial cells). It is about 50 times more active against *Staphylococcus* than bacitracin, but bacitracin is 20 times more active against *Streptococcus.* However, neomycin causes more allergic contact sensitivity than any other topical antibiotic.

Gentamicin, another antibacterial drug, is also effective against *Staphylococcus aureus* and group AB-hemolytic streptococci. While it may be used topically, it is no better than other drugs mentioned above and it may produce an allergic reaction.

antibiotic drugs   A group of drugs used to treat infections caused by bacteria. Originally prepared from molds and fungi, antibiotic drugs are now made synthetically. Antibiotics help fight infection when the body has been invaded by harmful bacteria or when the bacteria present in the body begin to multiply uncontrollably. More than one kind of antibiotic may be prescribed to increase the efficiency of treatment and to reduce the risk of antibiotic resistance.

Many bacteria develop resistance to a once-useful antibiotic. Resistance is most likely to develop if a person fails to take an antibiotic as directed during long-term treatment. Some drugs, known as broad-spectrum antibiotics, are effective against a wide range of bacteria, while others are useful only in treating specific types.

Antibiotics in Acne Treatment

Topical antibiotics (TETRACYCLINE, ERYTHROMYCIN, CLINDAMYCIN, and meclocycline) have an antibacterial effect when applied to the skin, in much the same way as BENZOYL PEROXIDE—except they are probably less effective. A preparation that combines erythromycin and benzoyl peroxide in a gel is probably more effective together than either preparation alone.

Systemic antibiotics can be very effective in the treatment of acne, despite the fact that acne is not a bacterial disease. In fact, 10 percent of all tetracycline sold in the United States is used to treat acne. It is believed that systemic antibiotic treatment probably prevents the development of additional inflammatory lesions. Erythromycin is as effective as tetracycline and does not have to be taken without food. Minocycline is also effective but is more expensive.

Types

Some of the most well-known antibiotics include the penicillins (amoxicillin, penicillin V, and oxacillin), the aminogylcosides (gentamicin and streptomycin), the cephalosporins (cefaclor and cephalexin), the tetracyclines (doxycycline and oxytetracycline), erythromycin, and neomycin.

Side Effects

Because these agents may kill "normal" bacteria naturally present in the body, fungi may grow in their place, causing oral, intestinal or vaginal candidiasis (thrush). Some patients may experience a severe allergic response, causing facial swelling, itching, or breathing problems.

anticoagulation syndrome (coumarin necrosis)   A condition characterized by lesions beginning between three and 10 days after the administration of a coumarin drug (such as dicumarol or warfarin) that occurs occasionally in young women. Coumarin is administered as an anticoagulant (blood thinner) to treat disorders in which there is excessive clotting, such as thrombophlebitis and certain heart conditions. Coumarin necrosis has been associated with protein C and protein S deficiency.

Symptoms and Diagnostic Path

The lesions begin as minute spots or blue or purple hemorrhagic patches (usually on the lower fatty areas of the body), quickly followed by tissue death, which can extend into the deep subcutaneous fat; the resulting ulcer may not heal for months.

Treatment Options and Outlook

Once the lesions begin to appear, their course is progressive regardless of whether the drug treatment is stopped.

There is no effective treatment. When the breast or penis is involved, amputation is recommended; other areas may require surgical debridement and skin grafts.

antifungal/anti-yeast agents   A group of drugs prescribed to treat infections caused by either fungi or yeasts (and sometimes both in one product) that can be administered directly to the skin or taken orally or by injection. They are commonly used to treat different types of TINEA, including ATHLETE'S FOOT, JOCK ITCH, and scalp RINGWORM. They are also used to treat THRUSH and rare fungal infections such as CRYPTOCOCCOSIS.

Side Effects

Agents applied to the skin, scalp, mouth, or vagina may sometimes increase irritation, and antifungal agents given by mouth or injection may cause more serious side effects, damaging the kidney or liver.

Types

Antifungal agents are available as creams, injections, tablets, lozenges, suspensions, and vaginal suppositories. The most common antifungals include AMPHOTERICIN B (IV only), cyclopirox, clotrimazole, naftifine, terbinafine, ECONAZOLE, GRISEOFULVIN (by mouth only), itraconazole (by mouth and IV only), fluconazole (by mouth and IV only), KETOCONAZOLE, miconazole, and TOLNAFTATE. While amphotericin B is the standard drug for treating fungal infections, it is usually given in the hospital because of the danger of side effects. On the other hand, itraconazole and fluconazole are the two most recently approved drugs to enter the antifungal arsenal. These two cause fewer side effects and can be taken orally on an outpatient basis.

Nonprescription creams such as Monistat 7 and Gyne-Lotrimin may be helpful in remedying candidal vaginal yeast infections, but fatal candidal infections affecting the brain, kidney, or other organs may occur in immuno-compromised patients in the hospital.

Anti-yeast agents, such as nystatin, do not kill most fungi, but most antifungals kill yeasts as well—except for griseofulvin. Drugs that are used for both systemic fungal and yeast infections include fluconazole, ketoconazole, amphotericin-B, and itraconazole.

antihistamines   A family of drugs used to treat allergic conditions, such as ITCHING and HIVES. The drugs work by blocking the action of HISTAMINE, a chemical that is released during an allergic reaction. Examples of antihistamines include diphenhydramine, promethazine, terfenadine, chlorpheniramine, and so on.

Without drug treatment, histamine dilates small blood vessels, causing redness and swelling; antihistamines block this effect, while preventing the irritation of nerve fibers that would otherwise cause itching. They are the most effective treatment for hives.

Side Effects

Older antihistamines caused drowsiness and dizziness, but new antihistamines such as Claritin do not enter the brain, and thus do not cause these side effects. Other possible symptoms include appetite loss, nausea, dry mouth, blurry vision, and problems in urination. Because older antihistamines have a sedative effect, they may also be used to induce sleep; patients taking these types of antihistamines should not drive or operate heavy machinery until the effects wear off.

anti-inflammatory drugs A family of drugs used to help decrease inflammation and pain. This class of drugs includes the nonsteroidal anti-inflammatory drugs (NSAIDS) and the CORTICOSTEROIDS, both of which fight inflammation.

NSAIDS

The NSAIDS are a group of chemically diverse drugs widely used to treat inflammation, which is one of the body's defense mechanisms in response to infection and certain chronic diseases (such as rheumatoid arthritis).

On their own, NSAIDs are not very toxic, but they should not be used by people with gastrointestinal disease, peptic ulcers, or poor heart function. They should not be taken with other nonsteroid painkillers or other anticoagulants (blood thinners), because bleeding time may be prolonged while on NSAIDs. Antacids and aspirin also may reduce the effectiveness of an anti-inflammatory drug.

Types

They include ibuprofen (Motrin, Rufen, Advil, Medipren, Nuprin), fenoprofen (Nalfon), meclofenamate (Meclomen), naproxen (Anaprox, Naprosyn), sulindac (Clinoril), indomethacin (Indocin), tolmetin (Tolectin), mefanamic acid, piroxicam (Feldene), oxyphenbutazone, and phenylbutazone.

CORTICOSTEROIDS

The corticosteroids are a group of drugs used primarily to treat inflammation that are similar to natural corticosteroid hormones produced by the adrenal glands. Skin diseases treated with these drugs include ECZEMA, ACNE, PEMPHIGUS, PSORIASIS, ALOPECIA, DERMATITIS, LICHEN PLANUS, ROSACEA, and ERYTHEMA MULTIFORME. Corticosteroids include CORTISONE, prednisone, prednisolone, hydrocortisone, dexamethasone, beclomethasone, and so on.

Side Effects

When taken in high doses for a long time, adverse effects can include tissue swelling, high blood pressure, diabetes mellitus, peptic ulcer, Cushing's syndrome, excess hairiness, and susceptibility to infection.

antimalarial drugs Also called antiprotozoals, this is a group of drugs used to treat malaria. The two most common used in dermatology are hydroxychloroquine and quinacrine. These drugs have been helpful in treating skin symptoms of malaria, LUPUS ERYTHEMATOSUS, PORPHYRIA, and skin lesions in DERMATOMYOSITIS.

Side Effects

Hydroxychloroquine and chloroquine may produce retinal damage; other possible side effects include aplastic anemia (a type of anemia caused by a decrease in bone marrow production of all types of blood cells). Quinacrine may produce yellowing of the skin. Any antimalarial drug may cause the hair to gray; some patients also experience a bluish-black discoloration of the inside of the mouth and skin under the fingernails that improves when the drug is stopped. Infrequent side effects include HIVES, exfoliative erythroderma, and a worsening of PSORIASIS.

antioxidant beauty products A wide range of beauty products contains antioxidants (molecules that can neutralize FREE RADICALS—a destructive form of oxygen that can cause wrinkles and sagging skin). Once activated, free radicals interfere with a wide range of body processes. Research suggests that antioxidants—especially the vitamins C and E, and beta-carotene—can neutralize free radicals before they damage skin.

Cosmetic companies reasoned that since free radicals damage skin, and vitamins C and E combat free radicals, spreading extra antioxidants on the skin should fend off the destruction. But while this may appear to make sense, skin care experts have yet to prove that capturing free radicals prevents skin damage. But because antioxidant research is still in its infancy, there is no research that proves it does not work. Early results suggest that VITAMIN C not only helps to reverse sun-induced skin damage but that it also works as a SUNSCREEN.

Most researchers do agree that taking a vitamin pill probably will not protect the skin, and that it is far less effective than applying the vitamins directly to the skin. To be effective in face creams, anti-oxidants must be present in significant amounts. But while the best concentrations are 10 percent for vitamin C and 2 or 3 percent for VITAMIN E, many cosmetic products contain less than a tenth of a percent of either one. In addition, it is not easy to make sure that vitamin C in creams penetrates into the skin.

antiperspirants Metallic salts designed to be applied to the skin to control excessive unpleasant odor by reducing the production of SWEAT. They contain aluminum or aluminum-zirconium salts that block the eccrine and apocrine sweat ducts, obstructing delivery of sweat to the skin's surface. These products also remove unpleasant odors because they create a drier environment that reduces the number of odor-causing bacteria. They are more effective than deodorants, which simply remove unpleasant odors. Some deodorants also contain antiperspirants.

Commercially available antiperspirants reduce underarm sweating by 20 to 40 percent; their effectiveness can be increased by applying in the morning and at bedtime. Antiperspirants should not be applied to moist or irritated skin, nor should they be used soon after shaving.

For those with extreme body odor problems, physicians may prescribe aluminum chloride hexahydrate, 20 percent solution in absolute alcohol (Drysol), for use on underarms, palms, or soles.

Drysol is applied at bedtime under a plastic film, but it may cause irritation if used often.

See also SWEAT AND THE SKIN; SWEAT GLANDS; SWEAT GLANDS, DISORDERS OF.

antipruritic agents Drugs used to treat ITCH-ING; however, generalized itching is not easy to treat unless the underlying condition is identified. Oral ANTIHISTAMINES are often prescribed, but they are most effective when the underlying condition involves the release of HISTAMINE (a chemical released during an allergic reaction that causes inflammation and itching, such as in HIVES).

Alternatively, some patients' itching may lessen with use of the drugs pramoxine and doxysin, or with a preparation containing menthol, phenol or camphor. Menthol eases itching because of the cooling feeling it produces; phenol temporarily numbs nerve endings in the skin. Camphor has a local anesthetic effect.

Less often, preparations of SALICYLIC ACID or COAL TAR may be used. Shake lotions of CALAMINE may also reduce itching.

Over-the-counter preparations containing benzocaine or diphenhydramine should be avoided, since either may produce an allergic skin contact response.

antiseptic cleansers Chemicals designed to prevent infection that are applied to the skin to destroy bacteria and other microorganisms. The use of antiseptics to prevent infection (antisepsis) is not the same thing as the creation of a germ-free environment (asepsis). Antiseptics are milder than disinfectants, which are used to decontaminate objects but are considered too strong for skin.

Antiseptic fluids are usually used to bathe wounds; antiseptic creams are applied to wounds before being bandaged.

Commonly used antiseptics include iodine and chlorhexidine compounds and HYDROGEN PEROX-IDE. Chlorhexidine is an antiseptic effective against many yeasts, fungi, and both gram-negative and gram-positive bacteria. Well tolerated by most people, it is quick-acting and effective for a long time. Antiseptic iodine compounds (such as the brownish yellow providone-iodine) are effective against bacteria, fungi, yeasts, viruses, and protozoa. However, they take longer to work than other antiseptics and may be ineffective in the presence of blood.

While HEXACHLOROPHENE has been widely used in the past (effective against many gram-positive organisms such as Staphylococcus), it has also been associated with neurotoxicity. Because hexachlorophene is less safe than other agents, such as chlorhexidine and iodine compounds, its use is regulated by the U.S. Food and Drug Administration.

antiviral agents A group of drugs used to treat viral infections; some of the best known of these drugs for use in skin infections are ACYCLOVIR, FAMCICLOVIR, and VALCYCLOVIR prescribed for the treatment of various forms of HERPES, and AZT (ZIDOVUDINE), prescribed for the treatment of AIDS. Until the development of acyclovir and AZT, no effective antiviral agents existed.

To this point, no drugs have been developed that eradicate viruses and cure the illnesses they cause. This is because viruses live only within cells; a drug capable of killing a virus would also kill its host cell. New antiviral agents interfere with viral replication or otherwise disrupt chemical processes of viral metabolism; some prevent viruses from penetrating cells. They are effective treatments for a variety of infections.

Antivirals including acyclovir, famcyclovir, and valacyclovir, are especially effective in treating herpes family infections. Antiviral drugs reduce the severity of the herpes symptoms and shorten the course of the infection, but the drugs cannot eliminate the virus completely.

Scientists have been testing several varieties of a vaccine that appears to lessen the severity of herpes attacks.

AZT (Retrovir) a drug still used in the treatment of AIDS, works by interrupting the replication cycle of the HIV virus, and has demonstrated effectiveness in delaying the progression of HIV infection.

Side Effects

Antiviral drugs have a variety of side effects. Creams and ointments may irritate skin, while oral antiviral drugs can cause side effects ranging from nausea and dizziness to bone marrow suppression and kidney problems.

aplasia cutis The medical name for the absence of small areas of skin that may occur any time from before birth to early childhood. These localized birth defects are typically found on the back of the scalp, although they may occur anywhere on the scalp (rarely, on the face, trunk, or limbs). At birth, the affected area may be covered by a tough, smooth membrane or it may be raw, ulcerated, and crusted.

The defect may be inherited, but is usually appears spontaneously. It is sometimes seen with the chromosome disorder trisomy 13.

Symptoms and Diagnostic Path

On the scalp, affected areas tend to be hairless with sharp margins that heal slowly, eventually replaced by a flat or hypertrophic scar. Occasionally, there may be a secondary infection or hemorrhage. There may be an underlying defect in the bone that will heal on its own during the baby's first two years of life.

Treatment Options and Outlook

There is no known treatment other than to cut out the hairless area or transplant normal skin and hair follicles.

APLIGRAF A type of ARTIFICIAL SKIN widely used by dermatologists as a skin substitute to cover skin ulcers on the foot. Like human skin, APLIGRAF consists of living cells and structural proteins. Manufactured from living cells, it is considered to be a medical device and has been approved for the treatment of leg ulcers and foot ulcers in diabetic patients.

Like human skin, APLIGRAF has two primary layers, a DERMIS and an EPIDERMIS. The epidermal layer is composed of human keratinocyte cells that form an outer protective layer. The dermal layer lies beneath the epidermis and is made up of human fibroblast cells. APLIGRAF does not contain Langerhans' cells, melanocytes, macrophages, lymphocytes, white blood cells, blood vessels, hair follicles, or sweat glands. APLIGRAF should not be used on clinically infected wounds and in patients with known allergies to bovine collagen.

See also COMPOSITE CULTURED SKIN.

apocrine glands   See SWEAT GLANDS.

apocrine bromhidrosis   See BROMHIDROSIS.

apocrine sweat   See SWEAT GLANDS.

arginosuccinic aciduria   A rare genetic disorder caused by a deficiency of the amino acid arginosuccinase.

This disorder is an autosomal recessive disorder, which means that a defective gene must be inherited from both parents to cause the abnormality. Generally, both parents of an affected person are unaffected carriers of the defective gene. Each of their children would have a one in four chance of being affected, and a two in four chance of being a carrier.

Symptoms and Diagnostic Path

This disorder causes sparse, dull, short, and fragile hair with frayed ends that looks like broom ends pushed together. Patients develop seizures and coma and subsequently die.

Treatment Options and Outlook

Some patients benefit from a low-protein diet with arginine supplements or additions of keto analogues of essential amino acids.

argon laser   A tube that contains argon gas energized by a power source (such as electricity). The resulting beam of light is up to 10 million times more powerful than the Sun, and is absorbed by different types of substances in the skin, including melanin pigment and hemoglobin in blood vessels.

The argon laser is the most effective and safest way to treat vascular lesions because the red color of the blood absorbs the blue-green color of the argon laser beam. PORT-WINE STAINS may be considerably lightened with this type of treatment, as will telangiectases, SPIDER ANGIOMAS, venous lakes, and certain pigmented lesions such as lentigines. It is also used to treat acne ROSACEA.

Until the late 1980s, the argon laser was the treatment of choice for port-wine stains; hemoglobin selectively absorbed the laser's light in the dilated blood vessels of these birthmarks. However, the therapy is limited by a substantial rate of scarring. The continuous laser energy dissipates into the surrounding dermis, causing thermal damage. Less-than-optimum treatment results in pale, immature port-wine stains. Moreover, the extent of clearing and rate of scarring are primarily dependent on the technique and experience of the operator.

However, more selective blood vessel damage can be obtained by using a wavelength that is more selectively absorbed by hemoglobin and delivered in a pulse shorter than the cooling time of the abnormal vessel, such as the PULSED DYE LASER.

There is some danger in using lasers. Because the beam generates heat, there is some risk of fire, especially on surgical dressings. Wet dressings placed around the surgical site will protect nearby normal tissue, reducing the chance of fire. Protective goggles during treatment are essential, and must be worn by the patient and all medical personnel. Very little discomfort is associated with most skin laser surgery.

Artecoll   A type of synthetic BIOLOGICAL IMPLANT developed as a SKIN FILLER in Europe, and approved for use as an implant material in Canada in 1998. Made from lucite beads called methylmethacrylate (MMA) suspended in COLLAGEN, it is similar to ZYDERM. Experts believe this implant may soon be approved by the U.S. Food and Drug Administration (as Artefill).

When injected into the deeper layers of skin, the collagen evenly disperses the microspheres of MMA; the collagen is absorbed over several months, and the microspheres remain in place to correct the defect. Because the correction is permanent, a series of injections is necessary to safely achieve the desired result. It is very effective at filling lines between the nose and mouth, but lumpiness is common when used to fill the lips.

Side Effects

Allergic reactions may occur in response to the collagen, and although MMA has been used for many years as a bone cement, redness, inflammation, and infection may occur, as with any other synthetic implant.

Although the incidence of complications has been reported by the manufacturer to be less than one in 10,000, inflammation, clumping, and granuloma formation have been reported in as many as half of patients having lip augmentation. Surgical excision of the material is the only effective treatment for these complications. Despite Artecoll's impending approval in the United States, the Swiss government has advised physicians in that country not to use it for augmentation.

artificial skin Synthetic skin, often used to treat burn victims, is capable of preventing infection and reducing fluid loss while not inducing an immune rejection response.

The concept of artificial skin dates back to at least the late 17th century, when water lizard skin was applied to open wounds. Since then, the need for an effective skin substitute has remained. Since those early days, many possibilities have been explored in the field of skin replacement.

In addition to using animal skins, researchers experimented with plastic sprays, sponges, and fresh skin from cadavers (ALLOGRAFTS). Cadaver skin proved to be the best temporary covering for large wounds, but it was hard to get and there were problems of potential disease transmission and rejection.

In the mid-1970s, scientists discovered how to culture epidermal cells to grow sheets of skin, and within 10 years this technique became commercially available. These grafts are helpful in temporarily covering wounds and in helping them to heal.

See also COMPOSITE CULTURED SKIN; PINCH GRAFT.

ascorbic acid deficiency See SCURVY.

ashy dermatosis Another name for ERYTHEMA DYSCHROMICUM PERSTANS.

asteatotic eczema See ECZEMA.

astringents Substances that cause skin tissue to dry and shrink by reducing its ability to absorb water. Astringents are widely used in skin tonics, but they may cause burning or stinging when applied.

While old-fashioned astringents were used to dry out the skin in the treatment of ACNE they also stripped the skin of essential moisture (usually because of a high alcohol content). Today, there's a new type of toner that not only cleanses less harshly than some of the old products but can lightly exfoliate, soothe, refresh, and leave skin soft and hydrated instead of dry and taut. These products are often marketed under a variety of names, including "toners," "clarifiers," "refreshers," "lotions," and "purifiers." While all may be more or less interchangeable, in general toners tend to be lighter and less drying than astringents because they usually contain lower concentrations of alcohol.

Many dermatologists advise patients to avoid alcohol, which dries the skin and actually increases oil production as glands are stimulated to compensate for excess dryness. Still, while alcohol may dry the skin temporarily, it does not cause any longer-term damage.

Those astringents or toners without alcohol rely on natural ingredients to cleanse and refresh the skin, using "botanicals" (naturally derived elements). Botanical extracts may include lavender, grapefruit seed, and orchid, and serve different functions, soothing, or stimulating the skin.

ataxia telangiectasia See LOUIS-BAR SYNDROME.

athlete's foot A common fungal condition causing the skin between the toes (usually the fourth and fifth toes) to itch, peel and crack, resulting in diffuse scaling and redness of the soles and sides of the foot.

Athlete's foot is usually caused by a fungal infection and is called *tinea pedis;* secondary infection in skin cracks is caused by bacteria.

Symptoms and Diagnostic Path

It is sometimes associated with thickening and crumbling of the nails. Linked to wearing shoes and sweating, the condition is rare in young children and in places of the world where people do not wear shoes.

Itchy skin on the foot is probably not athlete's foot if it occurs on the top of the toes. If the foot is red, swollen, sore, blistered, and oozing, the condition is more likely the result of some form of contact dermatitis, although inflammatory fungal infections can sometimes look like this.

Treatment Options and Outlook

The condition may clear up without any attention, but it usually requires treatment. An untreated fungal infection can lead to bacteria-inviting cracks in the skin. It is important to keep the affected area dry, wearing dry cotton socks or sandals. Even better—the foot should be kept uncovered.

Most infections can be cured by applying the nonprescription antifungal cream Lotrimin two or three times daily. Possible side effects include occasional skin irritation; antifungal oral drugs cause few side effects and are helpful in severe cases or when the nails are involved.

When the acute phase of the infection passes, dead skin should be removed with a bristle brush in order to remove the living fungi. Any bits of the skin should be washed away. In addition, toenails should be scraped every two or three days with an orange stick or toothpick.

Risk Factors and Preventive Measures

Disinfecting the floors of showers and locker rooms can help control the spread of infection. Once an infection has cleared up, antifungal cream should be used now and then—especially during warm weather. Plastic or too-tight shoes (or any type of footwear treated to keep out water) should be avoided. Natural materials (cotton and leather) and sandals are the best choices; wool and rubber can make a fungal problem worse by trapping moisture.

Shoes should be aired regularly in the sun, and wiped inside with a disinfectant-treated cloth to remove fungi-carrying dead skin. Insides of shoes should be dusted with antifungal powder or spray. Individuals who perspire heavily should change socks three or four times daily, and wear only natural white cotton socks, rinsed thoroughly during washing. Individuals should air dry feet after bathing and then apply powder, and always wear sandals or flip-flops in public bathing areas.

See also DERMATITIS, CONTACT.

atrophic papulosis, malignant See DEGOS' DISEASE.

atrophie blanche Unusual types of white scars with red macules and spidery red veins resembling chili peppers. This type of scar, which is usually found on the tops of the feet, ankles and legs, is the final result of lower leg ulcers.

Treatment Options and Outlook

Combinations of aspirin and dipyridamole, which affect the formation of platelets, have been helpful in the treatment of some cases of atrophie blanche. Other treatments have included phenformin, ethylestrenol, and pentoxifylline.

See also LIVEDO VASCULITIS.

attar of roses An extract of roses used to perfume products. This extract may cause allergic reactions in sensitive consumers.

atypical nevi (dysplastic nevi) An unusual MOLE that is a marker for an increased risk of MALIGNANT MELANOMA. Researchers suggest that almost 7 percent of Caucasians in the United States have atypical nevi, and half of their close relatives may also be affected.

There are two types of atypical nevi: familial and sporadic. The significance of familial nevi is clear: Those who have atypical moles *and* a family history of melanoma (two or more close blood relatives) have an almost 100 percent lifetime risk of developing melanoma.

No one knows the true significance of sporadic atypical moles. Although such patients with large numbers of atypical moles also appear to be at higher risk for developing malignant melanoma, the risk appears to be less than for those in the familial group (an estimated lifetime melanoma risk of 6 percent). Experts believe that about 50 percent of the populace has at least one of these lesions.

Melanoma warning signs include moles that are often asymmetrical (one half looks unlike the other), have irregular or hazy borders, are variegated and of irregular color, with a diameter slightly larger than that of a pencil eraser.

Although atypical moles continue to develop as the patient grows older, the lesions tend to remain stable. Only a small number of these spots ever undergoes malignant transformation.

Symptoms and Diagnostic Path

Atypical moles are found most often on the back, chest, abdomen and extremities, but they also may occur on unexposed areas (scalp, buttocks, groin, or breasts). They differ from ordinary acquired moles in several ways: first, atypical moles tend to occur in larger numbers than ordinary moles—often more than 100. In addition, these moles are often larger than the ordinary variety, and they will often measure more than a half inch. Although ordinary moles usually stop appearing by early adult life, atypical moles continue to develop into adulthood.

Atypical moles also may look different from ordinary moles. They tend to have irregular contours with irregular pigmentation. In addition to shades of brown, atypical moles may be red or pink—colors not normally found in ordinary moles. When these atypical characteristics are pronounced it may be difficult to tell the difference between an atypical mole and a superficial spreading malignant melanoma.

Treatment Options and Outlook

The most abnormal-looking lesions should be excised and examined microscopically. If very unusual, other odd-looking moles should be removed.

Risk Factors and Preventive Measures

If a doctor diagnoses atypical moles, the patient should discuss the family history and have close relatives examined for any sign of moles or melanoma. Patients who have both atypical moles and close family members with malignant melanoma should have regular skin exams (as often as every four to six months) and supplement medical checkups with self-examinations; full-body photographs may help an individual to more easily spot changes in moles. Patients should reduce sun exposure and use sunscreens with a high SPF and consider an eye exam, since moles also may affect the eyes.

augmentation mammoplasty   See MAMMOPLASTY.

aurothioglucose   An oil-based form of gold salts used in GOLD THERAPY for the treatment of PEMPHIGUS.

Side Effects

Side effects of gold salts can occur any time during treatment or months after treatment has been stopped. The most common adverse reaction is inflamed skin; ITCHING can be a warning of a skin RASH. This drug can cause grayish blue discoloration of the skin, a metallic taste, and mouth sores. Because gold salts can cause serious kidney and bone marrow problems, all patients require regular blood and urine test monitoring.

Injectable gold may cause flushing, dizziness, and fainting immediately after the injection. Rarely, patients can have severe allergic reactions resulting in shock.

See also GOLD SODIUM THIOMALATE.

Auspitz's sign   Pinpoint bleeding that occurs when the scale of a lesion in a patient with PSORIASIS is forcibly removed.

autograft   Tissue graft taken from one part of the body and placed on another part of the same patient; burn repair is often done by grafting strips of skin taken from elsewhere on the body (usually the upper body or thigh, called the "donor site"). Unlike ALLOGRAFTS, autografts are not rejected by the body's immune system.

See also PINCH GRAFT; SKIN GRAFT.

Autologen A type of custom COLLAGEN used as a COSMETIC SURGERY filler to correct skin-contour defects. This dispersion of intact collagen fibers and collagen tissue matrix is made from a patient's own skin, obtained by a cosmetic surgical procedure. Excised skin is placed in sterile containers and sent to laboratories on ice by express mail. "Custom collagen" is then created and sent back to the physician's office to be used on the same patient. Collagen can then be made at some future date. Because it is part of the patient's own tissues, allergic reactions are considered impossible. Theoretically, these injections should last longer than other biological fillers, from nine months to one year. Autologen does not require approval for cosmetic corrective use.

See also SKIN FILLERS.

autologous fat transplant A type of natural SKIN FILLER for wrinkles and other cosmetic procedures that is produced from the patient's own fat via LIPOSUCTION. No allergy testing is required before this procedure is done, but harvesting the fat is an involved, complicated process. There is no consensus on longevity, but most experts agree results last from months to years. Autologous fat transplants do not require approval by the U.S. Food and Drug Administration (FDA).

The procedure is being done to "fill-in" areas in the body where there is a lack of soft tissue, such as hollow cheeks, filling the lines between nose and mouth, and with depressed ACNE scars. It is also used to recontour the face, enhance the cheek and chin, correct facial or body deformities. More recently it has been done as a way to augment the breast.

Procedure

Both the donor site and the area to be treated are anesthetized and a needle attached to a syringe is inserted into a thick layer of fat at the donor site (such as the thigh, buttocks, or abdomen). Depending on the procedure, the syringe may or may not be attached to a high-powered suction device.

Fat cells are drawn into the syringe and then carefully reinjected into the area to be treated. The process is repeated until the defect has been corrected. A pressure bandage is applied to the donor site and sometimes to the recipient site to prevent bruising and swelling.

Risks and Complications

No significant complications have occurred. Because the fat is transplanted within the patient's own body, problems of rejection or allergic reactions do not occur. Scarring from the injections is minimal, because the injections are given within the creases of the body.

Outlook and Lifestyle Modifications

Fat transplants can be done under local anesthesia and is an outpatient procedure. Healing time is only a couple of days.

azathioprine (Imuran) An anti-cancer drug used to treat severe autoimmune diseases when other drugs fail to slow the progression of the disease or to improve symptoms. It is particularly effective in conjunction with CORTICOSTEROIDS such as prednisone or CORTISONE in the treatment of blistering disorders such as PEMPHIGUS.

The drug works by reducing the efficiency of the body's immune system by preventing lymphocytes (white blood cells) from multiplying. Lymphocytes destroy proteins not usually found in the body, but in autoimmune disorders they attack proteins that the immune system interprets as foreign.

Side Effects

Side effects include abnormal bleeding and increased susceptibility to infection as a result of reduced blood cell production. There may be nausea and vomiting, diarrhea, fever, HAIR LOSS, and skin eruptions. In animals, this drug causes birth defects. Temporary chromosomal abnormalities when using this drug also have been reported.

Long-term use increases the risk of skin cancer, a frequent side effect in kidney transplant patients.

azelaic acid A depigmenting agent originally identified as the cause of a lack of pigment (HYPOPIGMENTATION) associated with the fungus infection TINEA VERSICOLOR (a common skin condition producing pigmented flaking skin patches). Azelaic acid kills abnormal MELANOCYTES, melanin-producing cells. It is also being studied as a possible treatment for malignant melanoma, a deadly form of skin cancer. It is also an effective acne treatment when applied to the skin. Azelex is a recently developed topical cream that helps mild acne when applied to the affected area twice daily.

See also MELANOMA, MALIGNANT.

azulene A chamomile extract used in face and body creams, SUNBURN remedies, burn ointments, and bath salts.

B

bacterial skin infections Also known as pyodermas, this type of infection can be caused by a wide variety of bacteria. Most cases are caused by either staphylococci or steptococci. The most common of all the skin infections is IMPETIGO, a highly contagious infection of the topmost layers of the skin causing itchy, red, and blistering patches and honey-colored crusts. Most often appearing in childhood, impetigo is usually caused by *Staphylococci.*

Staph organisms also cause FOLLICULITIS, an infection near the openings of hair follicles that resembles ACNE and that can spread if untreated. It often occurs after repeated trauma to the area of skin from shaving, or following soaking in contaminated hot tubs and whirlpools.

When bacteria cause infection in deeper layers of the skin, they may result in BOILS hot, inflamed lesions that may look like an infected pimple appearing on the face, scalp, underarms, and buttocks. Larger and deeper than boils are CARBUNCLES, abscesses filled with pus and bacteria that are often extremely painful. Boils and carbuncles should never be squeezed, since the bacteria may be forced into the blood, causing widespread blood poisoning.

A most serious skin infection is CELLULITIS, usually appearing on the legs and characterized by high fever, weakness, shaking chills, pain, lymph gland swelling, and spreading warm redness. If deep swellings appear on the face, the condition is diagnosed as the potentially fatal ERYSIPELAS.

In general, bacterial skin infections usually respond well to oral antibiotics. Strep infections respond very quickly to penicillin and its derivatives, but staph infections may not; for this reason, physicians usually prescribe dicloxacillin or ERYTHROMYCIN to treat staph infections. All types of antibiotics usually require a 10-day course for a complete cure.

In addition to oral antibiotics, topical treatments may include applying warm compresses of tap water or BUROW'S SOLUTION to the affected area, or using topical over-the-counter antibiotics.

See also GROUP B STREPTOCOCCI INFECTIONS IN INFANTS; NECROTIZING FASCIITIS.

Bactroban See MUPIROCIN.

bags under eyes Loose, baggy skin under the eyes is the result of a gradual loss of skin elasticity due to aging, or because of an irreversible inherited condition called blepherochalasis. Puffy lower eyelids also can be caused by lack of sleep, stress, or illness.

The swelling can be reduced by applying dampened cotton pads, CHAMOMILE teabags dipped in cool water, or cucumbers, and lying down for 10 minutes.

Once the bags have formed, they can be covered up with makeup or surgically removed in a surgical procedure called BLEPHAROPLASTY.

baking soda A water-soluble powder used in baths as a soothing soak for irritated or itchy skin. Mixed with a bit of water into a paste, it can ease the pain of insect stings.

baldness Absence of hair on the scalp.
See also ALOPECIA AREATA.

baldness, female-pattern A typical pattern of loss of hair in women caused by hormones, aging, or heredity.

Hair grows from the hair follicle at an average rate of a half inch a month. Each hair grows for two to six years, then rests, and finally falls out. A new hair then begins growing in its place. At any time, about 85 percent of the hair is growing and 15 percent is resting.

Baldness occurs when the hair falls out but a new hair does not replace it. While the cause of the failure to grow a new hair in women is not well understood, it is associated with genetics, aging, and levels of male hormones (androgens). Changes in the levels of the androgens can affect hair production.

Symptoms and Diagnostic Path

The typical pattern of female-pattern baldness (more accurately known as female-pattern thinning) is different from that of male-pattern baldness. In women, the hair thins all over the head, but the hair in front of the head remains. There may be a moderate loss of hair on the crown, but this almost never progresses to total or near total baldness as it may in men.

In addition, hair loss can occur in women for reasons other than female-pattern baldness. These may include

- temporary shedding of hair (telogen effluvium)
- breaking of hair from styling or twisting (traction alopecia)
- ALOPECIA AREATA—an immune disorder causing temporary hair loss
- certain oral medications
- certain skin diseases

Treatment Options and Outlook

The hair loss of female-pattern baldness is permanent and usually mild to moderate. No treatment is required if the person is comfortable with her appearance. The only drug approved by the U.S. Food and Drug Administration (FDA) to treat female-pattern baldness is MINOXIDIL (Rogaine), which is applied to the scalp. It may help hair grow in 40 percent of women and may slow the loss of hair in 90 percent. Treatment is expensive, however, for the recommended twice-daily use. Hair

loss recurs when the drug is stopped. Minoxidil is available in a special formulation for women.

Hair transplants consist of removing tiny plugs of hair from areas where the hair is continuing to grow and placing them in areas that are balding. This can cause minor scarring in the donor areas, which is easily covered by the remaining hair. The procedure usually requires multiple transplantation sessions and is relatively expensive.

Suturing of hairpieces to the scalp is not recommended as it can result in scars and infections. The use of hair implants made of artificial fibers was banned by the FDA because of the high rate of infection.

Hair weaving, hairpieces, or hairstyle changes may disguise the hair loss and improve the cosmetic appearance. This is often the least expensive and safest method of treating female-pattern baldness.

baldness, male-pattern The most common cause of hair loss in men, which is caused by a normal response to male hormones (androgens) in men who are genetically predisposed to the condition. A quarter of all men start losing their hair by their third decade of life, and about two-thirds are bald or have a balding pattern by the time they are 60.

Balding can start at any time after puberty; men who begin balding at an early age are more likely to lose more hair. Caucasian men are the most likely to become bald (some estimates are as high as 80 percent) while Chinese men are about half as likely to lose their hair.

Symptoms and Diagnostic Path

The specific pattern of balding varies from person to person. "Classic balding" is where the hairline creeps from the front toward the top of the head, but there are other patterns. For example, some men lose hair only on the top of their head while others may only keep the hair on the sides of their head. Experts refer to seven basic types of pattern baldness, depending on which areas of the scalp are losing hair. Type I represents the least hair loss and Type VII the most. For instance, men with type IV pattern baldness have a moderately receding hairline and a small bald spot on the top of the head while those with type VII pattern balding only have hair on the sides of the head. No matter how severe the baldness in this condition, the hair on the sides and back of the head is never lost.

Male pattern baldness depends on the presence of male hormones, which are usually high after puberty. Testosterone, one well-known male hormone, can be converted into a more potent hormone called dihydrotestosterone (DHT) by an enzyme found in skin cells and hair follicles. Men with male-pattern baldness have high levels of DHT in their skin. When this hormone binds to a hormone receptor on the hair follicle, it slows down hair production. The follicles also produce weaker, shorter hair and may stop making scalp hair altogether.

However, male-pattern baldness does not affect all hair at the same time; some hair is more sensitive to hormones than others. For instance, a man is more likely to lose the hair on the temples than on the top.

Treatment Options and Outlook

There are a variety of treatments for male-pattern baldness, including HAIR TRANSPLANTS, scalp reduction, tissue expansion, and medication.

In transplantation, tiny plugs of hair from the back of the scalp are implanted to bald or thin areas. The process usually takes several sessions.

Alternatively (or in combination with hair transplants), some men prefer to undergo scalp reduction, in which the skin on the head is stretched and surgically removed by a dermatologic surgeon, hair transplant surgeon, or plastic surgeon. Then hairy areas on either side of the head are stretched over and sewn together. If the skin is too tight, tissue expansion is first performed.

In tissue expansion, tiny balloons are implanted under the scalp in areas with dense hair, which makes the areas up to a third larger. Over two or three months, the balloons are slowly inflated to stretch the skin. Then the skin is removed as in a scalp reduction, and the sides are pulled up to the top of the head (because hair on the sides of the head is more resistant to balding than hair on the crown).

Drug treatment may be a better choice for men who are reluctant to undergo invasive procedures, or who have early thinning. There are currently two different medications to treat this condition: FINASTERIDE and MINOXIDIL. Two drugs contain finasteride (Propecia and Proscar), which work by preventing the enzyme from converting testosterone into DHT, the primary cause of male-pattern baldness. Proscar is prescribed specifically for men with prostate enlargement. Propecia (the same medication at a lower dose) can stop hair loss and actually reverse the balding process. It normally takes at least three months to see any results from using this drug. Between 80 percent and 90 percent stop losing hair while more than 60 percent grow a significant amount of hair, and new hair will be lost within one year after medication is stopped.

The other drug used for baldness is minoxidil, known popularly as Rogaine. This drug is considered a hair loss prevention drug by the U.S. Food and Drug Administration. In this case, the liquid form of the drug is rubbed on the hairless patches of the scalp twice a day. According to clinical trials, minoxidil slows hair loss in more than 60 percent of men, but only regrows hair in one-third of men who use it. Hair loss will begin again within a few months after minoxidil is stopped.

balneotherapy Method of disease treatment by bathing (usually in mineral hot springs), once considered as fashionable "water cures."

bamboo hair Also known as trichorrhexis invaginata, this condition can sometimes develop in normal hair as the result of overprocessing. More likely, it is a congenital defect that is often a symptom of another disease, such as NETHERTON'S SYNDROME. Netherton's syndrome is usually present at birth, causing flaking skin, red rashes, and sparse hair growth with fragile bamboo hair. This syndrome is probably caused by an autosomal recessive gene that may be involved in keratinization of the hair. Examination of hair fibers has shown that the cuticle is normal but the internal structure is not completely keratinized at sporadic points along its length.

Symptoms and Diagnostic Path

This condition of the hair shaft is characterized by rough hair fibers with nodules that make the fiber look like bamboo. The nodules are defects in the fiber where a cup-and-ball shape has developed.

Treatment Options and Outlook

Bamboo hair often improves spontaneously as the child gets older; most treatments are aimed at preventing further trouble by avoiding overprocessing.

barber's itch The common term for sycosis vulgaris (inflammation of the beard area). The condition is caused by infected hair follicles (usually with *Staphylococcus aureus*) picked up from infected razors and towels.

Symptoms and Diagnostic Path

PUS-filled blisters or boils develop around the follicles, sometimes causing severe scarring unless treated.

Treatment Options and Outlook

Treatment usually involves antibiotic drugs; growing a beard may help prevent recurrence.

See also PSEUDOFOLLICULITIS BARBAE.

basal cell Small round cell found in the innermost part of the top skin layer (EPIDERMIS) where the rest of the epidermal cells are formed.

basal cell carcinoma The most common form of SKIN CANCER, affecting more than 800,000 Americans each year. One out of every three new cancers is a skin cancer, and 83.5 percent of these is a basal cell carcinoma. If untreated, the growth invades and grows deeper into surrounding tissues, but fortunately this type of cancer almost never spreads to other parts of the body.

Until recently, those most likely to get basal cell carcinoma were older people (especially men) who spent a great deal of time outdoors. Today, skin cancer affects men and women in almost equal numbers.

The incidence increases significantly in those with outdoor occupations and those who live in sunny climates; in Queensland, Australia, more than half the local white population has had a basal cell carcinoma by age 75. The number of new cases has risen sharply in recent years because of the thinning ozone layer and popularity of sunbathing. In addition, younger and younger people are being diagnosed with the disease.

Chronic overexposure to sunlight is the cause of 95 percent of all basal cell carcinomas. In a few cases, contact with arsenic, exposure to radiation, and complications of burns, scars, or vaccinations are contributing factors. People who have fair skin, light hair, and blue, green, or gray eyes are at highest risk. Those whose occupations require long hours outdoors or who spend lots of leisure time in the sun are in particular danger.

On the other hand, dark-skinned individuals are far less likely to develop skin cancer.

Symptoms and Diagnostic Path

More than 90 percent of this type of cancer is found on the face, often at the side of the eye or on the nose or other exposed area of the body, although it can appear in any location. The five most typical characteristics of basal cell carcinoma are very different from each other, and often two or more features are found in one tumor. Basal cell carcinoma may be

- an open sore that bleeds or oozes, remaining open for three or more weeks
- a reddish patch or irritated area (often on the shoulder, chest, arms, or legs) that may itch or hurt, or cause no sensation at all
- a smooth growth with an elevated, rolled border and indented center, developing tiny blood vessels on the surface as it grows
- a shiny bump that is pearly or translucent, often pink, red or white, tan, black, or brown
- a scar (white, yellow or waxy) with poorly defined borders; the skin itself looks shiny and taut. This last sign is less frequent but may indicate an aggressive tumor.

A diagnosis of basal cell carcinoma is made after physical examination and biopsy (removal and examination of a small piece of tissue).

Treatment Options and Outlook

If tumor cells are found, the growth can be removed by surgery or destroyed by radiation. The treatment is based on type, size, and location of the tumor and on the patient's age and health, but it can almost always be performed on an outpatient basis. Local anesthetics are used and not much pain is felt.

Surgical removal The most common treatment is simple excisional surgery. The physician removes the entire growth and an additional border of normal skin as a safety margin. The site is then stitched closed and the tissue is sent to the lab to determine if all malignant cells have been removed.

Alternatively, the surgeon may perform *electrosurgery* (CURETTAGE AND ELECTRODESICCATION) in which cancerous tissue is scraped from the skin with a curette (sharp ring-shaped device) and an electric needle burns a safety margin of normal skin around the tumor at the base of the scraped area. This technique is repeated twice to make sure the tumor has been completely removed.

With CRYOSURGERY, the physician does not cut the growth but instead freezes the lesion by applying LIQUID NITROGEN with a special spray or a cotton-tipped applicator; this method does not require anesthesia and produces no bleeding. It is easy to administer and is the treatment of choice for those who have bleeding disorders or are intolerant to anesthesia.

Laser surgery is used to focus a beam of light onto the lesion either to excise it or destroy it by vaporization. The major advantage of this technique is that it seals blood vessels as it cuts. In removing skin cancer, incisional laser surgery offers no real advantage over scalpel surgery.

Mohs' surgery (microscopically controlled surgery) involves the removal of very thin layers of the malignant tumor, checking each layer thoroughly under a microscope. This is repeated as often as necessary until the tissue is free of tumor; this method saves the most healthy tissue and has the highest cure rate; it is often used for tumors that recur and for tumors in areas where basal cell carcinomas are known to recur after other treatment techniques (nose, ears, and around the eyes).

Radiation therapy In radiation therapy, X-rays are directed at the malignant cells; it usually takes several treatments several times a week for a few weeks to totally destroy a tumor. Radiation therapy may be used with older patients or with those in poor health.

Drug treatment Researchers are now studying the possible use of interferon, a genetically engineered product of the human immune system, as a possible treatment of some basal cell carcinomas. Interferon interferes with viral multiplication and increases the activity of natural killer cells (types of lymphocytes that make up part of the body's immune system). Basal cell carcinoma has a better than 95 percent cure rate if detected and treated.

The larger the growth the more extensive the treatment. While this type of skin cancer almost never metastasizes, it can destroy surrounding tissue. Since removal of a tumor scars the skin, large tumors may require reconstructive surgery and skin grafts.

If a patient is diagnosed with one basal cell carcinoma, there is a greater chance of developing others over the body in the future. Even though a basal cell carcinoma has been removed, another can develop in the same place (or nearby), usually within the first two years after surgery. Basal cell carcinomas on the scalp, nose, and sides of the nose and around the ears are particularly problematic. If the cancer recurs, the physician may recommend a different type of treatment the second time, most likely Mohs' surgery. Therefore, it is important to examine the surgical site periodically.

Bazex syndrome A rare eruption of the nose, ears, and extremities associated with cancer of the lungs, esophagus, and tongue or the gastrointestinal tract.

Symptoms and Diagnostic Path

Symptoms begin on the hands and feet with scaling bluish red plaques; severe nail problems may include flaking and shedding of the nail itself, followed by involvement of the ear, nose bridge, elbows, and knees. The skin symptoms, which look much like PSORIASIS, may appear before a tumor is diagnosed and can predict the malignancy with almost 100 percent accuracy.

Treatment Options and Outlook
The skin lesions fade away when the tumor is removed. Symptoms may also be treated with keratolytics and topical steroids.

Beau's lines Temporary horizontal depressions across the nails that appear during certain acute infections such as MEASLES and MUMPS or inflammatory conditions such as inflammatory bowel disease or lupus, or after a heart attack. The depression first appears at the cuticle a few weeks after the underlying disease begins and slowly moves out to the end of the nail as the nail grows over a period of months. When this condition appears during a systemic disease, all of the fingernails and toenails are likely to be affected. If only one or two nails are affected, the condition is probably caused by trauma or cold.

bedbugs Flat, wingless brown insects that live in floors and furniture (especially beds) during the day, coming out at night to bite their human hosts. While they rarely transmit disease, their bites may become infected. Usually the bug sucks blood from several nearby sites, resulting in a group or cluster of lesions.

Soon after the bite, the patient experiences an itchy, burning wheal with a central red mark, which helps differentiate this from an ordinary wheal. The bedbug lesion may become firm or develop into a blister (especially in children). The wheal may subside soon, or it may last for several hours. They appear most often on the back, neck, face, ankles, wrists, buttocks, or wherever the body touches the bed.

Bedbugs can be killed with a variety of insecticides, including malathion, lindane, or pyrethrins.

bedsores A type of ulcer (also known as decubitus ulcers or pressure sores) that develops on the skin of bedridden, unconscious, or immobile patients. They often affect patients with stroke or spinal cord injuries; constantly wet skin caused by incontinence also may be a factor. Common site of breakdown includes the shoulders, elbows, lower back, hips and buttocks, knees, ankles, and heels.

Actor Christopher Reeve, a quadriplegic and an outspoken advocate for the disabled, died 10 years after his horseriding accident as a result of complications of a pressure sore, which indicates how serious these wounds can be. Although people living with paralysis are especially at risk, anyone who is bedridden, uses a wheelchair, or is unable to change positions without help can develop pressure sores.

Symptoms and Diagnostic Path
Bedsores begin as red, painful areas that turn purple before the skin breaks down, eventually turning into open sores. Once the skin is broken, the sores often become infected, enlarge, deepen, and are very slow to heal.

Pressure sores fall into one of four stages based on their severity, according to the National Pressure Ulcer Advisory Panel, a professional organization dedicated to the prevention and treatment of pressure sores.

Stage I A pressure sore begins with an area of red skin that may itch or hurt, and feel warm to the touch. In people with darker skin, the mark may look flaky or ashen, with a blue or purple cast. Stage I wounds are superficial and will fade away after the pressure is relieved.

Stage II The pressure sore now looks like an open sore, more like a blister or abrasion, affecting either the outermost or deeper layer of skin (or both). Surrounding skin may look red or purple. If treated promptly, stage II sores usually heal fairly quickly.

Stage III Characterized by a deep, craterlike wound, pressure ulcers at this stage extend all the way through the skin layers down to the muscle.

Stage IV In the most serious and advanced stage, there is damage to muscle, bone, and supporting structures such as tendons and joints, along with the overlying skin. Stage IV wounds are extremely difficult to heal and can lead to fatal infections.

Treatment Options and Outlook

Deep chronic ulcers may require treatment with antibiotics, packing with plastic foam, and sometimes even PLASTIC SURGERY.

Risk Factors and Preventive Measures

It is a far better idea to prevent a bedsore from developing than to try to treat one already in existence. Once a bedsore has developed, it will heal only if the pressure on the damaged skin is minimized.

To prevent sores, a patient's position should be changed at least every two hours; it is important to wash and dry pressure areas carefully (especially if there is incontinence). Barrier creams also may further protect the skin.

A ripple bed mattress may help prevent bedsores by stimulating circulation; this rippling effect is created by pumping air in and out of the mattress. Cushions and pillows may relieve pressure (place them between the knees and under the shoulder). A sheepskin under the buttocks and booties on feet also may also relieve pressure.

bee and wasp stings   More than half of all deaths due to venomous animals are a result of stings by bees and wasps. The Hymenoptera order includes three families: honeybee and bumblebees; wasps, hornets, and yellow jackets; and several species of ants.

Symptoms and Diagnostic Path

After being stung, the patient may have either an immediate reaction within two hours or a delayed reaction. Immediate reactions are the most common, and include local swelling, reddening, pain, and ITCHING, which usually subsides within a few hours.

However, in some patients with hypersensitivity to venom, the local reaction is marked by more severe and prolonged swelling and redness, with systemic reactions ranging from mild to fatal. Anaphylactic reactions (with breathing problems and internal swelling) usually occur within the first 10 to 30 minutes after the sting. The faster a reaction materializes the more severe it will be.

Treatment Options and Outlook

Ice, elevation, and oral antihistamines minimize local pain and swelling. In the case of a delayed local reaction appearing after 24 hours, a five-day course of systemic steroids may help. In honeybee stings, the stinger and attached venom sac must be scraped from the skin; forceps should not be used, because pressure on the sac can inject more venom.

Highly allergic individuals should carry an emergency kit including a tourniquet, syringe, epinephrine, and antihistamine. Those who have had several severe reactions should consider hyposensitization; IMMUNOTHERAPY with venom is 95 percent effective in eliminating serious allergic responses.

beeswax   A substance secreted by bees to build the walls of their cells in the hive; it is also used by cosmetic manufacturers as an emulsifier to soften and protect the skin. Without emulsifiers, the cosmetic would separate, leaving the solids at the bottom and the liquid ingredients at the top. Beeswax has caused allergic reactions in some sensitive people.

Behcet's syndrome   A rare disorder causing skin rashes and recurrent mouth ulcers among many other symptoms. Attacks often last for several weeks and recur frequently. Eye involvement many cause blindness; central nervous system involvement may be fatal. The syndrome was first described by Turkish dermatologist Hulusi Behcet (1889–1948).

Rare in the United States, the disease is more often found in some Middle Eastern countries and Japan, and is five times more likely to occur among men. The syndrome may become chronic in some patients.

Its cause is unknown, although some experts believe the disease could be triggered by a virus, a clotting problem, an autoimmune disorder, or heredity.

Symptoms and Diagnostic Path

Behcet's disease generally begins when individuals are in their 20s or 30s, although it can happen at any age, and it tends to occur more often in men than in women. A variety of skin lesions throughout the body have been associated with the disease (PAPULES, VESICLES, PUSTULES, ABSCESSES, subcutaneous thrombophlebitis, and nodular lesions). Other symptoms of the syndrome include genital, mouth or intestinal ulcers; eye inflammation; arthritis; venous thrombosis; blood clots; or neuropsychiatric symptoms.

Treatment Options and Outlook

Oral and genital ulcers may be treated topically, although this will not prevent new ulcers from forming. Topical CORTICOSTEROIDS may cut down on inflammation; topical anesthetics may ease pain. In severe cases, systemic anticancer drugs, corticosteroids, or immune suppressors (especially azathioprine) may be prescribed, but treatment is difficult. Colchicine or levamisole are sometimes effective. The disorder can be fatal depending on which organ system is involved; affected eyes and the central nervous system pose the greatest risk. Behcet's disease is a lifelong disorder that comes and goes. Permanent remission of symptoms has not been reported.

benign skin cancer See SKIN TUMOR, BENIGN.

benzoic acid A preservative used in skin care products that generally is not considered to be irritating, although it may cause an allergic reaction in consumers who are sensitive to similar chemicals.

benzoyl peroxide An antibacterial agent considered to be the most effective nonprescription ACNE treatment, markedly suppressing the bacterium *PROPIONIBACTERIUM ACNES* associated with acne. This extremely effective topical antibacterial agent draws peroxide into the pore where it releases oxygen, killing the bacteria that can aggravate acne. Benzoyl also suppresses fatty acid cells that irritate pores and helps to unplug blackheads. It is most effective for patients with inflammatory acne; by inhibiting bacteria, it decreases the inflammation in the skin.

Benzoyl peroxide is available in a cleansing bar, cream, gel, lotion, and facial mask. It is sold in strengths ranging between 5 and 10 percent, but dermatologists usually advise patients to start with a 5 percent product, since the lower concentration is just as effective and less likely to cause irritation. Most over-the-counter products contain benzoyl peroxide in a lotion base; the prescription items contain the chemical in a gel base. A fairly new prescription preparation combining 3 percent erythromycin with a 5 percent benzoyl peroxide in a gel base may be more effective than either component by itself.

Because the skin absorbs benzoyl peroxide, it should not be used by pregnant or nursing women unless directed by a physician. Its safety for children under age 12 has not been established. Because benzoyl peroxide is a bleach, it will discolor most fabrics and hair.

Over-the-counter cleansers that contain benzoyl peroxide include Fostex 10% Wash (liquid), Fostex 10% (bar), Oxy 10 Wash, Pan-Oxyl 5% and Pan-Oxyl 10%. Nonprescription lotions include Acne-10, Benozyl 5, Benozyl 10, Clearasil 10%, Dry and Clear (5%), Loroxide (5.5%), Oxy 5, Oxy 10, and Vanoxide (5%). Nonprescription creams include Acne-Aid (10%), Clearasil Maximum Strength (10%), Cuticura Acne (5%), Dry and Clear Double Strength, Fostex (10%), and Oxy 10 Cover. Gels include Clear by Design (2.5%), Del Aqua-5, Del Aqua-10, Fostex 5%, Fostex 10%, Xerac BP5, and Xerac BP10.

Side Effects

While most people experience some mild burning, itching or peeling, benzoyl peroxide can produce a stronger reaction in some people with very sensitive skin (especially those with very fair skin). It is normal to experience a warm or stinging feeling, with some dryness or peeling, but if the skin turns very red, or there is pain, a lot of scaling and swelling, then an adverse reaction has occurred and the product should be discontinued.

The stronger the preparation, the greater the chance of a reaction. Benzoyl peroxide should never be applied near the eyes, where it can cause swelling and irritation; some patients are also sensitive around the nose and mouth. Hands should be washed thoroughly after using the product; eyes should never be rubbed with contaminated fingers.

Some studies have reported that benzoyl peroxide may be carcinogenic, although this conclusion is controversial and inconclusive.

berloque dermatitis   See DERMATITIS, BERLOQUE.

bergamot oil   See OIL OF BERGAMOT.

beta-carotene   A plants substance that the body can convert into VITAMIN A; it acts as an antioxidant and immune system booster. Some experts suspect it may be possible to shield the body's immune system from harmful UVA rays and reduce the risk of skin cancer by supplementing the diet with beta-carotene.

Most, but not all, beta-carotene in supplements is synthetic, consisting of only one molecule. Natural beta-carotene found in food is made of two molecules. Researchers originally saw no meaningful difference between natural and synthetic beta-carotene, but this view was questioned when the link between beta-carotene–containing foods and lung cancer prevention was not duplicated in studies using synthetic pills.

Beta-carotene is found in green and orange-yellow vegetables. The most common beta-carotene supplement intake is probably 25,000 IU (15 mg) per day, though some people take as much as 100,000 IU (60 mg) per day.

Excessive beta-carotene (more than 100,000 IU, or 60 mg per day) sometimes tints the skin yellow-orange. Individuals taking beta-carotene for long periods of time should also supplement with VITAMIN E, as beta-carotene may reduce vitamin E levels.

beta hydroxy acids   A topical exfoliant used (sometimes in combination with ALPHA HYDROXY ACIDS) as ingredients in skin-care products designed to reduce the signs of aging in the skin.

Both AHA and BHA-containing cosmetics are derived from the chemical peels that dermatologists and plastic surgeons have used for years to help remove undesirable signs of skin aging, such as discoloration, roughness, and wrinkling. The chemicals cause the skin to peel off, revealing a fresher-looking layer of skin. Known as chemical exfoliation, the procedure is done in aestheticians' salons at low concentrations and at higher, more effective strengths in doctors' offices.

Cosmetic manufacturers began to market similar but milder versions of these chemical peels containing AHAs and BHAs for salon and at-home use around 1989; today, every cosmetic company has AHA and BHA in their products.

Some in the cosmetic industry have suggested that AHA and BHA products are more than simple cosmetics, coining the term COSMECEUTICAL to describe them instead. The U.S. Food and Drug Administration (FDA) has a particular concern about them because, unlike traditional cosmetics, they seem capable of penetrating the skin barrier and altering skin function.

While both AHAs and BHAs act as exfoliants, it has been claimed that BHAs are effective in reducing the appearance of fine lines and wrinkles and improving overall skin texture, without the occasional irritation associated with the use of AHAs.

BHA ingredients may be listed as

- SALICYLIC ACID (or related substances, such as salicylate, sodium salicylate, and willow extract)
- beta hydroxybutanoic acid
- tropic acid
- otrethocanic acid

Today, the most common BHA in cosmetics is salicylic acid. Rarely, citric acid is also cited as a BHA is cosmetic formulations, but more often it is considered an AHA.

The safety of salicylic acid used as a cosmetic ingredient has been evaluated by both the cosmetic industry and the FDA. Products containing salicylic acid should either contain a sunscreen or bear directions advising consumers to use other sun protection, according to the COSMETIC INGREDIENT REVIEW (CIR) Expert Panel, the cosmetic industry's independent body for reviewing the safety of cosmetic ingredients.

The long-term safety of salicylic acid in cosmetics also is being evaluated in studies initiated by the FDA and sponsored by the National Toxicology Program. These government-sponsored studies are examining the long-term effects of both glycolic acid (an AHA) and salicylic acid on the skin's response to ultraviolet (UV) light. These studies have determined that applying glycolic acid to the skin can make people more susceptible to the damaging effects of the sun, including sunburn.

Until these safety assessments are completed, the FDA advises consumers that similar precautions be taken for the use of cosmetics containing BHAs. Consumers should test any product that contains an AHA or BHA on a small area of skin before applying it to a large area. Cosmetics with these substances that cause skin irritation or prolonged stinging should not be used. Consumers should not exceed the recommended applications and avoid using AHA- or BHA-containing products on infants and children.

biologic agents Substances made from a living organism used to prevent, diagnose, or treat disease. Scientists have begun to focus on the successful treatment of skin diseases such as PSORIASIS and PYODERMA GANGRENOSUM using biologic agents designed to inhibit immune responses that are central to these conditions.

Biologic agents include alefacept, etanercept, and infliximab. These agents bind to and inhibit a molecule central to the immune response that drives psoriasis and other inflammatory skin diseases. They hold promise for revolutionizing the treatment of skin diseases.

biological implants A type of SKIN FILLER material used to correct wrinkles, soft tissue defects, and depressed scars that is readily available in a variety of shapes, sizes, and quantity, and are less likely to become infected or displaced than synthetics. Disadvantages to this type of skin filler include the possibility of allergic reactions and the theoretical risk of disease transmission from the donor of the material.

Examples of biological implants include bovine COLLAGEN (ZYDERM), human collagen (Cosmoderm and Cosmoplast) synthetic or naturally derived HYALURONIC ACID (RESTYLANE and Hylaform), or acellular dermal grafts (ALLODERM, CYMETRA).

biotin deficiency A lack of this water-soluble vitamin important in amino acid metabolism may cause fissured lips; red, tender tongue; and reddening and dryness of mucosal surfaces. In infants, a lethal form of biotin deficiency may cause a generalized SEBORRHEIC DERMATITIS or ICHTHYOSIS; a different form of infant biotin deficiency may cause diffuse reddening, scaling, and crusting at skin junctions and mucosal surfaces together with hair loss.

Although rare, biotin deficiency can occur when raw egg whites are eaten or with tube or injection feeding without biotin supplements.

Treatment Options and Outlook

The intravenous administration of biotin is an effective treatment for this condition.

birth control pills (the Pill) Contraceptive medications have been linked to a number of skin problems, including ACNE, hair loss, and blotchy pigmentation. Their use also can be associated with ERYTHEMA NODOSUM, an inflammatory skin disease characterized by red-purple swellings.

Many varieties of the birth control pill (such as Norlestrin, Norinyl, Ovral, and Loestrin) can aggravate acne and can also increased sensitivity to the sun, resulting in swelling of skin that has been exposed to the ultraviolet rays. Because of hormonal changes, hair may be lost while taking the Pill or after the Pill has been stopped. Women who develop skin problems while using birth control pills may be able to have their prescriptions changed to a different type of pill.

Pills with slightly higher estrogen levels, such as Demulen and others with 50 mg of estrogen, may actually improve acne.

Between 5 and 30 percent of women taking the Pill develop a blotchy, heightened skin color on their face, regardless of whether their prescription contained primarily estrogen or progesterone. This darkening, called melasma or CHLOASMA, is often seen during the last trimester of pregnancy, although it also appears in women who are neither pregnant nor taking birth control pills. Exposure to the sun will make this darkening worse.

When the Pill is taken for longer periods of time and at higher dosages, skin changes are likely to be noticeable.

birthmarks　An area of discolored skin present at birth; the most common birthmarks are MOLES (nevi), which are malformations of pigment cells. STRAWBERRY BIRTHMARKS are bright red, spongy and protuberant; PORT-WINE STAINS are purple-red, flat and often cover large areas. Both strawberry marks and port-wine stains are malformations of blood vessels.

True strawberry (superficial) HEMANGIOMAS all disappear by age seven, although they may leave an unsightly scar.

Port-wine stains never go away. In a few cases (referred to as STURGE-WEBER SYNDROME) port-wine stains are associated with abnormalities in the blood vessels of the brain.

Treatment Options and Outlook

Unattractive moles can be removed at any time from late childhood through adulthood. Port-wine stains can be lightened significantly using LASER treatment.

The PULSED DYE LASER is highly effective at lightening port-wine stains; treatment should be started within the first few weeks of life.

bisulfites　A substance contained in the mildest permanent waving solution used for body waves and color-treated hair.

bites and infestations　Fly and mosquito bites may cause swelling and ITCHING for several days and may lead to infection if sores are scratched open.

Treatment Options and Outlook

Because flies and mosquitoes can spread disease, the bite area should be washed with soap and water followed with an antiseptic. A nonprescription antihistamine, CALAMINE lotion, or ice packs can control itching. Itching also can be controlled with a paste to spread over the bite made out of: salt and water; baking soda (1 tsp. in a glass of water, place on bite for 20 minutes); or epsom salts (1 Tbs. in 1 quart of hot water).

Risk Factors and Preventive Measures

Many mosquitoes and biting insects are especially likely to bite around dusk and dawn. It is important to apply repellent during these times. However, in many parts of the country, there are mosquitoes that also bite during the day. The safest decision is to apply repellent whenever individuals are outdoors.

Consumers should follow the directions on the repellent to determine how frequently it needs to be reapplied. Sweating, perspiration, or getting wet may mean that it needs to be reapplied more often. If a person is not being bitten, it is not necessary to reapply repellent.

Repellents containing a higher concentration of active ingredient (such as DEET) provide longer-lasting protection. DEET (NIN-diethyl-m-toluamide) is the most effective of all bug repellents. A product containing 23.8 percent DEET provides an average of five hours of protection; 20 percent DEET provides almost four hours of protection; 6.65 percent DEET provides almost two hours of protections; and 4.75 percent DEET and 2 percent soybean oil are both able to provide roughly one and a half hours of protection. Consumers should choose a repellant that provides protection for the amount of time that they will be outdoors. A higher percentage of DEET should be used if the person will be outdoors for several hours. It may be used on children but should not be applied to infants. It should be kept out of eyes. New preparations combine SUNSCREEN and a bug repellent in one cream.

blackhead　A dark semisolid plug of greasy SEBUM blocking the outlet of an oil-producing gland in

Cross Section of Blackhead

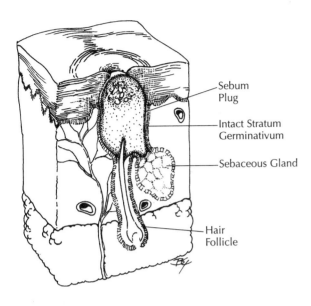

Sebum Plug

Intact Stratum Germinativum

Sebaceous Gland

Hair Follicle

the skin, most commonly found on the face, chest, back, and shoulders. It is associated with increased sebaceous gland activity in adolescents, and often appears as part of ACNE. The black color is not dirt, but a reaction that occurs when the plug mixes with air and skin pigment.

Treatment Options and Outlook

SALICYLIC ACID and Retin-A are particularly effective treatments for blackheads, but BENZOYL PEROXIDE also may be effective. Blackheads may be gently squeezed; cosmetologists also may remove them.

See also ACNE, TREATMENT FOR.

bleaching creams Nonprescription cosmetic bleaching creams do not change the color of the skin that has darkened as a result of hormonal imbalances, chemicals, sun exposure, and so on. Instead, they prevent the formation of MELANIN.

A variety of substances has been used in the past to bleach the skin, including lemon juice, tea, and salicylic acid. AMMONIATED MERCURY was used until 1974, when the U.S. Food and Drug Administration barred the sale of creams containing this substance because of its toxicity and the incidence of allergic reactions.

The agent HYDROQUINONE can sometimes be successful as it both helps to prevent new melanin production and bleaches existing pigment. It may be purchased over the counter in concentrations of 2 percent or less. Higher prescriptions require a prescription. Hydroquinone may be prescribed in combination with RETINOIC ACID (to enhance penetration) and a CORTICOSTEROID (to reduce irritation). It may require several months' treatment before a good response is achieved. Rarely, hydroquinone can trigger an allergic response or irritation in some people or produce a mottled appearance.

Monobenzoyl ether of hydroquinone (Benoquin) should never be used to bleach the skin because it destroys melanocytes and leaves permanent disfiguring white spots (it should only be used for patients with extensive VITILIGO in an effort to bleach their remaining unaffected skin so that they will be uniformly colored).

Prescription products containing hydroquinone include Eldopaque Cream, eldoquin, Eldopaque Forte (4 percent hydroquinone), Solaquin Forte (4 percent hydroquinone, PABA ester, benzophene), Lustra (4 percent hydroquinone and glycolic acid), Glyquin (4 percent hydroquinone and glycolic acid), Lustra AF (4 percent hydroquinone, glycolic acid, and sunscreen), Alustra (4 percent hydroquinone and retinol), and Melanex (3 percent hydroquinone).

Nonprescription products include Esoterica Cream, Altra HCQ Kit (4 percent hydroquinone, 1 percent hydrocortisone) and Ambi (2 percent hydroquinone, PABA ester).

Combined medications include hydroquinone 4 percent and salicylic acid 2 percent; hydroquinone 2 percent or 4 percent, hydrocortisone 2 percent, and tretinoin cream 0.05 percent applied sequentially; hydroquinone 4 percent, tretinoin 0.1 percent, and dexamethasone 0.1 percent applied sequentially.

Trichloroacetic acid may be effective in light-skinned people, but it should not be used on black skin. This highly caustic agent must be used with great caution to avoid instant tissue necrosis and permanent SCARS. In mild concentrations, it can be painted on pigmented lesions, which produces a mild lightening. The best concentration of this acid is one which produces lightening without excessive injury to the skin.

Alternatively, gentle freezing with LIQUID NITROGEN to treat localized colored spots may be effective by decreasing the amount of color. Melanocytes are particularly sensitive to destruction using this technique. This process does not work in those with dark or black skin, however, because of the risk of permanent depigmentation.

bleb A tiny blister usually formed by injecting a small amount of fluid under the outer layer of the skin, such as in a tuberculin test.

bleomycin An antibiotic obtained from a soil fungus used to treat certain cancers, such as KAPOSI'S SARCOMA and WARTS that have not responded to other treatment.

Side Effects

Painful injections, localized swelling and the development of a bleeding scab, bone marrow suppression, or anemia.

blepharoplasty See EYELID LIFT.

blister A raised oval or round collection of fluid within or beneath the outer layer of the skin. Blisters larger than a half inch in diameter are sometimes called bullae; small blisters are also called VESICLES. Blisters that have been inadvertently pierced may be susceptible to infection. If there is redness, swelling, heat, increased pain, or the drainage has an odor or is not clear, then the blister has become infected.

A blister appears after minor skin damage when fluid leaks from blood vessels in underlying skin. The fluid is usually sterile, and the blister provides valuable protection to the damaged tissue.

Blisters often appear after burns, SUNBURN, and friction (such as damage to hands from using a

rake without gloves, or as a result of wearing tight shoes). There are a number of skin diseases that also can cause blisters, including ECZEMA, IMPETIGO, EPIDERMOLYSIS BULLOSA, PORPHYRIA, ERYTHEMA MULTIFORME, and the bullous diseases of PEMPHIGOID, PEMPHIGUS, and DERMATITIS HERPETIFORMIS.

In addition, small blisters develop in the early stages of many viral infections, including CHICKEN POX, SHINGLES, and HERPES SIMPLEX. These blisters contain infectious particles capable of spreading the infection.

Treatment Options and Outlook

A blister should not be disturbed, but left to heal on its own. It may be pierced at the edge using a sterile needle, allowing the fluid to slowly seep out. A blister should not to be unroofed, as the roof protects against infection. Left intact even after the blister has been drained, the skin flap will act as a type of Band-aid; it will eventually harden and fall off by itself. However, patients with large, troublesome or unexplained blisters should seek medical advice; some experts believe that a large blister on a weight-bearing area almost always has to be pierced.

Otherwise, a patient should try applying a moleskin pad (available at drug stores) cut to resemble a doughnut with the blister in the middle; the moleskin will absorb the friction of daily activity.

Triple antibiotics (such as Neosporin) may eliminate bacterial contamination, whereas iodine or camphor-phenol slow down healing.

Risk Factors and Preventive Measures

People should always wear socks with shoes, and gloves on hands when working with tools. Feet should be powdered when wearing new shoes. If an individual is worried about getting blistered feet, blister-prone areas can be coated with PETROLEUM JELLY or DIAPER RASH ointment (such as A&D ointment) to cut down friction.

While there is controversy over the kind of sock material that best prevents blisters, current research suggests that acrylic spun fibers may actually be better than cotton in the presence of water. Wearing two sets of different materials on each foot with properly fitted shoes helps prevent blistering.

blistering disorders Blistering (or bullous) diseases are not common, but they are very dramatic and can be quite serious. Many of these diseases are triggered by problems in the immune system. Some are inherited; these can be diagnosed during pregnancy.

Among the blistering disorders are PEMPHIGUS, DERMATITIS HERPETIFORMIS, and the PEMPHIGOID group (bullous pemphigoid, HERPES GESTATIONIS, cicatricial pemphigoid, epidermolysis bullosa acquisita and linear IgA dermatosis).

Treatment for these disorders varies according to cause and severity. Creams are sometimes effective, but sometimes systemic treatment is needed.

Bloch-Sulzberger syndrome A disorder of pigmentation (also known as *incontinentia pigmenti*) probably transmitted as an X-linked dominant disorder that is usually lethal to male fetuses, and that occurs in baby girls of all races who carry the trait. It is sometimes associated with multiple defects of the central nervous system within the first month of life. Most affected individuals have numerous skin symptoms, as well as malformations of the eyes, teeth, bones, nails, heart, central nervous system, and hair. Mental deficiency is usually associated. The syndrome is divided into two forms: incontinentia pigmenti type I and type II. Type II is lethal in males.

Symptoms and Diagnostic Path

Streaks of red papules or vesicles over the arms, legs and trunk in a swirled or marbled pattern. Over a period of weeks, the swirls evolve into papules that eventually heal, leaving a brown-gray hyperpigmented discoloration.

Treatment Options and Outlook

There is no effective treatment; the child rapidly passes through the stages of the disease, and the lesions are usually gone by the age of two. The unusual pigmentation usually fades by age 20.

blood vessel disorders and the skin The blood supply in the skin is delivered by an interconnecting network of small arteries, veins, and tiny capillaries that connect the arteries to the veins. In the embryo, certain cells are responsible for stimulating blood vessel development. The blood vessel network is the first organ to begin developing in the embryo, which continues until adulthood.

Some blood vessel disorders are the result of the overproduction of blood vessel cells. For example, a HEMANGIOMA that often appears soon after birth goes through a period of rapid growth in which the blood vessel cells multiply too much. As the tumor shrinks and the skin eventually returns to a near-normal appearance, the cells gradually die off.

Other blood vessel disorders occur from malformations between the fourth and 10th week of pregnancy.

Malformations of blood vessels, such as PORT-WINE STAINS, are usually present at birth, although some appear years later. They tend to grow along with the patient, although periods of more rapid development can occur.

During pregnancy, hormonal influences can cause blood vessel changes. As a result, some women develop many tiny dilated blood vessels in the skin's surface layer (spider ANGIOMAS). They typically blanch under pressure; when released, the blood returns quickly. Many of these blood vessels fade away after pregnancy, when hormone levels return to normal. If they do not, laser treatment is available to eradicate them. Lasers have revolutionized the treatment of many blood vessel growths.

Bloom's syndrome This inherited syndrome is characterized by an intense sensitivity to light beginning in infancy, which causes reddening, blistering, and eventually persistent areas of reddened skin and TELANGIECTASIA on the face and hands. At birth, there is proportionate dwarfism; adults are short, with normal intelligence and sexual development, although males often have small testes.

The condition is found most often among Ashkenazi Jewish men originally from southeastern Poland and northwestern Ukraine. While Bloom's syndrome is characterized by many chromosomal abnormalities, the basic genetic defect is not known. More than 100 cases have been reported in the United States.

Treatment Options and Outlook

Bloom's syndrome has no specific treatment. Redness and photosensitivity, and resistance to infections, improve with age. Various types of leukemia develop at about age 22; patients who survive beyond age 22 typically develop solid tumors at an average age of 35 years. Fortunately, these tumors are sensitive to chemotherapy and radiotherapy. Infection gradually improves with age. There is a higher risk of premature death in the 20s or 30 because of secondary infection due to malignancies.

Because of the sensitivity to sunlight, the risk of SKIN CANCER increases significantly with this syndrome.

Risk Factors and Preventive Measures

Topical SUNSCREENS will prevent the SUNBURN reaction and decrease sun damage.

blush An involuntary reaction to unwanted attention, or embarrassment, that sends blood rushing to the face, neck, upper chest, and ears. When a person is embarrassed the body experiences this as stress, and involuntarily heats up. As a result, the hypothalamus (the body's temperature regulator) directs heat to the face, the site of the most capillaries (tiny blood vessels that let heat escape). The result is a red blush.

Some women during menopause also experience blushing due to changes in hormonal activity; facial flushing also occurs with the carcinoid syndrome (a rare condition characterized by facial flush, diarrhea, and wheezing caused by an intestinal or lung tumor).

Four out of five people have the tendency to blush, but how easily this occurs also depends on a person's genetic makeup. One way to stop a telltale blush is to sip cold water to head off the body's response to heat.

This nonverbal sign of embarrassment is understood in all human cultures. Studies have shown that those who appear embarrassed often appear to be more likeable.

Researchers conclude that those who do not show signs of embarrassment after a blunder send a disturbing message—either they are unfazed because they are accustomed to their own incompetence or because they do not care about the rules of behavior.

blusher A type of colored cosmetic designed to give the face a healthy-looking glow. Blushers come in four basic types: powder, cream, liquid, and gel.

Powder blushers have a soft finish and can be used to produce as much or as little color as desired. Powdered products work well on any skin characteristic, especially for those with oily or combination skin. Powder blushers should be applied with a fluffy brush over foundation or directly on bare skin.

Cream blushers are good choices for those with normal or dry skin; they camouflage fine lines and wrinkles better than powder products. However, creams must be applied carefully or they will streak. A bit of moisturizer is blended into the blusher, then smoothed onto cheeks using a moistened cosmetic sponge for more control. It should be applied in a soft arc along the cheekbones, blending edges until there is no obvious line. It should never be applied in a circle, because the color will look artificial.

Liquid blushes (also called "color rubs") are sheer and can be used to color cheeks or as an all-over facial tint. They work best for dry or normal skin, where they should be blended onto the skin with fingertips, working quickly for even coverage and a sheer finish.

Gel blushers are more transparent than liquid products, and work best on normal or dry skin. They must be applied gently with fingertips because they streak easily; they also can be used for total facial tint.

For an idea of where to apply blusher, the consumer should place index and middle fingers in a "v" formation over the cheekbones. Individuals should avoid applying too much blusher close to the nose or too close to the eyes. Blusher too high or too low on the cheek can look unnatural; it is always easier to add more than take some away.

The color of blusher should complement skin tone. Fair-skinned blondes look best with beige-pink to coral shades; fair-skinned brunettes are better in rosy to pale pink shades. Olive skin looks best with reddish bronze, soft rose, or coral shades, and black skin is best with a sheer tint of soft pink, pink-mauve, or blue-red (dark mauve blush tends to emphasize ashiness).

Bockhart's impetigo   See IMPETIGO, BOCKHART'S.

boil   An inflamed PUS-filled section of skin (usually an infected HAIR FOLLICLE) found often on the back of the neck or moist areas such as the armpits and groin. A large boil is called a CARBUNCLE.

Boils are usually caused by infection with the bacterium *Staphylococcus aureus*, which invades the body through a break in the skin, where it infects a blocked oil gland or hair follicle. When the body's immune system triggers the production of white blood cells to kill the germs, the resulting inflammation produces pus.

Symptoms and Diagnostic Path
A boil begins with a red, painful lump that swells as it fills with pus, until it becomes rounded with a yellowish tip. The boil may either continue to grow

Cross Section of Boil

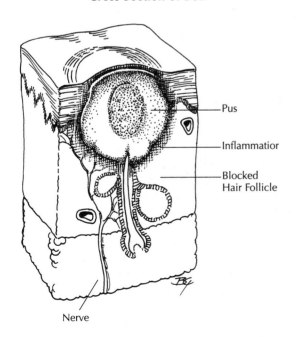

Pus

Inflammation

Blocked Hair Follicle

Nerve

until it erupts, drains and fades away, or it can be reabsorbed by the body. Recurrent boils may occur in people with known or unrecognized diabetes mellitus, or other diseases involving lowered body resistance.

Signs of a spreading infection include generalized symptoms of fever and chills, swelling lymph nodes, or red lines radiating from the boil.

Treatment Options and Outlook
Bacteria from a boil may find its way into the blood, causing blood poisoning; for this reason, doctors advise against squeezing boils that appear around the lips or nose, since the infection can be carried to the brain. Instead, patients should apply a hot compress for 20 minutes every two hours to relieve discomfort and hasten drainage and healing. The compress should be changed for a new hot one every five minutes during the 20-minute intervals. After treating a boil, hands should be washed thoroughly before cooking to guard against staph infection getting into food.

It may take up to a week for the boil to break on its own. To further reduce the chance of infection, patients should shower (not bathe). If the boil is large and painful, a physician may prescribe an antibiotic or open the boil with a sterile needle to drain the pus. Occasionally, large boils must be lanced with a surgical knife; this is usually done using a local anesthetic.

Risk Factors and Preventive Measures
For patients prone to boils, some experts recommend washing the skin with an antiseptic soap to prevent infections.

borate   An abrasive sometimes used to remove superficial ACNE lesions, although it probably is not effective since acne is deeply rooted in the follicles, according to the U.S. Food and Drug Administration. The PDA ruled it had not received enough clinical evidence to support the effectiveness of BORIC ACID and sodium borate as acne treatments.

borax   A white odorless mineral that is a mild cleanser and antiseptic. It is most often used as an emulsifier in COLD CREAM, but it also is included in mouthwashes, vanishing creams, bath salts, eye lotions, cleansing lotions, and scalp lotions. It has not been found to cause allergic reactions.

boric acid An antiseptic, bactericide, and fungicide prepared from sulfuric acid and natural BORAX that should not be ingested or inhaled, and should not be used on babies. Boric acid had been used in talcum powders in the past, and was once used as a dressing for WOUNDS and BURNS. However, after a number of people died following excessive absorption of boric acid in extensive wounds, borax fell out of favor as a salve for burns. Borax is no longer included in the manufacture of baby products.

Botox (botulinum A toxin) A purified form of the toxin that causes botulism, now used to reduce facial lines in people 18 to 65. Botox is the brand name for a purified form of the deadly toxin botulinum Type A, which is produced by a bacterium called *Clostridium botulinum*—the same one that causes botulism. The product called Botox contains only tiny quantities of the isolated toxin, with no intact bacteria. This means there is no chance of getting botulism from the injections.

When carefully injected in very low doses, botulinum toxin is a modern tool that can reduce the signs of aging. When a person frowns, the tissue between the eyebrows is gathered into a fold. Eventually, over many years, this muscle motion causes a chronic furrow. Tiny injections of Botox can paralyze certain facial muscles beneath the skin, wiping away forehead creases and wrinkles. Injecting botulinum toxin into the skin is a quick and easy almost painless office procedure that takes less than 30 minutes.

Procedure

Injecting Botox is a very different way of removing wrinkles than has been used in the past. Unlike COLLAGEN or fat injections that work by filling in the furrows of a person's face, Botox weakens the muscles above the brow and removes wrinkles naturally. While it is most effective for the frown

lines between the eyebrows, it also can be used to lessen the horizontal wrinkles in the middle of the forehead. When Botox is administered by a trained medical professional directly into an overactive muscle, it interferes with the release of a neurotransmitter that causes muscles to contract. This paralyzes the underlying muscles so the skin is not pulled down. As the relaxed muscles release the skin, the wrinkles slowly disappear. After several weeks, the muscles beneath the skin shrink and start to waste away. Botulinum toxin has revolutionized the treatment of aging skin, especially frown lines. Since botulinum toxin decreases the patient's ability to frown or squint, it also safely and effectively prevents the progressive worsening of these lines over time.

Botox was first used (and has been approved by the U.S. Food and Drug Administration [FDA]) to treat lazy eye (strabismus) and uncontrolled eye blinking and neck spasm. It was approved in 2002 by the FDA for cosmetic use.

Botox is the first botulinum toxin approved for marketing in the United States. Because of its safety, low cost, and simplicity of use, it is one of the fastest-growing new procedures for treating wrinkles. Myobloc (botulinum exotoxin B) was recently approved for eye and neck spasm and is now being used to treat facial frown lines.

Botulinum toxin has also been successfully used before and after skin resurfacing procedures, including lasers, chemical peels, and DERMABRASION, to maintain good results. When injected prior to the procedure, botulinum toxin allows smooth healing of resurfacing by preventing movement. Injected after resurfacing, botulinum toxin prevents the reappearance of movement-induced wrinkles.

Botulinum toxin has also been approved to treat individuals who suffer from HYPERHIDROSIS (excessive sweating) not managed by topical products. Botulinum toxin can be used to decrease sweating on the palms or soles, underarms, or forehead by injecting the toxin into the affected areas. Once injected, botulinum toxin paralyzes the sweat glands of the skin that are responsible for excessive perspiration.

A single treatment of botulinum toxin injected directly into the affected skin can provide up to six months of relief to patients who have tried antiperspirants, oral medications, and even surgical approaches to control severe sweating. These procedures can be performed in an office environment without anesthesia and can be repeated once or twice a year to maintain dryness.

Risks and Complications

In small doses, there is no scarring and no side effects. However, if Botox migrates from the injection site it can cause a droop of the eyebrow or upper eyelid for a week or two. For this reason, patients should not massage the injection site for 12 hours after treatment. Allergy to Botox is very rare, and no serious side effects have been reported in thousands of patients in 10 years.

botulinum A toxin   See BOTOX.

bouba   See YAWS.

Bowen's disease   A precancerous condition also known as SQUAMOUS CELL CANCER in situ, causing a scaling, reddish-pink slightly raised growth usually on the face or hands. The disease is more often found among men with fair skin; chronic sunlight exposure is the primary cause. Chronic ingestion of inorganic arsenicals also causes Bowen's disease, although this is rare today. About one-third of these patients have multiple lesions.

Symptoms and Diagnostic Path

Squamous cell cancers that occur as a result of Bowen's disease are usually more aggressive than those from ACTINIC KERATOSES. It is not uncommon for the cancer developing from Bowen's disease to spread to the lymph nodes. In addition, some studies suggest that patients with Bowen's disease may develop other premalignant and malignant tumors, such as actinic keratoses, BASAL CELL CARCINOMAS, and adnexal carcinomas.

Bowen's disease lesions on mucosal surfaces have a different appearance and biologic potential; when they occur on the penis they are called erythroplasia of Queyrat (usually in uncircumcised males); they occur less frequently on the vulva. These lesions are bright red with a velvety, glistening surface. While microscopically identical to Bowen's disease, these lesions have a higher rate of malignant transformation and the resulting squamous cell carcinomas are more aggressive than those arising from ordinary Bowen's disease.

Treatment Options and Outlook

The condition is treated by surgically removing the diseased patch of skin. Once removed, these skin conditions do not return. The most accurate and tissue-sparing form of excision is Mohs' surgery, rather than the vertical sections of standard surgical excision.

breast enlargement   See MAMMOPLASTY.

breast lift   See MAMMOPLASTY.

breast reduction   See MAMMOPLASTY.

bromhidrosis   A condition caused by sweat that has become foul-smelling because of bacterial decomposition.

See also SWEAT GLANDS.

bromoderma   A pustular skin eruption due to ingestion of bromides. Bromides, once prescribed as a sedative, are no longer administered because of their unpleasant side effects—including ACNE. The acne fades once bromides are discontinued.

brown recluse spider bites   The bite of these spiders of the *Loxosceles* family cause severe skin tissue death and extensive sloughing of the skin at the site of the bite, which also may be accompanied by generalized symptoms.

The United States species of this deadly spider, *L. reclusa* (or the Missouri brown spider), lives in about half of the states, although it is most often found in the central and south-central area of the country. Ounce for ounce, the venom of this spider is more deadly than that of many poisonous snakes. The venom of the female is more deadly than that of the male.

It is believed that the spider was mistakenly imported to this country in fruit crates and vegetables within the last 50 years; since then it has been making its way steadily north and west. The secretive spiders get their name from their fondness for dark, secret storage spaces, under boxes and in closets. While these spiders are not aggressive and will try to escape when cornered, if trapped they will bite. Its brown to fawn-colored body is about a ½ inch long, with a dark brown violin-shaped marking.

Symptoms and Diagnostic Path

Reaction to the brown recluse bite varies considerably from one person to the next, depending on the amount of venom injected, the patient's age, and health. The bite can cause a skin injury ranging from a small papule to a huge necrotic ulcer, together with a systemic reaction. Severe systemic reactions and death occur most often in children, but even this is rare.

The bite of this spider causes little pain at first, but within eight hours the pain becomes severe, and the area of the bite will get red. The local skin reaction may be minor, with mild ITCHING and a plaque or a small area of dead tissue that heals by itself within five days.

However, brown recluse spider venom contains a substance that is very destructive to tissue; in more severe cases, a blue-gray halo appears at the bite site, followed within 18 hours by a small blister and surrounding area of redness and swelling. Eventually, the blister ruptures, and within a week the skin cells in the area begin to die, creating a thick black scar on the base that slowly separates over several weeks. In a small number of patients; the ulcer does not heal for months.

The bite can also cause systemic reactions including fever, chills, weakness, nausea and vomiting, joint pain, and a generalized rash. In fatal bites, the patient usually dies within the first 48 hours as a result of kidney failure.

Treatment Options and Outlook

If a brown recluse bite is suspected, a physician should be consulted at once. There is no specific antivenin, although antivenin for other species of brown spiders of South America could give protection. Small bites may require only cold compresses, elevation, painkillers, and a tetanus shot.

DAPSONE may prevent tissue death, and although CORTICOSTEROIDS are sometimes used for larger lesions, their usefulness has not been proven. Antibiotics may prevent infection. In addition, antihistamines and muscle relaxants may provide some relief.

Exchange transfusions in which nearly all the patient's blood is replaced by a donor's blood may be attempted.

Immediate excision of the bite area may be the only way to prevent the massive necrosis caused by this spider, although not all experts agree on this treatment. Most physicians will not touch the lesion until all the destruction has occurred, which may not happen until 40 weeks after the bite.

Skin grafts may be necessary to heal the ulcer.

bruise A deep blue or black discoloration on the skin following trauma, caused by bleeding under the skin. Initially the bruise looks blue or black; as the hemoglobin begins to break down, the bruise turns yellow. While most bruises occur after a bump, they may also follow a period of heavy exercise; exercise sometimes causes tiny tears in blood vessels below the skin, allowing blood to seep out.

Easy bruising also may be a sign of disease, especially blood disorders such as anemia. In addition, some drugs (such as aspirin and other blood thinners) may lead to increased bruising; other drugs, such as anti-inflammatory agents, antidepressants, or asthma drugs may interfere with blood clotting under the skin. AIDS can cause purplish bumps that *seem* to be bruises that do not fade. Substance abusers also may find they have an increased susceptibility to bruising.

Some studies suggest that patients who lack vitamin C in their diets tend to bruise more easily and their wounds heal more slowly. This may be due to the fact that VITAMIN C helps build supportive COLLAGEN around blood vessels in the skin, which helps protect the vessels from rupture. For those who bruise easily, some experts suggest 500 mg of vitamin C three times a day to help build collagen (although vitamin C is not toxic, patients taking high doses of vitamin C should consult with their physician).

Treatment Options and Outlook

The discoloration of a bruise can be minimized by immediately applying cold, to keep down the swelling and constrict blood vessels, which helps to decrease the internal bleeding. An ice pack should be applied at 15-minute intervals immediately after the bump for the first 24 to 48 hours. Patients without access to ice can use a clean cold soda can, applying it for five to 10 minutes every 15 minutes. After 24 hours, heat should be used to dilate the blood vessels and improve circulation.

Risk Factors and Preventive Measures

Because vitamin C helps build up supportive tissue around blood vessels, those who bruise easily may find that 500 mg of vitamin C taken three times a day to build collagen may be effective. Although vitamin C is not considered to be toxic, experts advise patients to get their physician's approval before using high doses of vitamin C.

bubble bath Detergent cleansers containing ingredients capable of making bathwater foam can be irritating to mucous membranes and the skin if used in too great a concentration, especially in people with dry skin or ECZEMA, because these detergents tend to dry out the skin. Consumers should swirl the bubble bath throughout the water, and use a moisturizer after the bath. The drying or irritating effect of bubble bath can be prevented by adding bath oil (such as Nivea oil or Lubriderm oil) to the bath water.

bubo A swollen and inflamed lymph node (particularly in the axilla or groin) due to BUBONIC PLAGUE, tuberculosis, or SYPHILIS.

bubonic plague The most common form of PLAGUE, also known as "The Black Death" or black plague, because of the black spots it produced on the skin. It is also characterized by the appearance of a swollen lymph node (BUBO) in the groin or armpit early in the illness.

Bubonic plague is primarily transmitted from rodents to humans by flea bites. Fleas become infected by feeding on rodents, such as the chipmunks, prairie dogs, ground squirrels, mice, and other mammals that are infected with the bacteria *Yersinia pestis*. Fleas transmit the plague bacteria to humans and other mammals during the feeding process. The plague bacteria are maintained in the blood systems of rodents. After the bite, the bacteria spread through the body to the lymph nodes, which became painful and enlarged. In the past, the death rate was 90 percent. In the worst case, the lungs became infected and the pneumonic form was spread from person to person by coughing, sneezing, or simply talking. Typically, the time of infection to death was less than one week. The three major epidemics of the black plague in the sixth, 14th, and 17th centuries killed more than 137 million people.

Symptoms and Diagnostic Path

Bubonic plague is characterized by enlarged, tender lymph nodes, fever, chills, and prostration. It is fatal between 50 and 90 percent of the time if untreated; it is fatal 15 percent of the time when properly diagnosed and treated.

A few cases of bubonic plague still occur throughout the United States.

In the United States, the last urban plague epidemic occurred in Los Angeles in 1924–25. Since then, human plague in the United States has occurred as mostly scattered cases in rural areas (an average of 10 to 15 persons each year). In North America, plague is found in certain animals and their fleas from the Pacific Coast to the Great Plains, and from southwestern Canada to Mexico. Most human cases in the United States occur in two regions—northern New Mexico, northern Arizona, and southern Colorado; and California, southern Oregon, and far western Nevada.

In the United States, people at risk are those exposed to rodent fleas, wild rodents, or other susceptible animals in western states. The highest rates occur among Native Americans (especially Navajo); other high-risk groups include hunters; veterinarians, and pet owners handling infected cats; or campers or hikers entering areas with outbreaks of animal plague.

Plague also exists in Africa, Asia, and South America. Globally, the World Health Organization reports 1,000 to 3,000 cases of plague every year.

Treatment Options and Outlook

Today, modern antibiotics are effective against plague, but if an infected person is not treated promptly, the disease is likely to cause severe illness or death.

bulla   A large fluid-filled BLISTER, usually two centimeter or more in diameter.

burns   Burn injuries have become much more common in recent years, and are now considered a health care problem more serious than was the polio epidemic at its peak. In the past several years the medical profession has revolutionized understanding of problems associated with burns.

In the 1950s there were fewer than 10 hospitals in the United States that specialized in burns. Since that time, there has been significant advancement in understanding the problem of burn injuries, and there are now about 200 special burn care centers in the United States.

Every year, about 2.4 million Americans are burned or scalded badly enough to require medical care; about 75,000 are hospitalized. This type of injury is most common among children and the elderly and are usually due to preventable accidents in the home. Because the skin is a living tissue, temperatures that even briefly reach 120° F will destroy its cells.

Burns can be caused by contact with hot substances, flames, chemicals, radiation (in sunlight, X-rays, or ionizing radiation). While most accidental burns are visible almost immediately after the accident, burns from SUNBURN may appear several hours to a day later. It may be 10 to 30 days before the full effects of ionizing X-ray irradiation burns appear.

Severity of Burns

The severity of a burn depends on two factors: how deep the tissue destruction has penetrated, and the amount of body surface that has been affected. Burn recovery is also influenced by the age and general health of the victim, the location of the burn and any other associated injuries.

Traditionally, physicians have characterized burns as first-, second-, or third-degree, depending on the depth of skin damage. By accurately estimating the extent of damage, the physician can best determine the appropriate treatment.

First-degree burns   This type of minor burn affects only the EPIDERMIS (top layer of skin), causing reddening but no blisters or swelling. Typically, pain ebbs within 48 to 72 hours, and the burn heals quickly without scars, although the damaged skin may peel off in a day or two. A sunburn is an example of a first-degree burn.

Second-degree burns   This type of burn destroys the skin on a deeper level, creating redness and blisters; the deeper the burn, the more blisters, which increase in size within a few hours after the injury. However, some of the DERMIS (deep layer of the skin) remains, so that this type of burn can usually heal without scarring as long as there has been no accompanying infection. Second-degree burns may be extremely painful. How well a second-degree burn heals depends on the amount of skin that has been damaged.

Degree of Burn

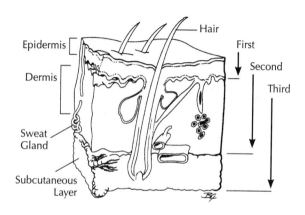

However, in very deep second-degree burns, the healed skin may resemble scars from a third-degree burn. These deeper burns take longer to heal—often up to a month or more—and the healing top skin layer is extremely fragile. In fact, some of the worst burn scars are caused by these very serious second-degree burns.

Third-degree burns This is the most serious type of burn, which destroys all the layers of the skin. If the burn is very deep, muscles and bones may also be exposed. The affected area will look white or charred, and even if the burned area is only small, it will require special treatment and skin grafts to help prevent serious scarring.

In this type of burn, there is no pain because the pain receptors have been destroyed along with the rest of the dermis and blood vessels, sweat glands, sebaceous glands, and hair follicles. Fluid loss and metabolic problems in these injuries are profound.

These burns always heal with scarring. Extensive third-degree burns require aggressive treatment in a hospital burn unit, and the death rate is significant.

Fourth-degree burns Occasionally, burns even deeper than a full thickness of the skin occur, such as when a part of the body is trapped in flame, or in an electrical burn. These deep burns enter the muscle and bone and are also called "black" or "char" burns (because of the typical color of the burn). If a fourth-degree burn involves more than a very small area of the body, the prognosis is very grave, since these deep burns can release toxic materials into the bloodstream. If the burn involves a small area, it should be cut away down to healthy tissue; a charred large area on an extremity usually requires amputation.

Electrical burns Electrical accidents can cause several different types of burns, including flame burns caused by ignited clothing, electrical current injury, or electrothermal burns from arcing current. Sometimes all three types of burns will be found in one victim.

Flame burns from ignited clothing may be the most serious part of the wound. An electric current injury is characterized by focal burns at the point where the current entered and left through the skin. Once an electric current enters the body, its path within the body is determined by tissues with

the least resistance. Bone offers the most resistance to electrical current, followed in descending order by fat, tendon, skin, muscle, blood, and nerve. The path the current takes determines whether the victim will survive, since current passing through the heart or the brainstem will result in almost instantaneous death from a disturbed heart rhythm. As current passes through muscle, it can set off severe spasms that can fracture or dislocate a bone. Although bone does not conduct the current well, it stores the heat from the electricity and can damage surrounding muscles.

Electrothermal (flash or arc) burns are heat injuries to the skin that occur when high-tension electrical current touches the skin, causing intense, deep damage. Damage is severe because the arc carries temperature of about 2,500° C—hot enough to melt bone.

Skin at both the entry and exit of the current is usually gray, yellow, and depressed; there may be some charring. All of these wounds must be debrided.

Extent of Burn

When a health care worker estimates a burned patient's injuries in a percentage ("a burn over 60 percent of the body," for example) the percentage is not simply a guess. Health care workers use a "rule of nines" to estimate the amount of body area affected by a burn. The percentage figure is computed by dividing the body into sections: 9 percent to the head and neck, 9 percent to each arm, 18 percent to each foot and leg, and 18 percent each to the front and back of the trunk. The remaining 1 percent makes up the perineum (the region of the body between the anus and the urethral opening). This rule is more accurate for adults, but less reliable in children, whose body proportions are different.

Effects of Burns

Because a burn destroys a large area of skin, it also disrupts fluid balance, metabolism, temperature, and immune response. Fluid is lost in part by oozing from BLISTERS (called a "weeping burn") and also from dilation of blood vessels that leak fluid into the area beneath the burned skin 36 to 48 hours after the injury. After this period, the fluid is slowly reabsorbed by the body. This fluid and salt loss can be significant, depending on the percentage of the burn.

While there is not much weeping from second- and third-degree burns, the underlying fluid loss is extensive; there may even be fluid loss from remote capillaries in unburned tissue (such as the lungs). If fluid loss is not reversed within an hour after the burn, the fluid loss begins to interfere with organ function and shock sets in. Once the fluid loss reaches a critical level, the circulatory shock becomes irreversible and nothing can be done to save the patient's life.

Burn patients also experience an increase in the metabolic and oxygen use rates. This metabolic increase is at first fueled by glycogen stored in the liver and muscles, but when these stores are depleted the body begins to break down its own protein structures. This metabolic response reaches a maximum level in burns of more than 40 percent.

Most burn patients die from infections of the skin, bloodstream, and lungs, in part due to a weakened immune system.

Treatment Options and Outlook

It is only since World War II that treatment of burns has made much progress. In fact, since ancient times physicians knew very little about proper burn management technique. EMOLLIENTS with unusual ingredients were often placed on the burn, and bleeding was a popular treatment for burns throughout the Middle Ages. Until the mid-1940s, the best treatment that could be offered was to wash the burn with soap and water, leaving it exposed to the air.

Generally, first-degree burns can be treated with proper first aid. Second-degree burns covering more than 15 percent of an adult's body, or 10 percent of a child's body, or burns of the face, hands or feet require prompt medical attention. All people with third-degree burns should get immediate medical help.

First/second-degree burn treatment First burns should be flushed with plenty of cold water for 15 to 30 minutes; if the burn was caused by hot grease or acid, the saturated clothing should be removed.

The grease should then be washed off the skin, and the burn should be soaked in cold water. If clothing sticks to the skin, it should not be pulled off. Instead, the victim should go to the emergency room.

If a first- or second-degree burn is smaller than a quarter on a child, or smaller than a silver dollar on an adult, the burn can be treated at home. Any burn on an infant, a person over 60, or a large burn, should be treated by a professional.

Butter should never be placed on a burn, since the fat can hold in heat and worsen the injury, possibly causing infection.

After rinsing with cold water, the burn should be wrapped in clean dry gauze and left alone for 24 hours. Antiseptics or other irritating substances should not be applied. A good way to remember how to treat a first-degree burn is not to put any substance on the burn that the patient would not put in an eye.

Third-degree burn treatment A third-degree burn should be seen by a doctor as soon as possible and treated in a specialized burn unit. These wounds should not be plunged into water, since cool water may worsen the shock that often accompanies a severe burn. Instead, the injury should be covered with a bulky sterile dressing or with freshly laundered bed linens. Clothing stuck to the wound should not be removed, and no ointments, salves, or sprays should be applied. The burned feet and legs should be elevated; burned hands should be raised above the level of the heart. Breathing should be closely monitored.

The doctor will either lightly dress these burns with an antibacterial dressing, or leave them exposed to enhance healing. Every effort is made to keep the skin germ free by reverse isolation nursing. If necessary, painkillers and antibiotics are prescribed, and intravenous fluids are given to offset fluid loss.

Extensive second-degree and all third-degree burns are treated with skin grafts or artificial skin to minimize scars. Extensive burns may need repeated plastic surgery.

Despite the widespread use of antibacterial agents, infection remains one of the most serious complications of burn wounds. Acute gastrointestinal ulcers often complicate recovery. Children are also prone to developing post-burn seizures, probably from electrolyte imbalances, low oxygen blood levels, infection, or drugs. Youngsters are also prone to high blood pressure after a burn injury, probably related to the release of certain stress hormones after the burn.

Common complications of burn grafts are the formation of fibrous masses of scar tissue called HYPERTROPHIC SCARS and KELOIDS, especially in dark-skinned individuals. Direct pressure on inflamed tissue reduces its blood supply and collagen content, which can head off the development of these scars. This pressure can be provided by wearing a variety of special burn splints, sleeves, stockings, and body jackets. Special cases may require body traction.

Scars are most common after effects of a serious burn and may require years of additional plastic surgery after skin grafting to release the contractures over joints. Unfortunately, despite modern cosmetic surgical techniques, burn scars are almost always unsightly and the results are almost never as good as the patient's preburn condition.

Burn scars should be carefully treated, even after they have completely healed. They should not be exposed to sunlight, and those areas of the skin exposed to the sun should be covered by SUNSCREEN. Since deep burns destroy oil and sweat glands, the patient may need to apply emollients and lotions to prevent drying and cracking.

Recovery from serious burns may take many years. Patients may require extensive psychological counseling in order to adjust to disfigurement and physical therapy to regain or maintain mobility in damaged joints. See also CHEMICAL BURNS.

Nevertheless, despite the best and most intensive treatment, between 8,000 and 12,000 patients with burns die, and approximately 1 million sustain substantial or permanent disabilities resulting from their burn injury each year.

Risk Factors and Preventive Measures
Burn accident statistics show that at least half of all burn accidents can be prevented. For example, one of every 13 structure fire deaths in the United States is caused by a child setting a fire. Children playing with fire account for more than one-third of preschool child deaths by fire.

Burow's solution One of the most common ASTRINGENTS used with wet dressings. This clear, colorless substance is also known as aluminum acetate.

burrow An excavation by parasites in the STRATUM CORNEUM (topmost layer of epidermis) of differing sizes and shapes.
See also SCABIES.

Buschke-Lowenstein tumor See WARTS.

Buschke-Ollendorff syndrome A genetic disorder, also known as osteopoikilosis with connective tissue moles, that is passed on to 50 percent of all offspring of an affected parent. It is characterized by multiple raised yellow-orange skin PAPULES, with a marked increase of connective tissue within these lesions. The condition usually appears in the 20s or 30s, with nodules or plaques on the thighs, buttocks, or abdominal wall. No treatment is required.
See also CONNECTIVE TISSUE NEVI.

butyl stearate One of the most common stearic acids used in cosmetics such as nail polish removers, lipsticks, and cleansing creams. Butyl stearate may cause an allergic reaction in sensitive consumers.

café-au-lait macule Pale, coffee-colored oval patches that may develop up to three inches across, anywhere on the skin. While a single such spot has no significance, the presence of six or more spots larger than 1.5 cm may be a sign of NEUROFIBROMATOSIS, a hereditary disease of the nerve fiber sheaths.

The hyperpigmentation is due to increased MELANIN in the skin. These spots are not related to ultraviolet radiation exposure, and may be present at birth or acquired later in life.

Treatment Options and Outlook
Laser therapy may fade these patches.

calamine A pink compound of ferric oxide and zinc oxide that is applied (as a lotion, ointment, or dusting powder) to the skin. Calamine cools, dries, and protects skin that is irritated or itchy because of DERMATITIS, ECZEMA, POISON IVY, INSECT BITES, or SUNBURN. It also may be combined with a topical local anesthetic such as benzocaine, or with CORTICOSTEROIDS or ANTIHISTAMINES, which reduce inflammation.

calcinosis cutis A condition in which abnormal amounts of calcium are deposited as nodules in the skin and connective tissue. Calcinosis is often associated with disorders of the connective tissue, such as DERMATOMYOSITIS or SCLERODERMA.

callus An area of thickening of the stratum corneum caused by regular or prolonged pressure or friction, or if body weight is carried unevenly. It is the body's protective response to repeat friction.

Symptoms and Diagnostic Path
Found most often on the feet, a callus may occur anywhere on the body that experiences constant friction.

A small focal callus with a hard core is called a CORN. Corns are often surrounded by callus. Initial thickening of the skin is a protective response, and the resulting callus is not painful unless very thick or fissured.

Some amount of callusing may be beneficial, especially for those who go barefoot a great deal or who perform a repetitive activity such as shoveling, gymnastics, or weight-lifting. Calluses protect the skin from heat, rough surfaces, and cuts.

Treatment Options and Outlook
Often, it is best to leave a callus alone because of its protective capability. A painful or troublesome callus on the foot may be treated by a dermatologist or podiatrist, who can pare away the thickened skin in layers with a scalpel. But calluses caused by foot deformities almost always recur unless the underlying problem is corrected either surgically or by using a molded shoe insole.

For patients with a lot of callused tissue, some experts suggest soaking the feet in diluted chamomile tea, which will soothe and soften hardened skin. Those with bad calluses should treat the area daily after a warm bath by abrading lightly with a callus file or pumice stone, followed by a moisturizing cream. This treatment should not be used on hard corns.

Patients with diabetes or those with reduced sensation in their feet should never treat themselves.

camouflage cosmetics Special types of cosmetics used for those with scars or discolored patches on the skin. The key cosmetic for camouflage is an opaque, heavyweight foundation (usually a cream) that is thicker than regular foundation and may be applied under regular foundation. Spread over an area with skin problem, it can make many disfiguring marks (including BIRTHMARKS, SCARS, and even discoloration left by SUNBURN) less noticeable. Both men and women can use these products that come in cream, powder, and stick formulas. Today, the use of opaque ingredients such as titanium dioxide allow consumers to use lighter, more "breathable" coverup products.

The key to using any corrective makeup is to blend the edges into surrounding skin; the best results come from using products that are precisely matched to skin color. However, for some people a slightly darker shade will hide a defect more completely. Opaque foundations (also called concealing creams) are available in shades from pale ivory to dark chocolate, and may be found at cosmetic counters in large department stores.

A coverup product used only on one small area, such as a birthmark, should be applied under foundation; once a translucent foundation is applied over it, it will seem as if the skin—not the makeup—is what is showing through.

Foundation cream is applied by first warming it in the hand and then applying with a finger or makeup sponge, using a pat/dab motion, beginning in the center of the area to be covered and blending outward. Rubbing causes an uneven application. After five minutes, a special translucent setting powder should be applied; after another five minutes, any excess should be brushed away.

When covering recent scars, always discuss the product safety with a dermatologist or surgeon first. Most people can begin applying makeup to cover bruising or disguise swelling as early as a day or two after surgery. To hide incision lines, a patient will need to wait until the stitches have been removed and the incision is completely closed. After a chemical peel or DERMABRASION, any crust must be completely gone before makeup can be used.

There are three basic approaches to camouflage cosmetics after surgery: concealing (hiding incision lines and bruises), color correcting (neutralizing color in reddened or yellowish skin), and contouring (disguising swelling and creating the illusion of highlights and shadows).

Camouflage cosmetics tend to be thicker and more adherent than everyday makeup, so it is important to remove them every night. A cleansing cream should be used to remove all makeup. Then a gentle, alcohol-free toner should be applied with a cotton ball to remove any cleanser residue. This is followed with a moisturizer formulated for skin type: oily, dry, or combination.

For women interested in concealing dark shadows under the eye, the key is to use as little coverup as possible. The best idea is to apply concealer under the dark circles, which are often caused by shadows cast by excess skin or fat below the eyes. Small dots of concealer is blended upward into the darker area with light strokes of the fingertips. White under-eye concealer should be avoided because it looks too unnatural.

It is also possible to change the color of the skin with these products. A delicate pale green base will neutralize a reddish complexion. To improve a yellowing complexion, a peach or lavender base should be used. A flesh-colored concealing cream or regular makeup base can then be applied over this.

If applied thickly enough, the opaque cream can also be an effective SUNBLOCK; a better choice is a cream that specifically includes a SUNSCREEN.

camphor A volatile fragrant compound derived from an Asian evergreen tree that is used as an antiseptic in some skin care products because it feels soothing to the skin. It also may help stop ITCHING and is a rubefacient (it reddens the skin).

Camphor is absorbed almost immediately in the skin, causing a feeling of warmth and then numbness. Camphor will not affect the outcome of an ACNE breakout, but it is helpful for chapped skin and as a counter-irritant in liniment rubs, where it warms and soothes sore muscles.

If inhaled for a long time, camphor can induce a severe headache.

cancer, skin See SKIN CANCER.

Candida albicans The yeast that causes the infection called candidiasis, often within the vagina or on other areas of mucous membrane (such as the inside of the mouth). The infection is also known as thrush or moniliasis.

See also CANDIDA INFECTION.

candida infection A type of YEAST INFECTION caused by *Candida albicans*. The infection is also known as "thrush," moniliasis, or candidiasis. Candida produces skin disease by invading the keratinized EPIDERMIS—rarely, in some forms of chronic infection of the skin and mucous membranes, the infection may invade the dermis and subcutaneous tissue.

The yeast that causes candidiasis naturally grows in both the vagina and the mouth, where it is usually kept under control by bacteria present in the body. However, the yeast may grow if the bacteria are destroyed, for example, as during antibiotic therapy, if the body's natural resistance to disease is affected (as in AIDS), or if a person is taking drugs that suppress the immune system. The fungus also may flourish in the presence of some disorders (diabetes mellitus), during hormonal changes of pregnancy, or while taking birth control pills.

Candidal infection of the penis, which occurs more often among uncircumcised males, may be transmitted from an infected partner. Similarly, it can also spread from the genitals or mouth to other moist areas of the body (such as the skin folds in the groin or under the breasts). It may crop up with diaper rash in infants.

Symptoms and Diagnostic Path

Infection of the skin of the mouth causes sore, white-colored raised patches which are usually asymptomatic. In skin folds or with diaper rash, it forms an itchy red rash with flaky white patches. There may be burning or stinging and itching in skin folds or other affected areas. The skin looks beefy red or scalded with an irregular margin; a chronic scaly form may occasionally occur.

Treatment Options and Outlook

Antifungal drugs (such as clotrimazole, miconazole, nystatin, or econazole nitrate) will usually clear up the infection, but it may recur. Those with a tendency toward this type of infection should keep the skin dry. However, primary irritation or allergy rarely may occur due to topical medications and worsen the skin condition. Compresses with BUROW'S SOLUTION, plenty of air, and infrared heat lamps to dry the affected parts may help.

Risk Factors and Preventive Measures

Yogurt (18 oz. daily serving), which contains lactobacillus acidophilus, reduces the colonization of the vagina and mouth and is effective in preventing recurrent yeast infections.

See also *CANDIDA* PARONYCHIA.

candida paronychia A yeast infection in the nail fold that is relatively common, usually among people with jobs requiring prolonged immersion of hands in water. Microorganisms, both *Candida* species and bacteria, invade the area under the nail fold. It usually affects the fingernails, and far less often affects the toenails.

Symptoms and Diagnostic Path

This infection is characterized by redness, swelling, inflammation, and sometimes PUS. The cuticle is lost and the nail plate surface develops irregular ridges and deformity. There may be some lifting of the nail (ONYCHOLYSIS), which can worsen the condition.

Swabs or scrapings of the nail fold for microscopic examination and culture may be helpful if the diagnosis is uncertain.

Treatment Options and Outlook

A topical imidazole (either as a cream or paint) is usually effective. It may require three to six months of treatment, until a new cuticle has formed. Combined topical preparations of an antifungal with a CORTICOSTEROID may be considered for infection with uncomfortable and severe inflammation, or if the patient also has ECZEMA. Systemic treatment is needed only rarely, if the patient does not respond to topical treatment. Severe, chronic candida paronychia may occur in people with a suppressed immune system; systemic treatment is usually necessary in this case. Antiseptics may be necessary to treat associated bacterial infection of the nail fold.

candidiasis See CANDIDA INFECTION.

canker sore A small painful ulcer on the inside of the mouth, lip, or underneath the tongue that heals without treatment. Canker sores are *not* the same type of skin lesion as HERPES simplex (also known as "cold sores" or "fever blisters").

The difference between canker sores and COLD SORES is their appearance and location. Cold sores often involve the skin of the lips, and cankers do not; cold sores often strike the gums, and cankers rarely do; cold sores are often accompanied by tender lymph glands in the neck.

Unlike cold sores, canker sores are not caused by a virus but are probably the result of bacteria or a temporarily malfunctioning immune system. Because hemolytic streptococcus bacteria have so often been isolated from canker sores, experts believe they may be caused by a hypersensitive reaction to the bacteria.

Other factors often associated with a flareup include trauma (such as biting the inside of the cheek), acute stress and allergies, or chemical irritants in toothpaste or mouthwash. More women than men experience canker sores, which are more likely to occur during the premenstrual period and are also more likely to occur if other members of the family suffer from them.

About 20 percent of Americans at any one time experience a canker sore, commonly between ages 10 and 40. They are particularly common in children who wear braces. The most severely affected people have almost continuous sores, while others have just one or two per year.

Symptoms and Diagnostic Path

A canker sore is usually a small oval ulcer with a grayish white center surrounded by a red, inflamed halo, which usually lasts for one or two weeks. A canker sore should heal within two weeks. If the sufferer cannot eat, speak, or sleep, or if the sore does not heal not within two weeks, medical help should be sought.

Treatment Options and Outlook

While the ulcers will heal themselves, topical painkillers ease the pain; healing can be hastened by using a CORTICOSTEROID OINTMENT or a tetracycline mouthwash.

Over-the-counter medications containing carbamide peroxide (Cankaid, Glyoxide, and Amosan) also may be effective in treating the sore, but none are effective in preventing them. Other treatments include liquid or gel forms of benzocaine, menthol, camphor, eucalyptol and or alcohol, or pastes (such as Orabase, or Zilactin, a mix of tannic acid and alcohol in a gel) that form a protective "bandage" over the sore. For short-term pain relief, a prescription mouthwash containing 2 percent viscous lidocaine can help. In severe cases, rinsing with topical corticosteroids after meals may be necessary.

Risk Factors and Preventive Measures

No treatments have been demonstrated to reliably prevent canker sores. Patients who are prone to canker sores should avoid coffee, spices, citrus fruits, tomatoes, walnuts, strawberries, chocolates, commercial toothpastes, and mouthwashes. Instead, patients should brush teeth with baking soda for a month or two, and rinse with warm salt water.

capsaicin The active ingredient in hot peppers that produces an irritating effect when used on the skin; it has been found to ease the incessant itch of PSORIASIS and the pain of herpetic neuralgia. Capsaicin is believed to interfere with the substance P, the chemical in the body that transmits both the pain and the "itch" impulses to the brain. When a patient applies capsaicin to the skin, the local nerves release a large amount of substance P, thus depleting the supply. The itch or pain subsides because the body takes some time to build up the stores of the chemical again.

While capsaicin does not cure the underlying condition, it can decrease the pain or itch.

The cream may burn or tingle when first applied to the skin, but this sensation should lessen over time.

See also ZOSTRIX.

carbenicillin (Trade names: Geopen, Pyopen) A synthetic penicillin, available by mouth or by intravenous injection, that is effective against a wide range of bacterial skin infections.

carbolic acid A caustic acid formerly used in CHEMICAL FACE PEEL. Carbolic acid is too caustic for this purpose and is therefore no longer used in skin care.

carbolic soap A disinfectant soap with about 10 percent phenol used to treat oily skin.

carbon dioxide (CO_2) laser A versatile laser that can be operated in either focused or defocused mode. When defocused, the target area is larger and the beam surface vaporizes the surface of the target and destroys cells instantly. The heating and destruction occur so quickly, in fact, that there is little heat conducted to adjacent cells, and the zone of injury is small and can be carefully controlled.

In the focused mode, the beam diameter narrows to just 0.1 mm; this intense beam is capable of cutting tissue, the depth and precision of which depends on the speed with which the laser beam is moved along the tissue. Because it produces heat, the laser actually sterilizes the cut as it goes, and seals blood vessels so that the surgical field is bloodless unless a large blood vessel is cut. Because the heat is concentrated on a small area, there is little tissue damage, so the tissue can be preserved, and examined later.

The CO_2 laser can be used to treat a variety of benign or malignant skin conditions. However, while warts also can be destroyed with this technique, the resulting plume of smoke may contain infectious wart particles.

Risks and Complications

There are some risks associated in the CO_2 laser treatment. Because the CO_2 beam is invisible, the potential for damage to eye is great; usually, a small red helium-neon laser is used with the CO_2 beam, so that its red light marks the area being struck by the CO_2 beam. Still, everyone in the room must wear special protective eye goggles.

Because the beam generates heat, there is also a risk of fire (especially on surgical dressings). Wet dressings placed over normal neighboring skin will reduce the chance of fire and of inadvertent damage to surrounding tissue.

carbuncle A cluster of BOILS (PUS-filled inflamed hair roots) commonly found on the back of the neck and the buttocks usually caused by the bacterium *Staphylococcus aureus*. Carbuncles usually begin as a single boil that spreads. They primarily affect patients with lowered resistance to infection.

Treatment Options and Outlook

Carbuncles are treated with oral and topical antibiotics and hot compresses. These may relieve the pain by causing the pus-filled heads to burst; if this occurs, the carbuncle should be covered with a dressing until it has healed completely.

Once the inflammation has been controlled, the lesion may be cut and drained. The cavity may then need packing with a PETROLEUM JELLY or iodoform dressing. In some cases, draining is not necessary if a 10-day course of antibiotics and topical antibiotics cures the infection.

Risk Factors and Preventive Measures

Recurrent carbuncles are usually caused by auto-inoculation (that is, patients carry the bacteria that causes carbuncles and constantly reinfect themselves). Regular washing with antibacterial soap (especially around rashes, irritations, shaving, or areas of heavy sweating) can help prevent reinfection. Hands and bedding should be washed often.

carcinoma, basal cell See BASAL CELL CARCINOMA.

carcinoma, squamous cell See SQUAMOUS CELL CARCINOMA.

carnauba wax A type of wax derived from the pores of the Brazilian carnauba palm tree used to give cosmetics a more solid consistency. This wax is included in depilatories, creams, and stick deodorants. It has not been shown to induce an allergic reaction.

carotenemia Yellowing of the skin resembling JAUNDICE caused by excess carotene in the blood, most commonly found on the palms, soles of the feet, and central third of the face, and in the sweat. Carotenemia does not usually affect the whites of the eyes, which helps distinguish it from jaundice.

This condition is caused by eating too much of certain vegetables and fruits rich in carotene, or is the result of therapy with BETA-CAROTENE for certain disorders (such as ERYTHROPOIETIC PROTOPORPHYRIA). Too much carotene in the blood also may be a symptom of hypothyroidism, diabetes mellitus, hypopituitarism, or anorexia nervosa.

Treatment Options and Outlook

When carotenemia is caused by beta-carotene therapy or excess dietary ingestion, the skin returns to normal several months after the diet or therapy has stopped.

cartilage-hair hypoplasia A genetic disorder characterized by thin hair shafts with little or no pigment, and short-limb dwarfism. Because of defects in the immune system, there may be other problems such as recurrent respiratory infections and severe SHINGLES. There is no known treatment.

See also HAIR, DISORDERS OF.

casein A whole-milk protein used in cosmetics as an emulsifier (especially in massage creams) that does not affect the skin's health in any way.

castor oil A vegetable oil derived from the castor bean. Used in many cosmetics as an emollient, it forms a hard film when dry. It is often used in lipsticks, but because of its unpleasant smell, it is not often found in other cosmetics. Because it is rarely associated with skin irritation or allergic reactions, it is used in some medical-grade creams and pastes, and several types of eyedrops.

catagen The brief stage of the hair growth cycle in which growth stops and resting starts.

See also HAIR, ANATOMY OF.

cat scratch disease A bacterial infection caused by *Bartonella henselae* as a result of being bitten or scratched by a cat. A small skin lesion typically develops at the point of injury, and lymph nodes (especially near the head, neck, and arms) become swollen. This may be followed by a slight fever. Kittens are more likely to be infected and to transmit the bacteria to people; about 40 percent of all cats carry *B. henselae* at some point. Although *B. henselae* has been found in fleas, so far scientists have found no evidence that a bite from an infected flea can transmit cat scratch disease (CSD).

Although CSD occurs all over the world, it is an uncommon disease. The Centers for Disease Control and Prevention estimates that there are 2.5 cases of CSD per 100,000 people per year in the United States.

Symptoms and Diagnostic Path

Between three to 10 days after a bite or scratch, the patient notices swollen lymph nodes, which may become painful or tender. After three to 10 days, a red round lump usually appears at the site of infection. A small infected blister sometimes develops at the original wound site. There also may be fever, headache, fatigue, and a poor appetite.

A biopsy of the swollen lymph node can be taken, and a skin test using cat scratch disease antigen may be performed.

Treatment Options and Outlook

Painkillers may be needed to relieve fever and headache; a severely affected lymph node or blister may have to be drained. In most cases, the illness fades after one or two months, and the cat does not need to be destroyed. Rare complications of *B. henselae* infection are bacillary angiomatosis.

Risk Factors and Preventive Measures

Cats that carry *B. henselae* do not show any signs of illness. People with impaired immune systems, such as those undergoing chemotherapy for cancer, organ transplant patients, and people with HIV/AIDS are more likely than others to have complications with CSD. Most people who contract CSD are under age 17 and are usually under age 12.

To prevent transmission of CDS, pet owners should avoid any activity that may lead to cat scratches and bites. The wound from any cat bite or scratch should be washed immediately and thoroughly with running water and soap.

causalgia   A persistent burning pain (usually in an arm or leg) with red and tender skin over the painful area; conversely, the skin may sometimes be cold, blue, and clammy. Experts are not sure of the cause. The pain may become worse during times of emotional stress or by normal sensations (such as touch).

Symptoms and Diagnostic Path

Typical features include dramatic changes in the color and temperature of the skin over the affected area, along with intense burning pain, skin sensitivity, sweating, and swelling.

Treatment Options and Outlook

Because there is no cure, treatment is focused on relieving painful symptoms. Doctors may prescribe topical painkillers, antidepressants, corticosteroids, and opioids to relieve pain, but no single drug or combination of drugs results in consistent long-lasting improvement.

Other treatments may include physical therapy, sympathetic nerve block, spinal cord stimulation, and drug pumps to deliver opioids and local painkillers into the spinal cord.

Full recovery may take many months. In some cases patients may have crippling pain without remission, in spite of treatment.

cavernous hemangioma
See HEMANGIOMA, CAVERNOUS.

cayenne pepper spots   Tiny red spots often associated with inflammation of tiny blood vessels (capillaritis). These spots are seen typically in a group of conditions called progressive pigmentary purpura.

cellulite   The so-called dimpling of the legs in women that describes an anatomically normal irregularity found in almost all women's skin. In fact, there is no such thing as "cellulite" itself; the appearance of dimpling simply occurs because the fat deposits in a woman's leg are different from those in a man's leg. In women, the subcutaneous fat appears in large channels, whereas men have connective tissue strands that hold in the fat, preventing the dimpling effect.

European clinics inject enzymes into the leg to "dissolve" this nonexistent substance, and topical aminophylline cream has recently been used in the United States, but there is no effective treatment for "cellulite" except to physically remove fat with liposuction or by decreasing the amount of fat in the legs with diet and exercise.

cellulitis   A bacterial infection of loose connective tissue (particularly subcutaneous tissue) usually caused by B-hemolytic streptococci and staphylococci. Untreated, the disease may lead to bacteremia, blood poisoning or GANGRENE; facial infections may spread to the eye socket. Very rarely, cellulitis develops after childbirth and may spread to the pelvic organs. Before the development of antibiotics, cellulitis was occasionally fatal. Today, any form of cellulitis is likely to be more serious in those with compromised immune systems.

Symptoms and Diagnostic Path

Affected area (usually face, neck or limbs) is usually hot, tender, and red, with associated fever and chills.

Treatment Options and Outlook

Antibiotics (penicillin, cephalosporins, or clindamycin) must be taken for up to two weeks to clear the infection.

cerate An ointment or cream made with wax and oil.

chalazion Also called a meibomian CYST, this is a round, painless swelling on the eyelid. It is caused by an obstruction of one of the meibomian glands responsible for lubricating the edge of the eyelid. A large swelling may exert pressure on the cornea at the front of the eye, blurring the vision.

Symptoms and Diagnostic Path

The cysts can occur at any age, but they are especially common in people with ACNE, ROSACEA, or seborrheic DERMATITIS. If the cyst becomes infected, the lid swells even more, becoming even more painful and red.

Treatment Options and Outlook

About one-third of the cysts fade without treatment. Compressing with hot compresses for 20 minutes, four times a day for several days is often effective. Large chalazions usually need to be surgically removed with local anesthetic.

chamomile An herb that scientists have found to have real value for hair and skin. A mild mixture of chamomile leaves produces an oily substance that is soothing to the skin, used most often by adding it to the bath. A solution of concentrated chamomile left on the hair for a few hours will lighten it by several shades.

chancre An ulcer (usually on the genitals) that develops during the first stage of SYPHILIS.

Symptoms and Diagnostic Path

Appearing first as a dull red spot between three to four weeks after exposure. It can also appear on the lips or in the throat if oral sex has taken place. The spot gradually develops in a painless ulcer with a clearly defined firm, heaped up edge and a rubbery base. If the chancre is the result of a sexually transmitted infection (which is very common) the ulcer may be painful.

Microscopic examination of a smear of the chancre will reveal the spirochete, which causes the disease; blood test results are usually negative early in primary syphilis.

Treatment Options and Outlook

Penicillin injections almost always prevent primary syphilis from developing into more serious stages of the disease.

chapped skin Red, dry and cracked painful skin caused by low humidity (especially during fall and winter).

Treatment Options and Outlook

Badly chapped skin should not be put in water; related washing removes the oil layer, allowing moisture in skin to evaporate. Instead of using soap, patients should rub on soap-free skin cleanser, working it into a lather and then wiping it off—or wash skin with bath oil. Warm, not hot, water should be used in the bath. Patients should always add oil to the bath, pat dry, then apply body lotion, such as Lubriderm, Complex 15, Moisturel, and Eucerin.

Chediak-Higashi syndrome An inherited defect of pigment characterized by partial ALBINISM, PHOTOPHOBIA, silvery hair, and susceptibility to infection.

The disorder has been observed not just in humans, but also in many different mammals, including cats, Aleutian minks, beige mice, and even killer whales.

Symptoms and Diagnostic Path

A few patients have white hair and skin, and some have nystagmus (involuntary eye movements). Most have blond or gray hair, blue eyes, and fair skin.

Skin infections occur frequently and may be fatal, ranging from a superficial PYODERMA (ulcer) to deep, slow-healing abscesses and ulcers that may cause scars.

Treatment Options and Outlook

There is no known treatment. The use of 500 mg. of VITAMIN C three times a day is controversial.

Patients should protect themselves against exposure to the sun, wearing protective clothing, ultraviolet blocking sunglasses, and sunscreens.

The disease is often fatal in childhood as a result of infection or bleeding; few patients live to adulthood, although survival into the 20s or 30s has been reported.

cheilitis Inflammation, dryness and cracking of the lips and corners of the mouth that can be caused by a downturned mouth, poorly fitting dentures, dental work, local infection, COSMETIC ALLERGY, SUNBURN, skiing, or windburn. Patients should apply Vaseline (or other lip balms in stick form) hourly to ease the pain until the underlying cause is identified and treated, and avoid licking the lips.

cheiloplasty Cosmetic surgery to reshape the lips.

chemabrasion See CHEMICAL FACE PEEL.

chemical burns Although most industrial chemicals are relatively weak and require prolonged contact before visible changes occur, some (such as concentrated sulfuric acid) can be quite harmful. Almost any substance encountered in the workplace may become an irritant if exposure is frequent enough. Workers are usually exposed to many different potential irritants, and skin BURNS may be the accumulation of multiple exposures.

Treatment Options and Outlook

The irritant agent must be identified, and exposure to the skin eliminated. Severe cases may be treated with an oral CORTICOSTEROID such as prednisone. Topical steroids, which reduce inflammation, may be applied to the skin. High-potency topical corticosteroids are more useful when inflammation is moderate to severe; gel and cream preparations absorb moisture and help to dry oozing, weeping, vesicular DERMATITIS.

chemical exposure and the skin Certain chemicals used in manufacturing are dangerous to the skin, but only to employees—not the general public. Workers should use appropriate protective clothing.

Another concern about chemical exposure is the effect of FREE RADICALS on the skin. Free radicals are unstable molecules that can disrupt healthy cells during metabolic processes, and are believed to speed up aging and even cause cancer. They are produced naturally in the body, but they also occur in cigarette smoke, nitrous oxide, ozone, and toxic wastes.

As a result of these concerns about pollution, skin care companies have devised a range of pollutant-fighting treatments, some which prevent oxidation and others that just shield the skin from pollution. But experts disagree as to whether these products are just a fancy marketing gimmick or whether they represent serious skin safeguards; none has ever been studied.

Until more research has been completed, experts advise consumers to wash with mild soap and apply moisturizer, which creates an extra barrier against dirt and debris.

chemical face peel A controlled burn using a caustic chemical to repair facial damage such as ACNE scars, wrinkles, or pigmentation caused by sun damage. A chemical peel is the means of regenerating elastin or COLLAGEN (the skin's supportive tissue) lost to age and sun exposure. There are two major types of peels: superficial and deep.

While it may sound like a facial, a chemical peel is in fact surgery, using potent chemicals (glycolic acid, lactic acid, trichloroacetic acid, phenol and or resorcinol) that actually dissolves the top layer of skin, erasing irregular pigmentation, mild acne scars, crow's feet, fine cheek wrinkles, and tiny vertical lines above the upper lip. The deeper the peel, the more effective it is.

After a deep peel, a thick crust lasts for a week, and the purple-red skin color may take six months to fade away. It is a painful, emotionally difficult process to endure, but after the skin heals the result is pinker, tighter, smoother and relatively wrinkle- and blemish-free skin, which may remain younger-looking for 15 years or more.

On the other hand, a "surface" or freshening peel is more like a superficial facial, leaving the skin glowing for a week or two, but not going deep enough to erase scars or wrinkles.

The procedure is not for everyone. Subjects with dark or olive skin may end up with a blotchy appearance, and those with poor liver, heart, or kidney function could be affected by the solution that strips away the upper layers of the skin, which is absorbed into the bloodstream.

Prospective patients of any peel, no matter how minor, should investigate the surgeon's ability and experience, since it takes a great deal of expertise to apply a good chemical peel. Consumers should ask whether the procedure comprises a large portion of the person's practice (one of the two or three procedures most often performed). Ask how many peels the doctor does a week, and how he or she learned the procedure.

The cost of a peel ranges from $200 to $3,000 depending on the area of skin to be treated, the depth of the peel and the area of the country in which the dermatologist practices.

Chemical skin peels have been around for thousands of years, with women using everything from sour milk to wine residue to freshen their complexions. Since the 1950s, American women have gone to plastic surgeons and dermatologists for peels using phenol or trichloracetic acid. While these products are still used for those who need fairly deep chemical peels, newer milder, products are now on the market.

These new products, called ALPHA HYDROXY ACIDS, are available over the counter in concentrations of less than 10 percent, in beauty salons in concentrations of up to 40 percent, and in dermatologist's offices in concentrations up to 70 percent. These milder peels improve the skin's appearance by speeding up the shedding of dead skin cells, clearing up acne-prone skin, softening tiny lines around the eyes and mouth, smoothing dry skin and fading dark spots caused by sun or hormonal changes.

See also DERMABRASION; GLYCOLIC ACID.

chemical pollutants and the skin The daily onslaught of smog, car exhaust, and acid rain take their toll on building facades in America's cities, and some dermatologists believe chemical pollution can also harm the skin.

Some experts blame toxics for a range of problems from minor irritation to premature aging, although there have been few controlled studies of the problem. Some experts believe the increase in airborne toxicants contributes to the rise of skin cancer; others believe that ozone in smog can penetrate and damage the skin's outer layer. Others point to the effect of FREE RADICALS, unstable molecules that can disrupt healthy cells in a process known as oxidation; they have been linked to premature aging and cancer. They are produced naturally in the body, but they are also found in cigarette smoke, nitrous oxide, ozone, and toxic waste. Critics of this belief point out that a person's skin was designed to keep *out* such harmful substances.

Experts advise patients to wash with mild soap and apply a moisturizer, which creates an extra barrier against dirt and debris. Washing the facial area thoroughly at the end of the day with soap or a soap substitute and water is also important.

chemosurgery See MOHS' MICROSCOPICALLY CONTROLLED EXCISIONS.

cherry angioma A common benign skin growth that appears as a small, smooth, cherry red bump. They are most common after age 40, and they can occur almost anywhere on the body but most commonly develop on the trunk. The size of the skin growth may vary. Although they are painless and harmless, cherry angiomas may bleed profusely if injured.

The cause is unknown.

Symptoms and Diagnostic Path
The bright red, smooth skin lesion is small, from about the size of a pinhead to about ¼-inch diameter.

Treatment Options and Outlook

Cherry angiomas do not usually require treatment. If cosmetically displeasing, however, they may be removed by surgery, freezing (CRYOTHERAPY), burning (ELECTROCAUTERY), or laser therapy. Cherry angiomas are benign and generally harmless, and removal usually does not cause scarring.

chicken pox A once-common childhood infectious disease characterized by a rash and fever that—prior to the development of a vaccine in 1995—affected about 3.9 million people each year in the United States. About 90 percent of cases occur in children under age 10, primarily in winter and spring. Since the vaccine was introduced, there has been a steady decline in cases of chicken pox. The availability of a safe and effective varicella vaccine has reduced the impact of the disease substantially.

High vaccination coverage levels among all age groups are necessary to ensure that children do not reach adolescence or adulthood without having immunity to varicella. By June 2004, 44 states had implemented child care or elementary school entry requirements for varicella. However, by March 2005, only 18 states included middle- or high school varicella vaccination requirements.

Chicken pox is also known as varicella, after the virus (varicella-zoster, or VZV) that causes the disease. VZV is a member of the family of herpes viruses and is similar to the herpes simplex viruses (HSV). The virus is spread by airborne droplets.

While an attack of chicken pox creates a lifelong immunity to the disease, the virus does not disappear. It remains dormant within a patient's nerve tissues after the attack. In later life, the virus can reactivate and cause an attack of herpes zoster (SHINGLES).

Most people throughout the world have had the disease by age 10, and chicken pox is rare in adults. When it does occur after childhood, it can be deadly. About 90 people in the United States die every year as a result of chicken pox, and another 9,300 must be hospitalized. The infection strikes hardest in infants, adults, and those with immune system problems. Adults are much more likely to be hospitalized than children.

If possible, a child with suspected chicken pox should not be brought into a doctor's office where others may be exposed to the disease; it can be very dangerous to newborns or those with suppressed immune systems. The virus can be spread both through the air and by direct contact with an infected individual. Instead, a physician should be contacted by phone and describe symptoms.

Symptoms and Diagnostic Path

The incubation period after exposure ranges from one to three weeks, and is followed by a rash on the body (torso, face, armpits, upper arms and legs, inside the mouth, and sometimes in the windpipe and bronchial tubes, causing a dry cough). The rash is made up of small, red, itchy spots that grow into fluid-filled BLISTERS within a few hours. After several days, the blisters dry out and form scabs. New spots usually continue to form over four to seven days. Patients are contagious five days before the rash appears and until all the skin lesions have crusted over (usually about a week after they appear).

Although children usually have only a slight fever, adults often experience fever, breathing problems, and severe varicella pneumonia. In rare cases, children may develop this type of pneumonia or Reye's syndrome; they may also develop bacterial infections. Occasionally, chicken pox can lead to varicella encephalitis (an inflammation of the brain). Immunocompromised patients who are susceptible to VZV are at high risk for having severe varicella infections with widespread lesions.

Treatment Options and Outlook

In most cases, rest is all that is needed for children, with chicken pox, who usually recover within 10 days. Adults take longer to recover. ACETAMINOPHEN may reduce fever, and CALAMINE, baking soda, or OATMEAL baths and oral antihistamines ease the itch. Compresses can dry weeping lesions. Scratching should be avoided, since it can lead to bacterial infection of lesions and increases the chance of scarring; children may need to wear gloves during sleep to avoid nighttime scratching.

Aspirin should never be given to a child who has been exposed to (or has recently recovered from) chicken pox. Aspirin in these cases has been linked to the development of Reye's syndrome.

The drug ACYCLOVIR may be prescribed for chicken pox patients. It is usually recommended for people with chronic skin or lung disorders, in severe cases of chicken pox, or for those with compromised immune systems. Unlike herpes simplex viruses, VZV is relatively resistant to acyclovir, and doses required for treatment are much larger than for other diseases. While the drug may decrease the length of the illness and mitigate symptoms, its high cost and marginal effectiveness have prompted the American Academy of Pediatrics not to recommend it as a routine treatment.

Risk Factors and Preventive Measures

The American Academy of Pediatrics recommends the chicken pox vaccine (VariVax) for all children, teens and young adults who have not had the disease. The vaccine, which has been used in Japan for some time, was approved by the Food and Drug Administration in April 1995. Although its approval had initially met with some controversy, pediatricians today recommend the vaccine for their patients. Since the chicken pox vaccine was licensed in 1995, several million doses of vaccine have been given to children in the United States. Studies continue to show the vaccine to be safe and effective.

The vaccine is made from a live, weakened virus that, once injected in a human patient, creates a mild infection similar to natural chicken pox—but without related complications. The mild infection spurs the body to develop an immune response to the disease; these defenses are then ready when the body encounters the natural virus.

The vaccine is considered to be safe. Proponents of the vaccine point out that it makes sense to vaccinate children because they are likely to suffer from chicken pox.

The American Academy of Pediatrics recommends a single dose of the chicken pox vaccine for all children between 12 and 18 months of age who have not had chicken pox. Older children should be immunized at the earliest opportunity, also with a single dose. For healthy children older than 13 who have not had chicken pox and have never been immunized against the disease, two doses of the vaccine are required, four to eight weeks apart.

Immunization with the chicken pox vaccine will prevent most children from getting chicken pox. If vaccinated children do get chicken pox, they generally have a much milder form of the disease. They have fewer skin lesions, a lower fever, and recover more quickly. In fact, the disease may be so mild that the skin lesions look like insect bites. Even so, vaccinated children with a mild case of chicken pox can still infect others at risk of getting chicken pox.

Currently, revaccination with the chicken pox vaccine is not recommended. However, studies are underway to determine how long protection from the vaccine lasts and whether a person will need revaccination in the future.

High-risk, susceptible patients may also obtain passive immunization with VZV immune globulin, which can abort or modify infection if administered within three days of exposure.

Rarely (in less than one person out of 1,000) there may be seizure caused by fever. Very rarely, pneumonia may result. Other serious problems, including severe brain reactions and low blood count, have been reported after chicken pox vaccination. These happen so rarely experts can not tell whether the vaccine causes them or not. If it does, it is extremely rare.

See also VARICELLA VIRUS VACCINE LIVE.

chigger bites　A bite from the chigger (or harvest mite) causes an intense, itchy swelling up to half an inch across. The swelling usually fades without treatment between three days to a week.

The female mites are attracted to warm moist areas of the body, such as the skin underneath sweat bands, where they burrow under the skin's surface.

The larvae of these mites of the genus *Trombididae* live outdoors throughout the southeastern United States, and they are especially active in the grass near trees in summer. They attach themselves to their patient's legs where they feed on blood. The swelling may progress to form a BLISTER, and the ITCHING can last for weeks.

Secondary infection may occur as a result of scratching.

Close-fitting clothing with shirts tucked in and pants tucked into socks will discourage chiggers.

chilblains An injury of the skin tissue caused by cold, but not freezing, temperatures. Also known as "pernio," chilblains are most commonly seen on the earlobes, nose, fingers, and toes of young women.

Symptoms and Diagnostic Path

Chilblains look like itchy purple lesions that occur after exposure to cold. These lesions may last from days to weeks, with burning, ITCHING, and pain. Repeated episodes of chilblains may lead to a chronic condition that persists throughout the winter.

Treatment Options and Outlook

Administration of vasodilating drugs may provide some relief.

Risk Factors and Preventive Measures

Chilblains may be prevented by wearing adequate clothing in cold temperatures. Severe lesions respond to bed rest and gentle rewarming in a 105 degree bath. The patient with chronic chilblains *must* avoid exposure to cold.

chin augmentation A surgical procedure often performed together with NOSE REPAIR (rhinoplasty) in order to rearrange the facial balance, accentuating and flattering the neckline.

Procedure

The incision may be placed either inside the mouth or under the chin, which creates a pocket in the chin into which an implant can be placed. The wound is then closed with stitches and a tape bandage applied to the chin.

Outlook and Lifestyle Modifications

If the incision is in the mouth, antibiotics are administered to prevent infection, and a liquid diet is required for 48 hours to avoid getting food in the wound. Elevating the head prevents excess swelling and bruising, and the bandage is removed after the fifth day. Stitches are removed a week after surgery, and swelling usually subsides in the second week.

chloasma Also known as melasma or the mask of pregnancy, this condition often appears during pregnancy in which blotches of pale brown skin pigmentation appear on the face. It may occur in women who have been exposed to too much sun. Chloasma also occurs as a side effect of taking contraceptive pills and injected depot contraceptive preparations. It may also be noticed in apparently healthy, normal, nonpregnant women where it is presumed to be due to some mild and harmless estrogen stimulation of pigment receptors in the skin. Occasionally, the skin darkening will appear in men or postmenopausal women. The tendency to develop chloasma may run in families.

Symptoms and Diagnostic Path

The pigmentation primarily appears on the forehead, cheeks and nose, sometimes merging to form the "mask of pregnancy." It is made worse by even brief exposures to sunlight. While it usually fades away over a period of time, in some patients it becomes permanent; it also tends to recur in successive pregnancies.

Treatment Options and Outlook

The condition may improve if the patient avoids sunlight or uses a strong sunblock and (if appropriate) changes the brand of (or stops using) BIRTH CONTROL PILLS. In addition, some patients may respond to hypopigmenting agents containing HYDROQUINONE or to the combination of TRETINOIN cream and hydroquinone. Chloasma in premenopausal women may improve after menopause, even without therapy.

chloracne An ACNE-like eruption caused by exposure to chlorinated hydrocarbon products. These lesions may occur in up to 95 percent of cases where toxic generalized symptoms (such as liver disease) are also present. Chloracne is caused when toxic materials cause the underlying sebaceous glands to atrophy, forming KERATIN-filled cysts. The hydrocarbon product most often associated with chloracne is 2,3,7,8-tetrachlorodibenzodioxin.

Chloracne has usually been associated with massive hydrocarbon exposure, such as in an industrial accident or contamination during the manufacturing process.

New chloracne lesions usually stop forming within six months after exposure, but existing lesions often take a long time to heal and may persist indefinitely.

Symptoms and Diagnostic Path

Symptoms include numerous closed BLACKHEADS with some inflammatory pustules and noninflammatory, straw-colored cysts. In addition to the usual acne areas, the ears also may be affected, and covered areas outside the usual acne distribution may be involved in severe cases.

Treatment Options and Outlook

Chloracne is often resistant to treatment, and does not respond well to systemic antibiotics and topical BENZOYL PEROXIDE. Topical derivatives of VITAMIN A, such as retinoic acid creams or gels (Retin-A) may help. Oral vitamin A sometimes helps and sometimes does not; anecdotal reports indicate that ISOTRETINOIN (Accutane) may be effective. In some cases, acne surgery is the only effective treatment.

chlorophyll A chemical in the cells of green plants that absorbs light so that plants can synthesize food. It is widely used as an ingredient in deodorants, toothpastes, and mouthwashes to protect against odor.

chromate, allergy to See ALLERGIES AND THE SKIN.

chromomycosis An invasive fungal infection of the top two layers of the skin in the feet and legs that almost always begins at the site of trauma, or penetration of a foreign object. It is most common in the tropics. Also called chromoblastomycosis, chromomycosis is characterized by a pile of warty sores, usually on the legs. The infection may remain local, involve the entire extremity or turn into a generalized infection.

This tropical infection is caused by a group of closely related molds found in the soil. It affects people involved in manual labor with soil or its products. While it is not clear why the infection occurs only in the tropics, it is believed that in colder climates, workers wear shoes, which protect feet from contracting the infection. Still, even in the tropics this disorder is not common.

The condition is chronic and may last for years or decades, leading to the necessity of amputation, the development of ELEPHANTIASIS, or SQUAMOUS CELL CARINOMA.

Symptoms and Diagnostic Path

The infection begins with itchy, watery PAPULES or an ulcer on the leg or foot, followed by foul-smelling plaques of the foot, ankle, knee, elbow, or hand. The papule or ulcer slowly enlarges over months to years; as it spreads, the central area becomes scarred. Many patients develop secondary bacterial infections.

Treatment Options and Outlook

Bed rest, elevation of affected body part, and antibiotic therapy to control secondary infections are recommended. Surgical excision of the affected area, destruction of the affected tissue or drug treatment (potassium iodide, flucytosine, thiabendazole, KETOCONAZOLE, and topical heat) may be successful.

chromosomal defects and skin disease Abnormalities in the human chromosome are often associated with prominent skin defects. Deletion of the short arm of chromosome 4 (4P) causes central scalp defects. An extra autosome (trisomy 8) causes short nails, excess skin on the back of the neck, and no knee cap. Trisomy 10 causes congenital scalp defect and trisomy 13 causes scalp defects. Down syndrome (trisomy 21) may include ELASTOSIS PERFORANS SERPIGINOSA, unusual creases on the palms, a shortened fifth finger, premature wrinkles, frequent hair loss, and fissured and furrowed skin. Turner's syndrome (deficiency of one X chromosome or presence of an abnormal X) may cause congenital and persistent lymphedema, moles, cystic hygromas, low hairline in back, and increased skin aging. Klinefelter's syndrome (XXY) may be associated with leg ulcers.

chrysotherapy   See GOLD THERAPY.

cimetidine (trade name: Tagamet)   An antihistamine developed for the treatment of gastrointestinal ulcers, cimetidine is occasionally effective in the treatment of chronic HIVES and has recently been studied as a treatment for multiple warts in children.

cinnamate   A SUNSCREEN that blocks both ultraviolet-B (UV-B) and, less well, UV-A sun rays. Cinnamate is one of more than 20 chemicals that the U.S. Food and Drug Administration recognizes as safe, effective sunscreen ingredients. The success of the product depends on how well, how often, and how consistently it is used. However, cinnamate can cause a rash.

ciprofloxacin (trade name: Cipro)   An oral antimicrobial drug used to treat skin infections such as cutaneous ANTHRAX.

Side Effects
Nausea and vomiting, diarrhea, abdominal pain, sun sensitivity, and headache.

citric acid   Chemical found in citrus fruits that is used as a grease-cutter in shampoos.

citronella   A strong-smelling substance obtained from the *Cymbopogon nardus* grass of Asia, used as an insect repellent and perfume. Some sensitive individuals may develop skin sensitivity to citronella.

clavus   See CORN.

clay   A mineral used in face and body powder, face masks and foundations that is particularly helpful for normal and oily skin, and ACNE conditions. It does not cause allergic reactions.

cleansing products   While it is true that skin problems such as ACNE have more to do with trapped oil and bacteria in the oil glands than oil on the skin's surface, cleansing agents can give a feeling of improvement because they do remove surface oil. Skin cleansing can remove dirt, cosmetics, cellular debris, body secretions, sweat, and microorganisms.

How often and how vigorously a person should clean the skin depends on skin type, daily activities, and the environment. Washing alone is the most effective method of skin cleansing; while water alone removes many types of dirt, a soap or detergent helps to remove oils. In the United States, soaps account for about 90 percent of the toilet bars sold.

People with normal skin should wash the face no more than twice a day with gentle cleansers. Very hot water should be avoided, and a low-alcohol astringent or an alcohol-free toner should be used after each washing.

Oily skin should be washed three times a day; "gentle" or "rich" cleansers should not be used. People with oily skin can use hotter water than people with other skin types; an astringent with a high alcohol content should be used after each washing. The skin should be exfoliated twice a week.

Combination skin requires the same regimen as those with normal skin; astringent on nose, chin, and forehead.

Sensitive skin should be washed once a day, with a very gentle cleanser and lukewarm water. Abrasives such as rough washcloths, grains, and toners or astringents with alcohol should not be used.

Abrasive cleansers/pads contain small gritty particles that mildly sand the skin. These are designed for people who want to scrub their acne away, but in fact most experts believe they are too irritating and are not that helpful.

Soaps, lotions, and cleansers work about as well as abrasives but they are not as harsh. All induce a mild exfoliation by helping to remove superficial skin cells, but they cannot really remove the oil in the follicles. In some cases, soaps can be excessively drying and irritating.

Soap-free cleansers or emollients may be used by those with sensitive skin.

Astringents, fresheners, toners, or refining lotions are usually composed of alcohol-in-water combinations used by those with oily skin to remove SEBUM or makeup. While many of these products are said to shrink pores, in fact it is impossible to permanently shrink pores. The pores may appear smaller as acne lesions are treated and oil and blackheads are removed.

See also SOAP AND THE SKIN; COSMETICS; MAKEUP.

climatotherapy The use of climate in the treatment of disease. This type of therapy is especially popular in the treatment of PSORIASIS, which responds well to hot, dry climates. Many patients often visit Hawaii, Florida, Mexico, and the Caribbean to clear their skin conditions by sunbathing, since the natural sunlight in regular doses will often clear most cases of psoriasis.

As yet there are no climatotherapy centers for psoriasis in the United States; the most organized centers for psoriasis are located in the region of the Dead Sea between Israel and Jordan.

clindamycin An antibiotic drug used to treat ACNE and serious infections that have not responded, or are resistant to, other antibiotics. Clindamycin is especially effective against most anaerobic bacteria, including *PROPIONIBACTERIUM ACNES*, which are often responsible for acne. It is also an excellent agent against *Staphylococcus aureus* and streptococcal species.

clofazimine A dye used primarily to treat LEPROSY. It is also effective in some patients with PYODERMA GANGRENOSUM, DISCOID LUPUS ERYTHEMATOSUS, ACNE FULMINANS, and GRANULOMA FACIALE.

This drug has a remarkable lack of toxicity, and although there is no evidence of birth defects, it does cross the placenta and cause pigmentation in offspring.

Administered by mouth, the drug should be taken with meals or milk; about 70 percent is absorbed within the small intestine. For most skin conditions, the drug needs to be taken for at least two months before any benefit is seen.

The drug should not be taken during the first three months of pregnancy, in patients prone to diarrhea or recurrent abdominal pain, and in those with kidney or liver disease.

Side Effects

The most obvious side effect is pink, red, or brownish black discoloration of the skin, especially in areas exposed to sunlight. Hair, sweat, sputum, urine and feces may also be discolored. These pigmentation side effects are related to dosage, however, and begin to fade when therapy is stopped. Other side effects include XERODERMA, ICHTHYOSIS, ITCHING, sensitivity to sunlight, and acnelike skin eruptions. There also may be nausea and vomiting, abdominal pain, and diarrhea.

clothes and sun protection A variety of clothing products can help protect consumers from the sun's rays, including laundry additives and clothing made from UV-protected fabric. Regular clothing has a SUN PROTECTION FACTOR of between 2 and 6. While most people think their clothing gives them adequate protection from the sun, that is not always the case. In fact, many white cotton T-shirts provide only an ultraviolet (UV) protection factor of 5, significantly less than the recommended SPF (SUN PROTECTION FACTOR) of 15.

Sun-protective clothing offers another way to protect skin from the harmful effects of the sun. Sun-protective fabrics differ from typical summer fabrics in several ways: They typically have a tighter weave or knit and are usually darker in color. Sun-protective clothes have a label listing the garment's Ultraviolet Protection Factor (UPF) value (that is, the level of protection the garment provides from the Sun's UV rays). The higher the UPF, the higher the protection from the Sun's UV rays.

The UPF rating indicates how much of the sun's UV radiation is absorbed by the fabric. For example, a fabric with a UPF rating of 20 only allows $\frac{1}{20}$th of the Sun's UV radiation to pass through it.

This means that this fabric will reduce the skin's UV radiation exposure by 20 times where it's protected by the fabric. Everything above UPF 50 may be labeled UPF 50+; however, these garments may not offer substantially more protection than those with a UPF of 50.

A garment should not be labeled "sun-protective" or "UV-protective" if its UPF is less than 15. Sun-protective clothing may lose its effectiveness if it is too tight or stretched out, damp or wet, and if it has been washed or worn repeatedly.

Rit, a producer of home dyes and laundry treatments, has created a laundry additive that washes UV protection into clothes to help block more than 96 percent of the sun's rays. Their product, Sun Guard, lasts for 20 washes on light-colored clothes.

See also SOLUMBRA; SUNBURN; SUNSCREEN; SUNTAN.

cloxacillin   A penicillin-type antibiotic used to treat staphylococcal infections. This drug should not be taken with acidic fruits or juices, or aged cheese. Taken with alcohol, this drug could cause stomach irritation. Use with birth control pills may impair the efficacy of the contraceptive.

coal tar derivatives   Thick, black substances commonly found as an ingredient in ointments and some shampoos, used to treat skin and scalp conditions such as ECZEMA, PSORIASIS, and certain types of DERMATITIS.

Crude coal tar or coal tar solutions are available as over-the-counter and prescription preparations, depending on strength. In the treatment of psoriasis, it may be applied directly to the affected area or may be added to bath water for a daily body soak. It also can be used with topical steroids, reducing the size and redness of itchy patches.

In addition, the coal tar may be used with ultraviolet light (UV-B), followed by exposure to radiation treatments in resistant cases of psoriasis. The tar is partially removed from the skin before exposing it to UV-B light and then to radiation therapy. The treatments are given daily for three to six weeks, or may be done at home with a portable machine or natural sunlight.

Cockayne-Touraine syndrome   A variant form of EPIDERMOLYSIS BULLOSA dystrophica, that usually occurs in infancy or early childhood. It is believed to be an inherited condition, which was first reported in 1895.

Symptoms and Diagnostic Path

It is characterized by recurrent, noninflammatory blistering eruptions mainly on the feet, less prominently on the hands. Symptoms typically begin after BLISTERS appear in early childhood, but they may also appear during adulthood, especially in warm weather. The lesions heal without residual scarring or other changes, such as thickening of the skin. They are occasionally associated with HYPERHIDROSIS (excessive sweating).

cocoa butter   An oil extracted from roasted cocoa nut seeds used to soften and lubricate the skin, often used instead of wax or harder creams. It has the same emollient properties as any other vegetable oil, and it has not been associated with allergic reactions.

coconut oil   A white saturated fat derived from coconuts that melts at body temperature and is used to smooth and lubricate the skin. Because it produces an excellent lather, it is often included as an ingredient in soap. Coconut oil can cause skin irritation in some sensitive individuals.

cold cream   A pharmaceutical and cosmetic product of animal fat or mineral oil and a sodium salt with a dispersing agent to enhance its vanishing quality.

cold sore   A small skin blister on the mouth usually found in a cluster, caused by the HERPES SIMPLEX VIRUS (HSV). The viral strain usually responsible for cold sores is herpes simplex Type I (HSVI); up to 90 percent of all people around the world carry this virus.

Cold sores tend to appear when the individual is under stress, exposed to sunlight, cold wind or another infection, or feels run down. Women tend to experience more cold sores during their menstrual periods, but some people are afflicted at regular intervals throughout the year. People with compromised immune systems may experience prolonged attacks.

Symptoms and Diagnostic Path

The first attack may not even be noticed, or it may cause a flulike illness with painful ulcers on the mouth or lips (called gingivostomatitis). An outbreak is often signaled by a tingling in the lips, followed by a small BLISTER that soon grows, causing ITCHING and soreness. Within a few days the blisters burst, encrust, and then disappear within a week. The virus then retreats along the nerve where it lies dormant in the nerve cell; in some patients, however, the virus is constantly reactivated.

Treatment Options and Outlook

For mild symptoms, the sore should be kept clean and dry so it will heal itself. For particularly virulent outbreaks, the antiviral drug ACYCLOVIR or idoxuridine paint may relieve symptoms or briefly shorten the length of the outbreak by no more than one day, but there is no evidence of acyclovir ointment is particularly helpful. Otherwise, there are a range of nonprescription drugs available containing a numbing agent (such as CAMPHOR or phenol) that also contain an emollient to reduce cracking. For patients with frequent outbreaks of HSV, acyclovir may be prescribed to be taken from seven to 10 days, as soon as the patient feels tingling. This usually prevents the outbreak, but does not prevent future outbreaks. In patients with very severe symptoms, daily acyclovir application is occasionally prescribed.

Some studies have suggested that ZINC may help prevent outbreaks because zinc interferes with herpes viral replication. Studies found that both zinc gluconate and zinc sulfate helped speed up healing time, but zinc gluconate was less irritating to the skin. Both zinc products are available at health food stores.

Sores can be protected with a dab of PETROLEUM JELLY (applied with a clean cotton swab); the swab that touched the affected area should not be dipped back into the jar.

collagen A tough natural constituent of connective tissue that is the body's major structural protein, forming an important part of tendons, bones, and connective tissues. The most common protein in the body, its tough insoluble nature is what gives skin its elasticity, and helps hold the cells and tissues together. Collagen makes up 77 percent of the fat-free dry weight of the skin. Injectable collagen is a natural animal protein made from the skin of cattle and injected into human skin to eliminate wrinkles or facial depressions. It has long been touted as a potent weapon against the appearance of aging.

To restore lost collagen, researchers have found that treating photodamaged skin with Retin-A resulted in an 80 percent increase in collagen, whereas patches treated with a placebo cream showed a 14 percent collagen reduction. However, researchers note that the results of improved collagen after treatment with Retin-A were observable only under the microscope; the increase in collagen was not readily apparent to the naked eye.

See also COLLAGEN DISEASES; COLLAGEN INJECTION; LUPUS ERYTHEMATOSUS; SCLERODERMA.

collagen diseases There are two groups of diseases called COLLAGEN diseases: the true collagen diseases, and connective tissue diseases. True collagen diseases are rare and are usually inherited; they are usually caused by faulty formation of collagen fibers. True collagen diseases are characterized by slack skin and poor wound healing.

Connective tissue diseases are caused by a malfunction in the immune system that affects blood vessels, producing secondary damage in connective tissue. For this reason, these diseases are sometimes called collagen vascular diseases, and include rheumatoid arthritis, systematic LUPUS ERYTHEMATOSUS,

PERIARTERITIS NODOSA, SCLERODERMA, and DERMATOMYOSITIS.

collagen injection One of the less painful, more conservative ways to temporarily remove wrinkles, now superseded by Retin-A treatments. The collagen framework is intact in young people, and the skin is moisturized and firm. Eventually, however, as the years pass the skin's support structure weakens and the skin loses its elasticity. As the collagen support wears away, the skin begins to lose its tone. Every time a person smiles, frowns, or squints, the collagen in skin is stressed. The effect of these constant facial movements builds up, and eventually facial lines begin to appear.

Creams that contain collagen that are applied to the skin surface cannot penetrate the skin because the molecules are too big. No moisturizer can reverse the cumulative damage caused by the breakdown of collagen, but creams containing retinoic acid can reverse sun-induced collagen damage and stimulate production of new collagen. Creams can keep the skin supple by slowing the rate of water loss from the skin.

Collagen injections can also replenish the skin's natural collagen. As the support structure of the skin is restored, the skin appears smoother and more youthful.

Zyderm and Zyplast are bovine-derived collagen products designed to replace lost collagen due to aging. Zyderm and Zyplast collagen are placed into the middle layers of the skin. However, 3 percent of people have allergic reactions to bovine collagen.

COSMODERM and COSMOPLAST are bioengineered human collagen products that are used in the same way as bovine collagen, but do not carry the risk of allergy and therefore do not require a skin test prior to the first treatment. The injections can fill in deep vertical wrinkles between the eyebrows, deep wrinkles running from mouth to nose, and forehead wrinkles. Results, however, last only between three and 18 months, averaging about six months. The price will vary depending on the part of the country where the procedure is carried out. Each nose-to-mouth crease requires a full syringe, and between a quarter to a half syringe of collagen is needed to fill furrows between the eyes.

Collagen injections are a good choice for someone who wishes to avoid the risks of surgery and is not ready for a moderate or deep peel, DERMABRASION, laser abrasion, or a full FACE-LIFT. Collagen injections are safe, and the least likely of all the wrinkle-removal methods to develop complications.

Procedure
Collagen should be injected into the skin only by a trained health care professional. By supplementing the skin's own collagen, collagen replacement therapy helps smooth facial lines as well as acne SCARS.

Tiny drops of thick collagen are injected with a fine needle underneath the skin to replace collagen lost by the body. During this injection, some patients may feel some stinging. The entire procedure may take between two and 10 minutes, and patients recover in about two to three hours.

After treatment, there may be some redness lasting up to 10 days; a few patients also experience bruising, temporary stinging, burning sensations, faint redness, swelling, or excessive fullness. Other patients have no reaction at all.

Risks and Complications
Because about 3 percent of the population is allergic to bovine collagen (developing a rash and swelling), physicians usually perform two separate skin tests and wait a month after each to be sure the patient has no allergic reaction. Other possible risks include contour irregularities, infection, or local ABSCESS.

Not everyone is a suitable candidate for collagen injections. They are not recommended for anyone with a history of immunological disorders such as LUPUS ERYTHROMATOSUS or rheumatoid arthritis. According to the U.S. Food and Drug Administration (FDA), more studies are required to establish whether or not collagen is linked to certain connective-tissue disorders.

collagenomas A rare connective tissue BIRTHMARK made of COLLAGEN, characterized by yellowish plaques up to several inches in diameter that usually occur on the upper trunk and sometimes the arms and legs. Usually present at birth or shortly after, no treatment is necessary.

See also CONNECTIVE TISSUE NEVI.

collodion baby An infant enclosed in a taut yellow-pink cellophane-like membrane at birth that may temporarily distort facial features (especially the ears, lips, and eyelids).

Symptoms and Diagnostic Path

A collodian baby is usually afflicted with LAMELLAR ICHTHYOSIS (a skin disorder characterized by rough, reddened, scaling skin). The membrane may be perforated by LANUGO (downy fetal hair) and scalp hair.

Shortly after birth, the membrane begins to crack and peel, revealing underlying red skin. It may take several weeks for the membrane to be completely shed so that a new membrane may form temporarily.

Infants born with collodion membrane rarely have normal skin after shedding. Patients with this condition will have lifelong scaling and dry, rough skin. However, 10 percent of these babies do have normal underlying skin (known as a "self healing" collodion baby).

Although often born prematurely, collodian babies are otherwise healthy. More severely affected babies may lose hair or nails, and have some problems in eating and breathing. These babies often have secondary bacterial and fungal infections because their skin must be softened by high humidity in their isolettes.

Treatment Options and Outlook

At birth, a baby with this condition is usually transferred to a neonatal intensive care unit where an incubator provides a humidified, neutral temperature environment. Other supportive treatments such as intravenous fluid and tube feeding are often necessary. It is important to keep the skin soft and attempt to reduce scaling. The collodion membrane should not be removed.

Treatment may include regular emollients such as petrolatum to keep the skin moist, pain relief, mild topical steroids to reduce secondary inflammation, and artificial tears if there is severe outward turning of the eyelid.

The life expectancy and difficulties that the collodion baby faces depend upon the particular underlying condition.

colloid milium A papular skin disease that usually occurs on the face that has been extensively overexposed to the sun. The condition consists of degenerated COLLAGEN.

comedo Another name for BLACKHEAD (open comedo). The plural of comedo is comedones.

composite cultured skin (CCS) A wound dressing made of living human cells taken from the skin of healthy donors, used to treat children with a rare skin disease called recessive dystrophic EPIDERMOLYSIS BULLOSA (RDEB). The cells are grown on a sponge made from cow COLLAGEN (a protein found in skin and bones). When applied to a wound, CCS serves as a temporary protective dressing that allows the body's cells to grow.

In RDEB, BLISTERs and sores appear on the skin, (especially the fingers and toes), which can produce SCARs that makes the fingers grow together so that the hand looks like a mitten. The child's affected hand is surgically rebuilt, using pieces of the child's own skin for grafts and flaps as needed. CCS may be used along with pieces of the child's own skin to cover wounds created during the rebuilding of the affected hand. CCS eliminates the need for taking skin from the patient's own body, lessening the chance of complications.

The new type of cultured skin product was approved by the U.S. Food and Drug Administration (FDA) in spring 2001.

Epidermolysis bullosa is such a severe disease that the FDA approved the use of artificial skin under special humanitarian rules that allow hospitals to use it to operate on carefully selected patients.

The product is similar to other artificial skin already used to treat hard-to-heal wounds; a competing product (see APLIGRAF) also is being studied as a possible treatment for EB.

concealing creams See CAMOUFLAGE COSMETICS.

conditioner Products whose ingredients change the surface structure of the hair, allowing it to be more manageable. These structural changes in the surface texture also provide softness and sheen.

Conditioners are made up of ingredients that cling to the hair cuticle; some conditioners penetrate and bind with the cuticle in a tight chemical bond. While shampoos and conditioners share many ingredients, their combinations and sequences vary widely.

Most conditioners contain basically the same ingredients: water, slip agents, and lubricants (dimethicone and cyclomethicone), quaternary compounds, thickeners, and more lubricants (stearyl alcohol, cetyl alcohol, protein, or balsam), humectants (propylene glycol, glycerin, sodium PCA, mucopolysaccharides, hyaluronic acid), preservatives, fragrance, and coloring agents. Many conditioners also add more exotic "natural" ingredients to appeal to consumers.

There *are* differences between conditioners, depending on the hair's condition, and there are differences in amounts of specific ingredients (some of which are better than others).

Beauty experts caution that most consumers apply conditioner improperly. Instead of applying near the top of the head and working it toward the ends, consumers should bend over and apply conditioner to ends first, using little or none on the roots. Sparing the roots helps to avoid weighing them down.

condylomata acuminata A type of GENITAL WART caused by infection with the human papilloma virus. Found throughout the world, the disorder is often diagnosed in sexually transmitted disease clinics, since the warts are usually spread by sexual contact.

Symptoms and Diagnostic Path

The WARTS primarily appear in the moist genital folds and creases, and while just one wart may appear, they are more commonly found in heaped-up bunches that form cauliflower-like masses. They are subject to injury and can bleed, although they are generally painless.

Giant condylomata acuminata can invade local tissue (Buschke-Lowenstein tumor), which may rarely develop into squamous cell carcinoma.

Treatment Options and Outlook

There is no known treatment to specifically eradicate human papilloma virus from the skin. The virus may survive even the most aggressive treatment, such as lasers. Recurrence, therefore, is common. Treatment is aimed at physically removing warts in the patient, and in affected sexual partners. Condoms should be worn to help reduce transmission.

Most lesions in moist areas can be treated with podophyllum resin in tincture of benzoin, which a doctor can paint on the lesion. It is then washed off four hours later. Extensive areas should not be treated at one time, since absorption of the resin can be toxic. For the same reason, pregnant women should not be treated.

The active chemical in podophyllum resin has been identified and is now available in the prescription product Condylax.

CRYOSURGERY (freezing) with liquid nitrogen is often effective, and it is nontoxic and does not require anesthesia. CURETTAGE AND ELECTRODESICCATION may also be successful.

While alpha interferon is available for treatment of resistant cases, it is not frequently recommended because of its high likelihood of toxicity, low effectiveness, and expense.

The CARBON DIOXIDE LASER and more conventional surgery may also be helpful in cases of extensive growths, especially for those who have not responded to other treatments.

In pregnant patients, cryotherapy is most effective. Birth control pills are believed to cause the warts to grow. Therefore, women taking birth control pills should stop taking the pills before the warts can be successfully treated.

Risk Factors and Preventive Measures

Because these warts are easily spread, sexual contact with affected individuals should be avoided.

See also PAPILLOMA VIRUS, HUMAN.

congenital absence of skin See APLASIA CUTIS.

congenital disorders of the skin A range of skin disorders can be present at birth. These include abnormalities of KERATIN such as ICHTHYOSIS; of pigment, such as CONGENITAL TISSUE NEVI and PIEBALDISM; of fat, such as lipodystrophy; of blood vessels, such as PORT-WINE STAINS and HEMANGIOMAS; of nerves, such as NEUROFIBROMATOSIS; and TUBEROUS SCLEROSIS.

connective tissue diseases See COLLAGEN DISEASES.

connective tissue nevi A group of rare conditions (sometimes inherited) characterized by lesions and tumors of the connective tissues of the skin. The lesions are usually normal or slightly yellowish colored. They include ELASTOMAS, COLLAGENOMAS, SHAGREEN PATCH and BUSCHKE-OLLENDORF SYNDROME.

Treatment Options and Outlook

No treatment is necessary for most connective tissue lesions, since they do not cause any severe cosmetic defects. Surgical removal is occasionally performed.

Conradi's disease Also known medically as "chondrodysplasia punctata," this genetic disorder is characterized by skin abnormalities in 30 percent of patients, together with facial abnormalities and congenital cataracts. At birth, the skin is dry and cracked, especially around hair follicles; some hair loss also may occur.

See also HAIR, DISEASES OF.

contact dermatitis See DERMATITIS, CONTACT.

contracture A deformity caused by shrinkage of scar tissue in the skin or connective tissue. They are common following extensive BURNS, and can restrict movement.

corn A small area of thickened skin (CALLUS) with a hard core, usually found on the toe, caused by the pressure of a tight shoe. Patients with high arches suffer most from corns, because the arch increases the pressure on the tips of toes while walking. "Soft corns" are caused by the rubbing of two bones from adjacent toes; they remain slightly softer than "hard corns" because of foot perspiration. Women with wide feet who wear pointed shoes are vulnerable to getting corns.

Treatment Options and Outlook

Different shoes may make the corn gradually disappear. Corns should not be pared with a sharp instrument.

Until the corn disappears, a corn pad may be used to cushion surrounding skin from pressure. The pad should be cut into the shape of a horseshoe, not an oval (which can make the corn bulge through the oval opening in the middle). The pad should be placed far enough behind the corn so it would not rub.

A nonprescription corn plaster (as a liquid, salve or disk) should be applied to the corn to shield it. Because the plasters contain harsh acids that may burn normal skin as well as the corn, patients should use them with caution. If irritation develops, they should not be used for a day or two.

At the first sign of pain, a bit of lanolin can be used to soften the corn; a pad on the area can relieve pressure. A few strands of lambswool or a toe separator/spacer can be placed between the toes to keep them from rubbing together.

corn oil A vegetable oil that can be used as an emollient. Corn oil is not usually associated with allergic reactions.

cornstarch A starch derived from corn kernels, used as a nonabrasive powder for irritated skin. Although cornstarch may encourage fungal skin infections (especially in people with diabetes), some experts suggest using a powder made of cornstarch instead of talcum powder. Reports have linked talcum powder with cancer and higher rates of ovarian cancer in women using talcum powder in the genital area, but experts at the National Institutes of Health conclude the data on talc are inconclusive.

corrosive chemicals Certain corrosive chemicals (such as oven cleaners, drain cleaners, and dishwasher detergents) contain alkalizers, which can cause serious BURNS on the skin. Alkalizers (which have a pH of 11.5 or more) include potassium, sodium, ammonium, and calcium; of these, potassium hydroxide is the strongest. When considering the danger from these products, the higher the concentration of these ingredients in the alkalizer, the more serious the burn caused.

While most people think of acids as corrosive, an alkalizer is even more so; acid walls off its burn, while an alkalizer actually *spreads* in the skin, dissolving tissue as it goes.

Treatment Options and Outlook

Any severe burn should be treated in a hospital emergency room. For a mild alkalizer burn, the affected area should be washed in lukewarm water for at least 15 minutes (preferably longer). Any contaminated clothes or jewelry should be removed. If eyes are involved, contact lenses should be removed immediately. If the alkaline substance is solid, the skin should be scrubbed to make sure all particles are removed; a weak acid (such as vinegar, lemon, or orange juice diluted with four parts of water) should be used to neutralize the alkaline that may have penetrated deeper in tissues.

Exception: calcium oxide, or quicklime. Quicklime tends to absorb water and creates slaked lime, which gives off heat. The quicklime should be removed *before* it comes in contact with water. The skin should be oiled before the lime is wet, and a stream of water should be applied at high pressure to immediately remove oxide particles. Any lime left on the skin can cause burns.

Corrosive burns also can be caused by *strong acids*, such as a toilet bowl cleaner (usually sulfuric or hydrochloric acid). Unfortunately, these acids are not usually listed on the container. If these products contact the skin, the area should be washed with large amounts of lukewarm water for 15 to 30 minutes. Salves and ointments should not be applied to the burn.

corticosteroids A group of hormones similar to the natural hormones produced by the cortex of the adrenal glands. Developed more than 30 years ago, the first topical corticosteroid revolutionized dermatologic therapy with its strong anti-inflammatory properties; stronger and stronger compounds have been developed ever since.

They are used both on the skin and internally to treat a wide variety of skin disorders from mild ECZEMA to widespread blistering disorders such as PEMPHIGUS. Their broad anti-inflammatory effects are the basis for both the therapeutic benefits and the adverse reactions associated with use of these drugs.

Applied in the form of creams, ointments, lotions, and aerosols, their absorption is increased if the drug is applied when the skin is moist (such as right after bathing). Absorption of topical corticosteroids also varies with body location; absorption is greater through the layers of skin on the scalp, face, and genital area than on the forearm; as a result, these areas are more susceptible to the side effects of the drugs than other sites. Excessive use of over-the-counter topical steroids (especially on large areas of inflamed skin) can lead to more side effects and decreased therapeutic effects.

Some skin problems may be masked or worsened by using topical corticosteroids. Infections and infestations (especially candidiasis, IMPETIGO, and SCABIES) may be either worsened or hidden, and ROSACEA may be worsened by topical corticosteroids.

Side Effects

The incidence of adverse effects depends on dosage, the form of the drug, and how long it was administered. Side effects are uncommon when given as a cream or by inhaler because only small amounts of the drug are absorbed into the blood. Infants and children have a greater risk of developing adverse effects, and should be treated with topical corticosteroids of low potency.

Acute side effects can include atrophy and thinning of the skin, especially when used on the skin of the face.

Tablets taken in high doses for long periods may cause tissue swelling, high blood pressure, diabetes mellitus, ulcers, HIRSUTISM (excess hairiness), and (rarely) psychosis. High doses also increase the susceptibility to infection by interfering with the body's immune system. Because long-term use of these drugs suppresses the production of natural corticosteroid hormones, sudden withdrawal of the drug may lead to collapse, coma, and death. Corticosteroid dosages should always be tapered off in decreasing amounts.

cortisone A synthetic CORTICOSTEROID drug used to reduce inflammation in severe allergic, rheumatic and connective tissue diseases, among other things.

Side Effects

High doses for long periods of time can cause swelling, high blood pressure, diabetes, excess hairiness, and inhibited growth in children. They can also interfere with the immune system, leaving the patient vulnerable to illness. Sudden withdrawal of the drugs may lead to collapse, coma, and death.

cosmeceutical Cosmetic products that have medicinal or druglike benefits. The U.S. Food, Drug and Cosmetic Act defines a "drug" as something that cures, treats, mitigates, or prevents disease or that affects the structure or function of the human body. Cosmetics are not considered to be "drugs" because they do not alter the function of skin.

However, many skin products (such as GLYCOLIC ACID and RETINOL) are quite effective at rejuvenating skin. Because they are not considered drugs but are more effective than cosmetics, the new designation "cosmeceutical" has been applied. However, the Food, Drug and Cosmetic Act does not recognize the term "cosmeceutical." While drugs are subject to a review and approval process by the FDA, cosmetics—and cosmeceuticals—are not approved by the FDA prior to sale.

cosmetic acupuncture A specialized type of acupuncture designed to help tighten facial muscles and stimulate good circulation in facial skin. This nonsurgical treatment is purported to reduce the signs of aging by inserting very thin disposable needles into the acupuncture points on the face, which increases local circulation to the face and stimulates COLLAGEN production. This may fill out the lines and gives firmness to the skin.

Acupuncture has been used for thousands of years to treat many conditions and illnesses. The effectiveness of acupuncture has been related to the manipulation of the energy points on the body to balance and to remove blockages in the meridians (channels of blood and energy) to stay healthy and prevent diseases.

A 1996 report in the international journal of *Clinical Acupuncture* reported that among 300 cases treated with cosmetic acupuncture, 90 percent had noticeable effects after one course of treatment. However, this work has not been reproduced.

Cosmetic acupuncture is said to take between five and 10 years off the face, helping eliminate fine lines and make the deeper lines look softer. It also supposedly helps to minimize dark circles, puffy eyes, double chin, sagging skin, and dropping eyelids, relax muscle tone, tighten the pores, and brighten the eyes. It also moisturizes the skin from inside.

Procedure

In this process, needles are inserted into acupuncture points on the face (and sometimes on the body), followed by a moisturizing facial massage. Several treatments are usually required for best results.

cosmetic allergy About 6 percent of all allergic skin reactions are linked to cosmetics, although this number is declining because of more sophisticated testing of cosmetic products.

While "HYPOALLERGENIC," "allergy-tested" or "dermatologist-approved" labels seem to indicate a safe choice for those allergic to cosmetics, in fact these labels are not regulated by the government and do not guarantee that the product has been any more extensively tested than any other cosmetic.

The U.S. Food and Drug Administration has not established a legal definition of such terms as "hypoallergenic" and while only a few products may actually be labeled "dermatologist tested," in fact most cosmetic safety testing is performed by dermatologists who work for private cosmetic-testing labs.

Experts do agree that even the best products labeled "hypo-allergenic" do not guarantee than *no one* will experience a reaction; the label simply means that these products are *less* likely to cause an allergic reaction.

Hypo-allergenic means that a manufacturer has tried to eliminate as many of the known common sensitizing ingredients as possible (such as flavorings, some preservatives, and fragrances) and has tried to cut out manufacturing by-products that might contaminate the final product. Manufacturers also work closely with dermatologists to find out the source of allergies to their products by providing samples of the individual ingredients for testing.

Those with highly sensitive skin should choose products that are labeled "fragrance free," since many studies have determined that it is the fragrance in a product that *most often* causes an allergic reaction. However, consumers should understand that "unscented" is *not* the same as "fragrance free"—an unscented product often contains masking fragrances to neutralize unpleasant odors.

As a general rule, all consumers should apply cosmetics carefully near the eye, since this area is the most vulnerable to an allergic reaction, due to the thin, sensitive nature of the skin here.

If consumers suspect they may be allergic to a product, they should bring it (along with package and ingredients label) to a dermatologist. The American Academy of Dermatology allows any board-certified dermatologist to obtain help from most cosmetic companies in determining the ingredients list of specific products.

Cosmetic Ingredient Review (CIR) Expert Panel
An unbiased panel of scientific experts that was established in 1976 by the COSMETIC, TOILETRY, AND FRAGRANCE ASSOCIATION (CTFA), to check the safety of ingredients used in cosmetics.

Although funded by CTFA, CIR and the review process are distinctly separate from CTFA and the cosmetic industry. The heart of the CIR program is the independent Expert Panel consisting of world-renowned physicians and scientists who review the available data. Expert Panel members must be free of any conflicts of interest and must meet the same conflict-of-interest requirements as outside experts to the U.S. Food and Drug Administration (FDA).

According to its 1999 Annual Report, CIR has found the following ingredients unsafe:

- *chloroacetamide* (a preservative), because of allergic reactions
- *ethoxyethanol* and *ethoxyethanol acetate* (a solvent), because of reproductive and developmental toxicity
- *HC Blue No. 1* (a hair coloring ingredient), because of possible carcinogenicity
- *p-Hydroxyanisole* (an antioxidant), because of skin depigmentation.
- *4-methoxy-m-phenylenediamine, 4-methoxy-m-phenylenediamine HCl,* and *4-methoxy-m-phenylenediamine sulfate* (hair dye ingredients), because of possible carcinogenicity.
- *pyrocatechol* (used in hair dyes and skin care preparations), because of carcinogenic and co-carcinogenic potential. (CIR describes this substance as unsafe for leave-on products and considers available data insufficient to assure safety for use in hair dyes.)

The seven CIR expert panel voting members include physicians and scientists who have been publicly nominated by consumer, scientific, and medical groups; government agencies; and industry. Three liaison members serve as nonvoting members representing the FDA, Consumer Federation of America, and CTFA. By uniting industry, consumers, and government, the expert panel creates a unique environment for discussions affecting public safety.

Working on the high-priority ingredients, CIR staff conduct extensive literature searches, compile data, and prepare draft reports. CIR staff organize the literature into chemistry, including physical properties and manufacture; use, including cosmetic and noncosmetic; general biology, including absorption, distribution, and metabolism; animal toxicology, including acute, short-term, subchronic, and chronic studies, as well as dermal irritation and sensitization; and a clinical assessment, which may include epidemiology studies along with classic repeat insult patch tests. In vitro test data are also gathered and incorporated into the review.

If the open, scientific literature does not contain enough information, the panel will order specific studies or provide previously unpublished data. After completion of a development process that includes multiple opportunities for public comment and open, public discussion of the report, a final report is issued. These final reports are available from CIR. Eventually, CIR final reports are published in the *International Journal of Toxicology*.

cosmetic ingredients, prohibited By law, the U.S. Food and Drug Administration does not have the authority to approve cosmetic products or ingredients, except for color additives. However, regulations prohibit or restrict the use of several ingredients because of safety concerns. In addition, cosmetic and fragrance trade associations have recommended avoiding or limiting the use of some substances.

Regulations specifically prohibit or restrict the use of the following ingredients in cosmetics:

- *Hexachlorophene:* Because of its neurotoxic effect and ability to penetrate human skin, hexachlorophene may be used only when an alternative preservative has not been shown to be as effective. The concentration of hexachlorophene may not exceed 0.1 percent, and it may not be used in cosmetics that in normal use may be applied to mucous membranes, such as the lips.
- *Mercury compounds:* Mercury compounds are readily absorbed through the skin on topical application and tend to accumulate in the body. They may cause allergic reactions, skin irritation, or neurotoxic manifestations. The use of mercury compounds as cosmetic ingredients is limited to eye area cosmetics at concentrations not exceeding 65 parts per million (0.0065 percent) of mercury calculated as the metal (about 100 ppm or 0.01 percent phenylmercuric acetate or nitrate) and provided no other effective and safe preservative is available for use. All other cosmetics containing mercury are subject to regulatory action unless it occurs in a trace amount of less than one part per million (0.0001 percent) and its presence is unavoidable under conditions of good manufacturing practice.

- *Chlorofluorocarbon propellants:* The use of chlorofluorocarbon propellants in cosmetic aerosol products intended for domestic consumption is prohibited.
- *Bithionol:* Prohibited because it may cause photocontact sensitization
- *Halogenated salicylanilides:* Prohibited because it may cause photocontact sensitization.
- *Chloroform:* Prohibited because of its animal carcinogenicity and likely hazard to human health
- *Vinyl chloride:* Prohibited as an ingredient of aerosol products, because of its carcinogenicity
- *Zirconium-containing complexes:* Prohibited in aerosol cosmetic products because of toxic effects on lungs
- *Methylene chloride:* Prohibited because of its animal carcinogenicity and likely hazard to human health

Color Additives

Color additives also are strictly regulated. In order to protect consumers from harmful contaminants, many cannot be used unless the color comes from a batch certified by the FDA and that batch is provided with its own individual certification lot number. Their uncertified counterparts are not allowed, and addition of the color to a product will make the entire product adulterated. While colors exempt from certification are not subject to such testing, manufacturers must assure that each color additive complies with the identity, specifications, labeling requirements, use, and restrictions of color additive regulations. With the exception of COAL-TAR hair dyes, all color additives, whether or not they are subject to certification, must be approved by the FDA for their intended use.

cosmetic labeling Federal regulations require ingredients to be listed on product labels in descending order by quantity. Consumers can check the ingredient listing to identify ingredients they wish to avoid. Based on the amount used, an ingredient such as water is usually found at the beginning of the product's ingredient listing, while additives and fragrances, used in small amounts, are normally seen at the end.

Cosmetic ingredients regulations apply only to retail products intended for home use. Products used exclusively by beauticians in beauty salons that are labeled "For Professional Use Only" and cosmetic samples such as those given out free at hotels and department stores are not required to include the ingredient declaration. However, these products must state the distributor, list the content's quantity, and include all necessary warning statements.

The Food and Drug Administration regulates only the labels that appear on cosmetic products themselves. Unfair and deceptive advertising that appears in magazines, in newspapers, or on television generally falls under the authority of the Federal Trade Commission.

cosmetics Preparations that are applied to the skin to enhance appearance. Since earliest times, women have been applying vegetable dyes and color pigments to their faces, pounding out preparations from leaves and flowers and natural ores. In 1992, Americans spent $3.5 billion on skin-care products alone—a 5.5 percent increase over 1991, according to the cosmetic consulting firm Kline & Co. At best, most cosmetics are only helpful in improving appearance; others may be actively harmful to the skin.

Cosmetics are not drugs, which are products that change the function or structure of the skin. For example, a deodorant is not a drug because it does not alter the body's sweating, it simply adds a perfume. But an antiperspirant *is* a drug, because it affects the function of the skin in order to decrease the amount of sweat.

While both cosmetics and drugs are regulated by the U.S. Food and Drug Administration, almost all of the FDA's time is taken up with drugs and very little is spent on investigating cosmetics. While cosmetics may be loosely regulated, they have been required to list their ingredients on the label since 1975, although they do not go into details regarding concentration or purity.

Ingredients

Cosmetics are made up of a variety of substances, including preservatives, stabilizers, emulsifiers, antioxidants, and so on. Preservatives are included in order to extend a product's shelf life. Most preservatives are divided into two types—antimicrobial agents and ANTIOXIDANTS. Antimicrobial agents, which work by inhibiting the growth of microbacteria and fungi in the cosmetic, include organic acids, alcohol, aldehydes, essential oils, ammonium compounds, mercury agents, phenolic agents, and acid agents. Antioxidants work by reducing oxidation and destruction of fats and oils in the product; they include both organic and inorganic agents. Preservatives are so important to the ingredients of cosmetics that preservative-free cosmetics would have to be kept in the refrigerator.

Cosmetics also contain some unusual ingredients. Squalene, used in moisturizers for its antibacterial qualities, originates in olives and sharks' livers. The red color found in many cosmetics is derived from carmine (crushed shells from a beetlelike slug). Some frosted eye shadows contain guanine (crushed fish scales). Ambergris (material coughed up by whales) was once coveted as a fragrance fixative, although cheaper fixatives are used today.

Contamination

Cosmetics should never be shared with anyone else. Bacteria, viruses, and fungi can all flourish in makeup. (There are no known cases of AIDS transmitted via cosmetics, however).

To counter the risk of infection, stores that once offered communal lipsticks and eye pencils are now using safer sampling products. For example, some companies now offer one-time-use tubes of mascara; other companies provide sterile swabs and sponges for consumers eager to sample the latest makeup shades. Some stores forbid their clerks to apply lipstick directly, even on someone's hand; instead, they use a new applicator for each customer. If consumers cannot find single-use makeup samples or fresh applicators, they should bring cotton swabs or applicators from home.

Choosing Cosmetics

Experts recommend that consumers should analyze their skin type before buying skin-care products. Consumers should always read labels to find out what ingredients are included. While HYPOALLERGENIC products have the simplest formulations, there is no guarantee that a reaction will not occur.

See also MAKEUP.

cosmetic surgery Operations performed to improve the appearance, instead of improving function or treating disease. Individuals seek out cosmetic surgery for a wide range of reasons, for example, to appear younger, to reduce too-large breasts, or resculpt a nose.

Cosmetic surgery can include operations of the brow and upper face and eyebrows to remove signs of aging; mid-face lift, to lift and restructure the mid-face; neck and chin (segmental meloplasty), to remove sagging excess neck skin and/or rebuild the chin; full FACE-LIFT (rhytidectomy) to lift the whole face; eyelids (blepharoplasty); nose (rhinoplasty) to reduce or reshape; abdomen (abdominal lipectomy) to remove excess fat tissue and skin; breast reduction/augmentation, to change the shape of the breast; ears (otoplasty) to pin back ears or change their shape; LIPOSUCTION, to remove excess fat; laser resurfacing chemical peels, and photorejuvenation to improve the appearance of the complexion.

Those who are contemplating cosmetic surgery should ask themselves the reasons why they want the operation, whether expectations for results are realistic, whether they can afford the procedure and whether they will be able to put up with the pain and other aftereffects.

Before a cosmetic operation, a responsible surgeon will ask a patient all the above questions, consult the persons medical history and ask about other surgeries. All options will be presented, and the surgery itself will be explained in detail.

See also ARGON LASER; CARBON DIOXIDE LASER; CHEMICAL FACE PEEL; COLLAGEN INJECTIONS; EYELID LIFT; FAT TRANSPLANTS; FIBREL; FREE-FLAP SURGERY; LASER TREATMENT; NOSE REPAIR; MAMMOPLASTY; LASER RESURFACING.

CosmoDerm or CosmoPlast Human-derived COLLAGEN used to repair wrinkles and other facial imperfections, and considered to be safer than bovine-derived collagen. Both products have been approved for cosmetic corrective use by the U.S. Food and Drug Administration.

CosmoDerm is used for minor skin defects, and CosmoPlast is used for defects that are more significant. This technique typically lasts between three and four months.

See also SKIN FILLERS.

coumarin (Coumadin) necrosis Another name for an anticoagulation syndrome, this severe reaction to the anticoagulant drug coumarin occurs infrequently, usually in young women. The reaction begins between three and 10 days after beginning treatment with a coumarin drug such as dicumarol or warfarin. Neither stopping nor continuing the drug changes the course of the lesions, once they appear.

They begin as tiny red spots or a blue-purple hemorrhagic patch, quickly followed by tissue death, which can extend deep into the subcutaneous fat and take months to heal. About 80 percent of the lesions occur on the lower body, such as the thighs, abdomen, and breasts (especially in areas filled with subcutaneous fat).

The condition has been associated with a lack of protein C, a vitamin K-dependent plasma protein that interferes with blood clotting.

See also HEPARIN NECROSIS.

Cowden's disease An inherited skin disease that appears in childhood or puberty, characterized by shiny PAPULES on the face, palms, tongue, and in the mouth area. There is also a strong association between Cowden's disease and the development of breast cancer in women, and thyroid and gastrointestinal cancer in males and females.

Cowden's disease is an autosomal dominant disorder, which means that only one defective gene (from one parent) is needed to cause the syndrome. Each child of an affected person usually has a one in two chance of inheriting the defective gene and of being affected, and a one in two chance of being unaffected.

Treatment Options and Outlook
Facial lesions can be removed with electrocautery by surgery or with laser therapy.

Risk Factors and Preventive Measures
Some experts suggest that bilateral preventive mastectomies should be carefully considered for women with a strong personal or a strong family history of Cowden's disease.

crab lice See LICE.

cradle cap A harmless, common skin condition in infants in which thick yellow scales form in patches over the scalp. It is a form of SEBORRHEIC DERMATITIS, which also may occur on the face, neck, behind the ears, and in the diaper area. Without treatment, it may persist for months but, when properly cared for, usually fades away within a few weeks.

Treatment Options and Outlook
The baby's hair should be washed with baby shampoo or a mild anti-dandruff shampoo once a day; after lathering, the scaly scalp should be massaged with a soft toothbrush for a few minutes. For very crusty conditions, olive or mineral oil should be rubbed into the baby's scalp an hour before a shampoo. The oil loosens and softens the scales, which can then be washed off. All the oil must be washed out, because if this is left in the hair it could aggravate the problem.

This treatment may need to be repeated for several days until all the scales are washed off. Baby's hair should be brushed daily with a soft-bristle brush to help loosen scales that can then be removed with a fine-tooth comb.

A physician should be consulted if the skin looks inflamed or the condition worsens. A mild corticosteroid solution or cream may be prescribed until the condition clears.

Risk Factors and Preventive Measures
Once the condition has improved, cradle cap can be prevented from recurring by frequent hair washing with a mild baby shampoo. Occasionally, a stronger medicated shampoo may be needed, but a pediatrician should make the decision. After the child's first birthday, the condition will not recur until puberty.

Sometimes, YEAST INFECTIONS become superimposed on the affected skin, most likely in the crease areas rather than on the scalp. If this occurs, the area will become extremely reddened and quite itchy. In this case, the pediatrician might prescribe specific anti-yeast cream containing the medicine Nystatin.

cream, cleansing An emulsifier that is really a soap, and therefore more alkaloid than the pH of the skin. Cleansing creams are all basically variations on old formulas containing borax, water, mineral oil, and bees-wax. Cleansing lotions and aerosol foams are basically variations of the same product in a different format.

Soap and water are better at removing oily dirt from the skin, but cleansing creams are better at removing oily makeup. Because of their alkalinity, cleansing creams can be irritating to sensitive skin.

See also COSMETICS; MAKEUP; SOAP AND THE SKIN.

CREST phenomenon Acronym for a condition that includes the symptoms of "calcinosis (abnormal calcium deposits in the skin), RAYNAUD'S PHENOMENON, esophageal dysmotility, sclerodactyly and telangiectasia." It is found in a group of patients with progressive systemic sclerosis.

Cronkhite-Canada disease An extremely rare disorder characterized by multiple benign growths in the intestines and stomach, loss of scalp hair, widespread areas of dark spots on the skin, and the loss of fingernails. The skin symptoms are thought to be due to protein loss and malabsorption.

Usually reported in older men, Cronkhite-Canada syndrome is relentlessly progressive, with a poor prognosis. However, cases of spontaneous remission have been reported following aggressive nutritional support.

Cross-McKusick-Breen syndrome A very rare disorder featuring lack of skin color.

Symptoms and Diagnostic Path

In addition to altered skin color, symptoms include mental retardation, short stature, writhing movements, and gingival fibromatosis.

Treatment Options and Outlook

Patients with this syndrome should avoid the midday sun and use UVA-UVB sunscreen. Sunglasses will help combat eye sensitivity to light. While neither BETA-CAROTENE nor PUVA can offer solar protection, beta-carotene may help improve skin color.

crotamiton cream (Trade name: Eurax lotion) A treatment for SCABIES that is not particularly effective. Experts suggest that five daily applications may be better than the two currently recommended, but current data are not conclusive. Its toxicity is unknown; it is applied to the whole body below the neck, left on for 48 hours, and then washed off.

cryosurgery The surgical destruction of tissue using below-freezing temperatures.

The standard agent for this type of surgery is liquid nitrogen at −195.6° C. Carbon dioxide is less often used. The liquid nitrogen is applied to the skin with a cotton-tipped applicator or via a Cryospray unit for five to 30 seconds, depending on the diagnosis. Cryotherapy precludes the need for anesthesia, which makes the procedure simpler than cold steel surgery. Dressings are usually not required after treatment. The area is washed twice daily with mild soap and water followed by application of an antibiotic ointment to prevent bacterial infection. Most lesions are red and scaly for several days to a few weeks, eventually crumbling away and leaving a smooth surface behind. A BLISTER may form and may cause mild discomfort.

Because it involves minimal scarring, it is especially helpful for cosmetic reasons.

The most common use of cryotherapy is for the treatment of lentigines (liver spots), SEBORRHEIC KERATOSES, ACTINIC KERATOSES, WARTS and MOLLUSCUM CONTAGIOSUM. Skin cancers, such as BASAL CELL CARCINOMA and some in-situ SQUAMOUS CELL CARCINOMAS, also may be treated with cryotherapy. Some lesions may require more than one treatment (usually spaced three weeks apart).

Risks and Complications

Complications may include HYPOPIGMENTATION or, less often, scarring.

Outlook and Lifestyle Modification

Some malignant lesions (basal cell or squamous cell carcinomas) treated with aggressive cryosurgery have reported cure rates of 95 percent.

cryptococcosis A rare FUNGAL INFECTION caused by inhaling *Cryptococcus neoformans*, found throughout the world, especially in soil contaminated with pigeon droppings. Although it usually affects adults, infection can occur at any age, especially among those already ill with cancer, such as leukemia or lymphoma, or those who have suppressed immune systems (such as patients with AIDS). Infection with this fungus is unusual in patients who are otherwise healthy. In the United States, 85 percent of cases occur in HIV-infected patients.

Symptoms and Diagnostic Path
While meningitis is the more usual and serious form of the disease, the infection also can cause a range of granular lesions, including ulcers, ABSCESSES, tumors, PAPULES, and nodules into the skin and lungs.

Treatment Options and Outlook
Fluconazole freely passes through the central nervous system and is the drug of choice; intravenous AMPHOTERICIN B and oral FLUCYTOSINE also may be helpful. If untreated, this infection may be fatal.

cucumber   As a fresh vegetable or in extracts, the naturally acidic cucumber contains VITAMIN C and CHLOROPHYLL; slices of cucumber can be helpful in soothing tired, puffy eyes. While the fresh cucumber can be beneficial, heavily processed commercial extracts do not usually contain any beneficial ingredients.

curettage and electrodesiccation   The removal of tissue with a sharp instrument called a curet, followed by electrosurgery in which tissue is destroyed by burning with an electric spark. Bleeding also can be stopped by electrodesiccation. Curettage is often used to remove WARTS, SEBORRHEIC KERATOSES, and BASAL CELL CARCINOMA.

Procedure
In the procedure, the bulk of a lesion is first removed with a curet under local anesthesia and the base is destroyed afterwards with electrodesiccation. Because the current does not penetrate very deeply, scooping out tissue with a curet increases the efficiency of the procedure.

For treating most basal and some SQUAMOUS CELL CANCERS, the procedure is usually repeated three times.

cutaneous atrophy   The medical term for thinning of the skin. It is a normal part of aging resulting in the loss of substance from the first two layers of the skin. In this condition, the skin is thin, easily wrinkled and fragile, with blood vessels showing through the skin. Multiple bruises (called Bateman's purpura) are also common, and minute tears in the skin on the backs of the hands and forearms may cause scars. This condition is most likely to occur in areas of aged skin exposed to excessive amounts of sunlight. Atrophy may also result from some inflammatory skin conditions or as a type of scarring.

cutaneous diphtheria   A bacterial infection common in the tropics, but also found in Canada and the southern United States. It is caused by the organism *Corynebacterium diphtheriae*, normally found in the mucous membranes of the nose and throat and probably on human skin.

Diphtheria is rare in the United States and Europe, where health officials have been immunizing children against it for decades. In the United States, fewer than five cases have occurred each year since 1980, according to the Centers for Disease Control and Prevention. Most cases of diphtheria occur in unvaccinated or inadequately vaccinated people. Diphtheria poses a threat to U.S. citizens who may not be fully immunized and who travel to other countries or have contact with immigrants or international travelers coming to the United States.

Symptoms and Diagnostic Path
Superficial ulcers on the skin with a gray-yellow or brown-gray membrane in the early stages that can be peeled off; later, a black or brown-black scab appears, surrounded by a tender inflammatory area.

Treatment and Options and Outlook
Antibiotics and specific antitoxins are useful. Oral penicillin V potassium is effective in mild cases. While the antibiotics will inhibit the growth of the bacteria, diphtheria antitoxin is required to inactivate the toxin. Complications and death are very rare.

Risk Factors and Preventive Measures
Today, diphtheria in the United States and other developed countries is extremely rare because the triple DPT vaccine (against diphtheria, pertussis,

and tetanus) is given routinely to children in the first year of life.

cutaneous focal mucinosis   See MUCINOSES.

cutaneous infections, noninvasive   See TINEA.

cutaneous tag   See SKIN TAGS.

cuticle   A layer of solid or semisolid material that covers the EPITHELIUM.

cutis   The skin.

cutis hyperelastica   The medical name for EHLERS-DANLOS SYNDROME.

cutis laxa   A group of genetic or acquired diseases of the connective tissue characterized by loss of normal skin elasticity, resulting in skin abnormalities that may either be generalized or localized.

Symptoms and Diagnostic Path

Generalized cutis laxa, also called generalized elastolysis, is characterized by loose folds of skin on the sides of the face, leading to sagging jowls and a bloodhound appearance. It appears around puberty or later. Changes appear in connective tissues in other parts of the body, leading to pulmonary emphysema, gastrointestinal tract and bladder problems, and multiple hernias. In its most severe form, the saggy skin over the entire body (not just sun-exposed areas) produces a striking appearance of old age.

Congenital forms of cutis laxa are characterized by loose, pendulous skin present at birth or shortly thereafter, giving the child a prematurely aged appearance. The skin can be pulled up but will not spring back when released. Multiple organs may be affected because of the defect in supporting structure.

Localized forms of cutis laxa may be hereditary, and may occur only in certain areas of the body as an independent disorder or as a part of the generalized form of the disease. The localized form may be the only expression of the disease, or it may be a precursor for later development of a more widespread form.

Blepharochalasis (abnormal looseness of the eyelids) may result from aging or may begin early in life. In the localized form, there may be coin-sized areas of loss of tissue in the skin, with out-pouching of underlying tissue. These patches may appear spontaneously, or after the skin has been injured by inflammation or disease (such as SYPHILIS, ERYTHEMA MULTIFORME, ACNE, HIVES, CHICKEN POX) Lesions will continue to appear throughout life, although most appear during childhood and adolescence.

Treatment Options and Outlook

There is no helpful treatment for either the generalized or the localized form of cutis laxa. Any attempt at surgical tightening is followed by prompt reappearance of the skin folds.

Patients with the localized form should avoid injury that could lead to inflammation and new lesions.

Unattractive lesions can be surgically excised, but the wounds may not heal well and the scars may spread and gape.

cutis marmorata telangiectatica congenita   Also known as van Lohuizen's disease, this congenital circulatory disorder causes an exaggerated network marbling (fixed LIVEDO RETICULARIS) of the skin of the trunk, legs and arms, face, and scalp.

Symptoms and Diagnostic Path

The demarcation between normal and abnormal skin is sharp and often seen at the midline. In addition, ulcers may appear on the affected skin. The condition usually improves with time.

Other symptoms include atrophy of the soft tissues and bones of the affected part. Other developmental abnormalities also can occur. HEMANGIOMAS and areas of nevus flammeus may be associated with this disorder.

This disease should not be confused with cutis marmorata, which is the term used to describe the normal transient physiological reaction of mottled blue skin in reaction to the cold that is seen in about half of all normal children and adults.

Treatment Options and Outlook
Only local treatment is needed if complications such as ulcers develop.

cyanosis Bluish discoloration of the skin due to an excess of deoxygenated hemoglobin in the blood, most easily seen in the nail beds of fingers and toes, and on lips and tongue. It occurs most often when blood flow through the skin slows down because of cold; however, this type of cyanosis is not serious and does not indicate any underlying disease.

In other instances, cyanosis can be a serious symptom of disease. It may indicate poor blood circulation in the extremities, in which fingers and toes turn blue even when the environment is fairly warm. Cyanosis also may be a sign of heart problems (such as heart failure) or fluid in the lungs.

Cyanosis present at birth could be a sign of congenital heart disease in which some of the blood does not reach the lungs to pick up oxygen but instead goes directly to the rest of the body.

cyclophosphamide (Trade names: Cytoxan and Neosar) An anticancer drug that has been used with some success in those with PEMPHIGUS and BULLOUS PEMPHIGOID. Other skin diseases that may respond to this drug include LUPUS ERYTHEMATOSUS, and PYODERMA GANGRENOSUM and in some types of vasculitis, such as Wegener's granulofosus. Patients with advanced forms of mycosis fungoides have been treated with chemotherapy combinations including cyclophosphamide.

Side Effects
Common side effects are hair loss, nausea, vomiting, and cystitis. Cystitis may be avoided if the patient drinks plenty of water shortly before and up to two hours after taking the drug orally followed by frequent urination. Less common side effects include mouth ulcers, increased discoloration of skin and nails, jaundice, clotting abnormalities, the complete absence of sperm, or lack of ovulation. This drug causes birth defects.

cyclopiroxolamine (ciclopiroxolamine) (Trade name: Loprox) A topical agent used to treat fungus infections that inhibits the growth of dermatophytes (microscopic fungi), *Candida albicans,* and the agent causing TINEA VERSICOLOR (a type of RINGWORM).

cyclosporine An immunosuppressant drug derived from soil fungus that suppresses the body's natural defense against abnormal cells. Introduced in 1984, it is used primarily to prevent and treat organ transplant rejection. It is also helpful in the treatment of skin diseases such as recalcitrant PSORIASIS, pemphigus vulgaris, GRAFT-VERSUS-HOST DISEASE, and BEHCET'S SYNDROME. Benefits from cyclosporine have also been reported in patients with severe atopic DERMATITIS, ALOPECIA, ICHTHYOSIS vulgaris, EPIDERMOLYSIS BULLOSA acquisita, PYODERMA GANGRENOSUM, systemic LUPUS ERYTHEMATOSUS, cutaneous T-cell lymphoma, and SARCOIDOSIS.

Side Effects
Because cyclosporine interferes with the immune system, patients treated with this drug are more susceptible to infection. Any flulike illness or localized infection requires immediate medical attention. Because cyclosporine is metabolized primarily by the liver, patients with liver disease may experience problems with this drug.

In addition, the drug has been found to cause kidney problems; therefore, regular kidney function monitoring is necessary for anyone being given this drug. If signs of kidney damage appear (such as protein in the urine), the dosage needs to be reduced or other drugs may be substituted. In many people, kidney problems disappear after the drug is stopped, but some people experience irreversible kidney damage from use of cyclosporine.

Other side effects may include high blood pressure, gastrointestinal problems, fatigue, development of secondary cancer (primarily lymphomas), and infections. Another fairly common side effect is swelling of the gums and hairiness.

Cymetra A micronized version of ALLODERM soft tissue filler that is rehydrated with the anesthetic lidocaine in the physician's office before injection so the procedure is much less painful. Cymetra is approved for cosmetic corrective use, but it is not recommended for use between the eyes or around the eye area. It is effective for nasal-labial folds and lip enhancement.

See also SKIN FILLERS.

cyst A closed cavity or sac containing a liquid or semisolid material beneath the skin. Cysts may be caused by a variety of reasons; those affecting the skin may be caused by a blocked duct leading from a fluid-forming sebaceous gland to the skin gland. While these cysts are benign, they may become unsightly and may be surgically removed.

Other types of skin cysts include DERMOID cysts, a type of skin cyst that may contain particles of hair follicles, sweat glands, nerves, and even teeth.

Dermoid cysts are found in parts of the body that fused during fetal development. Sometimes a dermoid cyst may appear after an injury. Treatment is surgical removal.

cytotoxic drugs, skin side effects of Anticancer drugs that kill or damage cells also may cause HYPERPIGMENTATION (darkening of the skin). While cytotoxic drugs primarily affect abnormal cells, they can also damage or kill healthy cells, especially those that multiply rapidly, such as in the skin.

Cytotoxic drugs that may affect the skin include BLEOMYCIN, which causes the skin to become deeply tanned because of pigment cell stimulation. In addition, cyclophosphamide and melphalan can cause bands of hyperpigmentation of the skin and in the nails.

cytotoxic drugs for skin diseases There are several cytotoxic drugs that can be used in the treatment of a variety of skin diseases. These include AZATHIOPRINE (Imuran), CYCLOPHOSPHA-MIDE (Cytoxan), HYDROXYUREA (Hydrea), and METHOTREXATE.

D

dandruff A harmless very common condition (also called SEBORRHEA) in which the scalp sheds dead skin, producing unattractive white flakes in the hair that often fall onto the collar and shoulders. When it worsens into an itchy, inflamed scalp rash, it is called seborrheic dermatitis (see DERMATITIS, SEBORRHEIC), and is also found on the face, back, and chest.

Treatment Options and Outlook

While no cure for dandruff exists, consumers find some relief with frequent shampooing; the more often, the easier it is to control dandruff. Because dandruff is often caused by an oily scalp, a mild nonmedicated shampoo may be enough to control the problem.

If the mild shampoo is not effective, an anti-dandruff product may work. Those with selenium sulfide or zinc pyrithione offer the quickest results by slowing down the rate at which scalp cells multiply, but no matter which type of anti-dandruff shampoo is used, the lather should not be rinsed off too quickly.

Products with SALICYLIC ACID and SULFUR loosen up the dandruff so it can be washed away, while antibacterial shampoos reduce bacteria on the scalp. Very stubborn cases may respond to tar shampoos, which work by slowing down cell growth; the tar lather should be left on the hair for up to 10 minutes so the tar can work. (Blond or silver hair may be stained by tar compounds.)

More and more dermatologists prescribe antifungal shampoos (such as Nizoral 2 percent shampoo) to curb flaking by controlling the growth of a yeast that occurs naturally on the scalp. Other choices include a corticosteroid cream or lotion to apply to the scalp.

dapsone (4,4'-diaminodiphenyl-sulfone) An antibacterial drug that has been used to treat resistant ACNE, LEPROSY, and DERMATITIS HERPETIFORMIS. Results with this drug, the most often-used of the sulfones, have been variable, but in some cases there have been excellent results. Its mechanism of action is unknown, although it does interfere with neutrophil function. Other diseases that may be treated with dapsone include bullous diseases and PYODERMA GANGRENOSUM.

The introduction of the sulfones in the 1950s had a dramatic impact on the treatment of leprosy. Of these, dapsone was the first safe and effective drug available, killing the bacteria (*Mycobacterium leprae*) and eliminating the need for patient isolation. Although resistance to dapsone is becoming widespread, it remains the drug of choice in the treatment of leprosy in conjunction with other medication.

Side Effects

The adverse effects of this drug tend to be dose-related, and adverse effects are uncommon with low doses. Concerns over safety may have been exaggerated by the high doses used in some early studies, according to some experts.

Severe allergic reactions may occur, including TOXIC EPIDERMAL NECROLYSIS and STEVENS-JOHNSON SYNDROME. Other side effects may include nausea, vomiting and rarely, damage to the liver, red blood cells, and nerves. There may also be sensory and significant motor nerve problems. During long-term treatment, blood tests are conducted to monitor liver function and the red blood cell level.

Neurological symptoms (such as psychosis) are believed to be dose-related; those with a history of psychiatric problems may be more likely to develop mental problems on this drug.

The cases of agranulocytosis (deficiency of blood cells due to bone marrow damage) seen among troops in Vietnam taking dapsone to prevent malaria could have been caused by concurrent use of other antimalarial drugs. According to reports, millions of patients have been successfully treated with dapsone for years with relatively low rates of toxic side effects.

Darier's disease Known medically as keratosis follicularis, this is a disorder of KERATINIZATION (the process whereby cells become horny as they approach the surface of the skin); it affects the skin, mucous membranes and nails. An uncommon inherited disease, this disorder usually begins in childhood or adolescence and gets worse following exposure to ULTRAVIOLET RADIATION.

Patients are also at risk for secondary bacterial infection and for serious, widespread viral skin infections usually due to the herpes simplex virus.

It is inherited in an autosomal dominant pattern, which means that a single gene from one parent causes the condition. The child of an affected parent has a 50 percent chance of inheriting the abnormal gene, but not all people with the abnormal gene will develop symptoms of the disease.

The abnormal gene involved in the development of Darier's disease has been identified as *ATP2A2*, found on chromosome 12q23-24.1. The exact way this abnormal gene causes the disease is still under investigation, but it seems as if the way skin cells join together may be disrupted if there is insufficient calcium.

Symptoms and Diagnostic Path

Itchy, greasy, foul-smelling brown papules form plaques on scalp, ears, face, neck, and upper trunk—these lesions are often induced by sunlight. Distinctive nail changes include fragile, short and relatively wide nails with notching, ridging, and red and white linear streaks. Darier's disease is diagnosed by its appearance and family history, but it is often mistaken for other skin problems. A skin biopsy may be required for a definitive diagnosis.

Treatment Options and Outlook

Patients with mild disease should avoid sun exposure and use SUNSCREEN. Secondary infections should be treated with antibiotics. Wet compresses and tap water soaks can help lessen odor and crusts, and DERMABRASION may be effective in mild cases. Synthetic retinoids (ACITRETIN or ISOTRETINOIN) often induce remission, but chronic use is often necessary to prevent relapse. Because many patients on long-term retinoids have developed diffuse skeletal abnormalities this chronic administration is rarely justified.

Deep dermabrasion followed by skin grafts may help some patients with severe problems.

While the disease comes and goes, there is a tendency for it to become more severe over time.

Darier's sign Itching and hives that occur after stroking or rubbing lesions of URTICARIA PIGMENTOSA.

Darier-White disease See DARIER'S DISEASE.

decubitus ulcer Another name for BEDSORES.

Degos' disease The common name for malignant atrophic papulosis, this is a rare disease, occurring most often in men.

Symptoms and Diagnostic Path

Symptoms include porcelain-white skin lesions (from five to more than 100) in the skin and gastrointestinal tract. Up to 60 percent of the patients with this disease develop these lesions in the gastrointestinal area, which results in loss of blood to the area and subsequent tissue death in weeks or years; these complications are usually fatal.

Treatment Options and Outlook

There is no effective treatment, but patients with skin lesions only have a good prognosis. Those with lesions in the gastrointestinal have a more serious and sometimes fatal outcome.

delusion of bromhidrosis The psychotic belief that a person's own body odor is profoundly offensive. This problem usually occurs during adolescence, often in conjunction with fastidious habits and no body odor. These patients usually show an ambivalent sexuality and little emotion.

Treatment Options and Outlook

There are no published data regarding the treatment of this disorder with pimozide, the drug used to treat Tourette syndrome and DELUSIONS OF PARASITOSIS. The patient's delusion must never be reinforced. Outlook is very poor for these patients, who often go on to develop serious mental illness.

delusions of parasitosis The erroneous belief that the skin is infested with parasites. Most patients also suffer from some type of mental disorder, such as psychosis or an obsessive-compulsive disorder.

Patients may report feelings of bugs crawling within the skin, and will go to extraordinary lengths to remove the bugs. They may try to rid themselves of "parasites" by washing often, applying insecticides or parasiticides, avoiding others to contain the "contamination." Some patients may paint their homes, destroy "infested" bedcovers, and call on pest control companies for help.

Also called acarophobia or parasitophobia, it is classified as a hypochondriacal psychosis. While treatment for parasitic delusions was once thought to be hopeless, a few patients have recovered.

Symptoms and Diagnostic Path

While there is no evidence of skin problems, these patients may insist there is; some puncture the skin with fingernails or needles to dig out the "parasites." These "insects" are then produced (usually bits of skin, hair, crusts, and other debris). Patients usually reject any suggestion that the parasites are not real with scorn or disbelief, and refuse to seek psychological counseling.

Chronic attempts to clean the skin may cause tissue breakdown; isolation to prevent "contamination" may result in psychological problems. Suicide is possible.

Treatment Options and Outlook

Some experts recommend confronting the patient with the delusion, but others counter that confrontation can be disastrous since the patient is absolutely sure of the infestation. The patient's belief should never be treated as factual, and antiparasitic lotions should not be administered. Depression or other psychological problems should be treated.

Pimozide (a drug used to treat Tourette syndrome) may help control, but not cure, the disorder, although side effects include irreversible body movements (tardive dyskinesia), EKG abnormalities, drowsiness, and sometimes death. Still, chronic administration of pimozide allows many patients to live normal lives.

Demodex folliculorum A mite found in the hair follicles and sebaceous secretions (especially in the face and nose). The mites usually cause no problems but may occasionally cause an inflammation of hair follicles called demodex FOLLICULITIS. Demodex are harmless and do not transmit diseases, but large numbers of demodex mites may cause ITCHING and skin disorders, referred to as demodicosis.

deodorant A modestly effective substance designed to be applied to the skin to control unpleasant odor, usually containing antimicrobial agents; it also may contain fragrance to disguise odor and antiseptics to destroy bacteria. Deodorant is a useful help against body odor caused by bacteria in decomposing sweat on the skin, but is less effective than ANTIPERSPIRANTS.

See also SWEAT GLANDS; SWEAT GLANDS, DISORDERS OF; DRYSOL.

depigmentation The removal or absence of skin pigment (usually MELANIN).

See also DEPIGMENTATION, CHEMICALLY INDUCED; and DEPIGMENTATION, POST-TRAUMATIC.

depigmentation, chemically induced A variety of chemicals (mostly derivatives of phenol or HYDROQUINONE) can produce DEPIGMENTATION of the skin that looks very much like VITILIGO. Progressive depigmentation beginning on the hands and spreading to other parts of the body may be caused by exposure to phenolic compounds, especially if the patient works in the plastics and rubber industries, or uses germicidal agents.

Treatment Options and Outlook

First, the patient should be protected from further exposure to industrial cleaning solutions, germicidal agents, rubber products, or depigmenting medications. It may be possible to repigment hair-bearing skin with PUVA.

Disorders of congenital depigmentation due to absence of melanocytes include PIEBALDISM, ALBINISM, and WAARDENBURG'S SYNDROME. Disorders involving acquired depigmentation caused by the absence of melanocytes include vitiligo, post-traumatic depigmentation, and chemically induced depigmentation.

See also DEPIGMENTATION, POST-TRAUMATIC.

depigmentation, post-traumatic Any physical, chemical, or infectious agent that destroys the outer skin layer (EPIDERMIS) will also destroy the PIGMENT CELLS along the basal skin layer. Normally, skin is repigmented as PIGMENT CELLS proliferate and migrate from hair bulbs and adjacent skin. If an injury destroys the hair bulbs or other nearby skin, the normal reservoir of new pigment cells is destroyed. That skin will probably remain permanently white.

Injuries that cause this type of depigmentation include BURNS, radiation, deep lacerations, or ABRASIONS. Likewise, any infections that leave deep scars (such as SHINGLES or CHICKEN POX) often leave depigmented areas. Many lesions of DISCOID LUPUS ERYTHEMATOSUS may be permanently depigmented.

Pigment cells are particularly vulnerable to injury from cold; freezing the epidermis by CRYOTHERAPY may cause a temporary depigmentation, but new pigment cells will eventually migrate into the area. Therefore, minor lesions in dark-skinned patients should be treated with cryotherapy with great caution.

Deep freezing to destroy basal cell epithelioma or SQUAMOUS CELL CARCINOMA may also leave an area of permanent depigmentation, since pigment cells in the hair bulbs are destroyed.

depigmentation disorder Any disorder that results in absence of PIGMENT CELLS from the skin, too few melanosomes, or improper MELANIN synthesis.

depigmenting agents The skin may lose pigmentation by using a range of agents, including HYDROQUINONE, monobenzyl ether of hydroquinone, or AZELAIC ACID.

See also DEPIGMENTATION, CHEMICALLY INDUCED.

depilatory A chemical agent (such as barium sulfide) for removing or destroying hair that is available in a cream or paste. Depilatories are used for cosmetic purposes and for the treatment of excess hairiness (HIRSUTISM). They dissolve the hair at the skin's surface but do not affect the hair's root. Hair grows back within a few days; therefore, they are only a temporary solution to hair removal.

Depilatories should not be used immediately after a hot bath or shower, since heat increases blood flow to the skin, opening skin pores and increasing the amount of chemical absorbed into the body.

Today, the most popular chemical depilatories are made of thioglycolates combined with calcium hydroxide. Earlier depilatories contained alkaline earth sulfides that had an unpleasant odor and irritated the skin. They are still used, however, by some African-American men to remove beard hair.

Although chemical depilatories offer a smoother skin surface than shaving, only about 1 percent of American women use them exclusively for hair removal; 8 percent of American women use depilatories in combination with other methods. Many consumers consider them expensive, slow, and irritating to the skin, with an unpleasant odor.

Side Effects

Chemical depilatories may cause an allergic reaction characterized by swelling and inflammation, and are not usually recommended for use on the face. Because the chemical structure of the KERATIN of the top-most skin layer resembles hair chemically, depilatories should not be left on the skin too long or they will cause irritation.

See also HAIR REMOVAL; ELECTROLYSIS.

dermabrasion Surgical removal of the surface layer of the skin by high-speed sanding to refresh the skin and reduce pitted scars of ACNE, improve appearance of raised scars, or remove tattoos. It is also used to smooth out WRINKLES and to remove pre-cancerous growths (KERATOSES). Dermabrasion is the most dramatic resurfacing technique that dermatologists can use, and it leaves the skin relatively smooth.

Procedure

The skin is numbed with a local anesthetic. Using an abrasive wheel or wire brush rotating at high speeds, the dermatologist removes layer after layer of skin to reach the smooth skin underneath scars, and remove precancerous lesions, broken blood vessels, wrinkles, and tattoos.

Risks and Complications

Age, skin type, coloring, and medical history all affect how well the procedure works. For example, people with dark skin may become permanently discolored or blotchy after a skin-refinishing treatment. People who develop allergic rashes or other skin reactions, or who get frequent fever BLISTERS or COLD SORES, may experience a flare-up. FRECKLES may disappear in the treated area.

Most surgeons will not perform treatment if the patient has had radiation treatments, a bad skin BURN, a previous deep chemical peel, or active acne on the facial skin.

Dermabrasion is normally safe when performed by a qualified, experienced board-certified physician. The most common risk is a change (either darkening or lightening) in skin pigmentation. Permanent darkening of the skin, usually caused by exposure to the sun in the days or months following surgery, may occur in some patients. On the other hand, some patients find

the treated skin remains a little lighter or blotchy in appearance.

Some patients may develop tiny WHITEHEADS after surgery that eventually disappear by themselves or with the help of an abrasive pad or soap; occasionally, the surgeon may have to remove them. Some patients may develop enlarged skin pores, although these usually shrink to near-normal size once the swelling has subsided.

Infection and scarring occasionally occur with dermabrasion. Some individuals develop excessive scar tissue (KELOID scars); these are usually treated with the application or injection of steroid medications. Patients can reduce these risks by choosing a qualified plastic surgeon and closely following the doctor's advice.

If the skin begins to get worse instead of better, becoming redder or itchier after starting to heal, it may signal the formation of abnormal scars, and the surgeon should be consulted immediately.

Outlook and Lifestyle Modifications

Right after the procedure, the skin will be quite red and swollen, and eating and talking may be difficult. There will probably be some tingling, burning, or aching; but any pain can be controlled with medications prescribed by the dermatologist. The swelling will begin to fade in a few days to a week or two.

After the procedure, a scab will form over the treated area as it begins to heal. This will fall off as a new layer of tight, pink skin forms underneath. The face may itch as new skin starts to grow; doctor-recommended ointments can ease the discomfort. If ointment is applied immediately after surgery, little or no scab will form.

The new skin will be a bit swollen, sensitive, and bright pink for several weeks. During this time, the patient can slowly start returning to normal activities, and may go back to work in about two weeks. The dermatologist will typically advise patients to avoid any activity that could bump the face for at least two weeks. More active sports (especially ball sports) should be avoided for four to six weeks. Swimmers should use only indoor pools to avoid sun and wind, keeping the face out of chlorinated water for at least four weeks. It will be at least three to four weeks before patients can drink alcohol without experiencing a red flush. It is most important to protect the skin from the sun until the pigment has completely returned, which may take as long as six to 12 months.

While pain is not considered to be a problem, many patients are bothered by the red, raw appearance of the skin for about 10 days after the procedure.

As with other types of facial peels, dermabrasion may cost several thousand dollars. A list of dermatologists qualified to perform dermabrasion is available via the toll-free hotline maintained by the American Society for Dermatologic Surgery.

dermal fillers   See SKIN FILLERS.

dermal stimulator   A substance that stimulates skin cells to make COLLAGEN, providing a slow correction of aging and WRINKLES over time. Poly-L lactic acid is a new dermal stimulator approved in 2005 by the U.S. Food and Drug Administration to fill the hollow cheeks from loss of fat seen in HIV-positive patients receiving treatment for AIDS. It is used to treat patients every month for four to five months until the full correction is achieved. These results should last for one to three years, experts suggest.

Although research studies of poly-L lactic acid for cosmetic use are just beginning, if proven effective, it could be a new option for patients looking for a safe, long-lasting fix for wrinkles, skin creases, and loss of cheek fullness with age.

dermaplaning   A process that scrapes away dead cells to smooth away SCARS. Dermaplaning is far less aggressive than DERMABRASION, which sands away the outer layer of skin (EPIDERMIS) and the superficial DERMIS to smooth down scars.

In dermaplaning, the physician uses an instrument called a dermatome, which resembles an electric razor whose blade moves back and forth to skim off the top layer of skin surrounding facial defects such as ACNE scars. The technique feels something like a fingernail scraping the skin.

dermatitis   The general term used to refer to a group of inflammatory conditions of the skin (*derm* meaning "skin" and *itis* meaning "inflammation of"). While people often use the terms ECZEMA and dermatitis interchangeably, eczema is actually dermatitis in its advanced stages, with BLISTERS, fissures, oozing, crusting, scabbing, thickening, peeling, and discoloration. While there are a wide variety of dermatitis conditions, the three main categories are atopic, contact, and seborrheic.

See also DERMATITIS, ASTEATOTIC; DERMATITIS, ATOPIC; DERMATITIS, BERLOQUE; DERMATITIS, CONTACT; DERMATITIS, EXFOLIATIVE; DERMATITIS, HAND; DERMATITIS, IRRITANT CONTACT; DERMATITIS, NICKEL; DERMATITIS, NUMMULAR; DERMATITIS, PERIORAL; DERMATITIS, SEAWEED; DERMATITIS ARTEFACTA; DERMATITIS HERPETIFORMIS; DERMATITIS PAPULOSA NIGRA; ALLERGIES AND THE SKIN; CRYOSURGERY; DIAPER RASH; DRY SKIN; GOURGEROT-BLUM SYNDROME; OIL OF BERGAMOT; SALYCYLIC ACID; SULFUR.

dermatitis, allergic   See ALLERGIES AND THE SKIN.

dermatitis, asteatotic   A disorder also known as "winter itch" first described in 1907 using the term *eczema craquele.*

There are many different factors that may lead to asteatotic dermatitis, including friction, frequent or prolonged bathing in hot water, use of soap and infrequent use of emollients, decreased sebaceous and sweat gland activity, radiation, nutritional deficiencies, ZINC deficiency, thyroid disease, medication side effects, and some cancers.

Symptoms and Diagnostic Path
The condition is characterized by itchy, dry, cracked, and fissured skin with irregular scaling found most often on the shins of elderly patients, although it may be present on the hands and trunk. The skin looks almost like cracked porcelain, and can lead to superficial bleeding and fissures as the EPIDERMIS loses water, splits, and cracks. The inflammation can be associated with asymmetrical leg swelling.

Although most cases get better, the condition can be chronic, with frequent relapses during the winter and times of low humidity. Men over age 60 develop asteatotic dermatitis more often than women, but the condition also can be found in younger people.

Treatment Options and Outlook

Patients should take short baths without hot water and little or no soap on the affected areas, followed by a good moisturizer such as a petrolatum-based emollient after bathing. Topical steroid ointments with or without polyethylene occlusion should be applied. Many patients will heal with mild topical steroids alone, depending on the severity of the skin lesions, how well patients comply with treatment, and if patients use little soap and hot water in the affected areas.

Asteatotic dermatitis responds well to therapy, but recurrences are common.

dermatitis, atopic   Also known as atopic ECZEMA, this condition is a chronic superficial inflammation common in infants, often appearing between two and 18 months of age. It typically occurs in those with an inherited tendency to develop allergy and is found in 10 percent of the population. It is usually associated with asthma, hay fever, or allergic rhinitis, and it may affect as many as seven to 24 of every 1,000 individuals. The highest prevalence is in children.

Typically, the condition begins in the first year of life in about 60 percent of cases, and before age five in 85 percent. The disease fades away in about 40 percent of individuals by adulthood, although patients with severe disease are more likely to have a persistent course.

Symptoms and Diagnostic Path

In acute cases, this form of eczema is characterized by a mild, very itchy rash on the face, neck, wrists, inner elbow creases, and behind the knees, with red, scaling skin and pimples. If scratched, the pimples leak a clear liquid, forming large weeping areas; infection may occur if the condition appears in the diaper area. ITCHING is often worse at night.

Atopic dermatitis tends to wax and wane; in chronic stages, there is scaling and skin color changes. Most patients improve during the summer and worsen during the winter, which is probably related to humidity and temperature.

Treatment Options and Outlook

Adequate hydration of the skin and avoiding irritants may be all that is required in those with mild cases. Irritant detergents include wool clothing, strong detergents, and water. Irritant detergents can be avoided by using a mild detergent (such as Ivory Snow flakes or Dreft), by avoiding wool, and adding bath oil to bath water. Emollients such as white petrolatum should be applied immediately after bathing, and topical CORTICOSTEROIDS and tar preparations are useful.

In acute cases, a medium-potency topical corticosteroid lotion or cream should be applied after bathing or after applying aluminum acetate or saline compresses.

For chronic cases, potent topical corticosteroids should be applied right after bathing; soaking or using compresses of water-soluble tar preparations may decrease the need for topical corticosteroids.

Adequate doses of antihistamines can control itching and prevent scratching, which could lead to secondary infection. With severe involvement, a short course of systemic corticosteroids may be needed; however, the risks of systemic corticosteroids limit their use in long-term treatment.

Oral antibiotics are helpful in infections of eczematous skin, a frequent complication in itchy children.

Although there is no cure, the long-term prognosis is good; spontaneous remission occurs in almost half of all patients by age 15. Those who may go on to struggle with persistent disease often have a family history of atopic dermatitis, associated asthma or hay fever, and late onset of severe disease.

dermatitis, berloque   A type of phototoxic contact dermatitis causing an irregular hyperpigmentation usually found on the neck. Berloque (French for "pendant" or "drop-like") dermatitis is caused by perfumes that contain OIL OF BERGAMOT, a naturally occurring photosensitizer (PSORALEN).

Symptoms and Diagnostic Path

After exposure to the sun, hyperpigmentation with sharp margins and streaks begins to appear, with very little reddening, on the neck or hands.

Exposure to certain concentrated plant juices (such as limes) that contain psoralens, followed by exposure to the sun, may produce a more severe reaction involving painful redness and blistering.

Treatment Options and Outlook

Patients with berloque dermatitis should use a daily SUNSCREEN with SPF 30 or higher to help keep the condition from worsening. Perfume should be be avoided on areas of the skin that are exposed to the sun. TRETINOIN (Retin-A) or Keralyt gel applied to the affected areas will improve this condition.

The reaction usually appears within 24 hours after sun exposure, peaking within 48 hours.

dermatitis, cement See ALLERGIES AND THE SKIN.

dermatitis, contact An inflammation of the skin caused by an allergic reaction to direct contact with a substance to which a person is sensitive. Usually an itchy or scaly rash erupts at the point of contact, which can be anywhere on the body. While the immune system normally protects against bacteria and viruses, an allergic response causes the immune system to overreact to usually harmless substances like dyes or metals.

Substances that are often implicated in contact dermatitis include metals (especially nickel); dyes and chemicals in clothing, furs, shoes, hair products, rubber compounds, paints, textiles, ink, and paper; cleaning products or detergents; cosmetics, perfumes, shaving lotions; POISON IVY; and insecticides. Formaldehyde is a potent antimicrobial that causes many cases of contact dermatitis, and is found in industry, medicine, the home (as a preservative) in permanent press clothes, newspapers, and so on. Formaldehyde-releasers are used as preservatives in cosmetics and industrial products and are often masked by other names.

Chromates Chromium (in the form of chromates) is the most common cause of contact dermatitis in men, usually from exposure on the job. Because chromates are common, they are often hard to avoid. A main source is cement, affecting those in the building trades. Leather that has been tanned with chromate may also cause contact dermatitis on the feet of sensitive individuals.

Symptoms, which often resemble NUMMULAR ECZEMA, are scaling, redness, and dryness. They may take years to improve, even after contact is avoided. In fact, most severely affected people never fully recover, probably because of the prevalence of chromates in everyday life. Workers with only a mild or moderate problems may remain on the job if they can avoid the substance, but a change in the work area does not guarantee the dermatitis won't recur. By adding ferrous sulfate to cement, the chromate becomes less sensitizing and this may be a breakthrough in preventing occupational chromate allergy.

Rubber A hypersensitivity to rubber may be suspected if the patient has a history of direct skin contact with a rubber product. There are many rubber chemicals that may produce allergy, especially those contained in disinfectants and preservatives in industrial processes (tetramethylthiuram disulfide and 2-mercaptobenzothiazole and thiourea derivatives). Because of the large number of different allergenic chemicals, it is not easy to perform patch testing for this problem. It is also common to find cross-reactions between related chemicals.

Topical medications About a third of all dermatology patients with a contact allergy will test positive for sensitivity to some type of ingredient in topical drugs or cosmetics. The most common include lanolin, neomycin, local anesthetics, formaldehyde, and preservatives (such as parabens or benzoisothiazides).

Lanolin, a skin cream product derived from sheep fleece, causes a reaction in some people. An artificial hypoallergenic lanolin derivative is now available.

Neomycin is a widely used topical antibiotic that may cause a contact dermatitis. The risk of allergy decreases when the antibiotic is used only for simple cuts or surgical wounds. It may be hard to diagnose neomycin allergy, since the dermatitis is not vesicular or bullous but appears to be an aggravation of preexisting dermatitis.

Parabens are widely used preservatives found in foods, drugs and one-third of all cosmetics. Considering how widespread they are, sensitization to the parabens is low. Although hypersensitivity usually occurs when a person contacts the ALLERGEN with any part of the body, parabens may be tolerated on normal facial skin but may cause dermatitis on eczematous skin.

Symptoms and Diagnostic Path

Contact dermatitis usually starts as an itchy red rash, evolving into blisters with cracking and peeling skin. The severity of this type of dermatitis depends on the particular substance, and how sensitive a person is. Symptoms should subside within a few days or weeks if the offending substance is avoided, although some kinds of dermatitis can become chronic.

Once an allergic reaction to a substance has occurred, a person can become sensitized; even the briefest subsequent contact will probably set off another attack.

Allergy patch tests may be helpful in determining the substances that are provoking the reaction. In the test, a physician exposes small areas of skin to a variety of known allergens, observing the skin for development of a reaction.

Treatment Options and Outlook

Mild cases of contact dermatitis do not require treatment, but frequent or severe outbreaks should be referred to a physician. Topical medications (CALAMINE, antihistamines, or over-the-counter cortisone creams) usually ease symptoms. Hydrocortisone cream (in 0.5 percent strength) is available without a prescription; stronger creams, which are necessary for cases of significant contact dermatitis, can have serious side effects and are available only with prescription.

It is a myth that patients with dermatitis should avoid bathing; *regular* bathing is as a way to reduce infection and soothe irritated skin (water should not be too hot or cold). Two cups of colloidal oatmeal (available in drugstores) or baking soda to the bath may help.

Individuals allergic to ANTIPERSPIRANTS—specifically the metallic salts (such as aluminum chloride, aluminum sulfate and zirconium chlorohydrate) that are the active ingredients—should avoid them. Sensitive consumers should look for products with anti-irritants such as zinc oxide, magnesium oxide, allantoinate, aluminum hydroxide, or triethanolamine.

In severe cases of weeping sores, cold milk compresses may help soothe the itching of contact dermatitis. CALAMINE LOTION with MENTHOL or phenol may be another good choice to help a dry oozing rash.

See also DERMATITIS, NICKEL.

dermatitis, diaper   See DIAPER RASH.

dermatitis, exfoliative   A severe, extensive inflammatory condition (also known as ERYTHRODERMA) that causes scaling and redness of all the skin of the body. An uncommon disorder, it is three times more common in men than women. Average age at onset is 50 years.

Drug reactions are the most common cause of exfoliative dermatitis, responsible for about 40 percent of cases. Common medications associated with this disorder include sulfonamides and penicillin; less commonly, antimalarials, barbiturates, allopurinol, nonsteroidal anti-inflammatory drugs, diphenylhydantoin, and gold are suspected to trigger this disorder. Once the offending drug is no longer administered, the skin lesions will often clear within weeks.

In 30 percent of cases, the disorder is due to preexisting skin conditions—most commonly, PSORIASIS or atopic dermatitis. Other associated skin conditions include LICHEN PLANUS, Reiter's syndrome, PITYRIASIS RUBRA PILARIS, PEMPHIGUS, allergic contact dermatitis, or stasis dermatitis. Most people suffering from this condition will usually find their exfoliative dermatitis clearing within weeks to months after effective treatment is begun, although recurrences are common.

Up to 20 percent of erythroderma is caused by cancer (usually either lymphomas and leukemias). Approximately 10 percent of cases have no known cause.

In those without a known cause, the disease lasts on average about five years. Intermittent flare-ups are frequent.

Symptoms and Diagnostic Path

While the causes of exfoliative dermatitis may vary, the symptoms are the same: generalized redness, warmth, swelling, itch, thickened and scaling skin that begins in one small area and spreads across the skin within days to weeks to months. While the mucous membranes are not usually affected, the palms, soles, scalp, and nails are often involved. Other common systemic complaints include chills or fever, dizziness on standing up, dehydration, enlarged lymph nodes, and swelling.

Because of the profound effect this disorder has on the metabolic system, the basal metabolic rate may rise by as much as 50 percent above normal, resulting in huge increases in exfoliation that may cause malnutrition (caused by the protein loss in the flaking skin).

Treatment Options and Outlook

Hospitalization may be required to stabilize fluid volume and temperature and to treat added infection. Nutritional supplements and medication to control itching may be required. Steroids, emollients, and moisturizing baths may make the patient more comfortable. Failure to implement these supportive treatments may require administration of methotrexate and retinoids.

Death rates in the past have been as high as 30 percent, and are related to infection. Death from erythroderma has become rare with medical advances.

dermatitis, hand   Also known as "hand ECZEMA," this condition is usually caused by exposure to detergents, cleansers, or dishwashing soap, although in some a specific cause may never be found. It is restricted to the hands, with little dermatitis elsewhere, and afflicts between 4 and 8 percent of the population.

There may be many different causes behind the development of this condition. *Contact dermatitis* is the most common type of hand dermatitis, which can produce an irritant or allergic eczematous reaction. *Irritant dermatitis* accounts for about 70 percent of contact hand dermatitis; detergents, soaps, and solvents are the most important causes.

Contact allergic hand dermatitis is seen in between 25 and 30 percent of cases. A preexisting irritant dermatitis can predispose an individual to the development of allergy. Contact allergic hand dermatitis usually evolves into chronically thickened skin that can not be distinguished from that caused by irritant dermatitis. The primary offenders behind the allergic type of hand dermatitis are nickel, chromate, rubber compounds, paraphenylenediamine, and parabens. Nickel allergy, affecting about 5 percent of the population (mostly women), is caused by costume jewelry, coins, handles, pens, surgical instruments, and kitchen utensils, any of which can be associated with hand dermatitis. Those with a chromate sensitivity can develop hand dermatitis from exposure at work (especially to cement, leather, paint, and photography dyes). Chemicals added to rubber (such as mercaptobenzothiazole and thiuram) cause rubber sensitization, producing hand dermatitis through contact with rubber gloves and tubing. Paraphenylenediamine is found in azo dyes, and often is a problem among hairdressers. Paraben-sensitive patients may find they are sensitive to many topical medications, cosmetics and foods.

Symptoms and Diagnostic Path

The condition is characterized by itchy BLISTERS up to an inch across on the palms, with dry cracked skin across the hands. The *acute* stage is characterized by dry blisters and redness; in the subacute stage the skin is red and scaly. Chronic hand dermatitis is characterized by thick, scaly, and dry skin with more and more skin markings.

Treatment Options and Outlook

The condition usually improves if the patient wears cotton gloves under rubber gloves when touching any possible irritant; the hands should be thoroughly dried after immersion in water and an unscented hand cream or white petrolatum should be applied several times a day. If the condition is severe, topical CORTICOSTEROIDS may be prescribed for inflammation and antibiotics may be needed to combat infection.

See also DERMATITIS, IRRITANT CONTACT; ECZEMA.

dermatitis, irritant contact Irritant contact dermatitis is a local inflammatory reaction (not an allergic reaction) caused by a single or repeated exposure to toxic chemicals.

Symptoms and Diagnostic Path

The appearance of lesions depends on the type of irritant, which can range from a blistering reaction to a scaly, red thickened skin. An *acute case* may result after only one contact with a highly toxic irritant. Easily diagnosed, it often occurs after industrial accidents.

A *cumulative case* is more common than acute dermatitis and is caused by repeated contact with mild irritants over a long period of time. The first signs are usually dry, cracking skin with redness, scaling, PAPULES, VESICLES, and thickening.

This type of dermatitis may involve a combination of irritants, set off by one highly toxic irritant (such as a caustic agent or a solvent). The irritation is sustained by subsequent use of detergents and soaps. The skin all over the body may become sensitized so that an acute condition on the hands can lead to increased sensitivity of the skin on the back. Because of the similarity between irritant and allergic contact dermatitis, patch testing can help distinguish between them.

Treatment Options and Outlook

Irritant contact dermatitis can be a difficult problem to treat, and may last for a long time. Moreover, it can lead to the development of allergic contact dermatitis. People who have experienced atopic dermatitis as children are more susceptible to developing irritant contact dermatitis as adults.

See also DERMATITIS, ATOPIC; DERMATITIS, CONTACT.

dermatitis, nickel An itchy skin reaction following contact with nickel, probably the most common form of dermatitis. Nickel, a shiny stainless metal, is often used in surface plating of metal objects, such as buttons, costume jewelry, and kitchen equipment. It is also an element in many alloys, and is widely used in dentistry.

It is found 10 times more often in women than men, and is often triggered by ear piercing. Having the ears pierced (using earrings with nickel posts) causes subsequent rashes to appear in other areas of the body whenever the person touches objects containing nickel. Necklaces, bracelets, belt buckles, and other jewelry that have never before caused a problem may suddenly cause a rash after the ears are pierced.

Nickel dermatitis is also associated with an increased risk of developing dermatitis of the hand. Those at high risk for developing an occupational nickel allergy include those in regular contact with the metal: restaurant workers, hairdressers, nurses, cashiers, and metal-industry employees.

Risk Factors and Preventive Measures

People with newly pierced ears or other body parts should wear only gold or steel posts until skin heals (about three weeks). Surgical steel is the best choice, and is available in some types of earrings specifically designed for sensitive skin.

Perspiration plays a big role in nickel dermatitis because it leaches out the nickel in nickel-plated jewelry. It is best to avoid the heat when wearing this type of jewelry. Only high-quality gold jewelry that is at least 14-karat gold should be worn; the lower the karat, the higher the percentage of nickel.

A few dermatologists go so far as to warn highly sensitive patients to avoid foods containing traces of nickel (such as coffee, beer, tea, apricots, chocolate, nuts, and so on).

See also DERMATITIS, CONTACT; DERMATITIS, ATOPIC.

dermatitis, nummular Also known as nummular ECZEMA, this stubborn, itchy condition usually occurs in adults, causing circular, scaly patches anywhere on the body, very similar to RINGWORM (tinea). The lesions may be clear in the center, resembling ringworm or a fungus. The condition tends to be chronic, with periods of waxing and waning.

While the cause is unknown, it is more common in the winter and is often associated with dry skin. Wool, soaps, and frequent bathing (more than once a day) often worsen the condition. Clothes washed or dried with liquid or sheet fabric softeners may also irritate the skin.

Treatment Options and Outlook

There is no cure, but there are effective ways of controlling nummular dermatitis. Vaseline, tar, and CORTISONE compounds applied to the skin are the best treatments. Weak cortisone salves can be used safely for years. When large areas of the body are treated or when strong cortisone preparations are used, however, periodic medical checkups are necessary. Strong cortisones shouldn't be applied to the face, armpits, groin, or anal area.

The skin should be lubricated, and a bath oil or Aveeno powder can be used in the tub. Patients should use lukewarm, not hot water, and should blot the skin afterwards so there is still some water left on the skin. Next, the patient should apply a moisturizer to all of the skin, such as Vaseline, Lubriderm, or Moisturel.

Wool or rough clothing should be avoided. Cotton (100 percent) clothes are best. Clothes should be laundered without any fabric softener or dryer sheets, and should be washed using dye-free, fragrance-free detergents.

dermatitis, perioral A rash of tiny pimples and pustules around the mouth usually found in women in their 20s and 30s. These lesions leave no scars.

Excessive use of corticosteroid creams, fluorinated toothpastes, moisturizing creams, cosmetics, and birth control pills have been linked to perioral dermatitis, but often the cause is unknown.

Treatment Options and Outlook

Oral tetracycline can cure the problem within two to eight weeks, although some patients need repeated courses of treatment. Recurrences are common. Alternatively, topical antibiotics such as clindamycin or erythromycin or topical SULFUR or SALICYLIC ACID may be prescribed.

dermatitis, pigmented purpuric lichenoid See GOUGEROT-BLUM SYNDROME.

dermatitis, radiation See RADIODERMATITIS.

dermatitis, seaweed A rash of bumpy red lesions caused by poisonous marine algae found in salt and fresh water around the world. The rash is usually caused by algae trapped underneath a bathing suit.

Epidemics of this seaweed-induced rash occasionally occur in the Pacific. In Hawaii, the highest number of cases occur during the summer, when persistent trade winds may dislodge the seaweed from the bottom. Fragments then drift into swimming bays and beaches.

Seaweed dermatitis should not be confused with SEA BATHER'S ERUPTION, an eruption caused by stings from larval forms of certain sea anemones and thimble jellyfishes, or SWIMMER'S ITCH, an eruption due to a bite from freshwater parasitic flatworms.

There are more than 3,000 species of algae; seaweed dermatitis is caused by direct contact with *Lyngbya majuscula* (also known as *Microcoleus lyngbyaceus*). The fine, hairlike, dark brown seaweed is found in certain tropical and sub-tropical shoreline waters at certain times of the year. The toxicity of this seaweed varies greatly depending upon region, season, and type. Not all strains of this seaweed are toxic. *Lyngbya majuscula* is a blue-green alga. It usually grows in clumps, looking like dark, matted masses of hair or felt. Most often this seaweed is blackish green or olive green, but it also grows in shades of gray, red, or yellow.

Symptoms and Diagnostic Path

Symptoms include an itching and burning sensation that begins anywhere from right away up to 24 hours after leaving the water. A red, sometimes blistering rash occurs, sometimes in a swimsuit pattern. It often occurs in men in the scrotum, and in females under the breasts, but this depends on the type of swimwear used.

Other symptoms include swollen eyes, irritation of the nose and throat, skin sores, headache, and fatigue. Symptoms typically last four to 48 hours. In more serious cases, skin sores may appear for several weeks. A rash also can occur on the face and in the eyes and mouth; some victims have swelling of eyes and mouth, but no rash.

Treatment Options and Outlook

The skin should be scrubbed with soap and water and flushed extensively with freshwater, rinsing with isopropyl (rubbing) alcohol.

Hydrocortisone cream 1 percent may be applied two to three times daily for itching, but should be discontinued immediately if any signs of infection appear.

CALAMINE lotion or, occasionally, systemic steroids are effective. If the wound shows any evidence of infection, such as redness, PUS, pain, foul odor, heat, or fever, antibiotics are usually recommended.

Antihistamines reduce itch, and topical emollients may provide relief from symptoms.

If the reaction is severe, oral steroids (prednisone) may be required. Irrigate exposed eyes with tap water for at least 15 minutes. Any difficulty breathing may signal an allergic reaction. If the skin shows any evidence of infection, antibiotics may be needed.

Risk Factors and Preventive Measures

The only sure way to avoid seaweed dermatitis is to avoid swimming in the ocean where seaweed blooms have been reported. Health authorities generally keep a close eye on algal blooms and report them through the media. In some countries, health authorities have powers to close public beaches.

After swimming in the ocean, individuals should shower with lots of soap and water as soon as possible. Swimmers also should thoroughly wash swimsuits, towels, and any associated swim gear to get rid of any attached algae.

dermatitis, seborrheic An extremely common form of ECZEMA that causes scaling around the nose, ears, scalp, mid-chest, and along the eyebrows, it is often misdiagnosed by non-physicians as DRY SKIN. However, the flaking from this type of dermatitis is *not* caused by dryness. It is believed to have a genetic link, although how the condition is inherited is not clear. It is most common in boys after puberty, and its incidence increases with age. Seborrheic dermatitis has also been observed in patients with Parkinson's disease, mental retardation, and a range of neurologic disorders. Use of some drugs (such as neuroleptics) has been associated with the skin problem.

Treatment Options and Outlook

Treatment is similar to other eczemas, with shampoos containing tar, sulfur, SALICYLIC ACID, or selenium daily. Hydrocortisone 1 percent cream will control the skin condition on the face and chest. If shampoos do not work, a steroid solution such as fluocinolone 0.01 percent may be applied to the scalp one or two times a day. Alternatively, ketoconazole 2 percent cream twice daily to the affected area may also be helpful, or systemic antibiotics may also be useful.

Untreated dandruff may progress to seborrheic dermatitis, with psoriasis-like plaques and secondary infections as a result of scratching.

dermatitis artefacta Any self-induced skin condition, ranging from a mild self-inflicted scratch to severe and extensive mutilation by a disturbed patient.

The problem occurs more often in women and is usually the result of psychological problems, often acting as an emotional release in situations of distress, or part of attention-seeking behavior.

The condition, also known as factitial dermatitis, usually affects women in their teens or early adulthood who tend to be emotionally immature or have psychosocial or interpersonal issues.

Various methods of causing lesions include applications of caustic substances (silver nitrate or phenol), injection of foreign material, BURNS, beating, or pricking the skin with a pin.

Symptoms and Diagnostic Path

Skin damage may range from ulcers, blisters or scratches, and often exhibits an asymmetrical or bizarre pattern that does not resemble any normal skin disease.

The well-defined lesions may include redness, blisters, ulcers, abscesses, swelling, superficial GAN-GRENE, and skin rash. The lesions are often shaped in bizarre ways, with irregular outlines in a linear or geometric pattern, and are usually quite different from surrounding normal skin.

The appearance of lesions varies depending on the methods used to injure the skin, which may be produced by a variety of mechanical or chemical means, including with fingernails, sharp or blunt objects, lit cigarettes, or caustic chemicals. Lesions do not evolve gradually, but appear almost overnight without any prior signs or symptoms. They are usually found on sites that are readily accessible to the patient's hands, such as on the face, hands, arms, or legs. The patient will usually deny that the rash is self-induced.

Treatment Options and Outlook

The treating health care expert is often regarded as an adversary, and treatment can be difficult because on a deeper level these patients do not really want to get better. Patients can be difficult, manipulative, evasive, untruthful, and ungrateful. Often, they are either unaware of, or they conceal, the real nature of their lesions.

Patients should not be directly confronted about the cause of their lesions. Instead this information should be conveyed indirectly. The doctor should create an accepting, empathetic, and nonjudgmental environment in which the patient can be closely supervised, which can lead to a doctor-patient relationship in which psychological issues may gradually be introduced. If appropriate, psychiatric referral may be recommended, although this is often refused. Medication (such as tranquilizers) has little effect. The prognosis is good in those patients who have suffered only a brief, traumatic experience, but is not good in those who are chronic sufferers. Resolution of the current underlying psychological problem will bring about a temporary cure, but dermatitis artefacta tends to wax and wane with the circumstances of the patient's life. To minimize future occurrences, a patient should continue to see the doctor for supervision or support, whether or not lesions are present.

dermatitis herpetiformis   Also known as Duhring's disease, this is a rare chronic skin disorder in which clusters of tiny red itchy blisters appear in a symmetrical pattern on various parts of the body, especially the back, elbows, knees, buttocks, and scalp.

The disease usually appears in people between the late 20s and early 40s, much more often in white males. It appears less often among African Americans and is quite rare among the Japanese.

About half of these patients also experience gastric hypoacidity and gastric atrophy. Males have a higher frequency of lymphoma (a type of cancer).

Treatment Options and Outlook

Oral DAPSONE or sulfapyridine usually improves the skin condition but has no effect on the problems occurring in the small intestine. Topical and systemic CORTICOSTEROIDS do not usually work. Removing foods containing gluten from the diet results in an improvement in skin condition and intestinal health, but this may take more than a year. Further, a wheat-free diet is expensive and especially difficult to maintain.

The skin condition also has improved following continuous treatment with PUVA (PSORLENS plus ultraviolet light A).

See also PUVA.

dermatitis papillaris capillitii   Another name for ACNE KELOIDALIS.

dermatitis papulosa nigra   Groups of small, very dark seborrheic KERATOSES that develop on the faces of African Americans. This disorder occurs earlier in life than seborrheic keratoses in fair-skinned patients.

In this disorder, the number of lesions increases as time goes on, although the lesions do not carry a risk of malignancy. Unlike warts, they do not spontaneously disappear.

Treatment Options and Outlook

The lesions may be removed by a variety of methods, but their removal may be followed by changes in pigment. Hyperpigmentation often results following CRYOSURGERY, since pigment-producing cells are easily destroyed. While cautery may be better tolerated, this technique must be performed carefully to prevent scarring. Hypopigmentation is also a risk. Light brown-skinned people often experience hypopigmentation after treatment. Sometimes physicians elect to treat only one lesion at first, to assess how the patient's skin responds to the treatment technique.

See also KERATOSIS, SEBORRHEIC.

dermatofibroma　A type of benign tumor arising from connective tissue cells, this skin NODULE is found most often on the arms and legs. Also known as histiocytoma cutis, it is composed of fibroblasts, COLLAGEN, capillaries, and histiocytes.

Many patients with this type of skin lesion report some type of preceding trauma, such as an insect bite, scratch, or a minor skin puncture. They occur at any age, although they usually appear in early adulthood through middle age.

Symptoms and Diagnostic Path

Most patients have only one or two lesions; infrequently, there are many tumors. Most of the lesions are slightly elevated and firm, although some may be depressed below the skin's surface. They may range in color from dusky pale to medium- or pinkish brown, with a smooth or rough surface. When squeezed, the skin over a tumor often dimples. Tumors may continue to grow slowly, once formed.

Treatment Options and Outlook

Because these tumors are completely benign, no treatment is necessary, although they can be excised if the patient desires.

dermatofibrosarcoma protuberans　An invasive tumor that occurs in the second layer of skin. After excision, it tends to recur in up to 75 percent of cases, although the malignancy rarely spreads to other parts of the body. More common in young men than in women, these tumors usually appear on the upper trunk and shoulder.

Symptoms and Diagnostic Path

The condition begins as a slow-growing firm nodule, ranging from brown to dusky red. The tumor begins as a very small bump on the surface of the skin, usually seen on the trunk, quickly undergoing a period of very rapid growth where the many small bumps form a larger, more noticeable mass. This mass swells and bulges outward, which is where it gets the name "protuberans." The area becomes tender and may bleed because the top layer of the skin is stretched so tightly. Dermatofibrosarcoma protuberans usually does not spread to other parts of the body, but grows locally.

Because the initial growth phase is so slow, it can be a few years before the patient notices the tumor and experiences enough discomfort to seek medical advice. To diagnose this condition, a doctor will biopsy a sample of the affected tissue to determine whether the cells and growth pattern in the sample are characteristic of dermatofibrosarcoma protuberans.

Treatment Options and Outlook

This condition has commonly been treated by removing the tumor and a significant amount of the tissue surrounding it. Mohs' microscopically controlled surgery is considered to be the treatment of choice. In this procedure, the tumor is removed and then the physician continues to remove the edges of tissue around the tumor site. After each bit of tissue is removed, it is examined under a microscope for signs of malignant cells. Tissue around the tumor site is continually removed until there is no longer any sign of malignant cells under the microscope. How the area is closed after wide excision or Mohs' surgery depends upon how much tissue must be removed.

Dermatofibrosarcoma protuberans has a high recurrence rate because the tumor has many projections beyond the main mass, which may be left behind when the tumor is removed. However, Mohs' surgery has proven very effective in reducing the recurrence rate. Chemotherapy is not an effective treatment because the tumor grows so slowly. Radiation therapy may be recommended for some patients.

If the tumor is going to recur, it will most likely happen during the first three years after surgery.

dermatoglyphics　Patterns of skin ridges on the fingers, palms, toes, and soles. On the fingers, ridges occur in patterns of loops, whorls, arches, and compounds (combinations of the first three). Fingerprint classifications are based on an analysis of these ridges. Fingerprints are accepted as a legal identification since no two individuals share the same pattern of ridges—not even identical twins.

dermatographia Literally "writing on the skin," in this condition, stroking or scratching the skin with a dull instrument produces HIVES that can last up to 30 minutes. This form of chronic hives may be inherited and usually persists for life. Antihistamines (especially hydroxyzine) may help.

dermatologic surgeon A DERMATOLOGIST who deals with the diagnosis and treatment of medically necessary and cosmetic conditions of the skin, hair, nails, veins, mucous membranes, and adjacent tissues by various surgical, reconstructive, cosmetic, and nonsurgical methods. A dermatologic surgeon repairs or improves the function and cosmetic appearance of skin tissue.

Most dermatologic surgeries are now minimally invasive and require only local or regional anesthesia. Dermatologic surgery procedures include anti-aging treatments, injectable and implantable soft-tissue fillers, correction of ACNE scarring, chemical peeling, tumescent LIPOSUCTION, vein therapy, hair restoration, laser surgery, skin cancer treatment, and reconstructive flaps and grafts.

dermatologist A physician who specializes in diagnosing and treating skin problems. Dermatologists spend at least one year after medical school in a hospital practicing general medicine, then go on to complete at least three years in advanced training in dermatology. Dermatologists are experts in all aspects of the skin, including hair, nails, and mucous membranes, and treat skin problems with medicine or surgery. They are carefully trained to understand how diseases of the skin can be related to many other, more general medical conditions.

Dermatologists treat common skin disorders such as ACNE, ECZEMA, and PSORIASIS. They also diagnose and treat skin growths, WARTS, cysts, and tumors. While all dermatologists treat SKIN CANCER, some have extra training in the surgical management of skin cancer and limit their practice to the treatment of this disease. Others have expertise in laser surgery, while still others specialize in skin resurfacing with chemical peels, DERMABRASION, or LASER RESURFACING.

Many dermatologists perform some COSMETIC SURGERY. For example, they can remove moles, destroy small capillaries on the face, and remove brown spots. Some inject COLLAGEN or fat to smooth out facial creases and WRINKLES. FACE-LIFTS or breast augmentations are sometimes performed by dermatologists.

Many dermatologists supply patients with lotions and creams that are tailored to each patient's skin care needs.

See also DERMATOLOGIC SURGEON.

dermatology The study of a vast field of knowledge about the physiology and pathology of the skin and hair, nails, SWEAT GLANDS, and oil glands. Robert Willan in England (1757–1812) was the first to publish and classify information about skin disease, which was further explored by Jean-Louis Alibert (1768–1837) in Paris, who considered each dermatosis as a specific branch of dermatology. But it was not until the discovery of the microscope that dermatologists were able to see the skin in all its structural and cellular detail. At the same time, the infant science of bacteriology revealed the secrets of infectious diseases such as IMPETIGO and BOILS. By 1906 the spirochete causing SYPHILIS had been isolated, and in 1914 PELLAGRA was shown to be a simple nutritional deficiency, although the missing vitamin (nicotinic acid) was not identified until the 1930s.

Today, the field of dermatology includes the investigation of disease (such as examining skin scrapings under a microscope), diagnosis, and treatment, ranging from application of creams and ointments to DERMABRASION, LIPOSUCTION, surgical excision, to laser surgery. In fact, dermatologists perform a wide variety of surgeries in the treatment of skin diseases, from sophisticated plastic surgical excisions to Mohs' technique for histological tracking of the furthest reaches of SKIN CANCER. The newest surgical techniques include

LIPOSUCTION for skin contour control, and the use of lasers for treating a variety of skin growths and marks, including tattoos and PORT-WINE STAINS.

dermatome A part of the mesoderm in the early embryo that forms the deeper layer of the skin (DERMIS). The entire surface of the body forms an interlocking web of dermatomes, the pattern of which is very similar from one person to another. Loss of sensation in a dermatome means that a particular nerve root has been damaged.

"Dermatome" also refers to a surgical instrument for cutting different thicknesses of skin for use in skin grafting.

dermatomyositis A rare (sometimes fatal) disease involving skin inflammation and a skin rash. One of a group of autoimmune disorders, dermatomyositis is sometimes associated with an underlying cancer of an internal organ. It is most often found in middle-aged women.

The average age at diagnosis is 40, and almost twice as many women are affected. About half the patients recover fully within two years; in about 30 percent of cases the condition persists, and the remaining 20 percent experience a progressive and sometimes fatal form of the disease that affects lungs and organs.

Symptoms and Diagnostic Path

Symptoms begin with a red rash on nose and cheeks, followed by purple discoloration on eyelids, and a red rash on the knees, knuckles, and elbows. As the disease progresses, muscles begin to weaken, becoming stiff and painful, and the skin over the muscles of the shoulders and pelvis becomes thickened. Other symptoms include weight loss, nausea, and fever. The role of sunlight in this disease has not been thoroughly examined, but in certain patients, exposure to sunlight may worsen skin symptoms and probably systemic symptoms as well.

Treatment Options and Outlook

CORTICOSTEROID and immunosuppressant drugs can control the skin inflammation and are used in combination with physical therapy to prevent muscles from scarring and shrinking. Death occurs in less than 10 percent of patients.

dermatopathology The study of the microscopic appearance of diseased skin.

dermatophagy The practice by amphibians and reptiles of eating their own skin. While scientists originally believed this was a rare practice, a new survey of more than 100 zoos and aquariums around the world has documented the practice in 285 species of frogs, lizards, salamanders, snakes, turtles, tuatara, and caecilians. Herpetologists believe the animals eat their skin for the extra protein, although some argue that the practice protects the vulnerable animals from predators by eliminating the evidence of their presence.

Because animals can eat their skin very quickly, there had been few reports of dermatophagy until researchers at the Smithsonian Institution sought help from animal caretakers for the new data. They note, however, that observations still need to be made in the wild, since captivity may affect the skin-eating behavior.

dermatophyte Superficial fungal infection that affects the skin, hair, and nails, usually caused by the fungi *Microsporum*, *Epidermophyton*, or *Trichophyton*. This type of infection can be spread by personal contact from person to person, to humans from soil, or from an animal to a person. It usually has a Latin name using the term TINEA ("RINGWORM") with the part of the body affected (such as "tinea pedis" for ATHLETE'S FOOT). Although there are many different kinds of dermatophytes, seven species cause more than 90 percent of all infections. The organisms are transmitted by either direct contact with an infected host (human or animal) or by direct or indirect contact with infected exfoliated skin or hair in combs, hair brushes, clothing, furniture, theater seats, caps, bed linens, towels, hotel rugs, and locker room floors.

Depending on the species, the organism may survive in the environment for up to 15 months.

There is an increased susceptibility to infection when there is a pre-existing injury.

See also TINEA BARBAE; TINEA CAPITIS; TINEA CORPORIS; TINEA MANUUM; TINEA NIGRA PALMARIS; TINEA VERSICOLOR.

dermatophytid A skin eruption caused by hypersensitivity to a type of fungus DERMATOPHYTE such as RINGWORM.

dermatophytosis A type of fungus infection (also called TINEA) caused by *Trichophyton, Epidermophyton* or *Microsporum* sp.

dermatosis cinecienta Another name for a progressive pigmented disorder called ERYTHEMA DYSCHROMICUM PERSTANS.

dermis The lower layer of the skin beneath the EPIDERMIS. The dermis is composed of fibers called COLLAGEN and ELASTIN, which are complex proteins responsible for the support and elasticity of the skin. It is collagen and elastin that enable the skin to snap back into shape after being stretched or pulled.

Also found in the dermis are tiny twiglike sensory nerve endings that allow a person to sense touch, temperature, vibration, and pain.

Each square foot of dermis contains 15 feet of small blood vessels that provide nutrients and oxygen; it is the constriction and dilation of these vessels in response to extremes of heat and cold that help regulate temperature throughout the body. It is also these vessels that are responsible for keeping the skin healthy and removing harmful metabolic wastes.

Interestingly, nutrients can *not* be easily supplied to the skin by applying substances to the skin surface. This means that slathering on fruits, vegetables, cream, lotion, or vitamins on the skin in the hope of getting the substance into the skin may be unproductive. Certain substances, however, can penetrate into the skin where they are biologically active.

dermoid Resembling the skin.

desquamation The continuous process of shedding of the skin. This is an important factor that limits the bacterial population on the skin, since epithelial cells colonized with bacteria are always being shed. The entire external layer of the skin is almost completely replaced every three to four weeks. Dead cells contain large amounts of keratin (a fibrous portion that forms the outer barrier of the skin).

developers Oxidizing agents (usually containing HYDROGEN PEROXIDE) that supply oxygen to the molecules of HAIR DYE so that a particular shade is achieved.

DHA See DIHYDROXYACETONE.

diaper rash Known medically as diaper DERMATITIS, this is a common condition of infancy caused by skin irritation from substances in feces or urine. It is probably worsened by friction from rough diapers and prolonged wetting of the skin.

While babies vary in their susceptibility to diaper rash, skin inflammation in some infants can be severe. In general, breast-fed babies have a lower incidence of diaper rash than bottle-fed babies, and the resistance continues long after the baby has been weaned. In some infants, diaper rash is the first indication of sensitive skin heralding a long series of later skin problems, such as ECZEMA.

Symptoms and Diagnostic Path
The skin appears reddened at first and, as the rash becomes chronic, the skin becomes dry and scaly. In chronic severe cases, the skin is covered with PAPULES, BLISTERS, and erosions that can be mistaken for bacterial infection or even BURNS. A long-term rash that will not clear may be caused by a candida (fungus) infection, PSORIASIS, or atopic eczema.

Treatment Options and Outlook
Some of the oldest advice is still the best in this case—expose the rash to air; take off the diaper and

lay the baby facedown (with face turned to one side) on towels over a waterproof sheet, as long as someone is there to watch the infant. Protective ointment (zinc oxide or "diaper rash ointment") will help prevent and clear the problem. In severe cases, a mild corticosteroid drug is necessary to control inflammation, often given in combination with an antifungal drug to kill any organisms that might cause THRUSH.

About half of all cases of diaper rash go away by themselves within a day. The other half of these rashes may last up to 10 days or more.

Risk Factors and Preventive Measures

Prevention of this skin condition is always better than trying to cure it once it appears. The aim in a preventive diaper rash program is to keep the baby's skin as dry as possible for as long as possible. Since a newborn breast-fed baby urinates about 20 times a day and has a bowel movement after each feeding, this can be a major undertaking! Still, diapers should be changed as often as possible followed by application of a water-repellent emollient with each change. (If possible, the diaper should be left off at least an hour a day).

Critics still disagree on the relative merits of cloth vs. disposable diapers and diaper rash, with each contingent asserting that only one type of diaper prevents diaper rash. Recent research has indicated that diapers containing absorbent gelling material significantly reduces skin wetness, leaving skin closer to the normal pH than either conventional disposable diapers or cloth products. Proponents of cloth diapers insist that the cloth allows for more air circulation to the skin and, because the cloth diapers do not hold as much water, these type of diapers tend to get changed more often than do disposable diapers.

While it is important to keep the diaper area clean, drying sensitive baby bottoms with a towel can be irritating to some infants. Experts suggest drying irritated bottoms with a hair dryer *set on low;* afterward, zinc oxide ointments (diaper rash ointments) can be applied. Since a baby's urine is sterile, the infant's bottom need not be cleaned after urination—only patted or air dried.

Parents who *do* use cloth diapers and wash their own should add one ounce of vinegar to one gal-lon of water during the final rinse water to help match the cloth's pH to baby's skin. The cloth diapers must be well rinsed. Diaper rash enzymes are most active in an environment with high pH (often found in cloth diapers after washing).

Cloth diapers provided by diaper services are usually very close to a baby's pH level, and are usually tested at regular intervals to ensure the products' pH level.

diascope A glass or clear plastic plate (usually a microscopic slide) placed against the skin to observe the skin after the blood vessels have been compressed. This diagnostic tool is used to blanch away any redness, which allows the underlying color of any lesion to be seen.

diet and skin Experts generally agree that a good healthy diet is beneficial to a good, healthy skin; they also stress that ACNE is *not* caused by a diet rich in oil, chocolate, or seafood.

A wide variety of studies has shown links with certain vitamins and healthy skin. VITAMIN A is important for healthy, normal growth of skin cells. Studies now being conducted with natural and synthetic derivatives of vitamin A may soon reveal that the vitamin holds the key to bolstering the skin's immune system, preventing acne and skin cancer. These derivatives, called retinoids, may someday be to skin diseases what antibiotics are to infections.

In addition, some B-complex vitamins and zinc deficiencies cause scaling and redness, especially around the mouth and nose.

Dietary deficiencies can also profoundly affect your skin. For example, VITAMIN C deficiency may result in SCURVY, causing bleeding gums, swelling skin, and large black and blue bruises over the body. (In fact, British sailors are nicknamed "limeys" because during the heyday of the great sailing vessels, they were fed limes and lemons to prevent scurvy). Vitamin C is also important in the production of COLLAGEN, the main supportive protein of skin.

A deficiency of vitamin A can cause acne and other skin problems. Extremely low levels of vitamin B$_2$ (riboflavin), B$_3$ (niacin) and B$_6$ are linked to skin inflammations and mucous membrane sores.

Severe malnutrition (such as experienced in Third World countries) can cause changes in color and texture of hair and skin, and low iron levels result in yellowish, pallid skin.

At the other end of the spectrum, too *many* nutrients can also cause skin problems. Excessive intake of iodine (from too much iodized salt or shellfish) can cause breakouts of deep pustules and cysts on the face and back. Too much BETA-CAROTENE (from some vegetables or carrots or supplements) can turn skin yellow; high levels of vitamin A can cause dryness and cracking skin and mucous membranes.

diethanolamine (DEA) A wetting agent used in cosmetics that may be linked to cancer in lab animals, according to the National Toxicology Program (NTP). The NTP completed a study in 1998 that found an association between cancer in lab animals and the topical application of DEA and some DEA-related ingredients. For the DEA-related ingredients, the NTP study suggests that the cancer is linked to possible residual levels of DEA. The NTP study did not establish a link between DEA and the risk of cancer in humans.

Although DEA itself is used in very few cosmetics, DEA-related ingredients are widely used in a variety of cosmetic products. These ingredients function as emulsifiers or foaming agents and generally are used at levels of 1 percent to 5 percent of a product's formulation.

While the U.S. government believes that at the present time there is no reason for consumers to be alarmed based on the use of these substances in cosmetics, consumers wishing to avoid cosmetics containing DEA or DEA-related ingredients should review the ingredient statement on the outer container label.

With the exception of color additives and a few prohibited ingredients, a cosmetic manufacturer may use almost any raw material as a cosmetic ingredient. The following are some of the most commonly used ingredients that may contain DEA:

cocamide DEA
cocamide MEA
DEA-cetyl phosphate
DEA oleth-3 phosphate
lauramide DEA
linoleamide MEA
myristamide DEA
oleamide DEA
stearamide MEA
TEA-lauryl sulfate
triethanolamine

dihydroxyacetone (DHA) A sunless tanning ingredient that works by reacting with the KERATIN protein in the top layer of the skin, providing a temporary tan. The DHA in sunless tanners is refined from a vegetable source such as sugar beets or sugar cane.

Discovered to be a temporary skin coloring agent back in the 1920s, DHA was first sold in an over-the-counter sunless tanning product in 1960 as Coppertone Quick Tan, also known as QT. In the 1970 the U.S. Food and Drug Administration added DHA to their list of approved cosmetic ingredients.

In the late 1980s cosmetic companies found a way to produce better results that were less orange and more brown with DHA by using an improved refining process yielding a higher quality, more predictable DHA. Since then, DHA has been further improved, leading to an explosion of self-tanning products.

DIN The European equivalent of SPF (SUN PROTECTION FACTOR), the rating system used for SUNSCREEN products. DIN stands for Deutsches Institut fur Normung, the institution that developed the European rating system. The DIN rating system uses lower numbers than the American SPF system for equivalent sun protection. For example, SPF 12 is equal to DIN 9; SPF 19 is equal to DIN 15.

diphenhydramine An antihistamine drug used to treat HIVES; it may be given as an injection to treat anaphylactic shock (a severe allergic reaction).

Side Effects

Possible side effects include drowsiness, dry mouth, and blurred vision.

discoid lupus erythematosus (DLE) A chronic type of lupus erythematosus that usually affects exposed areas of the skin. The more serious and potentially fatal form (SYSTEMIC LUPUS ERYTHEMATOSUS, or SLE) affects many systems of the body, including the skin, joints, kidneys, and nervous system.

This is an autoimmune disorder in which the body's immune system attacks a variety of tissues as though they were foreign, causing inflammation.

Symptoms and Diagnostic Path

In DLE, a rash starts as one or more red, circular, thickened areas that later scar. The lesions are reddened with follicular plugs, atrophy, scaling, and spidery veins. They may be found on the face, behind the ears and on the scalp, sometimes causing permanent hair loss. Lesions can also occur on other parts of the body. Individuals with DLE tend to be sensitive to light.

Although one-fifth of SLE patients also experience these discoid lesions, less than 5 percent of patients with DLE ever develop SLE.

Diagnosis of DLE usually requires a skin biopsy of a discoid lesion, which will reveal certain microscopic characteristics that allow it to be identified. If antibodies exist in the blood, or if other symptoms or physical signs are found, it is possible that the discoid lesions are a sign of SLE rather than DLE.

Treatment Options and Outlook

There is no cure; treatment aims at reducing inflammation and alleviating symptoms. It is essential to use SUNSCREENS, and avoid the sun whenever possible. The use of a potent topical CORTICOSTEROID or an injection into the lesion is appropriate, since these lesions often cause permanent scarring or hair loss if left untreated. Sometimes, short-term treatment with oral steroids will be used for particularly severe DLE outbreaks. Medications used to treat malaria are often used to treat DLE.

The prognosis for most people with DLE is excellent. While the lesions may be cosmetically unattractive, they are not life threatening. Only about 10 percent of patients with DLE will go on to develop SLE.

Risk Factors and Preventive Measures

DLE cannot be prevented, but flares can be lessened in patients with the disease by avoiding exposure to the sun and consistently using sunscreen.

dishpan hands See CHAPPED HANDS.

DLE See DISCOID LUPUS ERYTHEMATOSUS.

dressings Protective bandages over wounds that may be used to control bleeding, prevent infection, or absorb secretions. Dressings may be sterile or nonsterile. Sterile dressings are used to avoid infection, and should be absorbent enough so the skin around the wound does not become moist, which could encourage infection. Unless the wound must be cleaned often, the dressing should not be disturbed.

Skin dressings also are used to keep topical medications in place, and to relieve itching or pain. The *occlusive dressing* is a very effective means to increase the local skin temperature, enhancing the absorption of topical medication. Occlusive dressings also promote the retention of moisture, which stops the medication from evaporating. In an occlusive dressing, an airtight plastic film (such as plastic kitchen wrap) is placed over the medicated skin. Plastic surgical tape containing CORTICOSTEROID in the adhesive layer can be cut to size and applied to individual lesions. Occlusive dressings should be removed for 12 of every 24 hours in order to avoid local skin atrophy, bandlike streaks, telangiectasia (small red lesions caused by dilated blood vessels), inflamed hair follicles, nonhealing ulcers, and systemic absorption of corticosteroids.

Wet dressings are compresses soaked in water or saline, used for oozing, weeping, crusted, eroded, or ulcerated skin, that are usually applied for 10 to 30 minutes three or four times a day. Evaporation from the dressing soothes and dries by cooling the skin surface.

drug reactions A skin rash is one of the most common side effects of a wide range of drugs, and may be the first sign of a generalized toxic reaction. And yet, while skin symptoms of a drug reaction are quite common, scientists do not really understand the mechanism underlying most of the effects.

The risk of a drug-related rash is higher in certain groups: 35 to 50 percent more women than men, 50 to 80 percent of patients with infectious mononucleosis who take ampicillin. The risk of a drug rash is much higher in patients taking ampicillin and allopurinol together than either drug alone. Reasons behind the development of this rash are unknown.

Symptoms and Diagnostic Path

Skin rash is the most common adverse skin reaction to a drug, occurring in two to three percent of all patients. The rash is characterized by a fine, papular eruption that usually appears within the first seven to 10 days after the drug is begun. Antibiotics and allopurinol may induce rashes two or more weeks after they are started. Drug rashes often begin in areas of trauma or pressure, such as on the backs of bedridden patients or on the extremities of patients who are not bedridden. Drugs most frequently found to cause a rash are antimicrobial agents, blood products, nonsteroidal anti-inflammatory drugs (NSAIDs), and central nervous system drugs. According to one survey, drugs with reaction rates above one percent include trimethoprimsulfamethoxazole, ampicillin, amoxicillin, semisynthetic penicillins, penicillin, red blood cells, and cephalosporins.

Hives are the second most common allergic skin reaction to drugs, and are most often caused by antibiotics, blood products, radiocontrast agents, NSAIDs, and opiates. The hives usually last for less than 24 hours and are replaced by new lesions in new places.

Allergic contact dermatitis to medications used on the skin is common, featuring papules, blisters, and vesicles. Patch testing may be used to demonstrate contact hypersensitivity to a suspected topical medication. Substances found in topical medications that are often associated with allergic contact dermatitis include neomycin, benzocaine, ethylenediamine, diphenhydramine (in Caladryl), and parabens (preservatives found in many topical preparations, including some CORTICOSTEROIDS). Neomycin is the most sensitizing of currently-used topical antibiotics; approximately 5 percent of people have a sensitivity to it.

Most drug-related skin eruptions will fade away within two weeks after the drug is stopped, leaving no permanent scars or discolorations. However, some skin reactions may be life threatening, including anaphylaxis, toxic epidermal necrolysis, vasculitis, severe ERYTHEMA MULTIFORME, and exfoliative ERYTHRODERMA. Usually the wider the area of affected skin, the longer it will take for side effects to fade.

If a patient develops a rash following use of a certain drug, then continued use of the medication may induce a life-threatening eruption or an exfoliative erythroderma. However, patients who have developed rashes due to sulfonamides, penicillin, or carbamazine have been desensitized by withdrawing the drug until the rash resolves, and then restarting the medication gradually, increasing doses until therapeutic doses are achieved.

dry skin Also known as "xerosis," dry skin usually begins in the 30s and worsens as a person ages. Dry skin may come and go depending on the weather. It is worse in the cold, and it is related to a decrease in the relative humidity and dry air from central heating. If the dryness worsens, the skin may seem irritated to the point of developing into DERMATITIS, with redness and skin fissures. One of the worst aspects of dry skin is the itch, which may increase during stressful periods.

Treatment Options and Outlook

Daily bathing in lukewarm water with an added bath oil will also help to add water to the skin. The most effective emollients are often those people find least acceptable—semisolid oils that work to prevent evaporation, instead of moisturizers, which immediately soften the skin but can not seal the water into the EPIDERMIS. Studies have indicated that petrolatum and LANOLIN are very effective at abolishing dry skin within two weeks. There are many excellent MOISTURIZERS that, used daily, can prevent progressive dry skin. Moisturizers containing lactic acid, which helps to draw moisture from the dermis into the epidermis, may be effective.

Drysol (aluminum chloride hexahydrate) A prescription ANTIPERSPIRANT useful in patients with severe HYPERHIDROSIS (excessive sweating). Drysol is a 20 percent solution in absolute ALCOHOL. It can be used under the arms, on palms, or on soles. Drysol is reported to work in 80 percent of the people who use it for excessive sweating. Doctors generally recommend applying it to problem areas after drying the skin completely. Wearing it only at bedtime and then washing it off in the morning with plain water reduces the chance of skin irritation.

Treatment is typically repeated each night until sweating is under control. This may happen after just two or more treatments. Thereafter, it can be applied once or twice weekly, or as needed.

Drysol should not be applied to broken, irritated, or recently shaved skin, and it should not be used with regular daytime antiperspirants or DEODORANTS.

See also DEODORANTS.

duck bumps See GOOSEFLESH.

Duhring's disease See DERMATITIS HERPETIFORMIS.

dyshydrotic eczema See POMPHOLYX.

dyskeratosis congenita Almost all cases of this rare inherited disorder have been found in boys. By age five or six, the child experiences blistering of palms and nail beds, leading to a loss of nail plates and atrophy of the ends of the fingers and toes. There is a very high incidence of cancer and leukemia. In the teenage years, HYPERPIGMENTATION surrounding a central lack of pigment appears on the face and trunk and patients may be sensitive to light.

Treatment Options and Outlook

There is no treatment other than relieving the skin symptoms. Patients should avoid known cancer-causing substances, including ultraviolet light and tobacco.

dysplastic nevus syndrome See NEVUS SYNDROME, DYSPLASTIC.

ear repair   See OTOPLASTY.

eau de cologne   A light, fresh scent that can be reapplied often, and that is not as strong as pure perfume (parfum), because it is diluted with water. Eau de cologne has a 2–6 percent concentration of pure perfume, compared to eau de toilette (4–8 percent) and eau de parfum (8–15 percent).

See also FRAGRANCE.

ecchymosis   The medical term for a BRUISE, a blue or purple hemorrhage in the skin or mucous membrane.

eccrine gland   See SWEAT GLANDS.

econazole (Ecostatin)   An antifungal drug used to treat RINGWORM of the scalp, ATHLETE'S FOOT, JOCK ITCH, nail fungus, candidiasis, and others. Available in powder, cream, lotion, ointment, or vaginal tablet, the medication acts quickly (often within two days), killing fungi by damaging the fungal cell wall. The drug may take up to eight weeks to cure the infection. Rarely, the drug may cause skin irritation.

ecthyma   A deep ulcerative skin infection caused by bacteria (usually group A streptococci or staphylococcus) that often results in scarring, usually found on the legs and protected areas of the body. The condition begins with one lesion which enlarges and encrusts; beneath this crust is a pus-filled "punched ulcer."

Children are more commonly affected with echthyma, which is usually associated with poor hygiene, malnutrition, and minor skin injuries from trauma, insect bites, or SCABIES. The condition commonly occurs during unfavorable conditions, such as war or captivity.

Symptoms and Diagnostic Path
Echthyma may begin with a PUS-filled BLISTER, very much like IMEPTIGO, but in this case the infection penetrates through the outer layer of skin and into the deeper layer, developing into an ulcer with raised borders covered by a hard crust. Unlike impetigo, echthyma can sometimes cause scarring. Examination by a doctor is usually enough to diagnose echthyma. Lesions may be skin biopsied or cultured in some instances.

Treatment Options and Outlook
ERYTHROMYCIN or dicloxacillin can be effective. The lesions should also be soaked, and crusts removed. Full recovery is expected.

ectoderm   The outermost of the three primary germ (living substance capable of developing into an organ) layers of the embryo. From it are developed the EPIDERMIS and epidermal tissues (such as nails, hair, and skin glands), as well as the nervous system, the external sense organs (eye, ear, and so on), and the mucous membranes of mouth and anus.

ectodermal dysplasia (ED)   A group of genetic disorders that are identified by the absence or deficient function of at least two of these: teeth, hair, nails, or glands. At least 150 different (EDs) have been identified. Charles Darwin identified the first EDs in the

1860s, and today the number is believed to affect as many as seven out of every 10,000 births.

There is usually no reason to expect anything but normal intelligence with ectodermal dysplasia. Some of the extremely rare forms have been associated with mental retardation. As with the general population, some individuals affected by ED may be very bright, some may be average, and others may find challenges in learning.

Symptoms and Diagnostic Path

Individuals affected by EDs have abnormalities of sweat glands, tooth buds, hair follicles, and nail development. Some types of EDs are mild, while others are devastating. Many individuals affected by EDs cannot perspire. Air conditioning in the home, school, and workplace is a necessity. Other symptoms may include deficient tears and saliva, frequent respiratory infections, poor hearing or vision, missing fingers or toes, cleft lip and/or palate, poor immune system, sensitivity to light, lack of breast development.

Lifespan can be affected in some rare types of EDs, but there are very few documented examples of a death because of an inability to perspire.

There are four different types of ectodermal dysplasia: anhidrotic, anhydrotic, hypohidrotic, and hypohydrotic.

- *Anhidrotic* means "no sweating" and is derived from the Greek words *an* (none) and *hidros* (sweat). A person who does not sweat at all could be said to be anhidrotic.

- *Anhydrotic* means "no water" from the Greek *an* (none) and *hydro* (water). Those who are totally devoid of water could be said to be anhydrotic.

- *Hypohidrotic* means "deficient sweating" from the Greek *hypo* (under/deficient) and *hidros* (sweat) Someone whose sweat function is diminished (sweats little in response to heat or in response to stress only) could be said to be hypohidrotic.

- *Hypohydrotic* means "deficient water." Those who are partially or totally devoid of water could be said to be hypohydrotic.

As a baby is developing, three layers of tissue can be identified: an inner layer (the endoderm), a middle layer (the mesoderm), and an outer layer (the ectoderm). Defects in formation of the outer layer lead to ED. The reason that so many parts of the body are affected is because the ectoderm of the surface of the developing baby forms the skin, nails, hair, sweat glands, parts of the teeth, the lens of the eye, and the parts of the inner ear. Another portion of ectoderm forms the brain, spinal cord, nerves, the retina of the eye, and the pigment cells of the body.

Treatment Options and Outlook

There is no cure. Because most people with ED have missing or malformed teeth, dental treatment is necessary beginning with dentures as early as age two, multiple replacements as the child grows, and perhaps dental implants thereafter. Orthodontic treatment may also be necessary.

Precautions must be taken to limit upper respiratory infections, and care must be provided for the skin to prevent cracking, bleeding, and infection.

Professional care may minimize the effects of vision or hearing deficits, and surgical or cosmetic procedures may improve other deformities.

There is no evidence that the lifespan of a person diagnosed with one of the common ectodermal dysplasias is shorter than average, but a few rare syndromes may lead to a shortened lifespan.

ectoparasite A parasite that lives on the skin, getting nourishment either from the skin or by sucking the host's blood; various types of ticks, lice, mites, and some types of fungi may occasionally be ectoparasites on humans. (Parasites living *inside* the body are called "endoparasites.") Diseases caused by these parasites include SCABIES and PEDICULOSIS (louse infestation).

ectothrix A fungus that grows outside the hair shaft.

See also ENDOTHRIX.

eczema A superficial inflammation of the skin primarily affecting the outer skin layer (EPIDERMIS) that causes itching and a red rash often accompanied by BLISTERS that weep and then crust. This may be followed by scaling, thickening, or discoloration of the area.

Symptoms and Diagnostic Path

Eczema has many forms with two main divisions—eczematous dermatitis, which is caused by external factors, and endogenous eczema, occurring without any obvious outside cause.

Classification of endogenous eczema is based on its appearance and site. The five types are *atopic* (commonly found in childhood and sometimes associated with a family history of allergy, also called atopic dermatitis); *discoid* (small well-defined areas, also called nummular eczema or nummular dermatitis); POMPHOLYX (found on hands and feet, formerly called dyshidrotic pompholyx); *seborrheic* (scaly plaques in areas of the greatest sebum production, also called seborrheic dermatitis) and *varicose* (develops on the legs in association with poor circulation).

Other types of eczematous diseases include asteatotic eczema (due to overdrying of the skin) and polymorphic light eruption.

See also DERMATITIS, ATOPIC; DERMATITIS, HAND; DERMATITIS, NUMMULAR; DERMATITIS, SEBORRHEIC.

Treatment Options and Outlook

Treatment of eczema depends on the cause, but it usually includes the use of locally-applied CORTICOSTEROIDS. Creams, lotions, and antihistamines may help stop itching. Coal-tar ointments are often used when the problem has persisted for months or years and the skin has become thickened and leathery. To reduce scratching and irritation, soothing ointments should be covered by a dressing and absorbent, nonirritating materials should be worn next to the skin. Fabrics such as wool, silk, and rough synthetics should be avoided.

Children with atopic eczema should be bathed with a mild neutral soap no more than three times weekly. Bath oil may prevent excess skin drying, and fingernails should be clipped to decrease damage from scratching.

eczema, atopic See DERMATITIS, ATOPIC.

eczema herpeticum A rare skin condition caused by the HERPES SIMPLEX virus infection in a patient with a preexisting skin condition, such as DERMATITIS. It is characterized by extensive blistering, oozing, and crusting. The condition usually remains only on the skin.

Treatment Options and Outlook

Administration of acyclovir is effective. Symptoms can be treated by applying compresses and bathing.

egg Commercially produced skin care products containing egg do not help the skin, since the proteins in egg cannot be utilized by the skin in this way. However, a fresh egg mask can create a film on the face, locking in water and allowing the skin to build up a supply of water, which will temporarily soften dry skin.

Ehlers-Danlos syndrome A hereditary group of disorders in which there is a deficiency or defect of normal COLLAGEN (the most important protein in the body) that causes easily bruising, stretchy, thin skin. Known medically as "cutis hyperelastica," the disease is also characterized by paper-thin scars from wounds that have failed to heal properly.

Contortionists in circus side shows are often victims of Ehlers-Danlos syndrome, since the disease allows the skin to be stretched far beyond its usual length; the skin can still resume its original shape after distention.

The syndrome includes a family of 10 or more separate genetic disorders with varying inheritance patterns, some dominant, some recessive, and some X-linked. Four have been linked to specific enzyme deficiencies.

Symptoms and Diagnostic Path

Patients with this group of disorders do not become obviously distorted until late in life, when they may begin to experience significant cosmetic deformity caused by loose skin, joint changes, and scars resulting from the skin's fragility. Gaping wounds may develop from the slightest injuries, and surgical sutures do not hold well. Often, prominent scars appear on sites of frequent injury, such as the forehead, chin, knees, and shins.

Repeated tearing and bruises may cause skin to "outbag" and form pseudotumors. Joints may be hyperextendable; the fingers may often be able to bend 90 degrees backwards, and the thumb can be bent back to the wrist. Other characteristics include soft handshakes, high-arched palate, long neck, and sloping shoulders, with possible spine deformities. Common injuries include dislocations of the kneecap, hips, and temporal mandibular joints; eventually these can lead to arthritis of the large joints and spine.

Treatment Options and Outlook

There is no known treatment, but unnecessary injuries should be avoided. Surgery of various defects may be attempted, but there is a danger of bleeding and poor wound healing. Patients should protect fragile skin and joints, and avoid unnecessary injuries or extending skin, ligaments, or joints. Woman should understand that pregnancy carries a serious risk of hemorrhage.

Despite the lack of treatment, most patients have a normal life expectancy. Milder cases may correct themselves with aging, but other patients experience a progressive decline into severe arthritis and skin looseness over distorted joints. Death may result from a number of related internal organ problems.

elastic fibers   Connective tissue fibers that help to give the skin elasticity so that it returns to its normal position after stretching.

elastin   The protein that (together with COLLAGEN) is the primary substance in connective tissue. While collagen gives connective tissue strength, elastin gives skin its elastic properties, allowing the skin to stretch and spring back into place. Elastin becomes less elastic with age; as the skin and subcutaneous fat thins with age, the skin becomes looser. Elastin can be further damaged by extensive sun exposure, which can lead to wrinkling.

In cosmetic products, elastin cannot make the skin tighter. Used as a moisturizer it is thought to form a film on the skin that helps lock in moisture.

elastomas   A rare type of CONNECTIVE TISSUE NEVI characterized by overgrowth and distortion of the elastic fibers of the skin. Also known as "NEVUS ELASTICUS OF LEWANDOWSKY," this type of nevus is usually found as a collection of smooth skin-colored papules forming patches and plaques, most often on the trunk. No treatment is necessary.

elastosis   Degeneration of elastic tissue. It is most often seen as the result of long-standing sun exposure in photo-aged skin.

elastosis perforans serpiginosa   A rare disorder in which the skin is perforated, as though the body were trying to push out defective elastin, causing a circular or wavy indented lesion.

The syndrome may be inherited and usually appears during the 20s or 30s; male patients outnumber women four to one.

Symptoms and Diagnostic Path

EPS is a disease of the connective tissue that occurs in three different forms:

Idiopathic EPS: The cause of idiopathic EPS is unknown, but it may be inherited.
Reactive EPS: This form is associated with systemic, inherited, fibrous tissue abnormalities, such as EHLERS-DANLOS SYNDROME, Marfan syndrome, osteogenesis imperfecta, SCLERODERMA, and PSEUDOXANTHOMA ELASTICUM.
Drug-induced EPS: This form is caused by a side effect of D-penicillamine and occurs in about 1 percent of patients treated with the drug.

Lesions usually appear on the back of the neck or arms, although they may also appear on the face and lower extremities.

Treatment Options and Outlook

There is no satisfactory treatment for this syndrome; surgery may be attempted. In most cases, cutaneous

EPS is only a cosmetic problem. A rare systemic version is fatal, in which abnormal elastic tissue is found in the walls of ruptured blood vessels.

electrical injury An electric shock can damage the skin, if an electric current passes through the body. More than 1,000 people die from electrical accidents in the United States each year, and many more are seriously injured. Because the internal tissues of the body are moist and salty, they are good electric conductors. On the other hand, dry skin provides good resistance. For this reason, a shock to someone in a full bathtub will probably be fatal, whereas someone who is dry and standing outside the tub, wearing rubber-soled shoes (that do not conduct electricity), is far less likely to be hurt by the same shock.

All shocks except for the most mild are likely to cause unconsciousness, but the extent of tissue damage depends on the size and type of current. Skin tissues become charred where significant current enters and exits the body.

FIRST AID FOR ELECTRICAL INJURY

Rescuers should *NOT attempt any type of first aid until contact with the energy source is broken. The victim should not be touched with anything wet.*

The plug should be pulled out of the socket, or the rescuer should stand on a dry object and push the victim away from the source with a dry stick.

If the victim is unconscious and not breathing, CPR should be started.

If the victim is breathing, first-aid advice for burns and shock should be followed until an ambulance arrives.

---

electrodesiccation A dermatologic treatment method that destroys tissue by heat from a high-frequency electric current. The technique is used to treat a variety of skin lesions from SKIN TAGS, WARTS, and precancerous changes in the skin to skin cancers. It also may be used to destroy small tumors.

In the technique (which is usually performed with a local anesthetic), the physician applies an electric probe to the tissue for one or two seconds; the current flows to and through the lesion, destroying the tissue. While this may be enough

to destroy a small tumor, larger growths may also require curettage.

See also CURETTAGE AND ELECTRODESICCATION.

electrolysis A treatment in which an electric current is used to permanently remove excess body hair by destroying the hair's root bulb from which it grows. Although unwanted hair can be removed in a variety of ways (such as waxing, plucking, and so on), electrolysis is the only *permanent* hair removal method.

To remove a hair, a fine needle is inserted into the follicle along the hair shaft, destroying the root with a small electric current; the hair is then pulled out. The procedure may be slightly painful, but it is harmless when performed by trained operators. A number of sessions may be required until treatment is successful. At this point, there should be no more hair growth from that follicle, and minimal scarring.

Electrolysis can be performed on almost any part of the body, although it should be avoided on the lower margins of the eyebrows because the skin in this area is delicate and easily damaged. Some experts also disapprove of electrolysis in the armpits because of the danger of bacterial infection. Electrolysis is rarely used to remove leg hair because treatment of such large areas requires so many sessions that it is too time-consuming and expensive for most people.

Before selecting an electrologist, it is important to make sure the operator is fully trained, since incompetent electrolysis can cause permanent disfigurement.

electroporation A series of short electrical pulses that rearrange fatty layers in the outer skin layer to create temporary pores through which drugs may be administered. While the skin's outer layer of dead, flattened cells is an effective barrier to microbes, chemicals and other toxic agents, temporarily increasing the skin's permeability would be of benefit when it comes to administering certain medications.

Researchers at Massachusetts Institute of Technology successfully achieved a 1,000-fold increase in skin permeability using the technique, which delivers a series of millisecond electrical pulses every five seconds.

Before the technique can be used in drug delivery, researchers will need to answer questions about the technique's safety and effectiveness. The technique also may be used to transport fluids out of the body (such as a noninvasive way to take blood samples).

elephantiasis   A parasitic disease (also known as lymphatic filariasis) caused by microscopic, thread-like worms (*Wuchereria bancrofti, Brugia malayi,* or *B. timori*) that live only in the human lymph system (which maintains the body's fluid balance and fights infections). Elephantiasis affects more than 120 million people in 80 countries throughout the Tropics and sub-Tropics of Asia, Africa, and the Western Pacific, and parts of the Caribbean and South America. The worms do not occur in the United States.

When an infected female mosquito bites a person, she may inject the worm larvae into the blood, which reproduce and spread throughout the bloodstream, where they can live for many years. Often disease symptoms do not appear until years after infection. As the parasites accumulate in the blood vessels, they restrict circulation and cause fluid to build up in surrounding tissues.

Many mosquito bites over several months to years are needed to get lymphatic filariasis. People living for a long time in tropical or sub-tropical areas where the disease is common are at the greatest risk for infection. Short-term tourists have a very low risk.

Symptoms and Diagnostic Path

At first there are no symptoms, until after the adult worms die. At that point, the most common, visible signs of infection are excessively enlarged arms, genitalia, and breasts, although the legs are most commonly affected. The syndrome gets its name from the appearance of the skin of the legs, which resembles elephant hide.

Unfortunately, the disease is difficult to detect early, and improved laboratory tests are needed.

Treatment Options and Outlook

Medicines to treat lymphatic filariasis are most effective when used soon after infection, but they do have some toxic side effects. A vaccine is not yet available. People infected with adult worms can take an annual dose of medicine that kills the microscopic worms circulating in the blood. While this does not kill the adult worms, it does prevent infected people from giving the disease to someone else. Even after the adult worms die, however, lymphedema can develop.

To prevent the lymphedema from getting worse, patients should

- wash the swollen area with soap and water every day
- use anti-bacterial cream on any wounds to stop infections
- elevate and exercise the swollen arm or leg to move the fluid and improve the lymph flow
- apply elastic bandages to the affected parts, which may help

The disease usually is not life threatening, but it can permanently damage the lymph system and kidneys. Elephantiasis is a leading cause of permanent and long-term disability throughout the world. People with the disease can suffer pain, disfigurement, and sexual disability, and communities often shun those disfigured by the disease. Many women with visible signs of the disease will never marry, or their spouses and families will reject them, and patients often are unable to work.

emollients   Substances that soften and smooth the skin, helping to replace oils and prevent moisture loss. Common emollients present in almost all skin creams include LANOLIN, petrolatum, mineral oil, and squalane.

See also AGING AND THE SKIN.

emotion and the skin   Many experts believe that emotion plays a role in almost all skin diseases, whether or not the cause of the disorder is physical. Emotional factors sometimes cause skin disease, and often can either reduce or intensify itching and pain—even when the physical disease itself remains unchanged.

The psychological stress of illness or a variety of personal and family problems are often exhibited outwardly as skin problems. For example, even though SHINGLES or recurrent genital herpes are caused by a virus, and PSORIASIS is hereditary, negative emotions can trigger the onset of these diseases—or worsen a condition that already exists. Stress has also been linked with increased ACNE breakouts and worsening of HIVES.

One study evaluated more than 4,500 people to determine the link between emotional stress and skin disorders, as well as the time it took for the stressful event to trigger the disorder. Emotions were found to trigger ITCHING almost 100 percent of the time; hives, 68 percent; and psoriasis, 62 percent.

See also HERPES SIMPLEX.

endothrix A DERMATOPHYTE (superficial fungus) whose growth and spore production are confined primarily within the hair shaft, without forming conspicuous spores on the outside of the hair.

See also ECTOTHRIX.

entoderm The innermost of the three primary germ layers of the embryo, from which the epithelium of the pharynx, respiratory tract, digestive tract, bladder, and urethra are formed.

ephelis Another name for FRECKLE.

epidermis The surface layer of the skin. This layer covers the DERMIS and contains the basal cell layer, STRATUM SPINOSUM, STRATUM GRANULOSUM, STRATUM LUCIDUM, AND STRATUM CORNEUM.

There are two major zones of the epidermis—an inner region of moist cells and an outer layer of flattened dead cells known as the "stratum corneum" (or horny layer).

In the epidermis, there are three layers of living cells—the basal, spinous, and granular layers. The basal cells at the bottom of the dermis constantly divide, giving birth to daughter cells that begin to move toward the skin's surface, where they become part of the horny layer. It is this horny layer that protects against external chemical and antigen damage and inhibits injury from microbes, fungi, parasites, or insects.

epidermoid cysts A closed sac containing cheesy materia that may be common or benign. There are two types of epidermoid cysts—epidermal and pilar cysts. *Epidermal cysts* may be found alone or in groups, most often on the face, neck, upper chest, and back. As they enlarge, the skin thins and begins to look yellow white; if the cysts become infected the skin becomes red and tender. Ultimately, these cysts may rupture and drain PUS.

Pilar cysts involve hair follicles and are much less common than the epidermal variety. They are found most often on the scalp, although they may also crop up alone or in groups on the face, neck, and trunk. They look identical to an epidermal cyst, but they can be differentiated under the microscope by the appearance of the epithelium (tissue that covers the external surface of the body). Pilar cysts tend to run in families.

In the past, *pilar* and *epidermoid cysts* were wrongly known as *"sebaceous" cysts*. In fact, true sebaceous cysts are rare, and this term should only be used for a quite different type of cyst filled with a clear oily liquid made by sebaceous glands. Most cysts are either epidermoid (they originate in the epidermis and are filled with dead outer skin cells and keratin) or pilar cysts (originating in the skin lining hair follicles).

Treatment Options and Outlook

Both types of cysts must be completely removed or the epithelial sac must be destroyed; otherwise, the lesion may recur. Some lesions can be completely cut out in a wedge excision, while in other cases the sac may be removed through a small overlying incision after drainage of the cyst.

epidermolysis bullosa This rare inherited blistering condition loosens the outer layers of the skin, allowing the cells to be easily separated into its various layers. As a result, blisters form either spontaneously or after minor injury. The disorder is found primarily in young children and may range in severity from mild foot blistering in hot weather to widespread and severe blistering and scarring all over the body.

Epidermolysis bullosa is a group of inherited defects. Some are autosomal dominant (each child of an affected parent has a 50 percent chance of inheriting the defect); others are autosomal recessive (each of the children of two unaffected carrier parents has a one in four chance of inheriting the defect).

Treatment Options and Outlook

There is no specific treatment for this disorder. Even the slightest injury to the skin should be avoided. Wound care is essential once blisters or open sores develop. In mild cases, there may be gradual improvement, but more seriously affected children may experience serious disease.

epidermotropism   The infiltration of the top layer of the skin (epidermis) by lymphocytes.

epiloia   An acronym for TUBEROUS SCLEROSIS that designates "epilepsy, low intelligence, and ADENOMA SEBACEUM."

epithelioma   Any tumor derived from EPITHELIUM.

epithelium   The cells that cover the entire surface of the body. The skin consists of many layers of epithelium. The epithelium varies in cell type and thickness, according to its function in any particular area. There are three basic cell shapes: squamous (thin and flat), cuboidal (resembling a cube), and columnar (resembling a column). Because it is constantly subject to trauma, the outermost layer of cells are dead and constantly being shed.

epsom salts   Magnesium sulfate crystals used in baths to soothe the skin. It is effective in drying an oozing, inflamed area of skin and is also very effective as a soak for tired, sore muscles.

erysipelas   Formerly called St. Anthony's fire, this contagious infection of the facial skin and subcutaneous tissue is usually caused by group A streptococci. It is marked by rapid-spreading redness and swelling, which is believed to enter the skin through a small lesion. While this disease is contagious, it does not produce epidemics such as those of SCARLET FEVER. Erysipelas may affect both children and adults. The legs are affected in up to 80 percent of cases; the face accounts for up to 20 percent of infections.

Symptoms and Diagnostic Path

After a five- to seven-day incubation period, the skin feels tight, uncomfortable, itchy, and red, with patches appearing most often on the face, spreading across the cheeks and bridge of the nose. The patient also may notice sudden high fever (above 100° F) with headache, malaise, and vomiting. The lesions also occur on the scalp, genitals, hands, and legs. Within the inflammation, pimples appear, blister, burst, and crust over. The diagnosis of erysipelas is based on the characteristic appearance of the skin lesion; skin biopsies are usually not needed. Blood cultures rarely reveal the infection.

Treatment Options and Outlook

Penicillin and antibiotic relatives of penicillin are the usual choice of treatment, and should cure the infection within seven days. Bed rest, hot packs, and aspirin for pain and fever also may help.

Before the advent of antibiotics, this disease could be fatal (especially in infants and the elderly). Today, it can be quickly controlled with prompt treatment.

See also NECROTIZING FASCIITIS.

erythema   Redness of the skin caused by inflammation that may occur for a variety of reasons. Reddening of the skin is caused by an increased amount of blood in dilated blood vessels in the skin. Unlike a hemorrhage, the red skin color of erythema fades when the skin is compressed, since the blood is pushed out of the skin's vessels. (In a hemorrhage, the blood remains in the tissue outside the blood vessels so that compression does not remove the blood, and the red color does not disappear.)

A range of external factors may cause erythema, such as heat, sun rays, cold, and chemical irritants. Internal causes may include hot flashes, blushing, histamine release, fever, hot drinks, alcohol, or spices. Erythema also may be caused by a range of inflammatory skin conditions such as ACNE, DERMATITIS, ECZEMA, ERYSIPELAS, and ROSACEA.

In addition, erythema is a symptom of disorders including ERYTHEMA MULTIFORME, ERYTHEMA NODOSUM, LUPUS ERYTHEMATOSUS, and FIFTH DISEASE. Erythema often occurs with other primary skin lesions such as MACULES, PAPULES, NODULES, or surrounding blisters.

erythema ab igne   A skin reaction caused by chronic exposure to heat, such as by sitting too close to open fires or electric space heaters, or lying for long periods of time on a heating blanket.

In the past, it caused the typical telangiectasia (distended blood capillary vessels) and red-brown discoloration on the legs of those who sat in front of open fires or coal stoves in Great Britain and Europe. The condition became less common with the development of central heating. In the United States, the rising popularity of space heaters, wood-burning stoves, and fireplaces saw a resurgence in this syndrome. Erythema ab igne is also seen on the skin of glassblowers, bakers, and kitchen workers. Chronic use of heating pads may also lead to this problem.

Symptoms and Diagnostic Path

Limited exposure to heat that is not hot enough to cause a direct burn can cause instead this mild and transient lacy red rash. Prolonged and repeated exposure causes a marked redness and thinning. Rarely, sores may develop. Some patients may complain of mild itchiness and a burning sensation.

Treatment Options and Outlook

The dryness and itching may be eased by applying an EMOLLIENT; the redness will fade, although the telangiestasia and discoloration does not usually disappear completely.

Chronic exposure to heat must be stopped and avoided. If the area is only mildly affected with slight redness, the condition will improve on its own over a few months. If the condition is severe and the skin red and thinned, there is a possibility that SQUAMOUS CELL CARCINOMA may form after a period of years. Any persistent sore or lump within the rash should indicate the necessity of performing a skin biopsy to rule out the possibility of SKIN CANCER. Treatment with topical tretinoin or laser may improve the appearance, but abnormally pigmented skin may persist for years. Examples of this sort of heat-related damage have been reported throughout the world; "kangri cancer of India" is caused by holding pots of coal next to the skin; kange cancer of China is caused by sleeping on hot bricks; kairo cancer of Japan is associated with benzene-burning flasks next to the skin, and turf or peat fire cancer in Ireland is caused by sitting too close to a peat fire. These aggressive types of squamous cell cancers may appear after a latency period of 30 years.

erythema annulare centrifigum   One of a group of annular erythemas (ringlike rash) characterized by expanding ring-shaped plaques. The lesions, which are usually found on the trunk, enlarge slowly. While the disorder can occur at any age, most patients are young adults when stricken. Symptoms may last for only a short time, or they may persist for decades, depending on the cause.

This type of erythema may be associated with a DERMATOPHYTE infection, yeast infection (*Candida albicans*), parasitic bowel disease, or autoimmune disorders.

Treatment Options and Outlook

Eliminate the cause (that is, the fungus or parasite). Erythema annulare centrifugum caused by a yeast infection has been cured following treatment with oral and vaginal nystatin (an antibiotic effective against fungi).

erythema chronicum migrans   See LYME DISEASE.

erythema dyschromicum perstans   A progressive pigmented disorder of unknown cause that is one of the group of reactive ERYTHEMAS. It also has been called "ashy dermatosis" because of the characteristic slate-gray color of patients' skin.

Symptoms and Diagnostic Path

Other than the ashy appearance of the skin, there are few symptoms; patients usually are dark-skinned individuals of Latin American heritage.

Many slate gray MACULES and patches develop over the trunk, arms, and legs; the scalp, palms, soles, and mucous membranes are usually not affected. Some researchers suspect that the pigment changes represent a post-inflammatory hyperpigmentation. The condition is chronic and tends to spread.

Treatment Options and Outlook

There is no effective treatment, but makeup can cover cosmetically unattractive areas. Deliberate suntanning can also mask the lesions.

erythema gyratum repens   One of a group of disorders called annular erythemas characterized by a red ringlike rash (annula).

Symptoms and Diagnostic Path

Erythema gyratum repens causes reddened skin in a wood-grain pattern that is usually, although not always, associated with cancer, most often of the breast, lung, uterus, or upper gastrointestinal tract.

This rare reactive erythema begins with an itchy rash, found mostly on the trunk, arms, and legs, characterized by large lesions that flow together. The eruptions often look like coils of rope running parallel to each other, or growth rings on a tree. In about 60 percent of cases, the lesions occur before the cancer is diagnosed; in the other 40 percent of cases, erythema gyratum repens is diagnosed at the same time or shortly after the cancer diagnosis.

Treatment Options and Outlook

Treating the underlying cancer usually results in complete disappearance of the eruption. While topical therapy is of little benefit, emollients may help relieve the itch.

erythema infectiosum   See FIFTH DISEASE.

erythema marginatum   A type of reactive red skin color associated with rheumatic fever, a delayed complication of the upper respiratory tract caused by hemolytic streptococci, and characterized by rapidly changing ring-shaped red patches. The syndrome is becoming less common with the decline in rheumatic fever cases.

Symptoms and Diagnostic Path

The lesions tend to appear on the trunk, changing in size and shape, fading and reappearing over a matter of months.

In addition to the reddish lesions, patients usually have signs of active rheumatic fever including arthritis, fever, and so on.

Treatment Options and Outlook

The skin symptoms do not itch and do not require topical treatment, but rheumatic fever requires immediate attention.

erythema multiforme   A type of allergic reaction that occurs in response to medications, infections, or illness. Medications that can trigger erythema multiforme include antibiotics such as sulfonamides and penicillins, and anti-epileptics such as phenytoin and barbiturates. Associated infections include HERPES SIMPLEX and mycoplasma infections. This acute inflammation of the skin and mucous membranes characterized by a distinctive lesion called the "target lesion." Erythema multiforme literally means "skin redness of many varieties." Traditionally, the condition has been divided into major and minor forms (the latter is known as STEVENS-JOHNSON SYNDROME).

Erythema multiforme is most common in women in their mid-20s; the characteristic rash, which consists of a number of target lesions, is self-limiting, but may recur in up to 37 percent of cases, especially when caused by the herpes simplex virus.

The exact cause is unknown, but the disorder is believed to involve a hypersensitivity or allergic reaction to something that damages the blood vessels of the skin and skin tissues themselves. Approximately 90 percent of erythema multiforme cases are associated with herpes simplex or mycoplasma infections. The disorder occurs primarily in children and young adults.

Erythema multiforme may become noticeable with a classic skin lesion, with or without symptoms involving the entire body. In Stevens-Johnson syndrome, the systemic symptoms are severe and the lesions are extensive, involving multiple body areas, especially the mucous membranes. Toxic epidermal necrolysis (TEN syndrome, or Lyell's syndrome) involves multiple large BLISTERS that blend together, followed by sloughing of all or most of the skin and mucous membranes.

Alternatively, it may be associated with a viral or bacterial infection, radiation therapy, internal disease, chemical exposure, vaccination, or pregnancy. Herpes virus-associated erythema multiforme is found most often in teenagers and young adults; the minor form usually occurs 10 days after an acute eruption with either type 1 or type 2 herpes virus.

Half of all cases have no apparent cause.

Symptoms and Diagnostic Path

Erythema multiforme minor is usually preceded by malaise, fever, headache, sore throat, and cough for seven to 10 days. Target lesions then appear on the skin of palms and soles for three to five days and last up to two weeks. The target lesion may appear abruptly or slowly develop over two days, beginning as a pale central area surrounded by one or more rings of erythema; the center may occasionally blister. Lesions usually heal without scarring. Occasionally, erythema multiforme minor does not cause a target lesion, but instead produces hivelike plaques.

Erythema multiforme major is a more severe condition, beginning with an initial illness of fever, malaise, and prostration followed by an explosive eruption of target lesions over the body and mucous membranes, with severe ulceration, inflammation and bleeding in the eyes, mouth, nasal passages, and genitals. Appearance of these symptoms is a dermatologic emergency. Secondary infection is common; 20 percent of patients experience significant pain, eye problems, breathing problems, and difficulty maintaining oral fluid intake. Diagnosed most often among children, fluid and electrolyte imbalance or breathing problems can be fatal in 3 to 15 percent of patients. Involvement of the conjunctiva of the eyes may cause severe eye damage that can result in blindness. If the patient survives, there may be problems related to scarring in the eyes and other mucous membranes.

The diagnosis is primarily based on the appearance of the skin lesion and its typical symmetrical distribution, especially if there is a history of risk factors or associated diseases. A lesion biopsy and microscopic examination may help differentiate erythema multiforme from other disorders. Microscopic examination of the tissue may also show antibody deposits.

Treatment Options and Outlook

Suspected medications must be discontinued. In mild cases, no treatment may be required and the condition will fade away within two to three weeks. If no cause can be found, symptoms are treated and supportive care may include wet dressings or soaks and painkillers.

If possible, however, the underlying cause of erythema multiforme should be diagnosed and treated. Antihistamines are not effective against this condition.

Short courses of topical CORTICOSTEROID drugs are given to relieve the inflammation of erythema's minor form, although there is little support in the literature for this treatment.

Herpes virus–associated erythema multiforme is treated with daily doses of oral acyclovir.

The severe form of the condition is treated with painkillers, fluids, and sedatives. Lesions may be treated with wet compresses; extensive erosions should be treated as a third-degree burn. Use of corticosteroid drugs to treat the severe form is controversial, although often given despite a lack of controlled studies proving their effectiveness.

These patients usually respond to treatment, but they may become seriously ill if shock or systemic inflammation sets in. IV fluids and electrolyte replacement may be necessary; mouth lesions may be treated with a topical anesthetic, and petrolatum or other ointments may reduce cracking of dry lips.

Mild forms of erythema multiforme usually get better within two to six weeks, although the condition may recur. More severe forms may be difficult to treat. Stevens-Johnson syndrome and toxic epidermal necrolysis are associated with significant death rates.

erythema nodosum   An inflammatory skin disease associated with reddish purple swellings typically on the lower legs that also may be a result of another illness, such as SARCOIDOSIS, inflammatory bowel disease, COLLAGEN DISEASE, lymphoma, leukemia, or from drug hypersensitivity or infection. It occurs most often in women between ages 20 and 50, although the disease can appear in both sexes at any age.

Streptococcal throat infection is the most common underlying cause in the United States, although erythema nodosum is also frequently associated with tuberculosis and sarcoidosis elsewhere in the world. Frequent other associations include drug reactions from sulfonamides, penicillin, salicylates, and the birth control pill. About 30 percent of the time no cause can be found. The exact mechanism behind the disease is not known, although it is believed to be some type of immune reaction around large blood vessels in the subcutaneous fat.

Symptoms and Diagnostic Path

Shiny, tender swellings up to four inches across appear suddenly on shins, thighs, and sometimes arms. There is usually also fever and pain in muscles and joints, and there may be other symptoms, including chills, malaise, headache, or sore throat.

Pain may be severe and disabling, but permanent problems from this disease are rare. Lesions usually disappear within one or two months, although recurrences are common.

Treatment Options and Outlook

Treat any underlying illness; alter medication if condition is a response to drugs. Bed rest with the legs raised is important; for ambulatory patients, support stockings may help. Warm water compresses may be soothing and tenting the bedcovers may relieve discomfort from rubbing against material. Otherwise, treatment may include painkillers or sometimes nonsteroidal anti-inflammatory drugs to reduce inflammation. Some experts find potassium iodide to be effective, although the reason is unknown.

Even when the cause is unknown, the prognosis for recovery is good.

erythema toxicum neonatorum   A common, transient skin condition found in newborn infants during the first few days of life that usually disappears before the end of the first week and is characterized by PAPULES, PUSTULES, and pink MACULES. The skin condition may consist of only a few lesions or may cover the entire body except for palms and soles.

Less common in premature infants, the condition has been attributed to allergies, although its true cause is unknown.

Symptoms and Diagnostic Path

The condition usually develops in the second to fifth day after birth, but it may appear as late as two weeks post-partum. While a few infants may be born with the condition, it may in fact represent a different but similar disorder called transient neonatal pustular melanosis.

The typical skin lesion of erythema toxicum neonatorum is a white pustule on a red base; if pustules do not appear, there may be papules or macules or a splotchy red mark. While the condition may appear anywhere, lesions are usually found on the trunk. There may be one or two lesions or a generalized eruption.

Examination by a doctor during a routine well-baby exam is usually enough to make the diagnosis. No testing is usually needed.

Treatment Options and Outlook

The condition does not require any treatment and has no effect on future health. There are no complications.

erythrasma   A chronic bacterial infection of the toe web, groin, and underarms that causes mild burning and itching. More common in warmer climates, it is caused by *Corynebacterium minutissimum,* which produces porphyrins that fluoresce a coral red color that is observable under Wood's Light.

Symptoms and Diagnostic Path

Symptoms include sharply outlined dry, brown, slightly scaly, and slowly spreading patches.

The condition is diagnosed with a Wood's lamp test (when examined under this ultraviolet light, the lesions glow a coral red color) and with a culture of cells from the lesion.

Treatment Options and Outlook

C. minutissimum is very sensitive to a wide variety of antimicrobial drugs; extensive cases may also require oral administration of ERYTHROMYCIN, but topical treatment with antibiotics such as erythromycin or anti-fungals such as clotrimazole are usually effective.

Recurrences are common.

erythroderma   Redness over the entire body.
  See also DERMATITIS, EXFOLIATIVE.

erythromycin   An antibiotic used to treat a variety of infections, including some skin infections. It is often used as a systemic treatment for ACNE and in patients allergic to penicillin. In children under age 14 it is the alternative to TETRACYCLINE (an antibiotic that can permanently stain developing teeth and bones).

Because uncoated erythromycin is destroyed by acid in the stomach, the drug should be taken in enteric coated forms or as a compound. Otherwise, it could cause stomach distress.

Side Effects

Possible side effects include nausea and vomiting, abdominal pain, diarrhea, and an itchy rash. To reduce side effects, erythromycin may be taken with food to reduce the chance of irritating the stomach.

erythroplasia   Red plaque on the mucous membranes of the mouth that may be benign or malignant. Two types of erythroplasia are often malignant—smooth macular plaques and velvety red patches dappled with white.

erythropoietic protoporphyria   An uncommon subtype of PORPHYRIA that primarily affects the skin, causing it to be overly sensitive to sunlight. Beginning in childhood, areas of skin exposed to the sun (especially the face and hands) begin to itch, sting, and burn, lasting for hours to days after exposure. The skin becomes red and swollen in some cases, but usually heals without scarring. These signs and symptoms are often milder than the skin damage seen in other types of porphyria. No factors other than sun exposure are known to trigger symptoms.

Symptoms and Diagnostic Path

There may also be redness, swelling, and fluid-filled blisters in the exposed area. Chronic exposure to the sun may cause thickened skin and fine scars, most often seen on the upper lip and the backs of the hands.

While the exact incidence of this disease is not known, more than 300 cases have been reported worldwide. It begins (often in infancy) when children are first exposed to sunlight; they cry and begin to develop swellings in the exposed areas of skin. The skin may erode and scar, especially on the hands, nose, eyes, and ears. As the child ages, the skin over the knuckles appears thick and wrinkled.

Other internal findings include gallstones, mild hemolytic anemia, liver failure with jaundice, and cirrhosis of the liver.

Mutations in the FECH gene cause erythropoietic protoporphyria, but exactly how this gene is inherited is not yet fully understood. Experts suspect most cases are inherited in an autosomal dominant pattern, which means one copy of the altered gene is enough to trigger symptoms. Many people with one altered copy, however, do not ever develop signs and symptoms of the disorder. The condition shows autosomal recessive inheritance in a small number of families, which means two copies of the gene must be altered for a person to be affected by the disorder.

Treatment Options and Outlook

Oral administration of beta-carotene may reduce photosensitivity. Some patients have responded to treatment with iron or hematin, though this type of treatment has been found to worsen the condition of other patients.

Risk Factors and Preventive Measures
Patients with this condition should avoid sunlight and wear protective clothing when outdoors.

eschar A scab produced on the surface of the skin by BURNS, corrosive agents, some skin diseases, and infections or GANGRENE.

essential fatty acids (EFAs) Polyunsaturated fats necessary for healthy skin; a lack of these acids lead to dry scaly skin and HAIR LOSS. However, deficiency is quite rare, since just one teaspoon per day of a polyunsaturated fat (such as corn oil) provides enough EFAs.

While these acids are recognized as important in the diet, there is no evidence that they can be absorbed from the skin. Most experts believe that EFAs are important in slowing the evaporation of water from the skin's surface. One EFA, gamma linolenic acid (otherwise known as EVENING PRIMROSE OIL), is thought to be helpful in the treatment of atopic ECZEMA.

essential oils Oils extracted from flowers and herbs. This term is often more generally used to mean any perfumed oil that imitates a real scent.

estrogen A female sex hormone produced by the ovaries used in some facial creams designed for dry and lined skin. The U.S. Food and Drug Administration permits only low doses of estrogen in these creams, which do not alter the growth of skin cells but do enable the skin to retain water. Medical-grade estrogen is allowed to contain higher levels of estrogen than nonprescription products, and some experts believe that estrogen at this dosage level can improve skin tone on a limited basis.

etretinate (trade name: Tegison) A derivative of VITAMIN A used to treat severe PSORIASIS and some disorders of KERATINIZATION. Etretinate, like ISOTRETINOIN, is an analogue of vitamin A. It is more effective than isotretinoin for disorders of keratinization such as psoriasis and PITYRIASIS RUBRA PILARIS, while isotretinoin is more effective for ACNE. It is especially effective in treating pustular and erythrodermic types of psoriasis. Psoriasis requires long-term treatment with etretinate. Etretinate may be used alone, or together with more conventional psoriasis treatment (such as topical CORTICOSTEROIDS, tars, ANTHRALIN, PUVA, or METHOTREXATE).

Combining etretinate with photochemotherapy using oral PSORALENS and PUVA (called RE-PUVA) is popular in Europe as a treatment for extensive psoriasis. It has the benefits of reducing the amount of UVA exposure and the dose and length of etretinate therapy.

Side Effects
Dry skin and eyes, nosebleeds, hair loss, bone and joint pain. Etretinate is a very potent cause of birth defects and should never be taken during pregnancy.

evening primrose oil A type of ESSENTIAL FATTY ACID (also known as gamma linolenic acid). Taken in capsule form, this oil (alone or in combination with fish oil) is believed by some experts to significantly improve cases of atopic ECZEMA when taken in high doses. However these claims have not been proven and the long-term safety of high doses of the oil is not known.

Those who support the use of evening primrose oil do admit it takes six to eight capsules per day for at least six months before any results may be observed in patients. Experts also report cases of fake capsules, so consumers should avoid evening primrose oil available in no-name brands.

exanthem subitum The medical name for ROSEOLA INFANTUM, a viral disease caused by human herpes viruses 6 and 7 (HHV 6 and HHV 7).

excoriation Injury to the skin's surface caused by abrasion (scratching) or chemical reaction.

exercise and the skin Research suggests that exercise has especially important benefits for the skin. When comparing middle-aged athletes with a matched group of people who did not exercise, scientists found the athletes' skin was denser, thicker, more elastic, and stronger.

Researchers suspect that exercise flushes the skin, bringing oxygen-rich blood to the surface. It may also be that the production of COLLAGEN is enhanced by internally-generated heat (which is not the same as applying heat from the outside). Movement itself also seems to send messages to the cells in the body that manufacture the skin's elastic fibers.

When working out, individuals should never wear makeup, because blocking the evaporation of sweat by sealing the skin with makeup interferes with the process of cooling the body by perspiring.

Before exercise, the face and neck should be cleaned with lotion and water. Hair should be tied back, since sweat that is trapped against skin by hair is thought to be a cause of after-exercise skin breakouts. Harsh astringent should not be used before removing skin oils, because these natural skin oils can protect skin against the acid content of perspiration.

For exercise outside, a moisturizing SUNSCREEN should be applied.

exfoliation Removal of dead cells on the surface of the skin with a cosmetic buffing sponge or a grainy cleanser.

As the skin matures, the turnover of epidermal (upper-layer) skin cells slows down. Because the dead skin cells cling together on the surface, the complexion may appear dull and rough.

By exfoliating properly, some dermatologists say, it is possible to increase the epidermal-cell turnover, making the skin look smoother and pinker again. Exfoliation also helps stimulate the production of young epidermal cells.

However, the subject of exfoliation generates strong and differing viewpoints among dermatologists. Some believe this procedure may help skin look newer, fresher, plumper, and younger-looking, and encourage faster cell renewal. Others (including the American Academy of Dermatology) insist

the skin does not need any help in sloughing off dead skin and rank overcleansing as the biggest skin care mistake because it can overdry and irritate the skin.

Exfoliation supporters say the technique works best for those with healthy, normal, or dry complexions, and for those with dull, sun-damaged skin or skin with lots of BLACKHEADS. Even thin skin can be helped by milder exfoliants as long as there are no broken blood vessels. Patients who have had acne but whose complexions have improved may find that mild exfoliating keeps the pores unclogged and the complexion healthier.

Techniques

There are two types of exfoliation—mechanical and nonmechanical. *Mechanical* exfoliants include a wide range of techniques ranging from very mild (washcloths and sea sponges) through exfoliation sponges, loofahs—to the severe exfoliation methods utilizing pumice stones, cleansing grains, and scrubs.

Mechanical exfoliants stimulate the skin, but they may be too rough for sensitive skin or skin with broken blood vessels. People with this type of skin usually have fair, thin skin that reddens if touched. Dermatologists suggest that patients with acne not use mechanical exfoliation either, since the WHITEHEADS or closed comedones may rupture beneath the skin when rubbed, leading to more inflammatory acne.

Nonmechanical exfoliants include cosmetic masks that work on the skin surface cells, Retin-A, and chemical exfoliants (such as ALPHA-HYDROXY ACID). Masks never penetrate deeper than the dead superficial layer of the skin, and vary in strength according to the chemical used and its concentration. Depending on the concentration and the amount of time chemical exfoliants are kept on the skin, these can penetrate to living tissue. **They should be used only under medical supervision.**

Generally, it is not possible to exfoliate the same way all year; the skin changes depending on the season and the temperature. In the summer, skin has more moisture and in the winter tends to dry out.

The mildest exfoliations are the sea sponge, the face cloth, and cosmetic masks designed for sensitive or dry skin. A complexion brush moved in circular motions with some moisturizer can be a good exfoliator. For normal to thick skin, sea sponges or exfoliation sponges can be used effectively, but should be used no more than three times weekly in summer and no more than once a week in the winter.

Body exfoliation, on the other hand, is safe for all skin types, as long as any areas with inflammatory acne are avoided. It is especially beneficial for knees and elbows, especially when immediately followed by moisturizers. Self-tanning lotions also look best when applied after exfoliation.

exfoliative dermatitis   See DERMATITIS, EXFOLIATIVE.

exudate   Fluid containing PUS, cells, and protein that has been discharged from blood vessels into a tissue (or tissue surface) and is usually a result of inflammation.

eyelid lift   An operation (blepharoplasty) that removes wrinkled, drooping skin from the upper and/or lower eyelids. The outpatient operation is usually performed with a local anesthetic and sedation, and takes about one and a half to two hours. As a person grows older, the skin loses its elasticity and fat stores, becomes redistributed, causing the skin to look creased and droopy. This aging process, which can be accentuated by weight loss and stress and is accelerated by sun exposure, makes the eyelids look baggy. Removing the excess skin and redistributed fat can greatly improve appearance.

Procedure

During the operation, the surgeon removes a horizontal fold of skin from the center of the upper lids, so the scar will run in a natural crease line. Incisions in the lower lids are made either just below or just above the eyelashes to minimize the scar. Excess fat is removed from the upper and lower lid but extra skin is usually removed only from the upper lids.

After the operation, the patient can minimize swelling and bruising by applying ice packs to both eyes. Swelling usually subsides within three days, but bruising may last from two or three weeks.

Three to five days after the operation, the surgeon removes some of the stitches, and removes the remaining stitches within seven to 10 days.

Outlook and Lifestyle Modifications

The scars usually fade in time to unnoticeable marks within a year. Effects of the surgery can be expected to last between 10 and 20 years. Patients can go back to work within five to 14 days.

Actual cost may vary depending on the part of the country in which the surgery is performed.

Fabry's disease (Anderson-Fabry disease) The common name for angiokeratoma corporis diffusum, an hereditary disorder of fat metabolism resulting from an enzyme deficiency that causes widespread lesions (especially in the umbilical and knee areas), extremely painful neuralgias in hands and feet during hot weather, hardening of the arteries and kidney disease.

Symptoms and Diagnostic Path

Fabry's disease is an X-linked recessive disease caused by a defect on the X chromosome, usually leading to problems in males only. Women can be carriers of the defect; their male children have a 50 percent chance of being affected by the disease.

It is primarily characterized by the angiokeratoma, a 1- to 3-mm reddish purple raised skin lesion. Other skin symptoms include enlarged blood vessels, fingernail deformities, and reddened skin. Sweating may be inhibited.

Kidney problems can lead to kidney failure and high blood pressure. Tissue death in the brain or heart due to decreased blood flow is common.

Treatment Options and Outlook

Enzyme replacement may help slow the progression of the disease, and the pain in the hands and feet usually responds to anticonvulsants such as phenytoin and carbamazepine. Gastrointestinal hyperactivity may be treated with metoclopramide. Some individuals may require dialysis or kidney transplantation.

Kidney transplants can replace the missing enzyme and help ease pain and sweating. The angiokeratomas may be destroyed, but this does not often occur because they are small.

Patients with Fabry disease often survive into adulthood, but they are at increased risk of strokes, heart attack and heart disease, and renal failure.

face-lift (rhydectomy) Cosmetic surgery to improve the appearance by smoothing out wrinkles and lifting sagging skin in the lower third of the face.

A face-lift is usually performed on an outpatient basis using a local anesthetic and lasts between two and four hours. Loose skin is separated from underlying muscle and pulled upward and backward all around the face, going back 3 to 4 inches from the side of the face. When the skin is lifted well away from the face, it is pulled up and draped over the face. The excess skin that overlaps the incision line is removed, and the skin is sewn at the incision line.

Cotton and gauze pads are placed over the face and eyes, and the whole face (except nostrils and mouth) is wrapped in an elastic bandage. Pads are kept in place for 24 to 48 hours, and then removed. After less than a week, the entire bandage is removed.

Bruising is expected and there may be some discomfort, which is usually controlled with minor painkillers; within a few weeks, however, these signs of surgery disappear and the face begins to show improvement. The stitches are removed three days after the operation, and the scars are usually hidden by natural crease lines and the hair, fading within a year.

Patients may be back to work in 10 to 14 days, although bruising can last up to three weeks. After a face-lift, the face must be cleaned twice a day with a mild, neutral soap and creams should not be used because the pushing and pulling of creaming the face puts strain on the newly sewn tissue, which can cause the skin to sag again. Facial massage should never be applied after cosmetic surgery, since it will spread the scars and make them seem broader and thicker, and puts strain on newly sutured skin.

Risks/Complications

The two most significant side effects are oozing and infection. Occasionally, bleeding under the skin causes a blood clot that interferes with successful healing. An infection may lead to severe scarring that may require a SKIN GRAFT.

Outlook and Lifestyle Modification

Face-lifts cost an average of $4,000, although the exact amount will vary depending on the part of the country where the operation is performed. The results last for two to 10 years, and can successfully be repeated several times in a lifetime. Although many people believe that repeated face-lifts will cause a masklike expression, in fact a mask effect after a face-lift is an indication that the skin was tightened too much during the surgery.

See also PLASTIC SURGERY; PLASTIC SURGEON.

facial   A skin treatment of the face designed to clean, tone, and improve the skin's texture. Facials range from a simple mask applied at home to a sophisticated regimen in a beauty salon that may involve electrical currents, aromatic oils, or specialized creams. While the facial may moisturize or stimulate circulation in the skin, it cannot remove or prevent wrinkles.

A full facial in a salon usually begins with an examination of the skin itself, followed by cleansing and toning. Steaming may follow so that skin impurities can then be removed (using extraction or exfoliation, for example). The face may be massaged to increase circulation and to relax muscles before a mask appropriate to skin type is applied.

factitial dermatitis   See DERMATITIS ARTEFACTA.

famcyclovir (Famvir)   An antiviral medication that is the oral form of penciclovir, a drug similar to ACYCLOVIR, both used to treat herpes. However, famcyclovir lasts up to 10 times longer in the body than does acyclovir.

Famcyclovir reduces the severity of outbreaks and prevents the development of new blisters, and has also been shown to be effective for preventing genital herpes outbreaks.

Side Effects

Famcyclovir has few side effects; primary side effects are headache, fatigue, diarrhea, and nausea.

Farber's lipogranulomatosis   An inherited connective tissue disorder characterized by multiple subcutaneous nodules.

The disease is an autosomal recessive disorder, which means that a defective gene must be inherited from both parents to cause the abnormality. Generally, both parents of an affected child are unaffected carriers of the defective gene. Each of the children has a one in four chance of being affected, and a two in four chance of being a carrier.

The disease is caused by a deficiency in lysosomal acid ceramidase, which allows free ceramides to build up in tissues. This leads to the development of subcutaneous nodules.

Symptoms and Diagnostic Path

Infants typically have a weak, hoarse cry and swollen joints. Most patients die by age two, and almost none live beyond age 10. There is no known treatment.

fat atrophy   The presence of fat in the subcutaneous tissue under the skin provides a full, supple appearance. When fat cells are destroyed or removed, the surface of the skin appears to be depressed. The bony prominences of the body contribute to a gaunt appearance.

A group of rare disorders featuring localized or generalized fat atrophy are known as the lipodystrophies or lipoatrophies. They include partial lipodystrophy (Barraquer-Simmons disease), lipoatrophic diabetes (generalized lipodystrophy), and insulin lipoatrophy.

Symptoms and Diagnostic Path

Barraquer-Simmons disease is characterized by the partial loss of subcutaneous fat over a large part of the body over a course of several years, and is often triggered by a fever. The depletion of fat cells usually begins on the face and proceeds downward, and occurs four times as often in women.

Generalized lipodystrophy can be either present at birth or acquired (usually after a high fever). In both cases, the fat loss appears over the entire body. Symptoms also include a wide variety of other complaints, including insulin-resistant diabetes.

Insulin lipoatrophy is caused by repeated injections of insulin that reduce fat cells in a localized area. The depression appears about six months after injection, though rotating injection sites minimizes this problem. Spontaneous resolution of the depression may take up to 10 years.

Treatment Options and Outlook

Fat transfer (the technique of fat injection) allows fat to be removed from the patient's unaffected areas, cleansed, and then reinjected into the affected sites, where it appears to stay permanently.

See also FAT TRANSPLANTS.

fat transplants See AUTOLOGOUS FAT TRANSPLANT.

fever blisters Another name for a "cold sore."

Fibrel A freeze-dried gelatin extracted from pig connective tissue that, combined with a patient's blood and a chemical, stimulates the natural production of COLLAGEN at the site of the injection. Fibrel was approved in 1985.

Procedure

The material is injected until the SCAR or WRINKLE is elevated; the injections are given one or two weeks apart. As with collagen implants, overcorrection is necessary because there is some absorption by the body.

New collagen then begins to be deposited at the site of the Fibrel injection; it usually takes three months for the newly formed collagen to replaced the injected substance.

Risks and Complications

As with collagen injections, it is important to test for allergy before treating, although a positive reaction occurs in less than 1 percent of all cases. Fibrel is less allergenic than cow-derived collagen and longer-lasting than other liquid collagens (such as Zyderm). Still, redness, swelling, itching, and bruising can occur, and the injections are very painful.

See also SOFT TISSUE AUGMENTATION; BIOLOGICAL IMPLANTS.

fibroblasts Cells in the dermis (middle layer of skin) that produce COLLAGEN and elastin fibers.

fibrosis The deposition of fibrous tissue (SCAR) or connective tissue that may occur as a response to infection, inflammation, or injury. Fibrosis may also be caused by a lack of oxygen in a tissue because of reduced blood flow.

fibrous hamartoma of infancy See FIBROMATOSES.

fibroxanthoma of skin A typically benign tumor of the skin found most often on the sun-exposed areas of older people's skin. The lesion usually appears first as a small nodule that slowly gets bigger, though seldom exceeds 3 cm. This type of lesion rarely becomes malignant and is cured by surgical excision.

fifth disease Also known as "slapped cheeks" disease because of its dramatic symptom of a bright red rash across the cheeks, this is the least well known of the five common infectious childhood diseases—MEASLES, mumps, CHICKEN POX, and rubella (GERMAN MEASLES).

A parvovirus (B 19) usually occurs in small outbreaks among young children in the spring. Pet dogs or cats may be immunized against "parvovirus," but these are animal parvoviruses that do not infect humans. Therefore, a child cannot catch parvovirus from a pet dog or cat, and an animal cannot catch human parvovirus B19.

Although fifth disease is primarily an illness of childhood, an adult who is not immune can be infected with parvovirus B19 as well, and either have no symptoms or develop the typical rash of fifth disease, joint pain or swelling, or both. Usually, joints on both sides of the body are affected. The joints most frequently affected are the hands, wrists, and knees. The joint pain and swelling usually resolve in a week or two, but they may last several months. About half of adults, however, have been previously infected with parvovirus B19, have developed immunity to the virus, and cannot get fifth disease.

Parvovirus B19 has been found in the saliva, sputum, or nasal mucus of infected individuals before the rash appears, when they appear to have a cold. The virus is spread from person to person by direct contact with those secretions, such as sharing a glass or utensils. In a household, as many as half of susceptible persons exposed to a family member who has fifth disease may become infected. During school outbreaks, 10 percent to 60 percent of students may get fifth disease.

A susceptible person usually gets sick within four days to two weeks after being infected with the virus, but it may take as long as three weeks for symptoms to appear. A person infected with parvovirus B19 is contagious during the early part of the illness, before the rash appears. By the time a child has the characteristic reddened cheeks, for example, he or she is probably no longer contagious and may return to school. This contagious period is different from that for many other rash illnesses, such as MEASLES, for which the child is contagious as long as the rash is apparent. Once infected with the virus, people develop lasting immunity that protects them against infection in the future.

Symptoms and Diagnostic Path

The rash starts as rosy red spots on the cheeks that join into a red rash; within a few days, the rash has spread over the body, buttocks, and arms and legs. There is often a mild fever in addition to the skin rash, which may itch.

A physician can diagnose fifth disease by seeing the typical rash during a physical examination. If it is important to confirm the diagnosis, a blood test may reveal antibodies to parvovirus. If immunoglobulin M (IgM) antibody to parvovirus B19 is detected, the test result suggests that the person has had a recent infection.

Treatment Options and Outlook

Fifth disease is usually a mild illness that resolves on its own among children and adults who are otherwise healthy. Joint pain and swelling in adults usually resolve without long-term disability. Treatment of symptoms such as fever, pain, or ITCHING is usually all that is needed. Adults with joint pain and swelling may need to rest, restrict their activities, and take aspirin or ibuprofen to relieve symptoms.

The few people who have severe anemia caused by parvovirus B19 infection may need to be hospitalized and receive blood transfusions. Persons with immune problems may need special medical care, including treatment with immune globulin (antibodies), to help their bodies get rid of the infection.

However, parvovirus B19 infection may cause severe anemia in persons with sickle-cell disease or similar types of chronic anemia, and people who have problems with their immune systems may also develop a chronic anemia with parvovirus B19 infection that requires medical treatment. People who have leukemia or cancer, who are born with immune deficiencies, who have received an organ transplant, or who have human immunodeficiency virus (HIV) infection are at risk for serious illness due to parvovirus B19 infection.

Occasionally, serious complications may develop from parvovirus B19 infection during pregnancy.

Risk Factors and Preventive Measures

No vaccine or medicine will prevent parvovirus B19 infection. Frequent hand-washing is a practical and effective way to lessen the chance of infection. Keeping the patient with fifth disease home from work or school is not likely to prevent the spread of the virus, since people are contagious before they develop the rash.

filariasis A group of tropical diseases caused by a range of parasitic worms and larvae that transmit disease to humans. About 200 million people are affected by filariasis, which occurs in tropic and subtropic areas of Southeast Asia, South America, Africa, Asia, and the Pacific. When mosquitoes bite into the skin they inject the worm larvae, which migrate to the lymph nodes where they develop into mature worms in about a year.

Some of the species live in the lymphatic vessels, which become blocked, causing ELEPHANTIASIS (swelling of limbs with thickened, coarse skin). Another type of worm can be seen and felt just underneath the skin, which produces irritating and painful swellings called calabar swellings.

Symptoms and Diagnostic Path
Initial inflammatory symptoms occur between three months to a year after the mosquito bite, with swelling, redness and pain in arms, legs, or scrotum. ABSCESSES may occur as a result of dying worms and secondary bacterial infection. Repeated episodes of inflammation lead to obstruction of the lymphatic system, especially in the genital and leg areas. Chronic swelling stimulates the growth of connective tissue in the skin, causing massive permanent enlargement and deforming (elephantiasis).

Treatment Options and Outlook
Three weeks of the antihelminthic drug diethylcarbamazine cures the infection. Large doses are not given initially because reactions to large numbers of dying parasites are severe—fever, malaise, nausea, and vomiting—so doses are usually low at first. Oral antihistamines may help control HIVES and elastic stockings may help control swelling. No treatment, however, can reverse elephantiasis. Surgery may ease massive enlargement of the scrotum.

Risk Factors and Preventive Measures
In infested areas, filariasis can be controlled by taking diethylcarbamazine preventively, and by using insecticides, repellents, nets, and protective clothing.

filiform warts Slender fingerlike WARTS that are often found on the face (especially around the eyes and eyelids). They can be treated by cryotherapy, simple excision or ELECTRODESICCATION.

See also PAPILLOMAVIRUS, HUMAN; PLANTAR WARTS; GENITAL WARTS; FLAT WARTS.

fillers See SKIN FILLERS.

fingernails See NAILS.

fissure A crack or split in the skin.

flap A section of full-thickness skin that has been left attached at one end while the other end is surgically transferred to an adjacent part of the body. A flap differs from a graft in that a portion of tissue is attached to its original site and retains its blood supply. Flaps are used to cover wounds or repair defects caused by congenital deformity, accident, or surgery.

Because a flap retains its color and texture, it is more apt to survive than a graft. However, several operations usually are needed to move a flap. The major complication is necrosis at the base because of failure of blood supply.

Free flaps, on the other hand, are completely severed from the body and transferred to another site, when it receives its blood supply. The procedure is usually completed in only one surgery.

flat warts Multiple WARTS (also called juvenile warts) commonly found on the face, neck, forearms, knees, and the backs of the hands. These flat, flesh-colored papules may appear in groups of up to 100.

Symptoms and Diagnostic Path
They are often found in lines or streaks, as a result of scratching and passing on the virus. On the face, they can resemble ACNE, melanocytic nevi, or SEBORRHEIC KERATOSES. Flat warts on the arms or legs may resemble LICHEN PLANUS. About the size of a

pinhead, these growths are smoother than other kinds of warts, with flat tops; there can be as many as 100 flat warts in a cluster.

Treatment Options and Outlook
Flat warts are stubborn and require repeated treatments.

These warts may be treated by a variety of over-the-counter medications containing mild acids that help remove the dead skin cells on the surface of the wart, and irritate the skin, stimulating an immune response in the body that reacts against the wart. Alternatively, other physical methods are used. Warts may be removed by cryosurgery, in which liquid nitrogen is used to freeze the wart; this treatment is usually repeated every two to three weeks for a few months. This also irritates the skin, stimulating an immune response in the body that reacts against the wart. Electro-cauterization can be used to burn the wart away with electricity, although it must be done very gently to prevent a small scar. Laser treatments also can be used to remove warts.

See also FILIFORM WARTS; GENITAL WARTS; PAPIL-LOMAVIRUS, HUMAN; PLANTAR WARTS.

fleas There are several types of fleas that cause skin problems: the human flea (*Pulex irritans*), the cat and dog flea (*Ctenocephalides felis* and *C. canis*) and others found on mammals and birds.

Symptoms and Diagnostic Path
Flea bites cause wheals and red papules, depending on how sensitive the person is to flea bites.

As a person is repeatedly bitten, he becomes gradually sensitized (for example, infants do not respond to flea bites); however, those who are continually exposed eventually may become desensitized.

Treatment Options and Outlook
Itchy bites can be treated with topical steroid creams and systemic antihistamines.

Risk Factors and Preventive Measures
Elimination of fleas and larvae can be accomplished by spraying insecticides in crevices of fur-niture, under rugs, in beds, etc. Remove rubbish or sandpiles, and dust pets and pet bedding every two weeks with insecticides.

flesh-eating bacteria See NECROTIZING FASCIITIS.

flucytosine (Ancobon) A synthetic drug used to treat severe fungal infections caused by Candida or Cryptococcus. The drug is usually prescribed together with AMPHOTERICIN B or KETOCONAZOLE for the treatment of chromoblastomycosis or CRYPTOCOCCOSIS. Newer antifungals are replacing the agent.

fluocinolone A medium-strength CORTICOSTE-ROID prescribed as a topical agent either as a cream, solution or ointment to relieve skin inflammation, ITCHING and redness caused by disorders such as ECZEMA or PSORIASIS.

fluorescent lights and the skin Fluorescent bulbs emit small amounts of ULTRAVIOLET RADIATION, the type of solar radiation that has been blamed for SKIN CANCER.

In 1989, the National Institutes of Health said that the long-term effect of exposure to fluorescent bulbs is "an unresolved issue" and in 1990, the International Radiation Protection Association stated that ultraviolet radiation exposure from indoor fluorescent lighting should not be considered a malignant melanoma risk.

While the data remains inconclusive, those who are concerned can attach a plastic diffuser to their fluorescent lighting fixture (many lights come this way), which can eliminate or reduce the intensity of the ultraviolet emissions.

fluoroquinolones A group of antimicrobial drugs that are effective against many bacteria, including most *Pseudomonas* bacteria. Several of the fluoroquinolones are also active against *Mycoplasma, Chlamydia, Legionella* and a few other mycobacteria. Fluoroquinolones are not particularly effective against anaerobic organisms.

These drugs are used to treat many types of infections, including soft tissue infections and urethritis.

Fluoroquinolones include norfloxacin, ciprofloxacin, ofloxacin, enoxacin, pefloxacin, fleroxacin, lomefloxacin, and several other compounds.

Side Effects

The drugs have fewer side effects than many other antibiotics. The most common side effect is loss of appetite and sensitivity to light. Less common effects include nausea, abdominal pains, diarrhea, dizziness, rash, and so on. These drugs are not recommended for children or adolescents, since they may have toxic effects on developing cartilage.

fluorouracil An anticancer drug often used on the skin; also known as 5-fluorouracil or 5-FU. It is used to treat multiple ACTINIC KERATOSES and for flat, genital, and intraurethral WARTS, PSORIASIS, BOWEN'S DISEASE, and superficial BASAL CELL CARCINOMA or KERATOACANTHOMAS. It is of particular benefit when surgical removal of several tumors located together is difficult. It is applied according to various schedules—from twice a day two consecutive days a week for nine weeks, to daily or twice daily for four to six weeks. It is also injected within the lesion for patients with KERATOACANTHOMAS.

Side Effects

As treatment progresses, patients develop intense inflammation and irritation that is worsened by exposure to ultraviolet light. For this reason, patients with many lesions are often not treated until winter. Irritation is significant and occurs with all patients. It can be soothed by using moisturizers; occasionally, topical steroids are necessary.

Other possible side effects after systemic administration include nausea and vomiting, scars, diarrhea, hair loss, and impaired blood cell production. The drug applied as a cream may cause skin inflammation.

When treatment is stopped, the skin heals rapidly. It takes two to four weeks for healthy new skin to replace the skin destroyed by the 5-FU. After healing, the treated areas are often redder than normal and may feel more sensitive; this red-ness and sensitivity will gradually fade over a few weeks. Occasionally it persists for several months.

flush Transient redness and warmth (primarily of the face and neck) associated with certain medications and pathologic conditions.

See also ROSACEA; BLUSH.

Flynn-Aird syndrome A genetic disorder associated with skin ulceration in which subcutaneous tissue atrophies and forms ulcers, similar to conditions such as WERNER'S SYNDROME and SCLERODERMA.

Other symptoms include mental retardation, deafness, convulsions, baldness, and stiff joints, which may appear during the first or second decade of life. This disorder is transmitted as an autosomal dominant disorder, which means that only one defective gene (from one parent) is needed to cause the syndrome. Each child of an affected person usually has a one in two chance of inheriting the defective gene and of being affected.

focal dermal hypoplasia See HAIR, DISORDERS OF.

follicle See HAIR FOLLICLE.

follicular hyperkeratoses Disorders of KERATINIZATION characterized by thickening of the skin around and/or on hair follicles. These disorders include KERATOSIS PILARIS, disseminated and recurrent INFUNDIBULOFOLLICULITIS, and KYRLE'S DISEASE.

follicular mucinosa See MUCINOSES.

follicular orifice See PORE.

folliculitis Inflammation of a hair follicle. Folliculitis starts when hair follicles are irritated by friction from clothing, a blocked follicle, or shaving. In most cases of folliculitis, the damaged follicles are then infected with the bacteria *Staphylococcus*. While staphylococcal folliculitis can occur anywhere on the skin, it is most often found on hairy areas of the face, neck, armpits, thighs, or buttocks.

Symptoms and Diagnostic Path

Folliculitis is characterized by a shallow, superficial rash of pimples and PUSTULES around a hair follicle on the neck, under the arms, or in the groin.

A diagnosis is primarily based on the appearance, of the skin; a culture of the lesion may identify the bacteria or fungi.

Treatment Options and Outlook

Antibiotics cure staphylococcal folliculitis. Depending on the cause, it may also be necessary to avoid irritants or chemical exposure, minimize friction from clothing, avoid shaving the area, and keep the area clean. Hot moist compresses may help drain extensive areas of infection. Folliculitis usually responds well to treatment, but may recur.

Risk Factors and Preventive Measures

Because the infection may be spread from one person to the next in the same household, each family member should use separate towels and washcloths, bathe often and wash underclothes in boiling water to kill the bacteria.

Food, Drug and Cosmetic [FDC] Act of 1938 The primary law governing the composition of cosmetics (including all skin care products). The act was passed in the wake of a serious cosmetics-related injury in 1933, when at least one woman was blinded and others were injured by using Lash Lure, a tint administered in beauty salons to color eyelashes and eyebrows.

In addition to the FDC Act of 1938, cosmetics packaging and labeling is governed by the Fair Packaging and Labeling Act; both of these are enforced by the U.S. Food and Drug Administration (FDA). Because the FDA is severely hampered by its budget (only about 1 percent of which is spent on cosmetics regulation), in an average year, the FDA makes only about 400 on-site inspections of cosmetics manufacturers.

In 1977, regulations on cosmetics labeling were added to the FDC act. According to this law, the outside wrapper or container must tell the consumer the manufacturer's name, address, maker, or distributor, the product's weight, ingredients, and warn of any potential dangers. Ingredients listed must include any that are contained in the product in concentrations exceeding more than 1 percent in descending order of predominance. Ingredients should be listed only by their recognized names. If the cosmetic also qualifies as a drug, the drug ingredients must be listed as "active ingredients" at the top of the list. (For example, sunscreens are considered to be over-the-counter drugs, as are dandruff shampoos, acne medications, and so on.)

Fragrances can be listed only under the general heading "fragrance," and not under the specific ingredients from which the fragrance is derived—sometimes 10 or more substances.

Color ingredients can be listed in any order, no matter how much or little of the color they make up. Colors used in cosmetics are very strictly regulated, especially for products intended for use around the eye area. Many colors used in cosmetics are certified coal tar colors, which are prohibited for use around the eyes. Coal tar colors include any having the initials D&C or FD&C before the color name and number (such as D&C Yellow #10).

The FDA prohibits very few ingredients for cosmetics; those that are prohibited or restricted include bithionol, mercury compounds, vinyl chloride, halogenated salicylanilides, zirconium complexes, chloroform, chlorofluorocarbon propellants, and hexachlorophene.

There are significant differences in how the FDA handles the approval of a cosmetic and a drug. If a cosmetic is promoted as a way to improve appearance, a company can place it on the market without any pre-market approval from the FDA—provided the manufacturer understands that it is safe. If the FDA later discovers there is a safety concern with the cosmetic, officials can take action to remove it from the market.

For the purposes of the FDA, a drug is considered to be any product that purports to cure, treat, or mitigate a disease. Drug manufacturers must prove their medication is safe and effective before it is placed on the market.

Furthermore, a product that the FDA has considered to be a cosmetic may be relisted as a drug if the product subsequently is found to have a definite physiological effect on the body—even if the company did not market the product as a drug.

See also COSMETIC INGREDIENTS, PROHIBITED.

food reactions Allergies to certain foods can cause a wide range of reactions in up to 7 percent of the population, including specific skin symptoms such as ITCHING, HIVES, and swelling. If the reaction occurs immediately after the food allergen is eaten, the problem is not hard to trace. In cases where itching and redness do not occur until hours or even days after the food is eaten, the problem may be harder to track.

A range of common foods may bring on itchy skin symptoms, including citrus fruits, eggs, fish, cola drinks, artificial coloring, or milk. Infants prone to allergies may be particularly sensitive to milk and milk products, wheat, eggs, and citrus fruits. Acute hives usually result from an allergic reaction to foods such as shellfish, nuts, berries, tomatoes, eggs, citrus fruits, and pork.

Food *additives* also may cause problems. About 15 percent of people who are allergic to aspirin are sensitive to Yellow Dye #5 (tartrazine).

Many food allergies disappear with time, especially in children. About a third of proven allergies disappear in one to two years if the patient carefully avoids the offending foods.

A food allergy is diagnosed following a detailed food history, physical exam, and pertinent tests; skin testing may help identify cases of food allergy in cases of acute itching. However, skin testing is not usually helpful in diagnosing chronic itching due to food allergy. For these cases, a food diary and trial elimination of suspect foods may help.

Treatment Options and Outlook

Treatment involves eliminating or reducing the sensitive food. Drug therapy may be necessary for those with multiple food sensitivities that do not respond to elimination. Drug therapy involves the use of antihistamines, adrenergic agents, corticosteroids, and cromolyn sodium.

Treatment of an anaphylactic reaction to food depends on the severity of the reaction. If the person's heart was stopped, CPR should be started. Epinephrine is injected, and antihistamines and steroids may also be given to prevent recurrences of the reaction, and to control hives and swelling.

Risk Factors and Preventive Measures

Since severe reactions to food allergies were more likely to be caused by foods prepared away from home, the National Restaurant Association (NRA) and the Food Allergy Network began a program to help restaurant workers understand food allergies. The NRA provides free information to restaurants about the proper way to handle food allergy requests.

formaldehyde, sensitivity to Many people can develop a sensitivity to formaldehyde, which is used in industry and in medicine as a preservative or antimicrobial and, in larger amounts, in nail care products. Household products often contain formaldehyde as a preservative. Substances that release formaldehyde contained in cosmetics or industrial products may be listed under a trade name and not under "formaldehyde" on the product label.

Formaldehyde can be irritating to some people, and because of its toxicity the Food and Drug Administration limits its concentration in nail products to 5 percent.

See also ALLERGIES AND THE SKIN.

Fort Bragg fever See LEPTOSPIROSIS.

foundation This cosmetic product is generally applied first to the skin to even out skin tone. Choosing the right foundation requires finding the product that most closely resembles the consumer's skin color and that is appropriate for the person's skin type. Because foundation is worn next to the skin, it should not be too oily nor contain too much alcohol.

Dry skin benefits from foundations containing mineral oil, cream-formula, or oil-in-water emulsions. Products with a "matte finish" or those labeled "pore minimizing" are good choices for oily skin. Those with combination skin should choose an oil-free, pancake, or matte foundation.

Foundation should not be applied directly to skin without first applying a layer of lightweight, skin-matched moisturizer that absorbs easily. Even women with oily skin or breakouts should use this buffer layer, and tone down the shine with a dusting of loose translucent powder. Skin that is at all sensitive needs this protective shield of moisturizer to reduce the chance of developing a reaction from something in the foundation.

Because a person's neck skin is often a different color than facial skin, experts suggest matching the color of the foundation with the jawline. Foundation color should never be tested on the skin of the wrist or hand, because it won't match facial skin. Foundation should not be used to change skin color (to approximate a tan, for example) because the results will appear unnatural.

See also COSMETICS.

Fox-Fordyce disease Also known as apocrine miliaria, this is an uncommon chronic disorder of the sweat glands causing itchy lesions of the skin under the arms, in the pubic area, around the nipple parts of the genitalia, and sometimes on the chest and abdomen. It is characterized by retention of apocrine sweat leading to the formation of yellow PAPULES. There may also be hair loss in the affected areas. The ITCHING is often associated with emotional situations.

The disease appears after puberty, and is 10 times more common in women than men. Temporary improvement occurs during pregnancy. It is believed to be associated with an endocrinologic problem. Some women may find that the disease may regress after menopause.

Symptoms and Diagnostic Path
This disease often causes no symptoms.

Treatment Options and Outlook
This disease often requires no treatment. However, topical application of CORTICOSTEROIDS or TRETINOIN may help relieve symptoms, and birth control pills or estrogen alone are often helpful. The only permanent cure is to remove affected skin areas.

fragrance and the skin Modern fragrances usually contain about 50 different scent materials that may come from floral oils (flower petals), essential oils (such as citrus fruit peel), or animal perfumes (such as ambergris). By isolating the primary odor from a plant and combining it with chemicals, a new odor—or isolate—is formed. Fragrances may also contain manmade scents derived from petrolatum, coal tar, and so on.

Fragrance may be found in a variety of forms, including perfumes (alcohol solutions of 15–25 percent perfume concentrate), toilet water (3–5 percent perfume), or eau de cologne (about the same perfume concentration as toilet water, but whose scent blends the oils of lemon, bergamot and rosemary).

The odor of a fragrance depends on the chemistry of the wearer's skin, which is affected by genes, medication, diet, hormones, and skin type (oily skin traps fragrance and dry skin tends to let fragrance evaporate). Therefore, to test a fragrance, it is better to dab a few drops on the skin and wait a few seconds before sniffing it. However, the true "heart" of the scent will not be apparent for several hours.

Fragrances are created with different top, middle and end "notes" that change the scent gradually as it is worn over a period of hours. The top notes are the way the fragrance smells right after it is applied to the skin, and lasts for approximately 15 minutes after application. The middle notes take over for the next few hours, and are the heart of the scent.

To test a fragrance, it should be applied to the inside of the wrist. To prolong fragrance, it should be layered using several different preparations of the fragrance (oil or lotion, powder, and toilet water or perfume); cologne lasts for approximately two hours; eau de toilette lasts two to four hours, and perfume lasts four to six hours.

Keep in mind that dry skin does not hold fragrance as well as oily skin; soaking dry skin in bath oil before applying the same-scent fragrance or wearing body lotion can help the fragrance last. Pulse points (behind the ear, backs of the knees, wrists) are the best places to apply fragrance, since they tend to be warmer than other skin areas.

See also ALLERGIES AND THE SKIN; COSMETICS; MAKEUP.

fragrance, sensitivity to See ALLERGIES AND THE SKIN; FRAGRANCE AND THE SKIN.

frambesia See YAWS.

freckles Tiny round or oval patches of pigmented skin that are found on areas of the skin exposed to the sun. The tendency to freckle is inherited, and usually occurs in fair and red-haired individuals. Generally the more exposure to the sun, the more freckles appear. While freckles are harmless, those with highly freckled complexions should avoid excess sunlight and use SUNSCREENS.

Freckles (also called ephelids) are temporary—they come and go with the sun. On the other hand, LIVER SPOTS (lentigines) come and stay forever.

Freckles are caused by the skin's efforts to tan in spots where there is an uneven distribution of melanin, resulting in an irregular tanning pattern. Some people find they can prevent freckles by applying a sunscreen with a high SPF (SUN PROTECTION FACTOR); once freckles appear, however, they may take an entire season to fade away.

free-flap surgery A procedure by which flaps of skin are transplanted with blood vessels attached, thereby ensuring the health of the graft. In the past, when surgeons had to rely on simple SKIN GRAFTs in areas that had little blood supply or in which the blood vessels were impaired, blood flow could not be restored and the transplanted tissue would often die. Attempts to transplant additional blood vessels to the site required multistage operations that caused long recovery delays.

With free-flap surgery, physicians can transplant skin and blood vessels, using microscopes that magnify the operating field up to 40 times and sutures that are only one-third the width of a human hair. Employing a team approach during the operation allows donor and recipient sites to be operated on simultaneously.

Common sites for the donor skin and blood supply include the groin, scalp, armpit, forearm, thigh, or back.

When more than one of these tissues is needed in a special configuration unavailable naturally, the right kind of flap, called a prefabricated flap, can be pieced together gradually and then transplanted to its new home once the new structure is viable. For example, a new nose can be created on the forearm, where it is less conspicuous than on the face, and transplanted once it is complete.

Some uses for free-flap surgery include breast reconstruction, movement restoration in fingers, and so on.

free radicals A highly charged, destructive form of oxygen generated by each cell in the body that destroys cellular membranes through the oxidation process, contributing to premature aging, loss of elasticity, discoloration, and saggy skin. Rusting iron, crumbling stone, and flaking paint on a canvas are all the result of oxidation, an environmentally triggered free radical reaction.

Because free radicals are essential to many reactions in the body (they are generated by the immune system to fend off microbes and help the digestive system break down food), they should not be destroyed entirely. It is only when the levels become excessive that damage can occur.

Free radical damage to the skin can be offset by molecules called antioxidants, which neutralize free radicals before they can damage skin cells. They include beta carotene, selenium, the synthetic antioxidant molecule BHT, and phloroglucinol, a natural antioxidant extracted from algae. VITAMINS E and C are particularly potent antioxidants. While there is no guarantee regarding the effectiveness of the dietary supplements of antioxidants in preventing cell damage, many physicians believe and recommend the benefits of the antioxidants beta carotene, vitamins C and E to their patients. Still, the U.S. Food and Drug Administration and the National Academy of Sciences believe it is premature to recommend increases in vitamin C, E, and beta carotene intake. Other research groups and public health organizations are recommending daily doses of some vitamins and minerals that are four to 16 times higher than the current recommended daily allowances. No one is suggesting that vitamin supplements should take the place of a healthful diet and lifestyle, however.

While vitamins C and E are particularly good antioxidants, taking these vitamins orally may do a better job of protecting against free radicals in the body than on the skin. For this reason, some researchers are recommending that consumers apply these molecules directly to the skin. Some cosmetics are incorporating antioxidants into their ingredients as a way to make antioxidants more available to the skin.

frostbite Damage to the skin caused by exposure to very cold temperatures for a long period of time. The areas most likely to be affected are the feet and hands, nose, and ears. While anyone can become frostbitten, those with circulatory problems are at greatest risk.

Although it is theoretically possible for tissue to freeze in temperatures at about 32° F, the body's local internal temperature must fall to levels lower than that before freezing occurs at a specific area of the body. The danger of frostbite increases if a person is without adequate food, clothing, or shelter; wind or wet skin also hastens the outward transfer of heat and increases the risk of frostbite.

Symptoms and Diagnostic Path

Frostbitten skin appears as firm, pale, cold white patches with a lack of sensitivity to touch, although there may be a sharp, aching pain on the affected area. As the skin thaws, it becomes raw and painful. Frostbite damage may be described as "superficial" (FROSTNIP), involving skin and subcutaneous tissues or "deep" (true frostbite), affecting muscle, nerve, vessels, cartilage, and bone.

Treatment Options and Outlook

Normal body temperature should be restored before thawing any frostbitten flesh. A small area of frostnipped skin can be rewarmed by placing fingers or the heel of the hand over the affected area. Rapid thawing of the affected part in warm water baths is the current preferred treatment method for more extensive frostnip and for frostbite. If immediate emergency assistance is unavailable, severely frostbitten hands or feet should be thawed in warm, *not hot,* water (between 104–108° F) for 20 to 30

minutes. Other heat sources (such as heating pads) should not be used because the frostbitten tissue can still be burned by temperatures that under normal conditions would not harm the skin. If the skin tingles and burns as it warms, circulation is returning. *If numbness remains as the area is warmed, professional help should be obtained immediately.*

A frostbitten area should never be rubbed as it thaws. If feet are affected, the patient should not walk on them. In addition, frostbitten patients should not smoke cigarettes, since nicotine causes the blood vessels to constrict and may inhibit circulation. Neither bandages nor dressings should be used.

Thawing time is determined by the temperature of the water and the depth of freezing; it is complete when the extremity flushes pink or red. After rapid thawing, small BLISTERS appear, spontaneously rupturing in four to 10 days, followed by a black SCAB. Normal tissue may have formed below. Constant digital exercises should be performed to preserve joint motion. Further treatment is designed to prevent infection and preserve function of the affected part.

In severe cases, antibiotics, bed rest, and physical therapy may be necessary after the affected part has been warmed; cigarettes should be avoided during the entire recovery period.

The best chance of successful healing after frostbite occurs is when the affected part has not been frozen long, when thawing is rapid and when blisters develop early. The outlook is more uncertain when thawing is spontaneous at room temperature, when the part is frozen for a long time, or if the frostbite occurred in an area of fracture or dislocation. A poor outlook is indicated if thawing is delayed or occurs due to excessive heat, if blisters are dark, or if thawing is followed by refreezing. Refreezing almost always ends in amputation.

In mild cases, damage can be reversed, but if frostbite is severe the flow of blood to the area stops. Unless immediate treatment is begun, the area will be irreversibly damaged and amputation of the extremity may be required.

Major complications include infection, tissue death, sensory loss, persistent deep pain, and limited joint movement. Permanent effects may include fixed scars, small muscle wasting, deformed joints, arthritic bone changes, and increased sensitivity to cold.

Risk Factors and Preventive Measures

Frostbite is theoretically simple to prevent by wearing proper clothing in cold weather (dry and layered, warm and loose), especially on hands and feet. Nose and ears should be protected; tight apparel (boots, gloves or clothing) should never be worn. Conditions that increase the likelihood of frostbite include emaciation, fatigue, dehydration, and previous frostbite.

To stay warm, individuals should wear cotton blend socks (such as Orlon and cotton), not pure cotton socks. Clothes should be loose, and layered to help trap heat. The inner clothing layer should be made of a synthetic fabric, or a silk or wool blend that wicks away perspiration from the skin. The next layer should be something that insulates, like a wool shirt, for example. Waterproof, breathable boots and outer jacket are a good choice. Since the head is the source of greatest heat loss, a hat must be worn in cold weather; mittens are better than gloves because they trap heat from the whole hand.

Individuals who must go outside in cold weather should eat warm food (oatmeal, hot soup) to raise core body temperature, and drink plenty of fluids to stave off dehydration. Dehydration can worsen chills and frostbite by reducing blood volume. Caffeinated beverages, which constrict blood vessels and interfere with circulation, should be avoided. While alcohol may temporarily warm up hands and feet, it has a cumulative negative effect by increasing blood flow to the skin, reducing the core body temperature.

In any situation where freezing has occurred, thawing must be prevented if refreezing is a possibility. While it is possible to survive local freezing of an extremity, the body's *internal* temperature must be maintained, since loss of vital temperature can cause hypothermia and death.

frostnip   The earliest stage of FROSTBITE, this condition is reversible. In this stage, the skin suddenly turns white and frosty and becomes less sensitive.

Frostnip is treated by drying and gently rewarming the injured skin by placing it against warm skin (such as under the armpits or on the abdomen). If exposure to the cold continues, frostnip quickly deteriorates into full-blown frostbite, which causes permanent skin damage.

fucosidosis   A very rare genetic metabolic disorder caused by a lack of a lysosomal enzyme resulting in the accumulation of fucose between the cells.

There are three types of fucosidosis, but it is type III disease that causes skin symptoms, including pigmentary retinopathy (disorder of the retina) and (occasionally) lack of sweating (HYPOHIDROSIS) and purple nail beds. In addition, patients may have various neurologic problems, including seizures and recurrent pulmonary infections.

The disorder is an autosomal recessive disease, meaning that a defective gene must be inherited from both parents to cause the abnormality. Generally, both parents of an affected person are unaffected carriers of the defective gene. Each of their children has a one-in-four chance of being affected, and a two-in-four chance of being a carrier. There is no effective treatment.

Fulvicin   See GRISEOFULVIN.

fungal infections   Diseases of the skin (also called mycoses) caused by the spread of fungal organisms. Infection may range from a mild skin condition to severe disease with fatal symptoms. Fungal skin infections are either considered to be superficial (affecting skin, hair, nails) or subcutaneous (beneath the skin).

The *superficial* fungal infections include THRUSH (candidiasis) and TINEA (including RINGWORM, JOCK ITCH, and ATHLETE'S FOOT). *Subcutaneous infections* are rare; the most common is *sporotrichosis*, occurring after a contaminated scratch; most examples of this type of condition occur in tropical climates.

Symptoms and Diagnostic Path

Harmless fungi and yeasts are present all the time on the skin, but they do not multiply there because of competition among bacteria or because the body's immune system fights them off. Superficial fungal infections are extremely common, and occur in perfectly healthy individuals. Widespread or deep fungal infections of the skin are most common in those taking long-term antibiotics, CORTICOSTEROID, or immunosuppressant drugs, or in patients with an immune system disorder such as AIDS. Some people have a genetic tendency toward fungal infections.

There are two significant ways to determine the type of fungus causing the infection. The faster method involves placing a tissue sample in an alkaline solution of potassium hydroxide (KOH). The KOH changes the sample so that the fungus shows up more clearly under the microscope. Experts can often identify the fungus by the filaments it sends out through the skin sample. Another method involves growing a colony of fungus in the laboratory from a skin sample. This is more accurate but may take weeks. Finally, some fungi exhibit a fluorescent glow when exposed to ultraviolet light, which can also help to identify the fungus causing an infection.

Treatment Options and Outlook

One common antifungal drug taken by mouth (GRISEOFULVIN) is effective for treating TINEA CAPITIS, for example, but not for CANDIDA and certain mold infections. The drug KETOCONAZOLE (Nizoral) is effective against TINEA VERSICOLOR but not against other fungal infections.

Many broad-spectrum antifungal agents effectively treat a wide range of organisms, which means the patient can begin taking an antifungal drug without waiting for culture results. Three of these new antifungals are itraconazole (Sporanox), terbinafine (Lamisil), and fluconazole (Diflucan).

The treatment regimen is chosen based on the type and extent of the infection. Some work well in the short term, while others have a longer lasting effect. Some work well in small quantities, while others require larger doses to be effective. If only skin is involved, the treatment is relatively short (a few weeks). If the nails are affected, at least three months of treatment is required.

Occasional side effects of oral antifungals include nausea, diarrhea, abdominal pain, skin rashes, headache, and fatigue. The doctor may order a blood test to check liver function, especially during long-term therapy, if the patient has an already weakened liver or is using high doses of medication.

Risk Factors and Preventive Measures

A patient should receive effective follow-up care because fungal infections can recur and treatments are usually more successful if started early. It is possible to prevent fungal infection by not sharing hats, combs, brushes, or other objects. Wearing shoes in locker rooms, public showers, and around swimming pools can help reduce contact with athlete's foot fungus. Reducing moisture and humidity on the skin by drying it thoroughly and by changing sweaty clothes and socks also can help prevent fungus. Cleaning or discarding infected objects and garments also helps prevent recurrences.

See also TINEA BARBAE; TINEA CORPORIS; TINEA MANUUM; TINEA NIGRA PALMARIS; ATHLETE'S FOOT; JOCK ITCH.

Fungizone See AMPHOTERICIN B.

fungus A phylum of plants (including yeasts, rusts, molds, smuts, mushrooms, and so on) characterized by the absence of chlorophyll and the presence of a rigid cell wall. There are more than 100,000 different species of fungi around the world, most of which are harmless or beneficial to human health (such as molds used to produce antibiotics, yeasts used in baking and brewing, edible mushrooms and truffles, and yogurt cultures).

However, some fungi can invade and form colonies in the skin or underneath the skin, leading to disorders ranging from a mild skin irritation and inflammation to severe or fatal systemic infections.

See also FUNGAL INFECTIONS.

furuncle Another name for a BOIL.

furunculosis A bacterial infection characterized by tender, subcutaneous nodules usually capped with a small PUSTULE, and infected with *Staphylococcus aureus*. Furuncles (BOILS) occur when a few neighboring hair follicles become infected with *S. aureus*. If more follicles are involved, the furuncle becomes a CARBUNCLE. Furuncles most commonly affect the neck and upper back. Boils may also recur for years.

Treatment Options and Outlook

Surgical drainage of pus is followed by the application of warm compresses for 20 minutes four times a day. Bathing with antimicrobial soap decontaminates other areas. Systemic antibiotics are frequently required.

Risk Factors and Preventive Measures

The recurrence of furunculosis may be prevented by improving hygiene, by taking systemic antibiotics, and by ensuring that the source of infection is cleared.

Futcher's line See VOIGT'S LINE.

G

gangrene Death of tissue generally associated with loss of blood supply, followed by bacterial infection. It may affect either a fairly small area of skin or an entire limb.

In *dry gangrene,* an area of the skin dies because of a blocked blood supply, without bacterial infection; this type does not spread to other tissue. It may be caused by arteriosclerosis, diabetes mellitus, a stroke, blood clot, or FROSTBITE.

Wet gangrene follows bacterial infection of dry gangrene or a wound.

Gas gangrene is a particularly virulent form of wet gangrene caused by a deadly type of bacteria (*Clostridium welchii*) that destroys muscle while producing a foul odor. Gas gangrene has been responsible for millions of deaths during war.

Symptoms and Diagnostic Path

Pain occurs in the dying skin tissue, which becomes numb and black once it dies. If bacterial infection occurs, the gangrene will spread, giving off a noxious odor with redness, swelling, and oozing PUS around the blackened area. In cases of gas gangrene, symptoms may include persistent or severe pain, fever, gas in tissues beneath the skin, a sick feeling, and septic shock.

Gangrene can be diagnosed during a physical examination, but a number of tests and procedures also may be performed, including blood tests (a CBC may show a high white blood cell count), X-rays, scans, exploratory surgery, microscopic examination of tissue, or tissue or fluid cultures.

Treatment Options and Outlook

Dry gangrene: Improving circulation to the affected area can improve dry gangrene if it is begun early enough.

Wet gangrene: Once the tissue becomes infected, antibiotics are given to prevent wet gangrene from setting in. Once wet gangrene is diagnosed, amputation of the affected part, along with neighboring healthy tissue, is required in order to save the patient. The prognosis depends on the part of the body affected, the extent of the gangrene, its cause, and the patient's condition. Treatment delay can be fatal; significant involvement or other underlying medical conditions also can lead to death.

Gardner-Diamond syndrome This self-induced syndrome affects women almost exclusively, and is characterized by painful bruising of the skin after minor injury. These patients share a similar personality profile—masochistic tendencies, dependent relationships, and intense anger toward those closest to them.

Patients may first complain of tenderness, burning, or stabbing pain in the legs; skin lesions become bluish from within a few hours to three days later, and eventually come to resemble bruises. Recurrent lesions in groups are common. The condition is thought to be self-inflicted.

The prognosis for syndrome patients, even with extensive psychotherapy, is poor.

Gardner's syndrome A hereditary disorder featuring benign skin growths that appear during the first 10 years of life. The skin growths include epidermal and sebaceous cysts, lipomas, and fibromas.

The disorder is an autosomal dominant disease, which means that only one defective gene (from one parent) is needed to cause the syndrome. Each child of an affected person usually has a one in two chance of inheriting the defective gene and of being affected. It was discovered in the 1950s by Dr. Eldon Gardner, who noticed multiple symptoms among family members in two different families. Recently, the gene responsible for Gardner's syndrome, which affects the growth cells in the body, has been identified.

Symptoms and Diagnostic Path

The syndrome also causes thousands of polyps in the colon, as well as the stomach and upper intestine, together with bony tumors in the jaw and skull. The polyps associated with this syndrome usually appear around age 15 and eventually lead to cancer.

Treatment Options and Outlook

Since the inevitable outcome of this disease is colon cancer (typically about 10 to 15 years after the onset of the polyps), patients with documented Gardner's should have their colon and rectum removed. Although there is no recommended nonsurgical therapy for Gardner's, studies have shown that the colon polyps regress to a significant degree with use of sulindac (Clinoril), a nonsteroidal anti-inflammatory drug. Since other polyps may be present elsewhere, regular endoscopic examination of these areas is also a good idea.

All blood relatives of a person diagnosed with Gardner's syndrome should be screened with colonoscopy. There are also genetic tests to screen younger patients who may have not yet developed the polyps.

gastrointestinal bleeding, skin symptoms of If enough bleeding in the gastrointestinal tract occurs, the skin may appear pale. Cirrhosis of the liver may include skin symptoms of redness, spidery veins, or jaundice.

Gaucher's disease A hereditary disorder of lipid metabolism most often found among Ashkenazi Jews. A lack of the enzyme B-glucocerebrosidase, important to the metabolic process, leads to a buildup of fatty compounds (cerebrosides) in the liver, spleen, lymph nodes, and nervous system.

Gaucher's disease is an autosomal recessive disorder, which means that a defective gene must be inherited from both parents in order for the abnormality to occur. Generally, both parents of an affected person are unaffected carriers of the defective gene. Each of their children has a one in four chance of being affected and a two in four chance of being a carrier.

Symptoms and Diagnostic Path

The most common skin symptom is a yellow-brown discoloration appearing over exposed areas, mimicking MELASMA when it occurs on the face. If bone marrow or liver are involved, symptoms may include blue/purple hemorrhagic patches, purple papules, pale skin, or jaundice.

A biochemical assay is now available to identify carriers.

Treatment Options and Outlook

Researchers are studying the feasibility of replacing the deficient enzyme.

The disease is fatal in infancy, but a less severe form may become apparent only in adulthood.

gel A clear, jellylike, solid vehicle that becomes liquid when warmed or rubbed onto the skin. Gels usually contains volatile solvents that evaporate quickly when applied to the skin. Many gel products have been refined to eliminate oils, fragrances, color, or emulsifiers. Gel moisturizers and cleansers also have a higher water content than most creams and lotions, which makes them feel cool and soothing on the skin.

While most creams can leave the skin feeling greasy, gels are absorbed almost instantly, like water. Gels work well for women with normal to oily skin because they add moisture without adding oil. But for those with dry skin who may need more moisture, a better skin-care choice is an emollient-rich cream or lotion, because gels have a tendency to be drying.

genetic disorders of the skin There is a wide range of genetic diseases affecting the skin. Genetic hair defects that cause loss of hair include hidrotic ectodermal dysplasia, ANHIDROTIC ECTODERMAL DYSPLASIA, CARTILAGE-HAIR HYPOPLASIA, trichorhinophalangeal syndrome, biotin responsive carboxylase deficiency, marie unna hypotrichosis, congenital skin defect (APLASIA CUTIS), CONRADI'S DISEASE, incontinentia pigmenti, focal dermal hypoplasia, and Hallermann-Streiff syndrome. Other genetic hair disorders include low sulfur hair syndromes and hypertrichosis lanuginosa.

Genetic blistering disorders include EPIDERMOLYSIS BULLOSA; ACRODERMATITIS ENTEROPATHICA; tyrosinemia type II (RICHNER-HANHART SYNDROME) pachyonychia.

Genetic diseases associated with sensitivity to light include BLOOM SYNDROME, XERODERMA PIGMENTOSUM, DYSKERATOSIS CONGENITA.

Genetic diseases associated with premature aging and hardening of the skin include WERNER'S SYNDROME and PROGERIA. Those associated with abnormal skin elasticity include EHLERS-DANLOS SYNDROME, CUTIS LAXA, BUSCHKE-OLLENDORFF SYNDROME, FARBER'S LIPOGRANULOMATOSIS, and PACHYDERMOPERIOSTOSIS.

Genetic skin disorders involving multiple new skin growths include epidermodysplasia verruciformis and GARDNER'S SYNDROME.

Other genetic diseases include: ANGIOKERATOMA, arginosuccinic aciduria, GENODERMATOSIS, LENTIGINOSIS PROFUSA, lentigo simplex, and MULTIPLE LENTIGINES SYNDROME.

See also CHROMOSOMAL DEFECTS AND SKIN DISEASE.

genital warts A type of WART found in the genital area, anorectal region, and occasionally the urethra, bladder, and ureters, caused by infection with human papillomavirus (HPV) (see PAPILLOMAVIRUS, HUMAN). The disorder is readily spread by sexual contact.

The warts primarily appear in the moist genital folds and creases. While just one wart may appear, they are commonly found in heaped-up bunches that form cauliflowerlike masses. They are subject to injury and can bleed, and they are usually painless.

One out of 10 Americans have genital HPV infections, and between 500,000 and a million new cases of genital warts occur each year. Some studies show that about a third of all sexually active teen-agers have genital HPV infections. Because they do not have symptoms or recognize them, millions of others do not know they carry HPV.

Genital HPVs can spread whether or not warts are present, usually by vaginal or anal intercourse. Because genital HPV infections are often unseen, they can be spread by sex partners who don't know they're infected. It may also be possible by contact with the virus through such potential vehicles as toilet facilities, steam room benches, shared swimsuits, or underwear.

People most at risk for genital HPV infections are people who

- have weakened immune systems
- are sexually involved with a number of different partners
- have sex partners who are sexually involved with a number of different partners
- have infected partners

The majority of those now seeking treatment for genital warts are young women between the ages of 15 and 29.

Symptoms and Diagnostic Path

HPV infections cause a variety of problems, but there may be no symptoms of infection at all. Genital warts caused by HPV may be found on the vulva, in the vagina, and on the cervix, penis, anus, and urethra of infected women and men. They are only rarely found in the throat or mouth. Usually, the warts grow in more than one location, and may cluster in large masses. Genital warts usually are painless, but they may itch. If allowed to grow, they can block the openings of the vagina, urethra, or anus and become very uncomfortable. Depending on their location, genital warts can cause sores and bleeding.

Genital warts often grow more rapidly during pregnancy. An increase in the size and number of genital warts occurs when a person's immune system is weakened by diabetes, an organ transplant, Hodgkin's disease, HIV/AIDS, or other conditions. There are other genital HPV infections that cannot be seen with the naked eye. Some are more dangerous than genital warts because they are associated with cancers of the cervix, vulva, vagina, or penis.

Medical examination is the first step in determining if there is a genital HPV infection. Many times a woman does not notice warty lesions, but her physician may see something unusual while performing a routine gynecologic examination or Pap smear. Pap smear results can be used to screen for tissue changes in the cervix and help corroborate findings of other tests like colposcopy or biopsy. Colposcopy (viewing the cervix through a special microscope) may be used to identify subtle tissue changes. Colposcopy also allows a sample of any suspicious tissue to be taken by the examiner.

Treatment Options and Outlook

HPV is a persistent and hard-to-cure organism, so treatment must usually be repeated. Moreover, an infected woman should be monitored throughout her life for recurrence or development of precancerous changes, whether or not warts are apparent. Because the virus remains in the lesions it creates, treatment for HPV consists of controlling infection by removing visible warts or precancerous lesions.

They can be removed by surgery, freezing, or by locally applied chemicals. The method depends on the extent of infection, accessibility of lesions, and malignant potential. To ensure that as many lesions as possible are treated, colposcopy may be used during therapy to better view internal lesions.

Surgery is sometimes used to cut away warts if treatment without anesthesia would cause discomfort or warts are so extensive that simultaneous reconstructive surgery is required. Surgery may permit a more thorough removal of infected sites, although its cost must be weighed against potential benefits and risks. Surgery may either mean an excisional biopsy done as an outpatient procedure or as a more involved procedure performed under anesthesia.

In superficial cryotherapy, liquid nitrogen is applied by cotton swab to minor external warts. Extensive lesions can be frozen faster and to a greater depth with a cold cautery device that pinpoints warts. Cold cautery cryotherapy is usually performed within a week after menstruation, and it cannot be used in pregnant women. After cryotherapy women may experience cramping,

abdominal pain, infection, or rarely, cervical scarring. Painkillers given before cryotherapy will ease pain, and icepacks applied externally after the procedure will reduce any swelling or inflammation. Considerable watery vaginal discharge for 10 to 20 days after cryotherapy is normal, but fever, pain unrelieved by analgesics, or unusually prolonged discharge should be reported to the doctor.

Laser treatment involves a high-intensity beam of light that vaporizes lesions, particularly those that are external or in less accessible locations. In the hands of a well-trained physician, laser therapy is highly effective in removing multiple lesions. The procedure is usually more expensive than other types of treatment, and carries risks of removing too much tissue, and delayed healing, scarring, or pain.

Acids such as trichloroacetic acid (TCA) or bichloroacetic acid (BCA) may be painted on visible warts using a small cotton swab or wooden applicator. To be effective, TCA or BCA must be applied in proper concentrations, but these sometimes cause a burning sensation after treatment. Local and systemic painkillers will help relieve pain. Scarring and chronic pain are potential aftereffects.

5-Fluorouracil (5-FU) cream applied to the vulva on a regular regimen can help control external lesions. However, it should not be used by pregnant women and may cause serious skin irritation.

Interferon, a newer drug approved for injection into a muscle or select lesions, can be used, but it is expensive, has significant systemic side effects, and cannot be used during pregnancy. Podophyllin was once a popular treatment, but is used less often now because it cannot be used during pregnancy or for most internal lesion sites and because it may cause cancer or toxic reactions.

After any HPV treatment, the treated area should be kept clean and dry with cornstarch dusting, cotton underwear, and loose clothing. Sexual intercourse should be avoided until healing has occurred externally and internally, usually within two to four weeks. Follow-up colposcopy and Pap smears are usually scheduled at three-month intervals after treatment of HPV, and yearly thereafter. These tests monitor that the cervix remains free of precancerous or cancerous tissue. A woman with

HPV should notify any sexual partners of her infection, use latex condoms with every partner (unless in a mutually monogamous relationship), and urge that the partner be treated for HPV if his physician has identified HPV lesions.

Risk Factors and Preventive Measures

Condoms are recommended for all sexual contacts other than between monogamous partners. Condoms prevent transmission of infection to a partner and lower the risk of becoming infected with a different form of HPV or other sexually transmitted diseases. Applying spermicides with nonoxynol-9 to affected or treated areas may be helpful in reducing transmission of the virus. Everyone with genital lesions, and all partners of persons with genital lesions, should alert new sexual partners about HPV infection risk and take precautions to limit spread of HPV.

genodermatosis   Any genetically determined disorder of the skin, such as EPIDERMOLYSIS BULLOSA, PROGERIA, GARDNER'S SYNDROME, and so on.

See also GENETIC DISORDERS OF THE SKIN.

gentamicin   An injectable antibiotic sometimes given in combination with other antibiotics to treat serious gram-negative bacterial infections. It cannot be given by mouth because it is inactivated during digestion.

Blood tests are taken during treatment to reduce the risk of toxic kidney damage.

German measles   The common name for rubella, this viral infection, as MEASLES, causes a rash on the face, trunk, and limbs. Rubella causes a mild illness in children and a slightly more problematic one in adults, but is serious primarily when contracted by pregnant women in the early months of pregnancy. During this time, there is a chance the virus will infect the fetus, which can lead to a range of serious birth defects known as rubella syndrome.

Although rubella was once found throughout the world, it is now much less common in most developed countries because of successful vaccination programs. The United States has tried to eradicate the disease by vaccinating all school-age children. By 2002, there were only 18 cases of rubella reported, and people age 15 to 39 accounted for 72 percent of all reported cases. Most reported rubella in the United States since the mid-1990s has occurred among Hispanic young adults who where born in areas where rubella vaccine is routinely not given.

Symptoms and Diagnostic Path

The infection usually affects youngsters between the ages of six and 12 with a rash that lasts for a few days, a slight fever and enlarged lymph nodes. Sometimes the symptoms are so mild, the entire infection comes and goes without notice. Adolescents and adults may have slightly more pronounced symptoms. The virus is contagious from a few days before the symptoms appear until a day after symptoms fade.

Rubella may be confused with other conditions characterized by rashes, such as SCARLET FEVER or drug allergy.

Treatment Options and Outlook

There is no specific treatment for rubella, although acetaminophen may reduce the fever.

Risk Factors and Preventive Measures

Vaccination, which can provide long-lasting immunity, is administered in the United States to all infants at about 15 months of age as part of measles and mumps immunization. There is not usually any reaction to the vaccine. Infection by rubella virus also provides immunity to future infection.

Gianotti-Crosti syndrome   A condition known medically as papular acrodermatitis that is characterized by skin-colored or slightly pink papules on the face, arms, legs, and buttocks of children. The lesions do not usually itch. There is a frequent association with hepatitis B virus. Other viruses cause the eruption include hepatitis A virus, Epstein-Barr virus, coxsackievirus A16, parainfluenza virus, respiratory syncytial virus, and polio-vaccine enterovirus.

Symptoms and Diagnostic Path

The patient usually feels fairly well, but has diarrhea or an upper respiratory infection when the skin suddenly breaks out in crops of PAPULES lasting up to two months, which then fade spontaneously.

Treatment Options and Outlook

There is no specific treatment, but itching may be relieved with an antipruritic lotion, weak topical CORTICOSTEROID lotion, or sedating antihistamines.

ginseng The dried root of the *Panax schinseng* plant that is reported to contain hormones and vitamins. However, research has not found any evidence that ginseng can improve the appearance of the skin. Ginseng has been associated with allergic skin reactions.

glanders An infection found in Asia, Africa, and South America that afflicts horses and donkeys and that may be occasionally transmitted to humans. The infection, which is caused by the bacterium *Burckholderia mallei,* causes an ulcer or abscess where it enters a wound in the skin.

Symptoms and Diagnostic Path

The infection causes lesions at the site of infection that may become filled with PUS. If the mucous membranes in the nose or mouth are involved, extensive tissue death and damage to the septum and palate may occur. The disease is diagnosed in the laboratory by isolating *Burkholderia mallei* from blood, sputum, urine, or skin lesions.

Treatment Options and Outlook

There is no satisfactory treatment, although tetracyclines, streptomycin, and chloramphenicol may be effective. Immediate surgical removal of lesions followed by treatment with sulfonamide is recommended. Glanders may appear as an acute disease, in which it may be rapidly fatal, or as a chronic condition that may persist for months or years. Death may occur as a result of liver disease or continuing infections.

glomus tumor A small, extremely painful swelling usually found on the extremities, especially the hands. This relatively uncommon benign growth appears as a soft or firm blue-red papule.

There are two variants, solitary and multiple (also known as glomangiomas), each with distinct clinical characteristics. Single glomus tumors, especially those occurring under the nail bed, are more common in women; multiple lesions are more common in men. Solitary glomus tumors are more common in adults; multiple growths develop 10 to 15 years earlier than single lesions, with about a third appearing before age 20. Very rare congenital glomus tumors are considered a variant of multiple glomus tumors.

Symptoms and Diagnostic Path

Glomus tumors are characterized by a sensitivity to cold, localized tenderness, and excruciating intermittent pain, which is described as a burning or bursting feeling. The exact incidence of glomus tumors is unknown, but the multiple variant is rare, comprising less than 10 percent of all cases. Most likely, many of these tumors are misdiagnosed as HEMANGIOMAS.

Malignant glomus tumors (glomangiosarcomas) are extremely rare. There has been only one report of a malignant glomus tumor that spread elsewhere in the body.

Treatment Options and Outlook

Surgical removal is required. If the tumor is located under the nail, repair of the nail bed must be performed after the removal of the lesions. Removal of multiple tumors may be more difficult since there are so many of them, and should be limited to those causing symptoms.

Other possible treatments include argon and carbon dioxide lasers, or treatment with hypertonic saline or sodium tetradecyl sulfate (especially for multiple lesions).

Treatment of glomangiosarcoma is based on a few case reports. Wide local excision has been found to be adequate treatment and is probably the treatment of choice.

Excision of painful lesions usually cures the problem, although occasionally a solitary lesion will recur. Malignant glomus tumors are extremely rare and usually locally aggressive, with an overall good prognosis when treated with wide excision.

glutamic acid   An amino acid included in some expensive cosmetics that purport to improve the appearance of the skin. All amino acids combine to form proteins under certain chemical conditions, but because more than two different amino acids are needed to form useful proteins, simply including glutamic acid in a SKIN CREAM will not provide much benefit. Further, is not possible to rebuild the proteins of the skin with amino acids, and they are not absorbed when applied to the skin.

glycerin   A clear liquid made by combining water and fat that is used in many cosmetics and toiletries because it improves the consistency of creams and lotions, and helps them retain moisture. Glycerin, however, tends to draw water out of the skin, and can make skin drier. It has not been found to cause allergic reactions.

glycolic acid   One of a number of natural fruit acids (ALPHA HYDROXY ACIDS) available both as over-the-counter and prescription mild skin peels. This topical product improves the skin's appearance by accelerating the natural process of shedding dead skin cells. Used properly, the acids work gently, producing only a slight tingling or stinging sensation in some consumers. Glycolic acid is the alpha hydroxy acid most frequently used for facial treatments but citric acid and lactic acid (from milk) also are useful.

Derived from sugar cane, glycolic acid can clear up ACNE-prone skin, soften tiny lines around the eyes and mouth, smooth dry skin and fade dark spots caused by sun or hormonal changes (such as in pregnancy). Fastest results are usually obtained in a doctor's office, since higher strength products are available to dermatologists. Over time, the rate at which old cells are sloughed off the surface of the skin slows down, resulting in a surface layer of dead skin cells that make skin look aged. AHAs loosen the substances holding the surface skin cells to one another, allowing the dead skin to peel off.

The skin underneath has a fresher, healthier look with a more even color and texture. In high concentrations and after long-term use, AHAs eventually may affect the deeper layers of the skin.

By federal law, all alpha hydroxy acid products are considered to be cosmetics, not drugs, and are not regulated by the U.S. Food and Drug Administration (FDA).

Over-the-counter products manufactured by reputable companies are usually mild, containing less than 10 percent alpha hydroxy acid. Beauty salon operators use products up to 40 percent, and physicians use solutions of up to 70 percent for their in-office peels.

Reputable firms do not sell stronger products over the counter because of the danger to consumers and the accompanying liability threat. But the FDA is reviewing glycolic acid to see whether strength percentages should be established by law. Irritations and even burns have been reported by those who have used "bootleg" products.

gnathostomiasis   A rare infection usually caused by ingestion of the third-stage larvae of the nematode *Gnathostoma spinigerum* found in Southeast Asia, although several other species also cause human disease. The larvae may be found in contaminated water or in undercooked freshwater fish, chicken, snails, frogs, and pigs. Rarely, larvae penetrate the skin of those exposed to such meat or water. In humans, the parasite may live in body tissues for as long as 10 years.

Within one to two days after ingestion, larvae invade the gastric/intestinal wall and migrate through the liver. Their migration through the body begins from three to four weeks to several years after ingestion. Typically, episodes last for one or two weeks. With time, episodes occur less often, are less intense, and do not last as long.

There have been no reports of human cases of gnathostomiasis acquired in the United States, and it remains rare in those who are exposed abroad. Gnathostomiasis is an uncommon disease even in endemic areas of Southeast Asia (including Japan, Korea, Laos, Malaysia, Taiwan, and Thailand) and Latin America (mainly Mexico and Ecuador), although its incidence appears to be increasing possibly due to changing dietary habits. It is most common in Thailand and Japan. In Thailand, it is the most common parasitic infection of the central nervous system.

Symptoms and Diagnostic Path

The most common symptoms are painful or itchy migratory swelling in the skin. The parasites are a common cause of parasitic eosinophilic meningitis caused by their migration into the central nervous system. Gnathostomiasis can persist for 10 to 12 years and may cause significant long-term health problems. Random invasion of the central nervous system may lead to death in 8 percent to 25 percent of cases.

Treatment Options and Outlook

The best treatment is surgical removal of the worm, which is possible only when it is accessible. Medication may also be used, including the synthetic nitroimidazole albendazole. Mebendazole, a former drug treatment, should not be used because it is too toxic. CORTICOSTEROID therapy in central nervous system disease may also be useful.

Goeckerman regimen An intensive treatment regimen for patients suffering with PSORIASIS combining ultraviolet B light and tar ointments. This regimen has been a standard in-patient treatment for 50 years. It involves applying 2 to 5 percent crude coal tar ointment to the entire body at bedtime, which is then left on the skin overnight. Application for two hours before exposure to ultraviolet light is an effective alternative. In the morning, the excess tar is removed with mineral oil and the patient is exposed to UV light; afterwards, the patient bathes away remaining tar. The amount of UV light is gradually increased over successive treatments. Treatment is given in outpatient clinics or, more rarely, in a hospital. Treatment usually lasts for three or four weeks, and may result in remission for six to eight months.

A modified form of treatment involves applying topical CORTICOSTEROIDS at night instead of coal tar. In the morning the steroids are removed and the patient applies tar before UV treatment. Corticosteroids cannot be used for more than four or five days because of the danger of a rebound attack of psoriasis.

gold sodium thiomalate A water-soluble gold salt used in chrysotherapy (GOLD THERAPY) to treat rheumatoid arthritis. More recently, it has been used intramuscularly to treat PEMPHIGUS.

A few patients experience a specific reaction within minutes after treatment with gold sodium thiomalate, including flushing, redness, weakness, vertigo, and low blood pressure. Other symptoms that appear within a day after treatment include arthralgia, joint stiffness, myalgia, and malaise.

See also AUROTHIOGLUCOSE.

gold therapy The common term for chrysotherapy, this treatment is most often used to treat arthritis sometimes associated with PSORIASIS. PEMPHIGUS also has been treated with gold salts. Gold, which is administered orally, has an anti-inflammatory effect that can relieve pain and stiffness, and prevent further joint damage. Two different gold preparations are used: the water-soluble GOLD SODIUM THIMALATE and the oil-based AUROTHIOGLUCOSE.

Side Effects

Possible side effects of gold therapy to the skin include exfoliative dermatitis (see DERMATITIS, EXFOLIATIVE), macules or papules, or lesions resembling LICHEN PLANUS or PITYRIASIS ROSEA. The drug is usually stopped if ITCHING occurs. After gold therapy stops, the lesions typically fade away up to three or four months later. After that, most patients will tolerate further gold treatments without skin symptoms.

Other side effects of gold therapy may include the diffuse depositing of metallic gold within the skin (a condition known as chrysiasis). Patients who are going to be treated intramuscularly are usually given a test dose to gauge sensitivity, followed by gradually increasing doses. Patients with pemphigus may require a cumulative dose of 500 mg before noticing improvement.

Possible side effects unrelated to the skin include problems with the liver and kidney, liver and bone marrow changes, appetite loss, diarrhea, nausea, and abdominal pain, and sometimes anaphylactic shock.

Because of the risk of side effects, patients are usually monitored with serial complete blood counts, platelet counts, urinalysis, and liver function tests.

goose bumps See GOOSEFLESH.

gooseflesh Formation of temporary raised bumps of skin caused by the reaction of blood vessels to cold or to fear.

In the presence of the stimulus, blood vessels contract, which also contracts the small muscle attached to the base of each hair follicle, causing the hairs to stand up. This makes the skin look like the skin of a plucked goose—hence, the name "goose flesh" or "goosebumps." The medical name for goosebumps is cutis anserina.

Gougerot-Blum syndrome A condition characterized by pigmented papular lesions that coalesce into itchy plaques. Also known medically as pigmented purpuric lichenoid dermatosis, it is one of a group of skin disorders known as PIGMENTED PURPURIC DERMATOSIS that all feature reddish brown spots or patches. The syndrome occurs when inflammation of tiny capillaries causes blood to leak into tissues, triggering the rust-colored pigment changes and lesions. The exact reason why the capillaries should become leaky is not known for certain, but experts suspect the syndrome may be a hypersensitivity reaction to viral infection, food additives, or medications.

Symptoms and Diagnostic Path

The lesions are most often found on the lower legs but may also appear on the lower trunk, abdomen, and arms. The disorder is primarily a cosmetic problem, since the lesions do not usually itch and do not affect internal organs.

Treatment Options and Outlook

There is no specific treatment. Systemic corticosteroids may be effective, but their risk generally outweighs their usefulness. Topical CORTICOSTEROIDS may be helpful.

graft-versus-host disease (GVHD) The first symptom of this common complication to bone marrow transplantation is a skin RASH. The condition is caused by cells present in the transplanted bone marrow (graft) that attack the transplant recipient's tissues (host). The disease may occur soon after any organ transplant (acute GVHD), or it may not appear until months later (chronic GVHD).

Symptoms and Diagnostic Path

In addition to the skin rash, there may be diarrhea, abdominal pain, jaundice, inflammation of eyes and mouth, and breathlessness.

Treatment Options and Outlook

Treatment consists of suppressing the immune response without damaging the new bone marrow. Immune suppressants often used to treat cancer are also carefully used in decreased dosages to suppress or prevent graft-versus-host disease. Treatment of acute GVHD includes giving high-dose CORTICOSTERIODS and antibodies to T cells.

Sometimes treatment of the condition can lead to severe complications.

Risk Factors and Preventive Measures

Giving immunosuppressant drugs (such as cyclosporine) may head off the reaction. Once the disease develops, it is treated with corticosteroid drugs and other immunosuppressants.

granular cell tumor A type of skin tumor that, like neurilemmoma, is derived from Schwann cells. They are most common in people between the ages of 40 and 60. The tumors can be found on almost any part of the body, but are most commonly located on the tongue. Though usually appearing alone, multiple outbreaks may occur. Only about 3 percent of all granular cell tumors are malignant.

Treatment

Surgical excision is the typical treatment.

granulation tissue Red, moist granular tissue on the surface of an open wound or ulcer during healing. It gets its name from the appearance of the skin surface, which has numerous granules. It is made up of healing tissue consisting of numerous blood vessels, white cells, and FIBROBLASTS.

granuloma A grouping of cells associated with chronic inflammation that can occur in any part of the body. They are usually a reaction to certain infectious agents, although they may occur with no known cause.

They are typical of certain infections such as tuberculosis and LEPROSY, of disorders such as SARCOIDOSIS or Crohn's disease, and in reactions to foreign substances such as silicone, berylium, starch, talc, and some tattoo pigments.

See also GRANULOMA ANNULARE; GRANULOMA, LETHAL MIDLINE.

granuloma, lethal midline A rare disorder characterized by an inflammation of the skin of the nose and facial structures, which are progressively destroyed. The condition primarily affects middle-aged women. It may be subclassified into midline malignant reticulosis, idiopathic midline granuloma, and Wegener's granulomatosis. Recent research suggests that this disease is a manifestation of lymphoma.

Symptoms and Diagnostic Path

Ulcers and swelling within the nose spreads to tissue destruction in the facial sinuses, gums, and eye orbits, leading to extensive destruction of the face, sinuses, hard palate, and larynx. Death may result from infection or hemorrhage.

Treatment Options and Outlook

Radiation therapy usually stops the progression of the disease and may improve symptoms. Wegener's granulomatosis responds to CORTICOSTEROIDS and cyclophosphamide.

granuloma annulare A harmless skin condition characterized by a raised circular area of pink bumps found most often on children's knuckles or fingers, the upper part of the feet, the elbows, or ears. The raised area spreads to form a ring up to 3 to 5 cm wide, with raised edges and a flat center, before slowly disappearing.

Although GRANULOMA annulare is usually localized, it may become widespread (generalized granuloma annulare). This type is occasionally associated with diabetes.

Cause of this disorder is unknown. It may be caused by underlying diabetes.

Treatment Options and Outlook

In most cases, the skin eventually heals completely over a period of months or years. In cases where the appearance or ITCHING is bothersome, topical corticosteroids are occasionally helpful. Most cases (75 percent) are healed within two years.

See also GRANULOMA, LETHAL MIDLINE; GRANULOMA FACIALE; GRANULOMATOUS DISEASES.

granuloma faciale A fairly rare benign skin disorder characterized by a single persistent red-brown MACULE, plaque, or NODULE (usually on the face) with a smooth, intact surface. It usually appears in middle-aged white men.

Symptoms and Diagnostic Path

These lesions are usually a variety of colors and sizes, with a raised, soft appearance and a definite border. They are typically found on the face, although similar lesions have been found on other parts of the body such as the scalp, trunk, and arms and legs.

Diagnosis is confirmed by a skin biopsy, which is typically necessary to rule out other skin diseases that have similar findings.

Treatment Options and Outlook

Granuloma faciale is a chronic condition that comes and goes, but spontaneous healing rarely occurs. The disease appears not to have any relationship to internal disease, and treatment is mainly to improve the appearance. Various medical and surgical therapies have been used, but none have been consistently successful. Granuloma faciale also has the tendency to recur after treatment.

Treatment includes topical steroids, CORTICOS-TERIOD injections, antimalarial tablets, topical psoralen UV-A (PUVA), or radiation therapy. Surgery may be advised, but SCARS are possible. Other treatments include DERMABRASION, ELECTROSURGERY, CRYOTHERAPY, or 5 PULSED-DYE LASER.

See also GRANULOMA; GRANULOMA, LETHAL MIDLINE; GRANULOMA ANNULARE; GRANULOMATOUS DISEASE.

granulomatous disease A chronic disorder associated with an impaired immune system that is usually an X-linked hereditary condition. This means the disease is caused by a defect on the X chromosome that usually leads to problems in boys only. Mothers and sisters of most male patients may be carriers, and half of their sons may be affected. Carriers of this disorder are not more susceptible to serious bacterial infections, but do have characteristic skin lesions that slowly become red and painful.

While infection gradually becomes less of a problem in adulthood, the possibility of severe, life-threatening bacterial infections always exists for these patients.

Symptoms and Diagnostic Path
Patients with this disease have recurrent bacterial infections of the skin, with lesions of the scalp, mouth, nose, and ears. Minor cuts and bruises often lead to furunculosis and ABSCESSES.

Treatment Options and Outlook
All infections in these patients should be treated by broad-spectrum antibiotics after culturing lesions at the first sign of infection. Long-term treatment may be needed, since these infections often do not respond well to antibiotics, and recurrences are frequent. Human recombinant gamma interferon has helped some patients and is being studied as a possible prevention of infection.

See also GRANULOMA; GRANULOMA, LETHAL MIDLINE; GRANULOMA ANNULARE; GRANULOMA FACIALE.

green hair A common problem unique to swimmers is the greenish tinge that their hair may develop from long-term exposure to chlorinated swimming pool water. This reversible pigment change occurs only in swimmers with natural or tinted blond, gray, or white hair.

Green hair is actually not caused by chlorine but, rather, by copper ions, although the chlorine may act as a bleach. While this condition poses no serious medical concern, it can be emotionally upsetting for swimmers because the green tinge is so noticeable.

Without proper treatment, the green color will last as long as the hair is exposed to the pool water.

The hair tinge can be removed by applying a 2 percent to 3 percent HYDROGEN PEROXIDE solution and leaving it in the hair for 30 minutes. Also effective is the use of commercial chelating agents applied after swimming, which will solve the problem without bleaching the hair.

Grenz zone A border of connective tissue separating the EPIDERMIS from the mid-DERMIS.

Grenz ray therapy An outdated treatment for inflammatory skin disease once used for ECZEMA, PSORIASIS, LICHEN PLANUS, TINEA CAPITIS, and ACNE. While superficial MYCOSIS FUNGOIDES, SEZARY SYNDROME, KAPOSI'S SARCOMA, and superficial BASAL CELL CARCINOMA also respond to Grenz rays, soft X-rays are preferred because of their better penetration.

Grisactin See GRISEOFULVIN.

griseofulvin (Trade names: Griseofulvin, Fulvicin, Grisactin) One of the oldest antifungal drugs available in America, this antibiotic penicillin derivative is given orally to treat ringworm (TINEA) infections that have not responded to creams or lotions. It is particularly effective against superficial DERMATOPHYTE infections of the scalp, beard, palms, soles, and nails, as well as ringworm of the scalp (TINEA CAPITIS), ringworm of the body (TINEA CORPORIS) and ATHLETE'S FOOT. Even with prolonged treatment, many nail infections do not respond completely, or they recur. Griseofulvin has been replaced by newer antifungals that are safer and more effective: terbinafine, itraconazole, and fluconazole. Resistance may develop to this drug. It is not effective against bacteria, deep fungi, *Candida albicans*, and TINEA VERSICOLOR. It is less effective against fungal infections of the nail.

When griseofulvin is taken with a high-fat meal, it is better absorbed and tolerated by the patient.

Griseofulvin should not be taken by patients suffering with acute intermittent PORPHYRIA, since it may cause an acute abdominal attack. The drug may also interact with birth control pills, producing breakthrough bleeding or allowing pregnancy.

Side Effects

The most common side effects are headache and gastrointestinal problems; others include loss of taste, dry mouth, and increased sun sensitivity. Long-term treatment may cause liver or bone marrow damage.

group B streptococci infections   The most common bacterial infection in newborns that may cause skin abscesses. A small number of infants with *Listeria* poisoning have skin lesions (including PAPULES, PUSTULES, and VESICLES).

Treatment Options and Outlook

Antibiotic treatment should begin immediately, since blood poisoning is likely. Prognosis is poor if the case is advanced and there are many lesions on the body.

Grover's disease   The common name for transient acantholytic dermatosis, a KERATINIZATION disorder that is fairly common (especially in men over age 40). Despite its medical name, the lesions of this disease frequently persist. It is believed that sunlight and blocked sweat ducts may play a role in the development of this problem. Most cases last six to 12 months, although it may last longer.

Symptoms and Diagnostic Path

Reddened crusted papules or vesicles appear on the back and extremities. ITCHING may or may not be a problem.

Treatment Options and Outlook

There is no definitive treatment. Topical CORTICOSTEROIDS and retinoids (such as Retin A) clear up the condition temporarily, but the rash returns as soon as the drug is stopped.

Hailey-Hailey disease The common name for familial benign chronic PEMPHIGUS, a rare genetic blistering disease. It is characterized by the appearance of crusts with redness and blisters—on the neck, under the arms, in the groin, and sometimes on the scalp—that may itch or cause pain. Lesions tend to get bigger, although they may spontaneously fade away without scarring; recurrences are common. The disease usually appears between ages 15 and 35.

The disease is autosomal dominant, which means that only one defective gene (from one parent) is needed to cause the syndrome. Each child of an affected person usually has a one in two chance of inheriting the defective gene and of being affected. However, a positive family history can only be traced in 70 percent of patients. The development of lesions can be triggered by bacterial or yeast infections and may be exacerbated by exposure to sunlight. A hot, moist environment and sweating can contribute to the problem.

Symptoms and Diagnostic Path
While the disease is benign, it can be annoying and tends to last for a long time, with alternating periods of remission and active lesions. Some patients show improvement with age.

Treatment Options and Outlook
Treatment is aimed at controlling infection, relieving symptoms, and avoiding heat, moisture, and friction. Cold water compresses and antibacterial creams or ointments may be applied to the skin. Steroid creams may ease inflammation and discomfort; systemic steroids are not effective. Systemic antibiotic treatment (TETRACYCLINE or ERYTHROMYCIN) may help. Surgical removal of chronic lesions followed by SKIN GRAFTS may be required.

Risk Factors and Preventive Measures
Patients with a family history are urged to avoid heat, moisture, and friction, and to be careful to avoid bacterial or yeast infection when possible.

hair, anatomy of Hair is composed of KERATIN, the protein that makes up NAILS and the outer skin layer (EPIDERMIS). Each hair shaft sits in a hair FOLLICLE, and each has a spongy semi-hollow core (the medulla) surrounded by long, thin fibers (the cortex) with several overlapping cell layers on the outside (the cuticle).

There are about 100,000 hairs on a typical person's head, growing about 1/72 of an inch each day. At this rate, it takes about 75 days for scalp hair to grow an inch.

Growth Stages
Hair goes through distinct stages, growing for two to six years and then resting for three months. At any one time, about 85 percent of a person's hair is active, 1 percent is entering the resting phase, and about 14 percent is resting. In its growing phase, there is live tissue called the hair bulb at the tip of each hair that supplies keratin and melanin; this is the pale-colored swelling that may be seen if a hair is pulled out of the follicle. The hair is formed by the upward growth of KERATINOCYTES, which become keratin-filled.

Hair that is in the resting phase separates from the bulb, and is shed. The rate of shedding of a normal adult scalp is about 100 hairs daily (usually after brushing or shampooing). The hair loss is continuous, but is always in the process of being replaced.

Types of Hair
The first kind of hair, developed in the uterus at the fourth month of gestation, is called LANUGO, a

Hair Anatomy

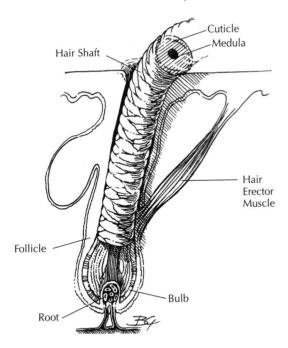

Hair Shaft

Cuticle

Medula

Hair Erector Muscle

Follicle

Bulb

Root

downy fuzz that is shed during the last month of pregnancy. After birth and until adolescence, fine, short, and colorless hair (vellus hair) covers most of the child's body. "Terminal hair" is thicker, longer and often pigmented, and grows on the scalp, eyebrows and eyelashes. At puberty, it also begins to grow in the secondary sexual areas such as the pubic area and the armpits, in addition to the face, chest, legs, and so on.

Appearance

The color of a person's hair is determined by the amount and type of pigment (MELANIN) in the hair shaft. Melanin is produced by special cells (melanocytes) in the base of the hair follicle. Red melanin causes red and auburn hair, and black melanin causes all other colors. White hair occurs when the cells receive no pigment.

Whether the hair is curly or straight depends on the shape of the hair's follicle. Straight hair grows from a straight follicle, whereas curly hair grows from a very curved follicle; wavy hair grows from a curved follicle.

Other Types of Hair

Eyebrows and eyelashes have a different growth period from scalp hair. Both eyebrows and eyelashes grow for about 10 weeks and then rest for nine months. This is why it takes so long to grow the eyebrows back after shaving them. Plucking the eyebrows, however, stimulates the follicles and makes them grow back faster. (This is the exception to the rule that cutting hair does not make it grow in faster).

See also HAIR, CARE OF; HAIR DYE; HAIR, DISORDERS OF.

hair, care of   There are a host of old wives' tales when it comes to hair. For example, it is not true that shampooing too often will harm the HAIR FOLLICLES, that massaging the scalp will prevent hair loss, or that shaving will make hair grow back faster or thicker.

There are two types of hair—terminal hair, which grows on the scalp, eyelashes, eyebrows and areas of sexual development; and vellus hair, the fine hair that covers the body until puberty. The same follicles can produce different types of hair at different times in a person's life.

In general, it takes two and a half months for scalp hair to grow an inch; it tends to grow for up to six years, and then rest for three months. When a new hair begins to grow below the old hair, it loosens and sheds. At any time, about 85 percent of scalp hair is growing, 1 percent is beginning to rest, and 14 percent is resting. It is this hair in the resting phase that ends up in a brush or in the bathtub drain.

As hair grows out, it is subject to weathering and injury to the overlapping cuticle scales that protect the inner cortical fiber of the hair. Once the hair is injured, it cannot be repaired because the shaft consists of dead cells. Cuticle scales near the scalp are smooth because they have not been injured; those near the ends of the hair have been repeatedly damaged and may be worn away, exposing the inner cortical fibers, and resulting in split ends.

Exposure to the sun or to chlorine from swimming pools can cause changes to the KERATIN, making the hair's texture change. While hair can tolerate changes such as permanents or dyeing if they are done carefully and not too often, these processes can cause alkaline oxidation damage.

Trauma

In addition, combing and brushing may cause a great deal of injury to the cuticle scales. Hair and scalp should be washed as often as necessary with shampoos to remove oily buildup, dead cells, microorganisms, cosmetics, and dirt. Because shampoos remove oil very well, those with oily scalps do not really need to choose a specially formulated shampoo. Most North Americans shampoo more often than is really necessary, but even daily shampooing is not really harmful nor is there evidence that frequent washing increases the production of SEBUM.

Dandruff Shampoos

While there is no cure for DANDRUFF, frequent shampooing is the most effective treatment and helps to alleviate symptoms in mild cases. SHAMPOOS that are effective against dandruff contain selenium sulfide, ZINC pyrithione, tar sulfur, or salicylic acid. It may help to rotate different antidandruff shampoos to get the best results. When using such a product, the shampoo should be applied immediately and then left on the scalp for five minutes to allow the ingredients time to work. Using a CONDITIONER afterward would not help avoid dandruff, but many improve manageability.

Acid-Balanced Shampoo

Researchers say that using a shampoo with an acid pH on normal hair or scalp does not provide any additional benefits. However, hair damaged by sunlight or dyes, bleaches, or straighteners may feel slimy when regular shampoo for damaged hair is used. An acid pH shampoo may make the hair feel more normal.

Baby Shampoo

These types of shampoos contain amphoteric detergents that irritate the eyes less, which make them useful for young children.

Conditioning Shampoos

While some products contain conditioners and shampoos, it is usually more effective to use a separate conditioner after shampooing.

Conditioners

Cream rinses are made up of quaternary cationic polymers, which form a layer on the hair shaft and lubricate it. This reduces the damage caused by combing or brushing. Because anionic detergent shampoos remove oil, the hair develops a static electric charge; conditioners help to dispel the charge. Rinses also allow the strands to be aligned and reflect light. African Americans in particular may benefit from using cream rinses because very curly hair does not align well and does not reflect light uniformly, which causes the hair to appear dull. Some cream rinses also have oils to increase lubrication. While damaged or treated hair can be improved by using conditioners, fine hair can be overconditioned and appear dull and greasy.

Silicone

One of the newest ingredients in hair care products is silicone (liquid plastic), which smooths the hair shaft and increases shine and manageability. Silicone works especially well for coarse or curly hair. However, regular use of silicone gels, shampoos, and serums can leave hair feeling sticky, dull, and hard to style.

Silicone works like clear NAIL POLISH, coating the hair so it reflects light and appears shiny. Since silicone does not dissolve in water, it helps prevent the hair from getting frizzy on damp days. However, because it does not easily rinse off, silicone tends to build up on the hair and when used too much, it causes the hair to look dirty and feel rubbery.

Fortunately, silicone will not permanently damage the hair, and it is not absorbed into the scalp. Experts recommend that consumers use a buildup remover shampoo weekly if silicone products are used. Some salons also offer special treatments to remove silicone buildup from the hair.

Setting/Permanent Wave Solutions

These chemicals work by breaking the chemical bonds that result in the hair's normal consistency, giving it more curl or straightness (depending on their purpose), and then forming new bonds to keep the hair in place. Neither setting nor permanent wave solutions badly weaken normal hair, but if they are too strong or left on too long they can cause minor problems such as split ends or dullness, or can lead to profound structural damage and hair loss. If too strong or if used too long, they cause breakage. Only rarely, however, do the chemicals actually damage the hair follicle itself. Therefore, chemically damaged hair will be replaced by normal hair eventually.

Bleaching

Bleaching products can damage the hair's protein if they are used for too long or too often, leaving the hair dull and almost colorless, and more susceptible to injury.

See also HAIR, ANATOMY OF; HAIR, DISORDERS OF; HAIR DYE.

hair, disorders of While many disorders of the hair may seem to be simply a cosmetic problem, in fact some may be evidence of an underlying disease. While brittle, unhealthy-looking hair may be caused by excessive blow drying, combing, or shampooing, it may also be a sign of a vitamin or mineral deficiency, or hypothyroidism. Very dry hair is probably caused by too much perming, tinting, bleaching, or use of hot rollers—but it could also be a sign of malnutrition.

Ingrown hairs are another hair condition that can cause problems, especially in people with very curly hair. In this condition, the free-growing end of the hair penetrates the skin near the follicle and can cause severe inflammation.

hair, gray In most people, what appears to be "gray" hair is actually a combination of pigmented and nonpigmented hair. Most people with some gray hair are not usually entirely gray, but have a mixture of white hairs among those of the normal shades of brown, blond, red, or black.

As a person ages, the body's production of MELANIN decreases. New hair contains less pigment and the shaft eventually grows in without any pigment at all. The only color left in the hair is the color of the KERATIN itself: yellowish gray. Eventually, more and more hair continues to grow in the same way until the entire head is filled with gray hair.

White hair is due to a lack of melanin granules in the cortex of the hair shaft; usually occurring with advancing age, this lack of melanin granules means the body is losing its ability to synthesize the pigments from enzymes and proteins. True gray hairs are quite rare, and are caused by a decrease—not a total lack—of the pigment content in the hair shaft. In most people, what appears to be "gray" hair is actually a combination of pigmented and nonpigmented hair. Some hereditary diseases also predispose a person to premature grayness.

Most people begin to develop a few gray hairs at about age 30, becoming progressively grayer over the next 20 years as more and more of their hair lacks pigment. By age 60 or 70, the hair often turns completely white, which means that all of the hairs on the head have lost their pigment granules.

Premature Gray Hair

Hair that turns gray prematurely (in the early 20s) may often be the result of genetic factors, since the tendency seems to run in families. Severe stress, mental illness, serious physical ailments, and traumatic experiences have been associated with premature gray hair and the acceleration of graying, although scientists do not know why. A few cases of premature graying are due to a deficiency of vitamin B_{12} (a disease known as pernicious anemia); this can be reversed by replacing the vitamin. Vitamin B is probably most effective for those whose grayness began after a severe strain, such as a long debilitating illness or severe stress.

Hair that begins to turn gray because of genetics and age is not reversible.

Throughout history, a number of famous individuals who experienced great stress were said to have turned gray overnight. Sir Thomas More and Queen Marie-Antoinette both were said to have suddenly gone gray when they got the news that they were to be executed.

Although hair strands do not actually change color within hours, a person's hair can seem to turn gray in a matter of days. The phenomenon is caused by ALOPECIA AREATA, thought to be an autoimmune disorder in which the body's immune system attacks the hair follicles. While scientists do not know why the antibodies begin the attack, severe psychological stress may play a role. Alopecia areata can cause varying degrees of hair loss, from small bald patches to the loss of every bit of hair.

When the hair goes gray quickly, it is believed that the antibodies are selective and concentrate on just the pigment-producing cells in the follicles, causing only pigmented strands to fall out. If this occurs in someone whose hair is in the process of going white, the sudden loss of darker hair will make the person look as if he or she suddenly "went gray." Because alopecia can disappear, rapid graying is not always permanent.

Treatment Options and Outlook

Once hair has started to gray, there is nothing that can be done to reverse the process. However, there are some hair dyes that are specifically used to color gray hair.

Some gray hair appears to have a yellowing tinge, apparently as a result of age-related changes in melanin production. This discoloration can be worsened by tobacco smoke, carbolic acid found in dry powder shampoos, setting lotions, and especially dandruff shampoos containing RESORCINOL. The easiest way to get rid of this tinge (from either external or internal factors) is to treat the hair with a bluing rinse; setting lotions or hair sprays, which have a tendency to turn gray hair yellow, should not be used.

See also HAIR, CARE OF.

hair dye Products used to alter the color of the hair is divided in two basic categories—permanent and semipermanent. Permanent dye can lift out the natural pigment and replace it with a different color. Each strand of hair is protected by an outer cuticle constructed of transparent overlapping scales much like shingles on a roof, and an inner cortex where the hair's natural pigment resides.

Permanent Dyes

Permanent dyes contain ammonia, which opens the scales of the cuticle to allow the dye to penetrate the hair shaft, and peroxide, which removes natural pigment from the cortex so the new color can be layered on like paint on a canvas. The color does not just wash away because once it is deposited in the cortex, the dye produces a color

molecule so big it gets trapped. The drawback to permanent dyes is that as the hair continues to grow, the natural color will begin to show up again in about 10 days.

Semipermanent Dyes

Semipermanent dyes penetrate into the hair shaft, but not as deeply as permanent dyes. Although semipermanent dyes do not rinse off with water, they do fade and wash out of hair after about five to 10 shampoos.

Vegetable Dyes

Vegetable dyes deposit a coating of dye on the cuticle of the hair shaft; HENNA is an example of a vegetable dye. These dyes only keep their color with repeated applications.

Synthetic (Aniline) Dyes

Synthetic dyes (including paraphenylenediamine) are popular because they are easy to apply and their color is stable. Because they react chemically with hair, however, they can also react with skin protein and trigger an allergic reaction. About 10 percent of people who use these dyes will develop an allergy to them, and break out in red splotches. This is why a sensitivity test must be performed on every person each time an aniline product is used. While the hair can protect the scalp skin from damage, unprotected skin that touches the dye may react. In allergic individuals, these dyes used in areas around the eyes, on the eyebrows or the eyelashes can cause blindness as a result of the severe allergic reaction. This is why hair dye should never be used on eyelashes or eyebrows, and why the U.S. Food and Drug Administration prohibits aniline dyes or derivatives in eyelash and eyebrow dyes.

Metallic Dyes

Metallic dyes (now only rarely used) can cause poisoning when the metal (silver, copper, iron, or lead) reacts with the sulfur in the hair. Also called color restorers, they are a progressive type of dye that is combed through the hair and after several days, gradually covers gray hair. Hair dyes with metallic products will not react well to waving, straightening, or to any other type of hair coloring.

Cross Section of Skin Showing Hair Folicle

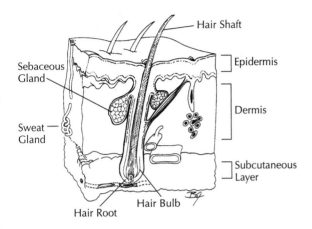

Hair Shaft

Epidermis

Sebaceous
Gland

Dermis

Sweat
Gland

Subcutaneous
Layer

Hair Bulb

Hair Root

Hair Dye and Cancer

There is no strong evidence of a clear cancer risk for people who dye their hair. Most of the previous studies that raised concerns about hair dye were relatively small, and looked at the former habits of people who had already gotten cancer. In general, result show that women who dye their hair—even those who have used hair color for more than 20 years—are at no greater risk than those who never colored their hair.

See also HAIR, ANATOMY OF; HAIR, CARE OF; HAIR, DISORDERS OF.

hair follicle A sheath of epidermal cells and connective tissue that surrounds the root of a hair.

hairiness See HIRSUTISM.

hair loss The gradual loss of hair, either as a result of a disease such as ALOPECIA AREATA or by hereditary and aging pattern baldness, occurs in about 30 million men and 20 million women every year. About 40 percent of all men will show some degree of hair loss by age 35; 25 percent of all women experience some hair loss by age 40, but about 60 percent of all women experience hair loss by the time they reach menopause. Contrary to common belief, hereditary hair loss is not caused by a sudden stop in hair growth. Instead, it is the result of the gradual miniaturization of certain HAIR FOLLICLES; as this progresses, hairs become shorter and thinner, eventually ceasing to grow.

Every human follows a genetically programmed schedule for growing, resting, and shedding hair. At any one time, as much as 85 percent of the scalp hair is growing up to an inch a month, and it may continue to grow for two to six years without stopping. When the growth phase ends, each hair begins a two-to-six month resting phase, and then begins a shedding phase. Only 10 to 15 percent of hair is in the resting phase at any one time; shedding occurs randomly. Eventually, a new hair begins to sprout from the root deep within the hair follicle, replacing the older hair above it as a new growth period begins.

It is normal to shed between 50 to 100 hairs daily—a loss that is not noticed, since most people have about 100,000 hairs on their head. Excessive shedding (more than 200 hairs) usually becomes noticeable within months, and can be caused in men and women by medical disorders (including malnutrition), medications, or (most often) heredity.

In most cases, hair loss is related to "androgenetic alopecia," or hereditary hair loss. Normal genes and androgens (especially testosterone) cause progressive shrinking of certain scalp follicles over time. The shrinking follicle produces a smaller, finer hair with each growth cycle. In addition to a smaller follicle, androgenetic alopecia is characterized by a shortened growth phase, which results in shorter hair.

The balding process is a gradual conversion of active, large follicles to less active, smaller follicles, resulting in short, thin hairs that are barely visible and eventually disappear completely. In men, hereditary baldness (also called "MALE PATTERN BALDNESS") is characterized by a receding hairline above the forehead and loss of hair at the crown. If male pattern baldness progresses to its final stage, the person is left with hair only around the sides and back of the head. This is also known as pattern thinning in women. Hereditary hair loss is a general or diffuse thinning of the hair over the top of the head—women rarely lose all their hair.

The second most common cause of hair loss is alopecia areata, which causes hair to fall out in clumps. This disorder often starts at a young age and may progress to the point where the person loses all scalp hair (alopecia totalis) or all body hair, including eyelashes and eyebrows (alopecia universalis). In some cases, alopecia areata follows a stressful event, such as divorce or death of a significant other. In most people, the hair will grow back, but the exact cause of the hair loss is not known. Most experts believe it may be caused by an immunological disorder in which antibodies are produced that attack the hair follicles.

Hair loss may be caused by medical disorders, such as a hyperactive or underactive thyroid gland, certain tumors, diabetes, severe infections, secondary syphilis, anemia, and systemic LUPUS ERYTHEMATOSUS. It may be caused by medications for gout, arthritis, high blood pressure, or depression, as well as high doses of VITAMIN A and chemotherapy drugs. Oral contraceptives may cause hair to fall out because of the increase of hormones. Hair loss due to medication is reversible once the medication is stopped.

Hair that is constantly damaged by excess bleaching, dyeing, or permanent waving may begin to break and fall out; over-teasing hair or excessive straightening with hot irons can also cause hair loss. Metal combs can damage hair and scalp as well.

Traction alopecia is caused by ponytails, braids, or cornrows that are pulled too tight, pulling the hair out by its roots. Friction alopecia is caused by constantly wearing snug-fitting wigs or hats.

Finally, poor diet low in protein or iron may cause abnormal hair loss.

Treatment Options and Outlook

Ever since ancient Egyptians anointed their bald spots with fats from ibex, lion, crocodile, serpent, goose, and hippopotamus to encourage hair growth, humans have been trying to treat hair loss. In 420 B.C., Hippocrates tried to fend off his hair loss by whipping up typical potions of opium, horseradish, pigeon droppings, beetroot, and spices.

Today there are several options for coping with hair loss, ranging from sophisticated styling and hair transplantation to medical treatment.

Concealing hair loss Concealing hair loss is easier for women. Women can work with their hairdressers to make their hair appear fuller through properly applied mousses, shampoos, perms, and dyes. Shorter hair styles hold a curl more easily and can help hide thin hair. Both men and women find that powdered eye shadow applied to the scalp provides a darkened background that can disguise thinning hair; wigs and hairpieces may completely cover the problem.

Hairpieces HAIR WEAVING and bonding are the most common methods of affixing a hairpiece to the head. Hair weaving ties the hairpiece with a tough nonshrinkable thread to clumps of existing natural hair that has been woven together to form anchoring places for the piece. Bonding uses a medical glue to anchor the piece to the natural hair. Both techniques must be performed by a trained hairdresser and require regular visits to have the piece washed and dyed. Periodic tightening is required.

Implants are another way to attach hairpieces, but they must be performed by a physician. By this method, the physician implants sutures or surgical threads into the scalp to which the hairpiece can be attached.

Surgical treatments Hair transplants, scalp reduction, and transposition flaps are also available. In a transplant, surgeons move skin from areas of the scalp that grow hair, such as the back and sides, to areas of the scalp that are no longer growing hair. After a period of about three months, the transplanted hair begins to grow. Hair transplant techniques have been refined in the past decade. Smaller grafts are now used for a more natural look.

Scalp reductions treat hair loss as too much scalp rather than too little hair. In this procedure, surgeons cut out areas of the scalp that no longer grow hair. The scalp is then pulled back together and help in place with sutures or surgical staples until it heals. Scalp reduction may also be successfully combined with hair replacement.

Transposition flaps are a variation of hair replacement, which involves transplanting an entire strip of hair-bearing skin instead of individual grafts. Used to cover a large area of hair loss, the flaps are a good choice for men. However, because they involve complicated multiple surgery and are expensive, the procedure is not often performed.

Medical treatment MINOXIDIL (trade name: Rogaine topical solution) is a medically proven product that will regrow hair in men and women. Clinical tests conducted by dermatologists at 27 U.S. medical centers involving more than 2,300 men with male pattern baldness resulted in regrowth in about half (48 percent) of male patients. An additional 36 percent had minimal regrowth; the rest (16 percent) had no regrowth. In other studies, almost two out of every three women were evaluated by physicians to have regrown some hair; 13 percent had moderate regrowth and 50 percent had minimal regrowth. The rest (37 percent) had no regrowth. Among subjects who did not use minoxidil, 39 percent also saw some regrowth.

Future Research

Scientists are studying the anti-androgens (drugs that would counteract the effect of the male hormone testosterone) that are responsible for signaling hair to fall out. Growth factors are also being studied to see if they can encourage growth in the tissue of the hair follicle.

hairpieces   Also called toupees, these products provide fodder for jokes, but a high-quality, well-fitted piece can be successfully worn by some men. The key to a natural-looking toupee is to buy a good quality, custom-made hairpiece that is carefully matched to individual hair color and texture. Lifestyle and hobbies should also be considered when making this purchase.

A hairpiece consultant can recommend ways the hair can be attached to the head. Hairpieces should be handled carefully and washed or cleaned periodically.

hair removal   Hair is usually removed from a part of the body for cosmetic reasons, although it may also be removed from a planned surgical site prior to an operation.

Shaving removes hair at the skin level and is suitable for hair on the legs, armpits, pubic area, and facial beard area in men. However, hair quickly grows back from shaved areas and shaving can cause irritation.

Depilatory creams dissolve the hair just below the skin's surface, creating a smooth effect, but the cream may irritate sensitive skin areas and should be used only on the legs.

Waxing is a technique used often in beauty salons as a way to remove hair from the legs or face. In this technique, warm wax is applied to the skin and then peeled off, pulling out the hair as it goes.

Plucking with tweezers is a good technique for stray eyebrow hairs and other small areas. After all of these techniques, hair will regrow in about three weeks.

Sugaring is a type of hair removal system that uses honey and special strips to eliminate hair. A thin coating of the honey hair-removal gel is applied in the direction of the hair growth; a cloth strip is then placed on the gel and stroked firmly two or three times in the direction of hair growth. Holding the skin taut with one hand, the consumer picks up the lower end of the cloth with the other hand and pulls quickly in opposite direction of the hair growth. Proponents of this method say that hair does not return for four to six weeks.

ELECTROLYSIS permanently removes hair through the use of an electric current to destroy the hair's root.

hair transplants   A surgical operation in which a person's skin is moved from areas of the scalp genetically programmed to grow hair (such as the back and sides) to areas of the scalp that are no longer growing hair. After a period of about three months, the transplanted hair begins to grow.

Transplants are less often performed in women because women tend to experience diffuse hair thinning all over the scalp, which complicates the identification of hair that is not genetically coded to fall out. In the past few years, techniques have been improved so that even women with thinning hair can benefit from this technology.

Transplantation is best done before an area is completely bald. This way, the appearance of "new" hair is more subtle and the procedure less obvious. Further transplants may be needed periodically as natural hair continues to fall out, but the hair that is transplanted will remain. Results of this procedure may be enhanced by reducing the size of the scalp area or stretching scalp skin with temporary inflatable bags, and then reducing the scalp area. Physicians charge either by the plug or for the entire procedure.

Transposition flaps, a variation of hair replacement, involves transplanting an entire strip of hair-bearing skin instead of individual grafts. Used to cover a large area of hair loss, the flaps are a good choice for men who have large bald areas. But because this technique involves complicated multiple surgery, the flaps are expensive and the procedure is not often performed.

hair weaving A procedure in which a hairpiece is tied with a tough nonshrinkable thread to clumps of existing natural hair woven and braided together to form an anchoring for the piece. This technique must be performed by a trained hairdresser, and requires regular visits to have the piece washed and dyed.

Results vary depending on hair style and texture; since the natural hair will continue to grow, regular sessions to tighten the braids will be needed. While the technique may be performed on both men and women, it is more commonly done for men. A weave generally lasts two to three years.

Implants are another way to attach hairpieces, but these must be performed by a physician. Implants are beneficial for those with little natural hair to anchor the wave. With this method, the physician implants sutures or surgical threads into the scalp to which the hairpiece can be attached.

haloderma Any skin eruption caused by the ingestion of halide.

haloprogin (Trade name: Halotex) A topical treatment for fungal infections available as a 1 percent cream or solution that is usually applied two or three times a day. It is effective against DERMATOPHYTES and, to a lesser degree, against *Candida* and *Malassezia furfur* (the cause of TINEA VERSICOLOR.)

Halotex See HALOPROGIN.

hand, foot, and mouth disease A common infectious disease of toddlers that produces blistering of palms, soles and the inside of the mouth, caused by the coxsackievirus. Toddlers sometimes exhibit no symptoms, but infants may develop flulike symptoms that last several days. The condition often sweeps through day care centers in the summer. The mild illness usually lasts only a few days; there is no treatment other than painkillers to relieve blister discomfort. There is no connection to hoof-and-mouth disease, which affects cattle and sheep.

hand cream A cream designed to soften and moisturize the skin of the hands that may contain alcohol, stearic acid, LANOLIN, and gum substances. Hand creams are usually not as greaseless as those designed to be used under makeup.

hand dermatitis See DERMATITIS, HAND.

hangnails Small torn pieces of skin on the sides or base of a nail that expose a raw, painful area. Hangnails may result after immersion in water, or from nailbiting. The raw area may go on to become infected and develop into a PARONYCHIA.

Treatment Options and Outlook

Trim a hangnail with scissors and keep it covered with a bandage until it heals. Hangnails can be prevented by using a moisturizing cream.

Hansen's disease See LEPROSY.

harlequin color change A phenomenon caused by vascular autonomic imbalance most often seen in premature newborns during the first week of life. When the infant is lying on its side, the bottom half of the body becomes red, in sharp contrast to the top half of the body, which is quite pale. The condition may last briefly or up to 20 minutes.

harlequin fetus   A rare genetic form of ICHTHYOSIS in which infants are born with very thick, hard skin with deep moist fissures that produce a grotesque appearance. The fissures appear most often over areas of movement, such as the joints, neck, underarms, and groin. Ears may be underdeveloped and flat, and hair and nails may be absent. Most are born dead, or die shortly after birth from respiratory failure and the inability to eat. However, recent treatment of children born with the syndrome with etretinate, a derivative of VITAMIN A, has showed them to have shed the armorlike thick skin and live, albeit with severe remaining icthyosis.

The condition, which can be diagnosed before birth, may be linked with a defect in lipid metabolism or abnormal protein metabolism. More than one genetic defect may produce this syndrome.

Hartnup disease   A rare hereditary metabolic disorder in which there is an eruption of lesions similar to PELLAGRA. Usually seen in children between age three and nine, the disease is an autosomal recessive trait, which means that a defective gene must be inherited from both parents to cause the abnormality. Generally, both parents of an affected person are unaffected carriers of the defective gene. Each of the children has a one in four chance of being affected, and a two in four chance of being a carrier.

The condition may be triggered by poor diet, sun exposure, sulfa drugs, or stress. Frequency of attacks lessens with age.

Symptoms and Diagnostic Path

Other physical symptoms include progressive dementia, spasticity, short stature, abnormal hair, and diarrhea.

Treatment Options and Outlook

Patients are treated with supplements of nicotinamide.

hats and the sun   A hat can help shield the skin from the sun's UV rays, as long as it is large enough to provide shade for all of the head and neck. For the most protection, individuals should wear a hat with a 7 cm brim (about three inches) that shades the face, ears, and the back of the neck. Baseball caps protect the forehead and nose, but leave the cheeks, chin, and neck exposed. Individuals should wear clothing that covers those areas, use SUNSCREEN with at least SPF 15, or stay in the shade to protect the skin.

For the best protection, hats should be made of a tightly woven fabric, such as canvas, which works best to protect the skin from UV rays. Individuals should avoid straw hats with holes that let sunlight through.

head lice   See LICE.

heat disorders   The body maintains its optimum internal temperature through the hypothalamus. When the temperature of the blood rises, the hypothalamus sends nerve impulses that stimulate the SWEAT GLANDS and dilate the blood vessels in the skin. The act of sweating does not cool off the body. The cooling effect is caused by the evaporation of the sweat from the skin. Dilation of the blood vessels increases blood flow near the surface of the skin, increasing the amount of heat that is lost by convection and radiation.

When the hypothalamus does not function properly, the body may progressively overheat, leading to a fatal heat stroke if untreated. Any malfunction or overload of the body's mechanisms for keeping temperature on an even keel may result in a heat disorder. Poor adaptation to heat may cause heat cramps, heat exhaustion, or heat stroke. High summer temperatures may cause PRICKLY HEAT, and an out-of-control infection can set off high fever, further damaging the body. Excessive sweating can cause an imbalance of salts and fluids in the body, which can lead to heat cramps or heat exhaustion throughout the day. To prevent heat disorders caused by excessive sweating, drink liquids (preferably water) throughout the day.

Risks Factors and Preventive Measures

Most environmental heat disorders can be prevented by acclimation to hot conditions over a three-week period, eating a light diet, avoiding alcohol, and wearing loose, lightweight clothes.

heat rash   A rash that occurs at high temperatures when sweat ducts are blocked by tight clothes made of fibers that do not breathe. Heat rash is most common on the chest and back, where perspiration is greatest, and is typified by widespread slightly raised red VESICLES or even PUSTULES. It settles down over a period of hours to days once the heat and sweating are eliminated. To protect against this rash, individuals should wear cotton clothing and use oil-free SUNSCREENS instead of heavier versions, which may trap perspiration.

helminthic infections   An infestation by any species of parasitic worms, most of which are not found in the United States. Several types of worms (or their larvae), ranging from microscopic in size to many feet long, can parasitize humans, although they do not usually multiply within the gastrointestinal tract.

There are two main classes, the roundworms and the platyhelminths, which include cestodes (tapeworms) and trematodes (flukes).

Worm diseases with skin symptoms include FILARIASIS and schistosomiasis.

hemangioma   A benign tumor or BIRTHMARK caused by an abnormal number of blood vessels in the skin. Hemangiomas may be either superficial, superficial and deep, or deep.

Symptoms and Diagnostic Path
Superficial hemangiomas, known as strawberry marks or capillary hemangiomas, are bright red and raised. These marks develop shortly after birth; at about the age of six months, the tumor begins to subside and the redness slowly fades; by age seven the hemangioma completely disappears.

Deep (or cavernous) hemangiomas are blue-purple growths that do not spontaneously clear.

Treatment Options and Outlook
Superficial hemangiomas do not require treatment for any medical reason, unless they interfere with

a vital function (such as those blocking the eyes, ears, mouth, nose, or anus). If the marks appear on the face, there may be psychological reasons to remove these superficial lesions. A hemangioma that bleeds frequently also may require removal, especially if located on the lip or tongue, or on the vulva or anus, where it could be disturbed by constant pressure. Superficial hemangiomas may be removed by PULSED DYE LASERS, which is most successful in young patients, or by surgical excision. Deep hemangiomas are best treated surgically.

hemangiosarcoma   See SARCOMA.

hemochromatosis   A disease also known as "bronze diabetes" in which too much dietary iron is absorbed, resulting in a bronzed skin color due to pigment deposited under the skin.

This is an inherited disease primarily affecting men; women rarely are affected because they regularly lose iron during their menstrual periods each month. While the disease is known to be genetic, its exact mode of transmission is not known.

Symptoms and Diagnostic Path
During middle age, the first signs of the disease are a loss of sexual desire and shrinking testes; left untreated, the iron overload causes chronic liver damage, impaired insulin production leading to diabetes mellitus, heart problems, and liver cancer.

Treatment Options and Outlook
The disorder is treated by removing some of the patient's blood once or twice weekly; once the iron level is normal, the procedure is done only three or four times yearly. Early treatment can prevent complications; for those who have already developed the disease, regular blood removal (called venesection) can head off problems. In some cases, chelation therapy (administration of chemicals that bind to iron and remove it from the body) may be used.

henna   The most popular of the vegetable dyes, this powdered substance is made from the crushed leaves of the *Lawsonia* shrub and is used primarily to give red-orange highlights to the hair. The color can be built up to give the hair body and added shine that complements brown hair particularly but does not cover gray very well. Henna can be very messy to apply, staining anything it touches and drying and stiffening the hair (making it a good choice for oily hair). Because henna builds up on the hair, it should not be used more than three times a year, and once it has been used, very little else can be done with the hair until it grows out. The color does not allow for permanent waving, straightening, or coloring with semi-permanent dyes. While henna has not been found to cause allergic reactions to the scalp, it can damage the hair.

Henoch-Schonlein purpura (HSP) A relatively rare condition in which inflamed blood vessels leak blood into the skin, joints, kidneys, and intestine. The disease is most common in childhood (especially among boys). In about two-thirds of the cases, HSP occurs after a respiratory infection. Incidence of the disease peaks between November and January.

It is suspected to be linked to an abnormal allergic reaction in response to infection.

Symptoms and Diagnostic Path
The disease usually starts with an acute and symmetrical rash on the skin around the ankle, the legs, the buttocks, and arms. After 12 to 24 hours, the lesions become dusky red and they may coalesce into larger patches. In children younger than three years the symptoms may be dominated by swelling of the scalp, the hands, and the feet. The joints are involved in up to 75 percent of the cases. About half the time there may be colicky abdominal pain or bloody diarrhea. Kidney problems may occur in as many as 80 percent of the cases.

Treatment Options and Outlook
With bed rest and mild painkillers, most children recover within a month. In severe cases, CORTICO-STEROIDS ease the joint pain and may sometimes affect the stomach problems, but they would not influence the long-term outcome of kidney disease. Plasma exchange has given encouraging results in individual cases but has not been confirmed in a larger series.

heparin necrosis Also known as anticoagulation syndrome, this condition is characterized by lesions at an injection site, and appears between four and 11 days after treatment with heparin (an anti-blood-clotting drug). The lesions quickly enlarge into large necrotic areas. There is no successful treatment, but the disease is self-limiting. Amputation is recommended for severe cases involving the penis or breast; other areas require excision and grafting.

See also COUMARIN NECROSIS.

herald patch The initial red, scaly eruption of PITYRIASIS ROSEA that occurs days before the disease spreads. It resembles a RINGWORM infection that is soon followed by multiple lesions, usually appearing first on the trunk.

hereditary disorders of the skin See GENETIC DISORDERS OF THE SKIN.

Hermansky-Pudlak syndrome A form of ALBINISM featuring white or pale yellow hair, many freckles, deeply pigmented nevi, eye problems, and heavy bleeding. Sufferers also have problems with lipid storage, which may cause complications such as pulmonary fibrosis and pulmonary insufficiency. The condition is found around the world, although it is most common in Puerto Rico and Brazil. The severity of the condition ranges from very mild with few symptoms to severe and disabling. Since HPS is an autosomal recessive disorder, both parents are expected to be carriers of the abnormal gene.

Symptoms and Diagnostic Path
People with the type of albinism found in this syndrome may have varied amounts of pigmentation. Some may have white or creamy skin; others may have sun freckling and yellow or light brown hair. A few with HPS may have dark brown hair and lightly pigmented skin. The visual problems inherent

in HPS is caused by the lack of pigment during eye development. This results in poor vision and frequently leads to legal blindness, light sensitivity, crossed eyes, and involuntary movement of the eyes (nystagmus).

Standard blood tests cannot identify the platelet defect in HPS. For proper diagnosis, the platelets must be examined under an electron microscope to observe the absence of dense bodies. Special laboratories are needed for this test.

Treatment Options and Outlook
Every person with albinism should understand HPS and inform a doctor of its possibility, especially before any medical or dental procedures. There is currently no treatment for HPS, although symptoms may be treated.

herpes gestationis A rare skin disorder occurring during pregnancy characterized by herpes-like BLISTERS on the legs and abdomen. Unrelated to the herpes simplex virus, it is named for the appearance of the eruption.

Unrelated to any disorders caused by the herpes simplex virus, herpes gestationis is an autoimmune blistering condition somewhat similar to bullous PEMPHIGOID.

Treatment Options and Outlook
Systemic CORTICOSTEROIDS are used to treat the disease. Experts debate whether herpes gestationis is associated with an increased incidence in maternal or fetal death. The condition usually fades after delivery but tends to recur in subsequent pregnancies.

herpes progenitalis See HERPES SIMPLEX INFECTION.

herpes simplex infection A group of inflammatory skin diseases characterized by spreading or creeping small clustered BLISTERS caused by the herpes simplex virus. Different forms of the virus result in either COLD SORES or the sexually transmitted disease genital herpes characterized by blisters on the sex organs. More than 25 million people in America are affected by the herpes virus.

There are two forms of the herpes simplex virus that are most common—type 1 and type 2. Herpes simplex, type 1 (HSV1) is usually associated with infections of the lips, mouth, and face, while herpes simplex, type 2 (HSV2) is usually associated with infections of the genitals, and in babies, who acquire the disease at birth.

However, there is a certain amount of overlap between the two, and conditions usually caused by HSV2 may be caused by HSV1 and vice versa. Both types are highly infectious, spread by direct contact with the lesions or by the fluid inside the blisters. Most people have been infected with HSV1 by the time they reach adulthood.

A person suffering an immunodeficiency disorder (such as AIDS) or someone taking immunosuppressant drugs who is exposed to the virus may experience a severe generalized infection that can be fatal.

Symptoms and Diagnostic Path
Before a blister develops, it is often preceded by a "prodrome"—burning, tingling sensation in the area where the blister subsequently appears. There also may be swollen and tender lymph glands. While the first infection by this virus may cause no symptoms at all, there may be a flulike illness in addition to ulcers on the skin around and inside the mouth for type 1 (oral) herpes. The first outbreak for type 2 also involves a sore, appearing three to seven days after exposure, but with type 2, the infection may be so severe as to cover the penis or vagina with blistering. It may be accompanied by high fever, tender swollen glands in the groin, and may last as long as two to six weeks before healing spontaneously. In women, the swelling from inflammation may be so severe as to impede urination. Exceptional pain, tenderness, high fever, and extensive blister may require hospitalization.

Afterward, the virus remains in the nerve cells. Many people experience recurrent reactivations of the virus (both type 1 and 2), suffering with repeated attacks of sores, especially during a fever or after prolonged sun exposure.

The virus may infect any other part of the body, but often affects the finger, causing painful blisters called a herpetic whitlow. In patients with a pre-existing skin condition (such as DERMATITIS), the virus may cause an extensive rash of blisters called ECZEMA HERPETICUM.

Treatment Options and Outlook

The antiviral drug ACYCLOVIR taken internally is effective in shortening the symptoms during the first attack. If taken as soon as tingling begins at the start of an outbreak, it can prevent it entirely. However, it does not prevent future attacks.

Risk Factors and Preventive Measures

Recently, scientists also have developed a therapeutic vaccine that reduces the frequency with which genital sores appear in patients infected with herpes. While it fails to outperform acyclovir, it sets the stage for a more effective treatment in the future.

herpes zoster   See SHINGLES.

heterograft   Also known as a xenograft, this is a living tissue graft transferred from one animal species to another, such as a heart valve transplanted from a pig to a human.

hexachlorophene   An antibacterial compound once widely used that is effective against many gram-positive organisms such as staphylococcus. However, it also has been associated with some unpleasant effects, including neurotoxicity in children and burn patients. Because it is not as safe as other antiseptics, such as chlorhexidine and iodine compounds, it is no longer commonly used.

Side Effects

Adverse reactions to compounds containing hexachlorophene may include DERMATITIS and sensitivity to sunlight. Sensitivity to hexachlorophene is rare; however, persons who have developed an allergy to the sun from similar compounds also may become sensitive to hexachlorophene. In those with highly sensitive skin, the use of hexachlorophene may at times produce a reaction characterized by redness or mild scaling or dryness, especially when it is combined with excessive rubbing or exposure to heat or cold.

See also ANTISEPTIC CLEANSERS.

hidradenitis suppurativa   Inflammation of an apocrine SWEAT GLAND, characterized by painful unpleasant-smelling lesions in the armpits and groin area. The lesions, which are most common in those with dark skin, appear in late adolescence and are related to bacterial infection.

Treatment Options and Outlook

This condition is very difficult to treat, and scarring is a frequent complication. Good hygiene is critical; skin should be washed with a mild antibacterial soap and cleansed fastidiously. If obesity is a problem, losing weight is essential.

Treatment with systemic antibiotics can help. In more severe cases, the dermatologist may consider administration of ISOTRETINOIN (Accutane) steroids, or surgery to remove affected tissue.

hidrocystoma   A benign cystic tumor in the SWEAT GLANDS, usually appearing on the eyelid. The CYST, which is relatively common among people in the United States, grows slowly and usually persists indefinitely.

The exact cause is unknown, but experts suspect it may be closely related to blockage of sweat duct apparatus, which leads to retention of sweat and a dilated cystic structure.

Symptoms and Diagnostic Path

The cyst is a dome-shaped bluish growth that may appear on the face, scalp, ears, or chest. Although it usually appears on the eyelid, it also may arise on other areas of the head, neck, and trunk; It also has been reported to occur on the penis, in the armpits, and in the anal region.

Treatment Options and Outlook

Surgical excision or carbon dioxide laser vaporization is the treatment of choice. Cysts are entirely benign and seldom recur. Vision usually is not affected.

hirsutism Excessive hairiness in women that grows thickly in a male pattern on face, trunk, and limbs. The condition is frequently seen in certain ethnic groups such as dark-haired Hispanics and women from the Mediterranean, and is usually of no medical significance. However, hirsutism some-times can be the sign of a hormonal imbalance or of an endocrine disease. In some cases, hirsutism is characterized by abnormally high levels of male hormones (such as polycystic ovary syndrome or congenital adrenal hyperplasia).

Treatment Options and Outlook
In cases where no medical cause is found, the unwanted hair can be bleached or removed.
See HAIR REMOVAL; ELECTROLYSIS.

histamine A chemical found in cells throughout the body that is released during an allergic reaction, resulting in inflammation. The effects of histamine can be offset by ANTIHISTAMINES. Histamine plays an important role in regulating the immune response. Its effects include redness, swelling, and HIVES.

histiocytoma cutis See DERMATOFIBROMA.

hives A skin reaction also known as *urticaria* (from the Latin word *urtica* for "nettle"), these raised, red, blotchy welts or wheals of various sizes can appear and disappear randomly on the surface of the skin. About one in five people experiences hives.

While the cause of the reaction is often unknown, hives may result from the release of histamine and other chemicals into the skin and/or blood. A wide variety of triggers have been known to cause hives, including food, pollen, animal dander, drugs, insect bites, infections, illness, cold, heat, light, or stress. Foods that have been linked with the development of hives include shellfish, fish, berries, nuts, eggs, and milk. Penicillin and aspirin also may cause hives in some susceptible patients.

In some patients, there may be a hereditary component in the tendency to develop hives. Termed HEREDITARY ANGIOEDEMA, this condition is characterized by nonitching swellings lasting three or four days that may be triggered by trauma or may appear to occur spontaneously.

Treatment Options and Outlook
The standard treatment for hives is antihistamines, but other drugs may also be used (including adrenaline or epinephrine, terbutaline, oral COR-TICOSTEROIDS, or cimetidine). In addition, sufferers should provide physicians with a detailed medical history, including a detailed diary of exposure to foods, chemicals, new products, and possible irri-tants over a period of two weeks to a month before onset of the hives.

Because hives may be triggered by such a wide variety of agents, it may never be possible to docu-ment the exact cause.

Physically uncomfortable but generally harm-less, they eventually disappear, leaving no lasting marks.

hives, sun-induced See SOLAR URTICARIA.

homograft See ALLOGRAFT.

hookworm A small, round blood-sucking worm that penetrates the skin, causing a red, itchy rash on the feet called "ground itch" (cutaneous larva migrans). The worms are of the species *Necator Americanus* or *Ancylostoma duodenale* (New and Old World hookworms respectively), and infest about 700 million people in tropical Third World countries.

In the United States, children can become infested when the common hookworm is passed through a dog's feces and is deposited into the soil. The parasites then stay in the soil where they will eventually hatch into larvae that can penetrate through the skin or be eaten. These worms are not usually affected by extreme environmental conditions, so they can be a problem in any area. A child can become infested by playing with an infected dog and coming into contact with the feces, or by walking barefoot in grass or sand where a dog has defecated. Younger children are at risk when they put dirt or sand into their mouths while playing. In children or adults who walk barefoot, the hookworm can penetrate the sole of the foot and cause a lesion. The larva will then begin to mature while it moves toward the intestines. As in dogs, the hookworm will attach to the intestinal wall.

Symptoms and Diagnostic Path

Humans who have become infected will show symptoms of intestinal bleeding, abdominal pains, anemia, severe diarrhea, and malnutrition. In minor infestations there may be no symptoms. In more severe cases, a red linear rash can be seen at the top of the sole of the foot or on the buttocks. Hookworms are diagnosed by examining a stool sample under a microscope. Counting the eggs in a specific amount of feces allows the health care provider to estimate the severity of the infection.

Treatment Options and Outlook

Antihelmintic drugs (such as mebendazole applied as a topical cream) kill the worms. Improved diet and blood transfusions also may be necessary.

Risk Factors and Preventive Measures

Human hookworm infection can be prevented in the United States by giving dogs and cats proper veterinary care and teaching children sensible personal hygiene.

See also LARVA MIGRANS, CUTANEOUS.

hordeolum   See STYE.

hormones and acne   Hormonal activity is important in the development of ACNE, since the condition depends on the stimulation of the hair follicles by male sexual hormones found in men and women. Some women with acne may have excessive levels of these hormones. This should be suspected if a woman has irregular periods or facial hair. The most frequent cause of androgen excess in females is polycystic ovarian disease.

horn, cutaneous   A hard, benign, pink or yellow growth most often seen in older persons. A slow-growing horn may develop on the former site of a WART, a sebaceous keratosis, ACTINIC KERATOSIS, or SQUAMOUS CELL CARCINOMA; left untreated, it may grow quite large and may protrude as much as three-quarters of an inch. Surgery can remove the growth.

See also KERATOSIS, SEBORRHEIC; KERATOSIS, SOLAR.

Horner's syndrome   A group of symptoms including absence of sweating (ANHIDROSIS), narrowing of the pupil of the eye, and drooping eyelids. The syndrome is caused by damage to the sympathetic nerve fibers (usually in the lower neck).

Symptoms and Diagnostic Path

Sympathetic nerve fiber injuries can result from a stroke in the brainstem, injury to the carotid artery, a tumor in the upper lobe of the lung, and cluster headaches. Rarely, Horner's syndrome may be present at birth and associated with a lack of pigmentation of the iris. Eye drops and certain medications may lead to this condition.

A neurological exam can diagnose the condition and find the cause by determining which, if any, other parts of the nervous system are affected. Tests may include an MRI of the head, carotid ultrasound, chest X-ray, CT scan of the chest, blood tests, an angiogram, and eye drop tests.

Treatment Options and Outlook

The treatment for Horner's syndrome depends upon the cause. In many cases there is no treatment that improves or reverses the condition. Treatment in acquired cases is aimed at eradicating the disease that produces the syndrome. Prognosis depends on whether treatment of the underlying cause is successful.

Howel-Evans syndrome   A genetic disorder of KERATINIZATION characterized by lesions of the palms and soles and cancer of the esophagus. It was first described in 1958, when two British families were reported to have a 70 percent incidence of esophageal cancer with related keratosis. No cancer was found in family members without keratosis.

The disorder is inherited in an autosomal dominant pattern, which means that only one defective gene (from one parent) is needed to cause the syndrome. Each child of an affected person usually has a one in two chance of inheriting the defective gene and of being affected.

No one knows why the cancer and the keratosis appear together.

HPV   See PAPILLOMA VIRUS, HUMAN.

human bites   Human bites (particularly on the hand) are common, and because of the bacteria found in the mouth, may often cause soft tissue infection. Septic arthritis or osteomyelitis may follow a human bite. *Staphylococcus aureus* and *Streptococcus* bacteria often contaminate human bites.

Treatment Options and Outlook

A human bite wound should be thoroughly cleaned, soaked, and elevated for 48 hours. It should be left open; oral antibiotics are often administered. Infected injuries may require local debridement, hospitalization, and intravenous antibiotics.

humectant   Substance that preserves the moisture or water content of the skin. Most dry skin lacks moisture rather than oil, and therefore humectants and MOISTURIZERS are needed instead of creams or oils. The most effective humectant is lactic acid, which when applied to the skin, draws water from the DERMIS into the EPIDERMIS.

Hunter's syndrome   A genetic metabolic disease that causes skin symptoms in 20 percent of cases. It is characterized by white or flesh-colored PAPULES or NODULES on the nape of the neck, the chest, and the upper arms and legs. Lesions may appear in children before age 10, spontaneously disappearing later in life.

Hunter's syndrome is an X-linked recessive disorder, which means that it is caused by a defect on the X chromosome and usually leads to problems in men only. Women can be carriers of the defect; if so, half their sons may be affected.

The condition is one of seven major types of mucopolysaccharidoses (diseases characterized by a lack of certain enzymes).

Symptoms and Diagnostic Path

Symptoms that do not involve the skin may include deafness, dwarfism, mental retardation, clawlike hands, and early mortality. There are also milder forms that allow the patient to live into adulthood.

Treatment Options and Outlook

There is no effective treatment for this disorder, although researchers hope one day the condition can be cured by replacing the missing enzymes.

Hutchinson's freckle   The common name for LENTIGO MALIGNA.

hyaluronic acid gel (Restylane and Hylaform)   A protective, lubricating, binding gel substance that is produced naturally by the body. It is used in some skin creams as a MOISTURIZER and is also used as a filler substance to fill out facial WRINKLES. Approved in March 2004, Restylane is injected into facial tissue to smooth wrinkles and folds, especially in the folds around the nose and mouth and to enhance the lips. Restylane works by temporarily adding volume to facial tissue and restoring a smoother appearance to the face for an effect that lasts for about six months.

It is injected by a doctor into areas of facial tissue where moderate to severe facial wrinkles and folds occur. The gel temporarily adds volume to the skin and can give the appearance of a smoother surface. Restylane and Hylaform will help smooth moderate to severe facial wrinkles and folds. In one study, most patients needed just one injection to smooth out the wrinkles.

Side effects of hyaluronic acid fillers include bruising, redness, swelling, pain, tenderness, and

ITCHING. These gels should not be used in patients with severe allergies marked by a history of anaphylaxis, multiple severe allergies, or severe allergies to gram-positive bacterial proteins. In addition, they should not be used for breast augmentation; implantation into bone, tendon, ligament, or muscle; or implantation into blood vessels, because they may obstruct blood flow.

See also SKIN FILLERS.

hydrogen peroxide A mild antiseptic sometimes used to treat skin infections. The solution combines with catalase (an enzyme present in the skin) to release oxygen, which kills bacteria and cleanses the infected areas. Currently, use of hydrogen peroxide is not recommended because it is a feeble germ killer.

Side Effects

Hydrogen peroxide sometimes causes soreness and irritation.

hydropic degeneration Damage to the cells of the basal layer, which produces tiny spaces in the cells.

hydroquinone (paradihydroxybenzene) This skin bleaching agent can reduce the intensity of pigmentation of FRECKLES, MELASMA, and solar LENTIGO. It suppresses PIGMENTATION by blocking the activity of an enzyme involved in the synthesis of MELANIN.

When applied to the skin over a period of several months, the skin temporarily becomes somewhat lighter. For continued and increased effectiveness it must be used for a longer term. Sun exposure (even through window glass) during treatment should be avoided because it reverses the effect of hydroquinone.

Hydroquinone is sometimes combined with TRETINOIN for better skin penetration and because tretinoin helps to lighten pigmentation, or with corticosteroids to reduce the irritation occasionally caused by tretinoin. Other ingredients often added to hydroquinone include GLYCOLIC ACID and RETINOL.

The medication was discovered when African-American workers who were handling rubber products containing hydroquinone noticed that the skin on their hands and other areas exposed to the chemical were getting lighter. Hydroquinone is prescribed in a 1 to 4 percent lotion, gel, or salve.

Side Effects

Occasionally, at higher concentrations a patient will have an adverse reaction to the agent and experience *increased* pigmentation or development of MILIA. Other adverse effects could include mild skin irritation or allergic reaction.

hydroxyurea (Trade name: Hydrea) An anticancer drug that inhibits DNA synthesis and that may be helpful for patients with extensive PSORIASIS.

Side Effects

Patients who have received prior radiation therapy before getting the drug may experience worsening of redness. Other side effects include skin eruptions, gastrointestinal disturbances, bone marrow abnormalities, and (rarely) neurologic symptoms. It may also cause temporary kidney problems. Because it causes birth defects in animals, it is not recommended for use during pregnancy.

hyperbilirubinemia A yellowish discoloration of the skin, sclerae, mucous membranes, and eardrums caused by high levels of bilirubin in the blood.

hypergranulosis An increase in the number of keratin-producing cells in the granular layer of the skin.

hyperhidrosis This disorder of excessive sweating begins at puberty, worsening in the summer and affecting the palms, soles, and armpits. It also may be caused by certain diseases, such as fevers, or the effect of using certain drugs. Excessively sweaty armpits and feet may cause unpleasant body odor.

The condition often improves when the patient enters the middle 20s to 30s.

The amount of sweat produced is regulated in the hypothalamus; overactivity of the hypothalamus or the sympathetic nerves can result in hyperhidrosis. Typically, hyperhidrosis first appears in childhood or adolescence; other family members may or may not also have the problem. An increase in air temperature, exercise, fever, anxiety, or spicy food may set off attacks of sweating, which usually lessen at night and disappear during sleep.

A few patients have hyperhidrosis as a consequence of a medical condition. Generalized hyperhidrosis may be due to drugs, cardiovascular disorders, respiratory failure, overactive thyroid, endocrine tumors, or Parkinson's disease. Localized hyperhidrosis may be due to a stroke, nerve damage, a brain tumor, or a chronic anxiety disorder.

Symptoms and Diagnostic Path

Hyperhidrosis is an embarrassing complaint and significantly interferes with many daily activities. Clothing gets damp and must be changed several times a day. Wet skin folds are prone to irritation. Patients find it embarrassing to shake hands and difficult to write neatly. Sweaty feet develop an unpleasant smell, ruin footwear, are prone to skin irritation or secondary infection, and require several sock changes a day.

Aluminum chloride with ethyl alcohol (DRYSOL) This prescription product is effective in some cases of excessive sweating of the hands, armpits, and feet, and is probably the least invasive of all treatment methods. It is typically the first type of treatment tried. The medication applied at night and left on the skin for six to eight hours. It is then washed off completely the following morning before the onset of daytime sweating. (Skin must be dry when Drysol is applied, or it will cause severe irritation.) About half of patients will develop some degree of skin irritation from this product, so it is important that the application directions be carefully followed.

Botox Botulinum toxin injections (BOTOX) into the armpits have revolutionized the treatment for this condition, since the injections can reduce or even stop sweating for three to six months. Botox is also effective for the palms and soles. Botulinum toxin may temporarily weaken the small muscles of the hands. Regional or local anesthesia is typically given in these sites because the injections are painful.

Iontophoresis This type of treatment involves using electrical stimulation (usually for patients with excessive sweating in the hands). Patients place their hands in a bath through which an electrical current is passed, which seems to stun the sweat glands and decrease the secretion of sweat for between six hours and a week.

Other medications Many medicines have been used with varying success, including sedatives (in those patients with stress-induced hyperhidrosis) and medications that affect the nervous system.

Surgery Surgery is typically considered only when less invasive medical treatments have failed. The surgical treatment of hyperhidrosis involves destroying or removing a specific portion of the main sympathetic nerve, which is part of a separate and parallel nervous system. The surgical therapy for hyperhidrosis entails removing or destroying the specific part that causes sweating in the underarm. Typically, the patient remains in the hospital for a period of 12 to 24 hours after surgery. Most patients need pain medication for between seven and 10 days after surgery.

This surgery will cure between 95 and 98 percent of excessive hand (palmar) hyperhidrosis and about 75 to 80 percent of armpit (axillary) hyperhidrosis. Approximately 25 percent of patients with hyperhidrosis of the feet (plantar) will notice some improvement, but surgery is not designed to treat plantar hyperhidrosis and should not be used if this is the only sweating complaint.

See also SWEAT GLANDS; ANTIPERSPIRANTS; DEODORANTS.

hyperkeratosis Thickening of the outer layer of the skin caused by too much KERATIN (a protein component of the outer skin layer). The most common types of hyperkeratosis are CORNS and CALLUSES (caused by pressure or friction). Hyperkeratosis often occurs in scaly conditions such as WARTS, ECZEMA, and LICHEN PLANUS.

hyperpigmentation Excess pigmentation that causes darker-than-usual skin. Darker skin (except for very black skin) often responds to trauma with hyperpigmentation, but the phenomenon occurs in all racial and ethnic groups.

Many chemicals can cause hyperpigmentation, but heavy metals can cause discoloration by being deposited within the skin. Arsenic, which some patients may ingest by drinking water from contaminated wells or by being exposed to insecticide sprays used in fruit orchards, can stimulate melanin formation within the EPIDERMIS, causing a brown hyperpigmentation. The hyperpigmentation is not caused by arsenic deposits within the dermis. Bismuth can also cause a brown hyperpigmentation; both bismuth and arsenic were once contained in medications.

hyperplasia An increase in the production and growth of normal cells in skin tissue. It can result in a thickened EPIDERMIS (outer layer of the skin). During pregnancy, the breasts grow in this fashion.

hypertrichosis Excessive hair growth in places not normally covered with hair. This excess hair growth is often caused by certain drugs (such as cyclosporine, minoxidil, and diazoxide). The condition is not the same as HIRSUTISM (excess hairiness in women).

hypertrophic scars An enlarged or thickened SCAR, remaining within the confines of the original wound in which excessive scar tissue rises above the skin during the healing process.

hypochondria, cutaneous See ACNE EXCORIÉE.

hypohidrosis Lessened or inability to sweat. This condition is a symptom of HYPOHIDROTIC ECTODERMAL DYSPLASIA, a rare inherited condition characterized by the decreased ability to sweat, dry wrinkly skin, sparse dry hair, small brittle nails, and cone-shaped teeth. Other causes of hypohidrosis include exfoliative dermatitis and some anticholinergic drugs.

See also DERMATITIS, EXFOLIATIVE.

hypohidrotic ectodermal dysplasia A rare, incurable genetic condition characterized by a decreased ability to sweat, dry wrinkly skin, sparse dry hair, small brittle nails, and cone-shaped teeth.

hypomelanosis of Ito A congenital disorder of pigmentation also known as incontinentia pigmenti achromicans.

The disorder has an autosomal dominant condition, which means that only one defective gene from one parent is needed to cause the syndrome. Each child of an affected person usually has a one in two chance of inheriting the defective gene and of being affected. Males are almost twice as likely to have the disorder as females.

Symptoms and Diagnostic Path
The condition is characterized by bizarre unpigmented areas that appear in whorls, streaks, and splashes on the skin of the trunk and extremities. The pigment changes are present at birth, and are often the first indication that the infant is not normal. In addition to skin symptoms, most patients also have other problems, including disorders of the central nervous system, eyes, hair, nails, teeth, musculoskeletal system, or internal organs. Up to 40 percent of these patients are also mentally retarded.

Treatment Options
As with other similar hypopigmentation disorders present at birth, there is no specific treatment for the skin problems with this disease. Topical application of methoxsalen and exposure to ultraviolet radiation may minimize the skin disfigurement.

hypopigmentation Decreased PIGMENTATION resulting in lightening of the skin that may be caused by a lack of pigment cells in an area of skin, or because the skin has too few MELANIN-producing cells.

Disorders of congenital hypopigmentation due to abnormal formation of melanin-producing cells include TUBEROUS SCLEROSIS, HYPOMELANOSIS OF ITO, NEVUS DEPIGMENTOSUS and CHEDIAK-HIGASHI SYNDROME. Oculocutaneous albinism is a congenital hypopigmentation due to problems with the synthesis of melanin. TINEA VERSICOLOR is an example of an acquired case of hypopigmentation caused by decreased synthesis of melanin. PITYRIASIS ALBA is an acquired type of hypopigmentation caused by the decreased transfer of melanin-producing cells.

Hypopigmentation also may follow an infection or inflammation. Many infectious and inflammatory skin disorders fade away while leaving hypopigmented macules and patches in the distribution and pattern of the original skin lesion. Dark skin that has been injured often exhibits hypopigmentation, but the phenomenon occurs among all racial and ethnic groups—the more common disorders that produce post-inflammatory hypopigmentation include PSORIASIS, eczematous dermatitis, atopic dermatitis, seborrheic dermatitis, tinea versicolor, CHICKEN POX, SYPHILIS, LICHEN PLANUS, PITYRIASIS ROSEA, pityriasis lichenoides chronica, and lichen striatus.

Drugs also can cause hypopigmentation. Chloroquine may cause hypopigmentation of the skin or bleaching of the hair; cosmetics and skin bleaches often available without prescription may cause hypopigmentation.

hypopituitarism and skin color The lack of melanocyte-stimulating hormones (MSH) can cause a generalized decrease in skin color.

See also DEPIGMENTING DISORDERS; PIGMENTATION DISORDERS.

iatrogenic atrophy Thinning of the skin, often produced by CORTICOSTEROIDS taken either by mouth or administered on the skin. This apparently occurs because the steroids interfere with the formation of COLLAGEN. The more potent the topical steroid, the faster and more severe the atrophy. Thinning of the skin associated with systemic corticosteroids affects the skin everywhere on the body. ("Iatrogenic" describes conditions that result from treatment.)

ibuprofen (Trade names: Motrin, Advil, Nuprin) A nonsteroidal anti-inflammatory drug (NSAID) used to ease pain and reduce inflammation in a wide variety of skin disorders.

Side Effects
Ibuprofen may cause skin rash, abdominal pain, diarrhea, nausea, heartburn and, occasionally, dizziness. However, it is less likely than other NSAIDs to cause peptic ulcers.

ice packs A treatment to reduce inflammation, bruising, and swelling of the skin. Cold causes the blood vessels in the skin to contract, reducing blood flow; it also numbs nerves and can reduce pain.

An ice pack can be made by wrapping ice in a wet cloth, applying to the skin's surface. Chemical ice packs may also be used; these are struck or shaken, which mixes the chemicals and produces a liquid with a very low temperature.

If no ice is available in an emergency situation, a chilled soda can, frozen meat, or other frozen food may be used as an ice pack. (It should be wrapped in material to avoid burning the skin).

ichthyosis Any of several generalized skin disorders characterized by dry, rough, scaling, darkened skin that occur because of an excess amount of KERATIN (the main protein component of the skin). The disorder's name is derived from the Greek word *ichthus* meaning "fish," because the appearance and condition of the skin resembles scales.

Symptoms and Diagnostic Path
This group of genetic diseases ranges from mild generalized dry skin (ichthyosis vulgaris) to severe widespread thickened scaly dry skin (LAMELLAR ICHTHYOSIS).

Ichthyosis vulgaris, which affects the thighs, arms and backs of the hands, usually appears at or shortly after birth and improves as the child grows older. However, in severe conditions, the infant is usually born dead, encased in skin as hard as armor plate.

Treatment Options and Outlook
There is no cure for any of the ichthyoses, but lubricants and ointments may help the dryness, and bath oils can moisten the skin. Washing with soap aggravates the condition. Ichthyosis improves in a warm, humid environment and worsens in cold weather.

icterus See JAUNDICE.

imiquimod cream (Trade name: Aldara) A topical drug that releases interferons that has recently been approved in the United States for the treatment of GENITAL WARTS, ACTINIC KERATOSIS, and BASAL CELL CARCINOMA, a slow-growing local type of skin cancer.

immersion foot Also known as "trench foot" during World War I, this condition causes the skin of the feet to turn pale, eventually becoming red, swollen, and painful. It occurs among shipwreck survivors and soldiers whose feet have been wet and cold for a long time, caused by death of skin tissue after prolonged immersion in water.

Treatment Options and Outlook

At the initial stage (where the skin is pale and there is no detectable pulse), the skin should be rewarmed gradually and carefully, since overheating may lead to GANGRENE (tissue death). If the condition has progressed to the latter stages, with red and swollen skin and a strong pulse, the foot should be gradually cooled. Even so, the feet may subsequently be overly sensitive to cold for several years.

Untreated, the condition can lead to severe muscle weakness, skin ulcers, or gangrene.

immunity and sunlight The sun has a detrimental effect on the body's immune system, decreasing its ability to recognize and destroy potentially lethal pathogens ranging from bacteria to cancer cells.

Ultraviolet-B light suppresses the function of T-lymphocytes, which are important in immune surveillance. There is evidence from animal research that this UV-B-induced suppression may decrease the immune system's ability to recognize and destroy malignant cells which initiate SKIN CANCER.

immunotherapy A preventive technique to combat allergy to substances such as pollen, dust mites, wasp, or bee venom. The treatment involves giving increasing doses of the irritating substance to make the patient's immune system less sensitive to the irritant.

Before immunotherapy begins, the patient and physician try to determine the trigger factors for the allergy with skin and blood tests.

A purified extract of a small amount of the allergen is injected into the skin of the arm once a week for about 30 weeks, after which injections can be administered every two weeks. Eventually, the injections can be given once a month. The therapy must be given for three to four years before the patient can be considered immune. The treatment increases a person's ability to tolerate the irritating substance.

Side Effects

Because there is a risk of a severe allergic reaction shortly after an injection, the technique requires close medical supervision.

See also BEE AND WASPS.

impetigo A superficial skin infection most commonly found in children, caused by streptococcal or staphyloccal bacteria (sometimes both).

Impetigo is spread through body contact and usually is found on exposed body areas such as the legs, face, and arms. Because impetigo is spread quickly through play groups and day care centers, children with the infection should be kept away from playmates and out of school until the sores disappear.

Symptoms and Diagnostic Path

The condition starts as tiny, almost imperceptible blisters on a child's skin, usually at the site of skin abrasion, scratch, or INSECT BITE. Most lesions occur on exposed areas, such as the face, scalp, and extremities. The red and itchy sores begin to ooze for the next few days, leaving a sticky golden crust. Untreated, the infection usually will last from two to three weeks but may continue indefinitely if not treated. It is most prevalent during hot, humid weather.

Impetigo is diagnosed by a simple examination.

Treatment Options and Outlook

Impetigo should be treated as soon as possible to avoid the spread of the infection to other children and to prevent a rare complication: a form of kidney disease called acute glomerulonephritis.

MUPIROCIN treatment is highly effective in simple uncomplicated impetigo and is the treatment of choice. In widespread disease, systemic antibiotics also can be used, such as dicloxacillin, cephalosporin, or erythromycin. With proper care this infection is quite manageable.

Risk Factors and Preventive Measures

Cleanliness and prompt attention to skin injury can help prevent impetigo. Impetigo patients and their families should bathe regularly with antibacterial soaps, and apply topical antibiotics to insect bites, cuts, abrasions, and infected lesions immediately. Impetigo in infants is especially contagious and serious. To prevent spreading, pillow cases, towels and washcloths should not be shared, and should be boiled after each use.

impetigo, Bockhart's A superficial form of FOLLICULITIS.

impetigo, bullous Also called "staphylococcal impetigo," this superficial skin infection is caused by *Staphylococcus aureus* bacteria and requires immediate attention. This disease has been more frequently diagnosed since the 1970s.

Symptoms and Diagnostic Path

Symptoms include thin-walled, flaccid fluid-filled BLISTERS that rupture easily; their fluid may be clear or full of PUS. After rupture, the base quickly dries to a shiny veneer, which looks different than the thicker crust found in common IMPETIGO. Lesions are usually found in groups, most often on the face or trunk instead of arms or legs.

This condition is diagnosed by a simple examination.

Treatment Options and Outlook

As with common impetigo, bullous impetigo is treated with dicloxacillin, cephalosporin, or ERYTHROMYCIN. It is important to wash the affected areas thoroughly twice a day with soap and water to keep the area as clean as possible. Blood poisoning complications are rare.

impetigo, staphylococcal See IMPETIGO, BULLOUS.

impetigo, streptococcal See IMPETIGO.

impetigo, superficial See IMPETIGO.

impetigo contagiosa See IMPETIGO; IMPETIGO, BULLOUS.

Imuran See AZANTHIOPRINE.

incontinentia pigmenti See BLOCH-SULZBERGER SYNDROME.

incontinentia pigmenti achromicans See HYPOMELANOSIS OF ITO.

infant acne See ACNE, INFANT.

infantile acropustulosis A recurring disease in infants that causes severe ITCHING, restlessness, and fretfulness, and that is typically diagnosed between 2 months and 10 months of age. First described in 1979, it is probably much more common than had previously been thought. Its cause is unknown, but many cases are preceded by SCABIES infestation. More often, however, cases occur despite scabies having been thoroughly ruled out. There appears to be no bacterial or viral cause, nor does it seem as if the immune system is involved. While initial reports suggested the problem was more common among African Americans, experts now believe it affects all races equally.

Symptoms and Diagnostic Path

Lesions begin as small itchy lesions that then form distinct VESICLES and PUSTULES that tend to heal with hyperpigmentation. Lesions always appear on the hands and the feet, usually on the palms of the hands and the soles of the feet, but they may also occur on the trunk, the scalp, and the face.

Children are fretful, irritable, and obviously uncomfortable, but otherwise healthy. Individual bouts last one to two weeks, recurring every two to four weeks.

Treatment Options and Outlook

Treatment is often unnecessary because of the self-limited nature of his condition. Topical steroids and oral DAPSONE have been used successfully in more persistent cases. Topical pramoxine preparations are available without prescription for the itch, and oral ANTIHISTAMINES may be useful.

The intensity and the duration of attacks diminish with each recurrence, and all cases spontaneously resolve in a few months to three years.

infant skin care   See SKIN CARE FOR INFANTS.

infant skin diseases   Infants are affected by a wide range of problems unique to their age group, and they also may show unusual symptoms of more common skin problems found in other patients. Because many skin problems of infants are related to systemic disorders, a complete physical exam is important to diagnosis.

Infant skin problems can include MILIA, SALMON PATCH, ERYTHEMA TOXICUM, PRICKLY HEAT, harlequin color changes, neonatal ACNE, HEMANGIOMAS, PORT-WINE STAINS, lymphatic disorders, transient neonatal pustular melanosis acropustulosis, APLASIA CUTIS, EPIDERMOLYSIS BULLOSA, INCONTINENTIA PIGMENTI, ICHTHYOSIS, bacterial infections (such as IMPETIGO, SYPHILIS, SCALDED SKIN SYNDROME), and viral infections (such as HERPES SIMPLEX, cytomegalovirus, RUBELLA, AIDS, toxoplasmosis).

Other problems include histiocytosis X, juvenile xanthogranuloma, MASTOCYTOSIS, and subcutaneous fat necrosis of the newborn. Pigmentary abnormalities may include CAFE AU LAIT SPOTS, BLUE NEVUS, and CONGENITAL MELANOCYTIC NEVI. Infants may also be affected by seborrheic dermatitis of infancy, DIAPER RASH, and neonatal lupus erythematosus.

Treatment for infant skin problems is difficult, complicated by the risks and toxicity of various medications that would be appropriate for an older patient.

inflammation   An essential part of the body's response to injury that results in redness, swelling, pain, and heat in the skin tissue because of either a chemical or physical injury, or an infection.

Inflammation occurs when skin tissue is damaged. A chemical called HISTAMINE is released, which increases blood flow to the damaged tissue, causing redness and heat; white blood cells enter the tissue and attack the bacteria and other foreign particles. Similar cells from the tissues remove and consume the dead cells, sometimes producing PUS. Histamine also makes blood capillaries leak, causing fluid to ooze out and create swelling.

Occasionally, inflammation is an inappropriate response (such as in autoimmune disorders) and results in conditions such as rheumatoid arthritis.

Treatment Options and Outlook

Inflammation may be suppressed with CORTICOSTEROID drugs or nonsteroidal anti-inflammatory drugs. These drugs work by reducing the production of prostaglandins (fatty acids that produce inflammation in injured tissue). The drugs also reduce the release and activity of white blood cells and normalize the size of blood vessels.

infrared light   Light in the part of the electromagnetic spectrum immediately after the red end of the visible light. Chronic exposure, such as in cases of bakers or furnace workers, can produce photoaging similar to that produced by longstanding sun exposure.

infundibulofolliculitis   Inflammation of a hair follicle above the opening of the sebaceous gland. Little is known about the cause.

Symptoms and Diagnostic Path

This uncommon itchy papular eruption affects the trunk, arms, and legs, and occurs almost exclusively in African Americans.

Treatment Options and Outlook

There is no cure but patients may try mild topical CORTICOSTEROIDS and emollients.

ingrown toenail   A painful nail condition in which one or both edges of the nail has grown inward into the skin around the nail bed, causing inflammation and infection. The condition is usually caused by wearing ill-fitting shoes, poor personal hygiene, or improperly cut toenails.

Symptoms and Diagnostic Path

Ingrown toenails cause pain, redness, swelling and, sometimes, an infection. The condition usually affects the big toe.

Treatment Options and Outlook

Antibiotics can relieve the infection; removal of the nail edge under local anesthetic may be necessary. Pain may be relieved by soaking the foot in strong, warm saline solution twice daily and covering the area with a dry gauze bandage.

Risk Factors and Preventive Measures

Toenails should be cut straight across, not angled down along the sides.

insect bites   Minute puncture wounds in the skin caused by any of a variety of insects, mites, mosquitoes, midges, gnats, sand flies, ticks, fleas, and bedbugs. Most insect bites are not terribly painful, and cause only a temporary itch for several days. They are extremely common, especially in children. Papular urticaria (hives) occurs most often in two- through seven-year-olds, usually in late spring or summer. Episodes last only two to three weeks, but can recur over a three- or four-year period.

Direct tissue injury may result from biting, stinging, or burrowing. Local hives may occur by venoms introduced with a bite or sting, or by contact with various secretions. Necrosis (tissue death) has been produced by the bite of certain spiders, such as the BROWN RECLUSE. Secondary abrasions or infections may occur. Insects may bite either on exposed areas of the skin or parts of the body where clothing fits tightly (in these areas, the movement of the insect is halted and it bites to feed or as a defense).

Treatment Options and Outlook

Itch and redness can be reduced with topical CORTICOSTEROIDS; CALAMINE lotion also helps the itch.

Topical antihistamines or anesthetics such as Benadryl and benzocaine should be avoided.

integument   A medical name for the skin.

interface dermatitis   See DERMATITIS.

interferon alpha (IFN-a)   A drug used to treat malignant melanoma and a number of other conditions. Interferon alpha is one type of interferon—natural proteins produced by the cells of the immune system in response to challenges by viruses, bacteria, parasites, and tumor cells. Interferon alpha is produced by many cell types, including T-cells and B-cells, and is an important component of the antiviral response. Interferon alpha is also active against tumors.

Interferon was scarce and expensive until 1980, when the interferon gene was inserted into bacteria using recombinant DNA technology, allowing mass cultivation and purification from bacterial cultures. Several different types of interferon are now approved for use in humans, and interferon therapy is used (in combination with chemotheraphy and radiation) as a treatment for many types of systemic cancer.

Interferon alfa 2b is used to treat malignant melanoma and for chronic myelogenous leukemia. Interferon alpha was approved by the U.S. Food and Drug Administration in 1991 as a treatment for hepatitis C. Several different forms of interferon alpha, including interferon alpha-2a, interferon alpha-2b, and interferon alfacon-1 are approved for the treatment of viral hepatitis.

See also MELANOMA, MALIGNANT.

internal malignancy, skin signs of   See MALIGNANCY, SKIN SIGNS OF INTERNAL.

intertrigo   Skin inflammation occurring primarily in obese people on adjacent surfaces of the skin, such as the neck creases, groin, armpits, folds of the abdomen, between fingers and toes, and the area beneath the breasts.

Symptoms and Diagnostic Path

Red, moist skin, with scales or blisters and an unpleasant odor. The condition, which worsens with sweating, is sometimes accompanied by seborrheic DERMATITIS or yeast infection.

Treatment Options and Outlook

Weight reduction, good personal cleanliness, dry skin, and CORTICOSTEROID or antifungal cream.

iododerma Any skin eruption caused by iodine or iodide ingestion.

isotretinoin (Trade name: Accutane) A synthetic oral form of VITAMIN A that has been used since the late 1970s to treat severe cystic ACNE that has failed to respond to other treatments. It is also effective in the healing of oral LEUKOPLAKIA and is also used to treat severe ICHTHYOSIS (disorders characterized by thickened, scaling skin). Roche, the maker of Accutane, estimates that nearly seven million Americans have taken its drug. Hundreds of thousands more have taken other brands of isotretinoin since they came on the market after Roche's patent expired in 2002.

Isotretinoin works by decreasing formation of oily plugs of SEBUM, reducing the formation of KERATIN (the tough outer layer of skin) and by shrinking SEBACEOUS GLANDS—so well that it can cause unpleasant side effects such as skin dryness and nosebleeds. Isotretinoin cures or greatly reduces severe disfiguring acne in up to 80 percent of patients. However, it can cause severe birth defects (including fetal brain, heart, and skeletal deformities); for this reason, pregnancy must be avoided during treatment and for at least two months after treatment has ended.

Currently, isotretinoin is given for four to six months for the first treatment; after treatment has ceased, the condition may continue to improve for at least two more months and sometimes for as long as one year, although the sebum production gradually returns to its original levels before treatment. More than 60 percent of patients with severe acne never again require treatment. However, about one-third of patients need a second course of the drug, which should be administered only after a six-month hiatus. This second course may require higher doses.

Side Effects

There are several serious side effects that have been associated with this medication, but the most serious of which are birth defects when the drug is taken by a pregnant woman. Isotretinoin causes the most severe birth defects if an expectant mother takes it during her first trimester, when she is least likely to know she is pregnant. It can lead to what is known as Accutane embryopathy, in which exposed fetuses typically have a pattern of brain abnormalities as well as major malformations of the head, ears, eyes, face, and heart.

In the beginning of 2006, the companies that make isotretinoin, together with the U.S. Food and Drug Administration, have imposed mandatory prescribing rules. Any woman of childbearing age who is given the drug must

- have negative pregnancy tests two months in a row before starting the drug during treatment
- either promise in writing to abstain from sex with a man or else use two forms of contraception, one of which must be a highly effective kind such as birth control pills or the injectable Depo-Provera
- take a pregnancy test each month during her treatment (usually five months)
- document every step she takes by logging onto iPledge, a national online database

By March 1, 2006, physicians and pharmacists also were required to register each isotretinoin prescription with iPledge to verify that they have done their part to ensure against pregnancy. The new rules are meant to prevent isotretinoin-related birth defects, but the rules are so strict that some doctors worry they might discourage many patients from using the drug, the only treatment that can erase severe acne.

Other less common side effects include dry skin and chapped lips, as well as fatigue, severe joint pain, headache, upset stomach, and blurred vision. Some suspect that isotretinoin may also cause depression or even suicide, although scientific studies have not demonstrated a connection.

Although the link between isotretinoin and depression has not been scientifically proven (the drug's manufacturer insists there is no such link), several people who have taken it claim they experienced depression, mood swings, and even suicidal feelings. Both the U.S. Food and Drug Administration and the drug company said depression is common among acne patients, whether or not they take isotretinoin. It appears that patients who are prone to depression may be at higher risk for developing depression while taking isotretinoin.

Other Symptoms

In addition to itching, thinning hair, and dry and flaky skin, isotretinoin occasionally may cause aching muscles and bones, increased lipid levels in the blood and, rarely, liver damage.

See also RETINA; RETINOIDS.

itching An intense tickling sensation on the skin that makes a person want to scratch. The precise reason for this response is not fully understood. Itching is the most prominent symptom in many skin diseases.

Skin that is too dry and scaly commonly causes itching. Many drug reactions result in itching (especially reactions to codeine, cocaine, and some antibiotics) and some types of rough clothing, soaps, and detergents can trigger an itching response in some people.

In addition, a wide range of disorders produce itching, including HIVES, ECZEMA, and FUNGUS INFECTIONS. PSORIASIS, LICHEN PLANUS, and DERMATITIS HERPETIFORMIS may also trigger bouts of itching.

Itching around the anus may be caused by hemorrhoids, anal fissure, or persistent diarrhea, or by too-rough cleaning after defecating. Worms are the most common cause of anal itching in children.

Itching around the vulva (pruritus vulvae) may be caused by candidiasis (a yeast infection), hormonal changes at puberty, pregnancy, or menopause, or the use of spermicides or vaginal suppositories, ointments, and deodorants.

Itchiness all over the body may be caused by diabetes mellitus, kidney failure, JAUNDICE, thyroid disorders, Hodgkin's disease, or blood disorders.

Infestations of lice and scabies cause severe itching, as can INSECT BITES.

Treatment Options and Outlook

Specific treatment depends on the underlying cause of the itching, but in general, cooling lotions (such as CALAMINE) can relieve the itching and irritation. EMOLLIENTS can reduce skin drying and help ease itching.

Because soap can irritate itchy skin (especially if the skin is dry or has a rash), it should only be used when really necessary. Mild cleansing solutions or water alone may be enough to keep itchy skin clean.

While scratching can temporarily ease the itch, it can actually make itching worse over time by overstimulation. The urge to scratch can be suppressed by using lotions, salves, or applying cool, wet compresses to the affected area, or systemic agents such as ANTIHISTAMINES.

Jarisch-Herxheimer reaction Also known as therapeutic shock, this reaction usually occurs within 12 hours of treatment with drugs used to kill *Treponema* bacteria, such as those that cause SYPHILIS.

The reaction is caused by the widespread death of spirochetes.

Symptoms and Diagnostic Path

The reaction is characterized by a flulike illness, including a rise in temperature (100°–102° F) with chills, malaise, and worsening of symptoms.

Treatment Options and Outlook

Although the reaction is benign in secondary SYPHILIS (it heralds a favorable response to treatment), in neurosyphilis this rare reaction may be severe. In these cases, oral CORTICOSTEROIDS may minimize the reaction.

jaundice Yellow discoloration of the skin caused by the accumulation in the blood of the yellow-brown bile pigment called bilirubin. Jaundice is a primary symptom of many different disorders of the liver and biliary systems.

Bilirubin is formed from hemoglobin as old red blood cells break down. The pigment is absorbed from the blood by the liver, where it is dissolved in water and excreted in bile. The process can be disrupted in one of three ways, causing one of the three types of jaundice—hemolytic, hepatocellular, and obstructive.

In *hemolytic jaundice,* the body breaks down too many red blood cells, producing too much bilirubin. A similar type of jaundice can develop in a newborn, whose liver has not yet developed the capacity to break down bilirubin. In adults, a type of jaundice much like hemolytic jaundice can develop as a symptom of mild liver disease.

In *hepatocellular jaundice,* the transfer of bilirubin from liver cells to bile is prevented, causing a buildup of bilirubin. This is usually the result of acute hepatitis or liver failure.

Obstructive jaundice is caused by a blockage of the bile ducts, which prevents the bile from flowing out of the liver. Obstructive jaundice can also occur if the bile ducts are missing or have been destroyed. As a result, bile cannot pass out of the liver, and bilirubin is forced back into the blood.

Treatment Options and Outlook

In all cases treatment is for the underlying disorder causing the jaudnice.

jellyfish stings The true jellyfish family includes about 200 species that drift along the shoreline, dragging tentacles capable of stinging when touched. While most stings from jellyfish may cause little harm, some jellyfish (and Portuguese men-of-war) can inflict severe stings, causing a victim to panic and drown. In the water, the shock of the sting often causes the victim to jerk away, which only stimulates the tentacles to release more poison. If stung by a jellyfish on dry land, more poison is released if the person tries to rip off the sticky threads of the tentacles.

Symptoms and Diagnostic Path

Stings can cause a severe, burning pain and a red welt or row of lesions at the site of the sting. There also may be generalized symptoms, including headache, nausea, vomiting, muscle cramps, diarrhea, convulsions, and breathing problems. The wound site becomes red and blistered and can leave permanent scars. One or two weeks after a sting, the victim may experience a recurrence of the lesions at the site.

The sting of the Portuguese man-of-war (a type of jellyfish) is rarely fatal, but causes hives, numbness, and severe chest, abdominal, and extremity pain. Death is usually the result of panic and drowning.

Treatment Options and Outlook

Because tentacles continue to discharge their stinging cells as long as they remain on the skin, the most important first aid intervention is to remove all of the tentacles.

First Aid   Alcohol, ammonia, or vinegar and salt water (*do not use freshwater*) can be poured over the sting site to deactivate the tentacles, which should then be scraped off with a towel or with sand held by a towel. TENTACLES MUST NOT BE REMOVED BY HAND. Alternatively, the tentacles should be pulled, not rubbed, away using an implement.

Baking soda in a paste can be applied to the sting to relieve pain; after an hour, it should be scraped off with an object to remove any remaining stinging cells. CALAMINE lotion will ease the burning sensation, and painkillers may help with the stinging pain. (Other popular remedies for pain include meat tenderizer, sugar, ammonia, and lemon juice. Some persons swear by the application of urine.)

Medications   If given early, the calcium blocker verapamil may be effective. Antivenin is effective against more dangerous species, but it must be given immediately.

Allergic reactions   Jellyfish stings also may cause an allergic reaction, which can be treated with Benadryl or CORTICOSTEROIDS. A severe reaction to the sting may require hospitalization.

jock itch   The common term for TINEA cruris, a fungal infection of the male genitals characterized by reddened, itchy areas spreading from the genitals outward to the inner thighs. It is uncommon in women.

Jock itch is caused by a tiny fungus that grows best in dark, damp conditions. This common fungus often infects men who are obese or who perspire heavily. It can be transmitted to the groin from the feet. The condition may occur at the same time as ATHLETE'S FOOT. It usually happens when a person has been perspiring heavily, during sports or hot, humid weather.

Treatment Options and Outlook

Over-the-counter antifungal drugs containing clotrimazole in topical forms such as lotion or cream can ease the itchy rash. Treatment should be continued for some time after the symptoms have passed to make sure the fungi has been eliminated, to prevent recurrence. Mild infections on the skin surface may require treatment for up to six weeks. Bathing too often or using too much medicated cream can worsen the condition.

Risk Factors and Preventive Measures

Avoiding rough, textured, or synthetic fabrics will help prevent jock itch. Loose cotton will let perspiration evaporate and skin breathe. The fungus that causes jock itch can be spread easily, so people should never share towels or clothes. An alkaline environment encourages the fungus to grow; since most soap is alkaline, too much scrubbing with soap will make jock itch worse.

When washing, patients should make sure to rinse all soap off the skin, drying well and keeping the area as dry as possible. Talcum powder reduces wetness and chafing.

Kaposi's sarcoma A condition characterized by skin tumors that is the most common malignant manifestation of acquired immunodeficiency syndrome (AIDS). Before the advent of the AIDS epidemic, Kaposi's sarcoma was a fairly rare skin condition that developed slowly and was seen almost exclusively in elderly Italian and Jewish men. Today, it is at least 20,000 times more common among immunosuppressed groups in the United States. About 95 percent of the epidemic Kaposi's sarcoma in the United States is found in homosexual and bisexual men, whereas other risk groups have an incidence of 3 percent. In patients with AIDS, Kaposi's sarcoma is highly aggressive and causes widespread tumors.

The cause of this disorder is unknown, although there is some evidence that it may be the result of a sexually transmitted infectious agent other than HIV, the virus that causes AIDS.

Symptoms and Diagnostic Path
Epidemic Kaposi's sarcoma may appear at anytime during HIV infection. Purple macules first appear anywhere on the body; in time, they may thicken into plaques or NODULES and are often seen in the mouth, on the hard palate, and the gums. In those with AIDS, tumors often affect the gastrointestinal and respiratory tracts, where they may cause severe internal bleeding. KS is diagnosed by an examination of the skin and lymph nodes. The doctor also may order other tests to see if the patient has other diseases.

Treatment Options and Outlook
Treatment should include an anti-retroviral agent such as zidovudine, which will not affect the tumors but will diminish the degree to which the immune system is suppressed. Antiretroviral agents may also boost the effectiveness of other drugs that do affect

Kaposi's. Localized lesions respond well to radiotherapy, cryotherapy, surgical excision, or injection with vinblastine, bleomycin, or INTERFERON ALFA. Oral administration of interferon alpha is effective in about half of patients with mild Kaposi's sarcoma. In more severe cases, chemotherapy is often required.

The outcome in adult patients with AIDS and Kaposi's sarcoma depends on the activity of the HIV disease, and the degree to which the person's immune system is suppressed.

Kawasaki disease An acute childhood disease of unknown cause featuring a measleslike rash over the body that usually occurs during the first years of life. Also called mucocutaneous lymph node syndrome, it was first observed in Japan during the 1960s. It is the leading cause of heart disease in children. The disease occurs more often among boys (more than 60 percent) and among those of Asian ancestry, but it can affect every racial and ethnic group. More than 4,000 cases of Kawasaki disease are diagnosed each year in the United States. Less than 1 percent of those are fatal.

Doctors do not know what causes Kawasaki disease, but it does not seem to be hereditary or contagious. Evidence strongly suggests it is caused by an infectious agent such as a virus. It is very rare for more than one child in a family to develop Kawasaki disease. Less than 2 percent of children have another attack of Kawasaki disease.

Symptoms and Diagnostic Path
The first symptom is a persistent fever, coupled with conjunctivitis, dry and cracked lips, swollen lymph nodes, red swollen palms and feet, and a measleslike rash. By the end of the second week, the skin at the tips of the fingers and toes peels and

the other symptoms subside. The disease can last for more than three months and can recur.

While most children recover completely, sudden death occurs in 1 or 2 percent of cases, usually due to coronary thrombosis during the acute phase of the illness.

Treatment Options and Outlook
Aspirin can reduce fever, rash, joint inflammation, and pain, and help prevent blood clots from forming. Intravenous gamma globulin can decrease the risk of developing coronary artery abnormalities when given early in the illness.

keloids   Large permanent and sometimes disfiguring scars that may develop after surgery or other injury to the skin. Occasionally they appear spontaneously (although they generally run in families). Similar in appearance to hypertrophic scars, keloids tend to grow indefinitely. They are particularly apt to occur in those of African or Asian descent, and are less common in Caucasians.

Symptoms and Diagnostic Path
Keloids are often found on the upper shoulders, the earlobes (after ear piercing), and the face, chest, and neck. Rare in infancy and old age, they appear more often in childhood, reaching a maximum outbreak between puberty and age 30. They slowly improve as patients get older. This relationship to age (and the fact that they sometimes appear during pregnancy) suggests a possible hormonal influence.

Treatment Options and Outlook
Treatment is usually not satisfactory, since keloids tend to recur after excision, at which point they can become even larger and more unsightly.

Small keloids may be treated by CORTICOSTEROIDS injected into the lesions. Large keloids can be debrided surgically but must be injected with corticosteroids immediately after surgery and four weeks later.

keratin   A protein containing high amounts of sulfur that is the primary component of the outermost layer of the skin, nails, horny tissue, and hair. Keratin is a tough substance that resists damage from a wide range of chemical and physical agents.

See also KERATINIZATION, DISORDERS OF; KERATINOCYTES.

keratinization   The process by which cells become tough and horny due to deposits of KERATIN placed within them. Keratinization (also called cornification) takes place in the EPIDERMIS (the outer layer of the skin), the hair, and the nails, where the cells flatten out, lose their nuclei, and become filled with keratin as they approach the surface of the skin.

keratinization, disorders of   Disorders usually characterized by obvious skin problems such as fissures, scales, or thickening of the top layer of the EPIDERMIS (stratum corneum). Disorders of KERATINIZATION include DARIER'S DISEASE, ICHTHYOSIS, epidermolytic hyperkeratosis, KID SYNDROME, NETHERTON'S SYNDROME, REFSUM'S DISEASE, CONRADI'S DISEASE, HARLEQUIN FETUS, lipid storage disease, FOLLICULAR HYPERKERATOSES, GROVER'S DISEASE, ACANTHOSIS NIGRICANS, POROKERATOSIS, PALMAR-PLANTAR KERATOSIS.

keratinocytes   Cells responsible for maintaining the skin's barrier that make up about 80 percent of the body's epidermal cells. The keratinocytes are made of the protein KERATIN; soft keratin is found in the epidermal cells and hard keratin is found in hair and nails.

The lowest layer of the EPIDERMIS is called the basal layer, where the cells of the epidermis are born; these cells reproduce rapidly and rise gradually toward the surface. These cells lie right next to the DERMIS, with its rich supply of blood vessels and glandular secretions. Their health and growth is dependent on the food and oxygen that the tiny capillaries of the dermis carry. As the cells in the basal layer are pushed up into the other layers, they undergo many changes, including the increase in the amount of keratin they produce. By the time the cells of the basal layer reach the top layer of the epidermis, they are no longer alive and they are entirely formed of keratin. This process of growth, maturation, and death is called keratinization. Problems in the speed and mount of keratin formation, as well as its disposal, lead to many different skin problems, such as thickened, cracked, and infected skin.

If the cells contain too little keratin, the appearance begins to look cracked and flaky as cells slough off. This can leave the lower layers exposed to infection and irritation. Keratin needs water to keep it pliable and healthy; when there is not enough water, the keratin crumbles and the cells cannot stay together. This is what happens when the skin becomes dry.

keratitis-ichthyosis-deafness syndrome See KID SYNDROME.

keratoacanthoma A skin NODULE that usually appears on the face or arm of elderly people that is often very difficult to distinguish from invasive SQUAMOUS CELL CARCINOMA. A biopsy may be necessary to tell the difference.

Initially small, it grows rapidly for two to three months, reaching a maximum size of about 2 cm across. The mature nodule has the slope of a volcano with bulging sides and a craterlike center.

Its cause is unknown, but it tends to be more common in those who have had years of exposure to strong sunlight and in those taking long-term immunosuppressant drugs.

Treatment Options and Outlook

Left alone, keratoacanthoma regresses completely, often leaving unpleasant scarring. It is best to remove it.

keratoderma A group of skin disorders characterized by thickening of the STRATUM CORNEUM on the palms and soles.

keratohyaline granules Deep, irregular grains in the outermost layer of the skin.

keratolysis Dissolution of the STRATUM CORNEUM.

keratolytic drugs Drugs that soften and loosen KERATIN (the tough outer layer of the skin) and remove scales. They include preparations of SULFUR, SALICYLIC ACID, and lactic acid, which are used in the treatment of skin and scalp disorders such as WARTS, calluses, ACNE, DANDRUFF, and PSORIASIS.

keratosis, seborrheic A skin lesion of unknown cause range from flat, dark brown rough patches to small, warty protrusions that are covered with a greasy, removable crust. Completely harmless but unsightly, it usually appears on light-skinned people after age 40.

While the lesions may appear alone, they are usually found in groups on the face, chest, back, abdomen, and extremities. As time goes on, the lesions become more deeply pigmented, become increasingly raised from the skin and develop a rougher contour. They are not caused by exposure to sunlight or by a virus.

Treatment Options and Outlook

When large, irritated or inflamed, they can be treated with a variety of techniques including CRYOTHERAPY, ELECTRODISSICATION, or CURETTAGE.

See also KERATOSIS PILARIS; DARIER'S DISEASE.

keratosis, solar See ACTINIC KERATOSIS.

keratosis follicularis See DARIER'S DISEASE.

keratosis pilaris A type of follicular HYPERKERATOSIS characterized by sandpaper-like skin with skin plugs that typically occurs on the upper outer arms. It may first begin in childhood or during adolescence, and is more severe in winter. An associated form of the condition causes a red halo around each plugged follicle. Less frequently, it may affect the thighs or the cheeks.

This disorder is chronic, but it improves during the summer months. While it is a nuisance, it is of no medical significance.

Treatment Options and Outlook

Emollients (such as Eucerin cream), agents containing lactic acid (Eucerin Plus), Lac-Hydrin or tretinoin (Retin-A) may be effective, but they must be used continuously for continuous effect. Most patients improve after being exposed to ultraviolet radiation.

See also KERATOSIS; DARIER'S DISEASE.

kerion An inflammatory fungal infection of the scalp characterized by a red pustular swelling, which lasts for up to two months. It may leave a scar and permanent loss of hair from the affected area.

Treatment Options and Outlook

Aggressive treatment with a systemic antifungal such as GRISEOFULVIN with systemic steroids is usually recommended.

See also TINEA.

ketoconazole (Trade name: Nizoral) An antifungal drug used to treat TINEA VERSICOLOR or yeast infection (THRUSH), superficial dermatophytoses, some systemic fungal infections, and seborrheic dermatitis.

Side Effects

Ketoconazole may cause nausea, but this may be avoided by taking the drug with food. It should not be taken at the same time as antacids, however, because ketoconazole requires an acidic stomach for absorption.

Other side effects include itching, headache, dizziness, abdominal pain, constipation, diarrhea, nervousness, rash, and liver damage. Occasionally, patients may experience hives and allergic reactions with the first dose.

Drug interactions with ketoconazole can be serious; this drug should not be taken with rifampin, isoniazid, warfarin, cyclosporine, or phenytoin.

kidney disease and skin symptoms While symptoms in the skin are not often associated with kidney disease, glomerulonephritis with kidney insufficiency can complicate the course of LUPUS ERYTHEMATOSUS and SYSTEMIC VASCULITIS and have prominent skin features. In addition, patients with progressive systemic sclerosis can also develop kidney failure.

Other skin symptoms associated with kidney disease include NAIL-PATELLA SYNDROME, which causes nail plate abnormalities and progressive renal disease; FABRY'S DISEASE, featuring small blue-black papules around the navel and kidney; generalized itching during hemodialysis; bullous dermatosis of renal failure, characterized by tense BLISTERS while on hemodialysis and sometimes in patients with chronic kidney failure; and skin lesions (WARTS, chronic HERPES, SQUAMOUS CELL CARCINOMA, ALOPECIA, bacterial and fungal infections) in kidney transplant patients.

KID syndrome The common name for keratitis-ichthyosis-deafness, this rare KERATINIZATION disorder leads to blindness and is associated with deafness and an unusual skin scaling. Patients with this condition have leathery skin texture, thickened palms and soles, and sparse hair.

Other associated health problems may include mental retardation, tight heel cords, tooth problems, and recurrent skin infections. The biochemical basis for this disease is unknown.

kissing bug bites Kissing bugs (members of the family Reduviidae), are also known as assassin bugs, cone-nose bugs, Walapai tigers, or Mexican bedbugs, and cause HIVE-like nodules or plaques with severe itching lasting up to a week. Sensitive individuals may experience hemorrhagic, giant hives or anaphylactic shock.

The bugs bite at night in small clusters on uncovered body parts such as the face or arms. They are generally brownish to black, medium-sized to large insects, usually found on foliage, although some occasionally enter houses. The adults often bite humans around the mouth; hence, its other common name, the kissing bug. The kissing bug can carry relapsing fever and Chagas' disease (American trypanosomiasis).

While most are found in South America, about 15 species are found in the southwestern United states. They usually live near rodents, armadillos, and opossums, but they can also be found in houses, living off humans. In the Southwest assassin bugs of the genus *Triatoma* are common, where they invade houses and may bite humans.

Klippel-Trenaunay syndrome A rare congenital disorder of blood vessel abnormalities characterized by port-wine BIRTHMARKS, VARICOSE VEINS, and other symptoms.

The cause is presently unknown, but is believed to be either genetic or the result of an intrauterine trauma between the third and sixth week of gestation.

Symptoms and Diagnostic Path

The most apparent symptom of Klippel-Trenaunay Syndrome (KTS) is the PORT-WINE STAIN, present at birth and typically covering a large area of the affected limb. The trunk can be affected, with the most typical pattern being from hip to toe, involving the buttocks on one side. The port-wine stain may be dark pink to purple and can be raised with nodules that bleed easily. Bleeding and skin infections are common with KT, and pain is a major concern with most patients.

In the past, KTS was sometimes called Klippel-Trenaunay-Weber syndrome but "Weber" has been dropped to avoid confusion with the Parkes Weber syndrome, a condition characterized by malformations of the arteries leading to overgrowth of arms and legs similar to KTS.

Treatment Options and Outlook

Laser treatment with a PULSED DYE LASER is available to lighten the port-wine stain in children and adults. Compression garments worn on the affected limb can ease pain and swelling. Sequential extremity pumps can help compress the limb. Antibiotics for CELLULITIS (skin infections) and iron supplements to combat anemia are helpful. Sclerotherapy (injecting alcohol into the veins) is used to clot veins in some patients. However, vein stripping

that was once standard treatment is less common today. Any surgical intervention should be very carefully considered.

Koebner's (Köbner's) phenomenon Lesions induced by scratching found in skin diseases such as PSORIASIS or LICHEN PLANUS.

koilonychia Also called "spoon nails," this is a condition in which nails are thin, dry, brittle, and concave (spoon shaped), with raised edges. In nail-patella syndrome, the nail may be split into two spoon-shaped parts.

Injury to the nail, iron-deficiency anemia, and LICHEN PLANUS are the main causes; the condition may be inherited.

kwashiorkor A severe type of malnutrition in young children occurring mainly in poor rural areas in developing countries, in which the child's skin flakes off, leaving a raw, weeping area beneath. Hair may lose its curliness, become sparse and brittle, and turn from dark to fair. The nails tend to be soft and thin. The illness begins when the child is suddenly weaned on a poor diet low in calories, protein, and essential micronutrients (such as ZINC, selenium and VITAMINS A and E).

Derived from the Ghanaian word meaning "disease suffered by a child displaced from the breast," kwashiorkor usually affects only those children between ages one and three.

Kwashiorkor may also be found among elderly people and in some patients with systemic diseases characterized by problems in absorbing or digesting protein.

Symptoms and Diagnostic Path

In addition to the skin and hair symptoms, growth is stunted, and there may be swelling. Behavioral symptoms in children include apathy, weakness, irritability, and inactivity. The liver becomes enlarged, and the child loses resistance to disease.

Treatment Options and Outlook

Warmth and fluids are important; infections should be treated. The child should first be fed milk and vitamin/mineral tablets, with the administration of zinc to prevent further skin flaking. When the child's appetite returns, a high-calorie, protein-rich diet should be given.

Most children treated for the condition recover, but those younger than age two are likely to suffer permanent stunted growth. Severe untreated cases can be fatal; blood poisoning kills about 30 percent of patients with kwashiorkor.

Kyrle's disease A disorder of KERATINIZATION known medically as hyperkeratosis follicularis et parafollicularis or en cutem penetrans.

Symptoms and Diagnostic Path

Symptoms include horny plugs surrounded by a red rim that may enlarge to form plaques. The lesions are found most often on the extremities, although they may occur anywhere on the body. A similar condition may appear in patients undergoing kidney dialysis.

Treatment Options and Outlook

Administration of a keratolytic agent or liquid nitrogen may be effective, but the disease is difficult to treat.

laceration A torn ragged wound.

LAMB syndrome See MULTIPLE LENTIGINES SYNDROME.

lamellar dystrophy of nails The splitting of nails into layers, also called onychoschyzia, often found in those who must immerse their hands in water. The condition may be caused by the constant absorption and evaporation of water from the nail plate. It is usually found in those whose hands are continually in and out of water, such as dish washers or laundresses.

lamellar ichthyosis A disorder of KERATINIZATION characterized by redness at birth with large, dark scales on the face, palms, and soles of the feet. This is usually a severe form of ICHTHYOSIS that can produce considerable disability and deformity throughout life.

This condition is a rare autosomal recessive trait, which means that a defective gene must be inherited in a double dose to cause the abnormality. Generally, both parents of an affected person are unaffected carriers of the defective gene. Each of their children has a one in four chance of being affected, and a two in four chance of being a carrier. It occurs in fewer than one child out of 300,000.

Symptoms and Diagnostic Path
The condition is always noticeable at birth, and is often a result of prematurity. Babies may be born encased in a membrane that is eventually shed. There is generalized severe dryness and scaling; in some patients, large dark scales appear over the entire body. Redness is noticeable in infancy and usually remains throughout life; hair loss occurs in some patients.

Treatment Options and Outlook
Infants should be kept in a continuous humid environment and the membrane encasing the child should not be removed. Moisturizing the skin is essential, moisturizers containing lactic acid are especially helpful. Systemic therapy with etretinate or ISOTRETINOIN is extremely helpful, but results only last as long as treatment continues. The side effects of high dose therapy are significant.

Right after birth, after the collodion membrane is shed, newborns are at risk for secondary infection and dehydration. As the child gets older, the condition can interfere with normal sweat gland function, which can lead to heat intolerance. Although the disorder is not life threatening, it is quite disfiguring and causes considerable psychological stress to affected patients. This disorder has no cure; therefore, treatment is directed at decreasing symptoms.

Langerhans cell A type of cell that makes up about 4 percent of all epidermal cells. It is an extremely important part of the body's immune system.

Langer's lines Lines of cleavage of the skin determined by the position and orientation of COLLAGEN bundles and elastic fibers.

lanolin A mixture of purified water and a yellow, oily substance obtained from sheep's wool that is used as an EMOLLIENT to treat dry skin. Lanolin is a common ingredient of bath oils and hand creams. It is also used to treat mild DERMATITIS. Occasionally lanolin can irritate the skin and in some individuals an allergic reaction develops.

lanugo The fine, downy hair on the body of a fetus that first appears in the fourth or fifth month and usually disappears by the end of the pregnancy. It can still be seen in some premature babies.

Lanugo hair (hypertrichosis lanugiosa) sometimes reappears on the skin of adults with cancer (especially of the breast, bladder, lung, or large intestine), in patients with anorexia nervosa, or as a side effect of some drugs (especially CYCLOSPORINE).

larva migrans, cutaneous Also known as creeping eruption, this disease is caused by HOOKWORM larvae that normally parasitize dogs, cats, or other animals. It is contracted by walking barefoot on soil or beaches contaminated with animal feces. The larvae penetrate the skin of the feet and move randomly, leaving intensely itchy red lines (sometimes accompanied by BLISTERS).

Because several different parasites produce similar symptoms, there may be difficulty in diagnosing specific disease such as many fall under the umbrella of "cutaneous larva migrans." Usually the term refers to disorders caused by cat or dog hookworm larvae.

Shaded, moist, and sandy areas—such as beaches, children's sandboxes, and areas underneath houses—are the most likely spots to harbor larvae. The eggs passed in the feces hatch into infective larvae that can penetrate human skin (even through beach towels).

Symptoms and Diagnostic Path

Skin lesions usually appear in areas that are in contact with soil, such as feet, hands, and buttocks. A red PAPULE appears within a few hours after the larvae penetrates the skin. After a latency period of a few days to a few months, the larvae migrate, causing a red, raised intensely itchy red line that may loop and meander all over the skin. Complica-

tions include bacterial infections, which can result from excessive scratching.

Treatment Options and Outlook

Thiabendazole is the drug of choice; its topical form is best for mild infections, applied to the tracks and normal skin around the traces. Systemic thiabendazole is also effective, but causes many side effects (dizziness, nausea, and vomiting).

About half of the larvae die within three months, even without treatment.

laser hair removal A nonsurgical cosmetic procedure using a low-energy laser that can permanently reduce unwanted facial or body hair. The laser passes through the patient's skin and is absorbed by the pigment in the hair follicle, which immediately and permanently disables a percentage of the follicles. In most cases, no anesthesia is necessary. The process can take from several minutes to several hours, depending on how much hair will be removed and the part of the body involved.

This noninvasive technique can remove unwanted hair anywhere on the body, leaving skin looking smoother. Because it can remove more than one hair at a time, it can be used to treat larger areas with minimal discomfort. National average cost of the procedure is about $355 per treatment, although fees vary considerably by geographic region, according to the American Society for Aesthetic Plastic Surgery.

Risks and Complications

Sometimes there is a temporary slight reddening of the skin or localized swelling.

Outlook and Lifestyle Modification

This type of hair removal should be considered to be an ongoing process that requires several sessions. After the treatments, clients may have to use specially formulated skin care products, or a prescribed skin care regimen. SUNSCREEN is recommended for any treated areas that may be exposed to the sun.

Patients with darker skin may not respond well, and blond, white or, gray hairs are less responsive to laser treatments and sometimes cannot be treated.

laser resurfacing A technique for removing medium to fine wrinkles and ACNE scars. Lasers produce an intense beam of bright light in one direction, which can vaporize wrinkles, scars, and blemishes and seal blood vessels. With its unique ability to produce one specific wavelength of light of varied intensity and length of pulse, the laser can be used for many different purposes.

There are several significant advantages that laser resurfacing, which can be performed in the DERMATOLOGIST's office, offers over traditional techniques. A relatively bloodless procedure, laser resurfacing offers more control in how deep the beam will penetrate the skin's surface, which allows the physician to direct the light with precision and safety in treating delicate areas around the lips and eyes, where it is an ideal technique to erase fine lines and wrinkles (especially on the upper lip, cheeks, and forehead). The treatment also can smooth and tighten eyelid skin, improve crow's-feet, soften frown lines, even out skin tone by removing brown spots and splotchy skin color, flatten scars, and repair smoker's lines. Depending on the type of laser and reason why it is being used, the treatment may call for a topical anesthetic cream, sedation, local anesthesia, or monitored intravenous sedation. There is not much discomfort during the procedure or throughout recovery.

There are two basic categories of lasers that can be used to resurface the skin: ablative and non-ablative.

Ablative Lasers

Ablative lasers remove the top layer of the skin, heating the next layers of the skin enough so that they regenerate COLLAGEN, the substance that makes up skin. This creates a wound that subsequently heals with smoother, more even skin. There are three types of ablative lasers used for resurfacing: carbon dioxide (CO_2), erbium:YAG (Er:YAG), and the long pulsed erbium:YAG. After ablative resurfacing, the treated areas usually are

kept moist with ointment or surgical bandages for the first few days. The skin is usually crusted pink or red, and depending on the type of laser and the patient's condition, the pink color may last for several days to several months. Makeup can be worn over the treated skin for one to two weeks.

CO_2 laser The newest pulsed CO_2 laser provides short bursts of extremely high-energy laser light that vaporizes skin tissue, revealing fresh skin underneath. Its highly focused beam allows the DERMATOLOGIST to gently remove the skin's surface with less risk of complications (such as scarring). It typically takes up to two months to heal completely.

erbium:YAG (Er:YAG) Once this high-powered laser gently penetrates the skin, it is absorbed by water in the tissue's cells, which scatters the heat so that the physician can more precisely remove thin layers of tissue while lessening the risk of damage to surrounding skin. This laser is ideal for patients with minor scars, superficial to moderate facial wrinkles, or skin discolorations. This laser also can rejuvenate sun-damaged delicate skin around the eyes and mouth without scarring, and also may be used for the neck or hands. The benefits of this laser include less redness, fewer side effects, and rapid healing.

Long pulse lasers More recently developed lasers provide results better than the CO_2 but not as dramatic as the Er: YAG. These lasers offer more wrinkle relief with less scarring risk, but their lower heat levels means results may not be as dramatic.

Non-ablative (Non-wounding) Lasers

These lasers have become quite popular, since this technique actually works beneath the skin's surface, meaning little recovery time is required. By directly treating the layers beneath the top layer of skin, the tissue can respond by regenerating skin as if it were repairing a wound. The process seems to stimulate collagen growth and tighten underlying skin, improving skin tone and removing fine lines and mild to moderate skin damage. However, non-ablative treatments require many sessions and may take several weeks for the final results to become apparent.

Non-ablative resurfacing treatments may take only a few minutes. Mild redness may last for a few hours with non-ablative techniques, and makeup may be applied afterward. Four to six treatments are usually necessary because the results from non-ablative techniques are generally less dramatic than those with Er:YAG and CO_2 lasers.

Risks and Complications

The most common complication of laser resurfacing is a darker-than-normal skin tone that may begin three to four weeks after surgery and can last several months. Patients with darker skin are at higher risk for developing this HYPERPIGMENTATION. Some patients may need to use BLEACHING CREAMS to help even out skin color after laser resurfacing.

Although there is some risk with all surgical procedures, scarring is not likely with the new Er: YAG and CO_2 lasers. Side effects are even more greatly reduced with the milder non-ablative lasers.

Medication given before surgery can help prevent COLD SORES, which sometimes flare up because of an existing herpes virus infection already present in the body.

Common side effects may include crusting, swelling, or discoloration at the treatment site. Other complications include ACNE flares and inflammatory of the skin. Newer surgical techniques and meticulous postoperative care have lessened the risks of pain, bleeding, swelling, and infection, but a reddened face for a few weeks is not uncommon, and occasionally may last for months.

Outlook and Lifestyle Modification

Laser resurfacing is not a substitute for a FACELIFT, and the procedure will not be able to tighten up loose facial skin or jowls. However, beneficial tightening of loose skin can occur from laser resurfacing, easing some facial folds and creases. In many cases, laser resurfacing is an alternative to traditional methods of skin rejuvenation, such as DERMABRASION and deep chemical peels. It can also work well together with chemical peels, eyelid surgery, LIPOSUCTION of the face and neck, collagen implants, and botulinum toxin.

laser treatment The acronym for "Light Amplification by Stimulated Emission of Radiation," lasers produce light of specific wavelengths in a nondivergent beam of monochromatic radiation that can mobilize immense heat and power when focused at close range. They can be used as a tool in both diagnosis and surgical procedures. A laser is a device that contains an active medium of either a gas, such as carbon dioxide or argon; a solid, such as ruby or neodymium: yttrium-aluminum-garnet (Nd:YAG); or a liquid, such as a dye that is powered by a source (such as electricity) to produce a beam of single-colored light up to 10 million times more powerful than the Sun.

Laser light is absorbed by different types of substances in tissue, depending on its wavelength, and it is the absorbed light which produces the effect on tissue. In a matter of seconds, this intense beam of light can hit a target and remove a skin problem, leaving little or no scarring. Most laser surgery can be done in the DERMATOLOGIST's office, and it is relatively painless, simple, quick, causes no blood loss, and is very effective.

Lasers have revolutionized the treatment of skin disease. Physicians wielding lasers can treat all sorts of skin problems, from precancerous growths to PORT-WINE STAINS. The color of the light a laser emits determines what kind of skin problem it can be used to treat.

Ruby lasers, which produce red light (694 nm), remove some tattoos and pigmented lesions such as CAFÉ-AU-LAIT MACULES and lentigines or liver spots. The Nd:YAG laser at 1064 nm (in the infrared spectrum) is also effective for tattoos and pigmented disorders. The CARBON DIOXIDE LASER also produces invisible infrared radiation (10,600 nm) and is used to remove benign skin growths, warts, and to resurface the skin. The PULSED DYE LASER is the best treatment for birthmarks such as the port-wine stain and hemangiomas, telangiectases, SPIDER ANGIOMAS, and venous lakes. Lasers are also effective in treating scars and stretch marks, for removing unwanted hair, and for reversing signs of skin aging.

Not all skin problems respond to laser treatment, however. While laser treatment of spider veins in the legs has improved over the past few years, they are still best treated by sclerotherapy, which involves injections of a saline solution or an agent called aethoxysclerol.

Dermatologists do not usually use lasers to remove malignant skin growths, unless the patient is taking blood thinners that could heighten the risk of hemorrhage during conventional surgery.

Lasers can be extremely dangerous when used around the eyes. A stray beam can hit the cornea or be absorbed by the retina and blind the patient. Protective goggles and eye shields are used to prevent eye damage.

Before consenting to laser surgery, patients should make sure the physician has had formal training and hands-on experience.

The American Society for Dermatologic Surgery or the American Society for Lasers in Medicine and Surgery can provide a list of dermatologists qualified to perform laser surgery.

latex allergy Natural rubber latex, the stretchy material used in everything from balloons and baby bottle nipples to surgical gloves and condoms, can cause an allergic skin reaction ranging from mild irritation to life-threatening anaphylactic shock. Those most at risk are health-care workers, rubber plant workers, and children with birth defects requiring multiple surgeries early in life.

In addition, the U.S. Food and Drug Administration has traced 16 deaths to a violent allergic reaction to an inflatable latex cuff used when administering barium enemas; the enema apparatus was later recalled by the manufacturer. Reactions to latex were rarely reported before 1970, but since the late 1970s many reactions were reported each year. Since then, latex allergy has become a major health concern as more and more people in the workplace have been affected. It appears that the increase in total exposure to latex and variations in manufacturing have led to a true increase in the number of persons with latex sensitivity.

Health care workers exposed to latex gloves or medical products containing latex are at especially high risk. It is estimated that between 8 and 12 percent of health care workers are now sensitive to latex. Workers in the latex manufacturing industry (such as glove manufacturing plants and latex doll manufacturers) are also at higher risk.

Between 1988 and 1992, the U.S. Federal Drug Administration (FDA) received more than 1,000 reports of adverse health effects from exposure to latex, including 15 deaths due to such exposure.

Any product containing latex may trigger a reaction. Medical products made with latex include adhesive tape, bandages, bulb syringes, dental devices, electrode pads, injection ports, face masks, latex gloves, mattresses on stretchers, PCA syringes, rubber syringe stoppers and medication vial stoppers, stethoscope and blood pressure cuff tubing, tourniquets, urinary catheters, and wound drains. Latex is also found in a wide variety of products around the house, such as balloons, buttons on electronic equipment, carpet backing, clothing (including underwear elastic), computer mouse pads, condoms, diapers, diaphragms, erasers, food handled with powdered latex, gloves, nipples and pacifiers, handles on racquets and tools, rubber bands, sanitary and incontinence pads, shoe soles, sports equipment, and toys.

In addition, certain fruits (such as bananas, chestnuts, kiwi, avocado, and tomato) may also trigger symptoms in latex-allergic individuals, perhaps because these foods are similar to a latex protein component. These foods have been responsible for anaphylactic reactions in latex-sensitive persons, while many other foods, including figs, apples, celery, melons, potatoes, papayas, and pitted fruits, such as cherries and peaches, have caused progressive symptoms beginning with ITCHING in the mouth. People with a history of reactions to these foods have a higher risk of developing a latex allergy. Those who are sensitive to latex should avoid foods to which they have had previous reactions.

While experts still do not know a great deal about food cross-reactions, it is clear that eliminating all of these foods would cause significant dietary restriction and is therefore not recommended to every latex-allergic persons.

Symptoms and Diagnostic Path

Airborne latex particles that stick to the cornstarch used to powder the inside of latex gloves are a source of sensitization and a significant cause of breathing problems in sensitive individuals. Once a person has become sensitized, allergic symptoms may appear during exposure to any product containing latex. About a third of patients who develop hives from contact with latex also develop other symptoms, including hay fever, asthma, and even anaphylactic shock. (In anaphylactic shock, a victim can develop shortness of breath, swollen lips, and throat, heart, and breathing difficulties within minutes). Death can result from anaphylactic shock without prompt treatment. Glove wearers may experience delayed hypersensitivity, skin irritation ranging from nonspecific itching to red, weepy skin. These symptoms are caused by the accelerators and chemicals used in the glove manufacture and not by the latex itself.

Direct skin contact with latex may cause an immediate hypersensitivity reaction of local or generalized HIVES within 30 to 60 minutes. Some persons have experienced anaphylactic reactions after having no previous symptoms. In fact, it is possible to have used latex gloves for years and to suddenly have a progression to systemic symptoms.

Risk Factors and Preventive Measures

Health care workers now use a new set of gloves for each patient they treat. More importantly, avoiding latex gloves or glove liners often can eliminate these symptoms entirely.

Powder-free gloves are now available because of new ways of treating latex that make gloves easier to put on than powdered gloves. Some newer glove products have very low protein levels, although there is a wide variation among different brands. Health care workers and patients allergic to latex must use nonlatex gloves. The National Institute of Occupational Safety and Health (NIOSH) recommends that nonlatex gloves be used for activities that do not involve contact with infections materials, such as food preparation, or routine housekeeping and maintenance.

Anyone sensitive to latex should carry an epinephrine auto-injection kit and wear Medic-Alert identification. Medical workers should carry extra pairs of nonlatex gloves for emergency medical or dental care.

See also ALLERGIES AND THE SKIN.

Lawrence-Seip syndrome A skin manifestation of insulin-resistant diabetes with both congenital and acquired types. Many of the cases have involved individuals of Portuguese or Norwegian ancestry, although Lawrence-Seip syndrome can affect any race. Males and females are affected equally in the congenital form, but more females are effected with the acquired form.

Symptoms and Diagnostic Path

The two forms of this syndrome have different symptoms. The congenital form of Lawrence-Seip syndrome is obvious from birth, while the acquired form usually can be diagnosed before age five years but certainly by age 15.

Congenital Lawrence-Seip The congenital type is typically diagnosed in the first two years of life, and is inherited in an autosomal recessive pattern. This means that the defective gene must be inherited in a double dose to cause the syndrome. These infants can be easily diagnosed because of an almost complete lack of subcutaneous fat. Although the baby will have a few smaller-than-normal fat cells, they contain little fat. Organs are enlarged, and toddlers may have a potentially dangerous overgrowth of tonsils and adenoids. These patients have well-defined muscles with prominent superficial veins. Wasting away of the clitoris or penis may be obvious. The earliest skin manifestations include excess hairiness of the face, neck, arms, and legs, and thick, tightly curled scalp hair that extends nearly to the eyebrows. There is no special growth of the pubic or underarm hair.

All patients with Lawrence-Seip syndrome have ACANTHOSIS NIGRICANS, a skin disease characterized by grayish warty pigmented lesions in body folds and under the arms, on the elbows, knees, and waist. Acanthosis nigricans can disappear with puberty. Gigantism with advanced bone age and advanced appearance of teeth is an early and constant feature. The growth rate is most marked in the first four years of life; these children may reach more than 90 percent of their adult height within the first 10 years of life. Growth eventually slows down and they reach short or normal height as adults. The abnormal distribution of fat in these patients does not affect female breast development at puberty, although females with this congenital syndrome have marked muscularity. Liver disease with cirrhosis is another constant feature, and an enlarged spleen tends to produce a protruding abdomen.

Diabetes mellitus usually begins in adolescence. Kidneys may be enlarged without apparent cause, and kidney failure may result. An enlarged heart is often observed with atrophied muscle and ventricular dysfunction. There may be heart murmurs and possibly high blood pressure. There also may be other problems with the heart, bones, and kidneys.

Acquired Lawrence Seip In this form of the syndrome, there may be a generalized problem with fat loss over the entire body, often following an illness or infection. The fat loss becomes obvious in adolescence or early adult life. Most of the features of the congenital form may occur, but in the acquired form there are not usually any heart, brain, or kidney problems. Bone age and genitals are normal. There may be some degree of acanthosis nigricans.

In this form of the disease, autoimmune disorders may be common, including hemolytic anemia and chronic inflammation of the kidneys. Patients with the acquired form of Lawrence-Seip syndrome also are prone to infection.

Treatment Options and Outlook

Patients with Lawrence-Seip syndrome must maintain a rigid special diet with four regular-sized meals a day, because of the limited ability to store energy as fat. In addition, some experts have treated this condition with leptin, a hormone secreted by fat cells, which may improve insulin resistance, high blood sugar, low fat stores, and liver problems.

Patients with the congenital form of Lawrence-Seip syndrome can live to young adulthood or early middle age, although childhood death as a result of massive gastrointestinal (GI) bleeding has been reported frequently. Kidney complications also are common causes of death in the congenital form.

Patients with the acquired form tend to die in middle age, often from gastrointestinal hemorrhage and liver failure.

leg ulcers An open sore on the leg that does not heal, usually caused by an inadequate blood supply from the area. Leg ulcers are most often found among the elderly.

BEDSORES (also called decubitus ulcers) develop on pressure spots on the legs as a result of poor circulation, pressure and immobility over a period of time. Leg ulcers may also be due to peripheral vascular disease (restricted blood supply to the extremities caused by thickening of the artery walls). Diabetes mellitus, which increases susceptibility to blood vessel disease and skin infection, may also lead to leg ulcers.

Treatment Options and Outlook

Treatment should be sought as early as possible. If an ulcer is filled with PUS, a wet dressing should be applied under a bandage. This should be changed only every three to seven days to avoid removing new skin from the area.

Risk Factors and Preventive Measures

Prevention is preferable to undergoing treatment. Anyone susceptible to leg ulcers should avoid obesity, leg injury, and immobility.

leishmaniasis A variety of diseases that affect the skin and mucous membranes caused by infection with single-celled parasites (called leishmania). The parasites are found in dogs and rodents in many parts of the world except Australia, Antarctica, the United States (with the exception of Texas), and large areas of Africa. Parasites are transmitted from the animals to humans via the bites of sand flies, which live on the fur of the animals. There are at least three types of the disease that affect the skin, one of which is common in the Middle East, North Africa, and the Mediterranean; the others are found in Central and South America.

Symptoms and Diagnostic Path

A persistent ulcer that may eventually heal but can leave an ugly scar forms at the sand-fly bite. In the South American form, there is more extensive tissue damage (often on the face), often causing severe disfigurement.

Treatment Options and Outlook

All forms of this disease are treated effectively with drugs (such as sodium stibogluconate or glucantime) given by injection into a muscle or vein. All types of this disorder with secondary bacterial infection also should be treated with antibiotics. Current treatments for leishmaniasis are expensive; some have serious side effects and may lead to the development of drug-resistant parasites.

Risk Factors and Preventive Measures

Studies are being conducted to develop a new human vaccine for leishmaniasis. The studies are being funded primarily through a $15 million grant from the Bill and Melinda Gates Foundation through the Infectious Disease Research Institute.

Because a new canine vaccine against visceral leishmaniasis has proven effective in early trials, experts hope that the high incidence of the disease in both dogs and humans can be reduced. Infected dogs are an important reservoir for continuing disease.

lemon A fruit that contains both citric acid and VITAMIN C, lemon is good at cutting grease and is one of the few natural ingredients that can retain its properties after chemical extraction. For best results, however, cosmetics should contain concentrated lemon juice and not just the essence for a lemony fragrance.

Fresh-squeezed and diluted lemon juice is an excellent rinse for oily hair.

lentiginosis profusa Also known as generalized lentiginosis, this disorder is characterized by the appearance of many small dark brown spots (lentigines). It is different from MULTIPLE LENTIGINES SYNDROME, which involves multiple lentigines and many other developmental problems, such as deafness and short stature.

See also LENTIGO; LENTIGO, ACTINIC; LENTIGO, MALIGNA.

lentigo A harmless flat, pigmented area of skin similar to a FRECKLE. They are more common in middle-aged and elderly people, and in those who have been exposed to the sun.

Lentigines (the plural of lentigo) may evolve slowly over years, or they may suddenly appear all at once. They are most often associated with either a single day of excessive sun exposure or from years of repeated sun exposure in fair-skinned individuals. In the United States, lentigines are seen in as many as 90 percent of Caucasians older than 60 years and in 20 percent of Caucasians younger than 35. Solar lentigines are more abundant in fair-skinned Caucasians; dark-skinned individuals do not usually develop lentigines because they have more natural pigment that provides some degree of protection from the sun. However, inherited patterned lentigines can appear in African Americans, particularly those with mixed American Indian heritage and those with relatives with red hair.

These lesions are significant because although benign, they may eventually become malignant. If the cells in the lesion look normal, the condition is called lentigo simplex. If the cells are abnormal, the condition is known as LENTIGO MALIGNA; these cells can turn into a malignant melanoma.

Symptoms and Diagnostic Path

This common condition is more common in middle-aged and elderly people, and in those who have been exposed to the sun. They occur equally among different races and genders, and can be found in all age groups. Unlike FRECKLES, lentigo lesions do not darken in response to sunlight exposure.

Treatment Options and Outlook

No treatment is necessary, but if cosmetically unacceptable it is best treated with cryotherapy or laser therapy.

See also MELANOMA, MALIGNANT.

lentigo, actinic Also known as a solar lentigo, age spot, or liver spot, this harmless small brown macule differs from a LENTIGO simplex by its larger size and by its appearance later in life on sun-exposed areas of skin, especially the face and the backs of the hands.

Symptoms and Diagnostic Path

Similar in appearance to a FRECKLE, lentigines do not clear once sun exposure is stopped. They may be found alone or in groups and are more common in middle-aged and elderly people and in those who have been exposed to the sun.

Treatment Options and Outlook

No treatment is necessary, but if raised, darker brown areas appear inside the lentigines, a physician should be consulted since these areas could develop into malignant melanoma. Lentigines can be relatively easily treated with liquid nitrogen or by laser treatment with either the Q-switched Nd:YAG laser, the Q-switched Alexandrite laser, or the Q-switched ruby laser.

See also LENTIGINOSIS PROFUSA; LENTIGO, MALIGNA; MELANOMA, MALIGNANT.

lentigo maligna Also known as a melanotic freckle of Hutchinson, this is considered to be a precancerous lesion that may transform itself into a malignant melanoma. It is different from an ordinary LENTIGO, which is benign. It is more common in women.

Symptoms and Diagnostic Path

A lentigo maligna may start out as small fawn-colored macule—usually on the face—very similar to a benign SEBORRHEIC KERATOSIS. As the patient ages, it becomes larger and irregularly shaped and colored. It gradually gets bigger until it forms an irregular patch with jagged or notched borders, irregularly colored from tan to dark brown or black. It may also be red or white. Scientists now believe that about 5 percent of these lesions turn into lentigo maligna melanoma.

The lesions are always seen on sun-exposed skin, and they are seen in patients older than those who are seen with melanoma.

Treatment Options and Outlook

Surgical removal, or cryotherapy, or radiation is effective.

See also MELANOMA, MALIGNANT.

LEOPARD syndrome See MULTIPLE LENTIGINES SYNDROME.

leprosy A chronic bacterial infection known medically as Hansen's disease that damages nerves in the skin, limbs, face, and mucous membranes. Untreated leprosy can lead to severe complications, which can include blindness and disfigurement. Contrary to popular belief, it is not highly contagious. While the disease still carries significant stigma, patient care has become integrated with routine health care, and anti-leprosy organizations have fought to repeal unfair laws and practices. Patients should no longer be referred to as "lepers."

Although leprosy is one of the oldest diseases in human history, it was not until 1873, when Armauer Hansen first saw the bacillus causing leprosy under a microscope, that the disease was discovered to be infectious instead of hereditary.

There were 678,758 new cases of leprosy reported in 2004 in 91 countries, primarily in Asia, Central and South America, and Africa; but probably fewer than 20 percent have access to treatment. India, Myanmar (Burma), and Nepal account for 70 percent of all cases. Africa is the second most common area. Brazil has 80 percent of all cases in South America. Most cases in the United States occur in California, Florida, Hawaii, Louisiana, New York, and Texas. There are about 100 new cases of leprosy each year in the United States, and 12,000 new cases each week around the world. Children represent about 16 percent of the new cases of leprosy.

Leprosy is caused by a rod-shaped bacterium, *Mycobacterium leprae,* that is spread in droplets of nasal mucus. A person is infectious only during the first phase of the disease, and only those living in prolonged close contact with an infected person are at risk. Leprosy is probably spread by droplet infection through sneezing and coughing. In those with untreated leprosy, large amounts of bacteria are found in nasal discharge; the bacteria travel through the air in these droplets. They can survive three weeks or longer outside the human body, in dust, or on clothing.

Although relatively infectious, leprosy is still one of the least contagious of all diseases. This—together with the fact that only 3 percent of the population is susceptible to leprosy—means that there is no justification for the practice (still prevalent in some countries) of isolating patients. Only a few people are susceptible because most people acquire a natural immunity when exposed to the disease.

Most of the body's destruction is caused not by bacterial growth but by a reaction of the body's immune system to the organisms as they die. In *lepromatous leprosy,* damage is widespread, progressive and severe. *Tuberculoid leprosy* is a milder form of the disease.

History

Ancient religious traditions associated with leprosy continued to influence social policy well into the 20th century. Leprosy was first mentioned as a curse in Shinto prayers of 1250 B.C.; it was also mentioned in some Egyptian legends to explain the exodus of the Hebrews. For hundreds of years, those with leprosy were taken to a priest, not a doctor, and were found "guilty," not sick.

These customs led to the forcible confinement of patients in "leprosaria," or leper colonies; their children, whether infected or not, were denied education in community schools. In eighth-century France, leprosy was considered grounds for divorce, and under the Roman Empire, was cause for banishment. Some countries passed legislation providing for the compulsory sterilization of leprosy patients, and others would not permit patients to handle the nation's currency. Others "steam treated" letters before allowing them in the mail, and some countries did not allow patients to vote. In medieval Europe, leprosy patients had to carry a "clapper" to warn others that a person with leprosy was approaching. Even as late as 1913, state Senator G. E. Willett of Montana was

forced to give up his seat after he was diagnosed with leprosy.

Religious customs also affected many treatments for leprosy. In 250 B.C., Chinese patients pricked their swollen limbs to let out the "foul air." Ramses II of Egypt believed that people with leprosy who used his water wells would be cured. And in medieval Europe, it was believed that leprosy could be cured by the touch of a king.

Historically, topical treatments ranged from turtle soup, whiskey, and various poultices (onion, sea salt and urine in Egypt; arsenic and powdered snake bones in China; water mixed with blood of dogs and infants under age two in Scotland; elephants' teeth; the flesh of crocodiles, snakes, lions, and bears). Other ingredients ranged from carbolic acid, creosote, phosphorus, mercury, and iodine, and plant extracts, including madar, cashew-nut oil, gurjum oil, or chaul-moogra.

The idea of caring for patients with leprosy became popular among missionaries following biblical directives and the teachings of Jesus; this service became fashionable about A.D. 1100 in Europe, after crusaders (including a king) returned with the disease. Special hospitals were built, operated and supported by cathedrals, but with the outbreak in the 1300s of bubonic plague, patients with leprosy began to be segregated again. Some countries seized the property of those with leprosy before burning them alive.

Leprosy is erroneously associated with the Old Testament, where references to "tsara'-ath," a term which most closely translates to "leprosy," actually refers to a broad spectrum of problems that affected cloth, leather, linen, and house walls as well as humans. Most medical historians doubt, and archaeologists have not found evidence to support, the idea that leprosy existed among the Hebrews in Moses' time. Biblical scholars also have problems with the translation of the Greek term *lepra* partly because the Greeks had a specific term for leprosy. The Greek word *lepra* was most likely used to refer to a variety of severe skin diseases. Greek medical writings later than the third century B.C. provide the earliest clinical references to modern leprosy. No mention of leprosy occurs in the New Testament after the Gospels.

Symptoms and Diagnostic Path

Damage is first confined to the nerves supplying the skin and muscles, destroying nerve endings, sweat glands, hair follicles, and pigment-producing cells. It first causes a lightening (or darkening) of the skin, with a loss of feeling and sweating. Some types of the disease produce a rash of bumps or nodules on the skin. As the disease progresses, bacilli also attack peripheral nerves; at first patients may feel an occasional "PINS AND NEEDLES" SENSATION, or have a numb patch on the skin. Next, patients become unable to feel sensations such as a light touch or temperature. Gradually, even hands, feet, and facial skin eventually become numb as muscles become paralyzed. Delicate connections between nerve cells and nerve endings are severed, and whole sections of the body become totally numb. For example, if the nerve above the elbow is affected, part of the hand becomes numb and small muscles become paralyzed, leading to curled fingers.

When a patient can no longer sense pain, the body loses the automatic withdrawal reflex that protects against trauma from sharp or hot objects, leading to extensive scarring or even loss of fingers and toes. Muscle paralysis can lead to further deformity, and damage to the facial nerve means eyelids cannot close, leading to ulceration and blindness. Direct invasion of bacteria may also lead to inflammation of the eyeball, also leading to blindness.

Treatment Options and Outlook

Several antibiotic agents are effective against leprosy and are best used in combinations of two or three. This multidrug therapy (MDT) is the current preferred treatment: it combines DAPSONE, clofazimine, and rifampin. The MDT was developed as leprosy bacilli became resistant to dapsone alone after decades of constant use. (Dapsone, a sulfone drug, was introduced during the 1940s). The most powerful of these is rifampin, a drug first used against tuberculosis and found to be effective against leprosy in 1968. Particular combinations of these drugs were recommended in 1984 by the World Health Organization as standard treatment for mass campaigns against leprosy.

MDT is often distributed in blister packs containing a month's supply of pills; dapsone is taken daily; clofazimine is taken every other day; and rifampin is taken monthly. There are now more than 1 million people receiving these drugs worldwide, and more than 1 million others have already completed treatment.

While the medication usually can cure leprosy within six months to two years, patients are no longer contagious within a few days after treatment begins. To prevent a relapse, treatment needs to be administered for at least two years after the last signs of the disease have disappeared. In the United States, patients are eligible for treatment by the Public Health Service at special clinics and hospitals, or at the Gillis W. Long Hansen's Disease Center in Louisiana, the only institution in the United States devoted primarily to treatment, research, training, and education related to leprosy. Eleven regional centers, located primarily in major urban areas, treat those with leprosy on an outpatient basis.

No vaccine for leprosy is available because scientists have not been able to grow cultures in lab environments. However, about 95 percent of the population is immune to leprosy, which occurs naturally in armadillos.

Ofloxacin causes a range of unpleasant side effects.

After leprosy is cured, patients must learn to watch for wounds and injuries they do not feel, and must learn to wear special shoes to protect insensitive feet.

leptospirosis A rare disease characterized by a skin rash and flulike symptoms caused by a spirochete bacterium excreted by rodents. Also known as Weil's disease, there are between 100 and 200 cases and a few deaths reported in the United States each year.

Outbreaks of leptospirosis are usually caused by exposure to water, food, or soil contaminated with the urine of infected cattle, pigs, horses, dogs, rodents, and wild animals. The disease is not known to be spread from person to person.

Leptospirosis is an occupational hazard for many people who work outdoors or with animals, such as sewer workers, veterinarians, dairy farmers, or military personnel. It is also a risk for campers or those who participate in outdoor sports in contaminated areas; the disease had been associated with swimming, wading, and whitewater rafting in contaminated lakes and rivers.

Symptoms and Diagnostic Path

After an incubation period of up to three weeks, an acute illness characterized by headache, fever and chills, severe muscle aches, and minute red spots and purple PAPULES appear. The kidneys are often affected, and liver damage and JAUNDICE are also common. The disease is diagnosed by blood or urine tests.

Treatment Options and Outlook

Antibiotics are effective, and in about one-third of cases the patients improve rapidly. Some patients go on to suffer a more persistent illness with slow recovery of kidney and liver function. The nervous system may also be affected, often producing signs of meningitis.

Risk Factors and Preventive Measures

The risk of this disease can be lessened by not swimming or wading in water that might be contaminated with animal urine. Those exposed to contaminated water or soil because of their job or recreational activities should wear protective clothing.

leukonychia A white discoloration of the nails that may involve the entire nail, a portion of it, or just a discolored band. Some patients inherit the condition; it may also be caused by certain treatments for leukemia (arsenic and antimetabolites). Patients with liver disease also may have complete discoloration. No treatment is available.

leukoplakia A smooth, opaque white patch found mostly on the mucus membranes of the lips and inside the mouth, primarily among the elderly. Some patches are benign, some are premalignant conditions, and others are malignant. Therefore, patients must see a DERMATOLOGIST or oral surgeon to confirm a diagnosis.

Leukoplakia in the mouth may be caused by tobacco smoke (especially pipe smoking), trauma from rubbing of dentures or a rough tooth. In some cases, it is genetic.

Symptoms and Diagnostic Path

The primary symptom of leukoplakia is a skin lesion that may occur on any mucosal surface (that is, skin in a cavity such as the mouth or vagina). It is typically found on the tongue, although it also may occur on the inside of the cheeks and occasionally, in women, on the genitals. Usually white or gray, the lesion may be red, with a thick, raised, and hardened appearance. The typical white lesion develops slowly, over weeks or months, until it eventually becomes rough and may be sensitive to touch, heat, spicy foods, or other irritation.

A biopsy of the lesion will confirm the diagnosis. There are two types of leukoplakia: benign and malignant.

Treatment Options and Outlook

Leukoplakia is usually harmless and lesions usually clear in a few weeks or months after the source of irritation is removed. However, about three percent of these lesions eventually become malignant. The lesion should be diagnosed and treated; eliminating the source of irritation may make the lesion disappear. Dental causes such as rough teeth, irregular denture surface, or fillings should be treated as soon as possible. Surgical removal of the lesion may be necessary. Treatment of leukoplakia on the vulva is the same as treatment of oral lesions.

Although some studies have suggested that VITAMIN A or VITAMIN E may shrink lesions, this should only be administered with close supervision by a health care provider.

lice Small wingless insects about the size of a sesame seed, with six legs and claws for grasping the hair. Lice are crawling insects that cannot jump or fly, and feed on human blood.

They are divided into three species: *Pediculus humanus capitis* (head louse); *pediculus humanus corporis* (body louse), and *Phthirus pubis* (the crab, or pubic, louse). All three have flat bodies that measure up to 3 mm across.

Head lice live on and suck blood from the scalp, leaving red spots that itch intensely and can lead to DERMATITIS and IMPETIGO. The females lay a daily batch of pale eggs called "NITS" that attach themselves to hairs close to the scalp. The nits hatch in about a week, and the adults can live for several weeks.

Head lice can be found among people of all walks of life. Children most often contract lice through direct contact, usually at school by sharing hats, brushes, combs, or headrests. Pets cannot contact head lice.

Symptoms and Diagnostic Path

Because lice move so quickly, it is the nits that will be seen on the hair shaft. Head lice and their nits can also be found on eyebrows and eyelashes. If one person in a family has head lice, all family members should be checked, but only those who are infested should be treated with lice pesticide.

Body lice live and lay eggs on clothing next to the skin, visiting the body only to feed. Body lice affect people who rarely change their clothes.

Pubic lice live in pubic hair or (rarely) armpits and beards. Pubic lice are commonly known as "crabs" because under the microscope they resemble a crab. Pubic lice cause incessant itching. They are visible to the naked eye and are easily transmitted during sex. It is also possible to pick them up from sheets or towels. They can live away from the host's body for up to one day, and the eggs can survive on their own for several days. Affected patients who do not wash underwear, sheets, and towels in hot enough water may be reinfected.

Treatment Options and Outlook

For *head lice,* lotions containing malathion or carbaryl kill lice and nits quickly. The lotion should be washed off 12 hours after application, followed by combing the hair with a fine-toothed comb to remove dead lice and nits. Shampoos containing malathion, lindane, or carbaryl are also effective if used repeatedly over several days. Combs and brushes should be plunged into very hot water to kill any attached eggs.

In 2004 the U.S. Food and Drug Administration (FDA) issued a Public Health Advisory concerning the use of topical formulations of LINDANE lotion and lindane shampoo for the treatment of scabies and head lice. The warning emphasizes that lindane products should be considered as a second-line therapy for the treatment of scabies and lice. While the FDA believes that the benefits of lindane outweigh the risks when used as directed, given the potential for neurotoxicity, patients should only be treated with these medications if other treatments are not tolerable or other approved therapies have failed. The new boxed warning also states that lindane lotion and shampoo should be used with caution in patients who weigh less than about 110 pounds. These products are not recommended for infants or premature infants.

These warnings are based on reports to the FDA's voluntary reporting system, which described that about half of reported adverse events occurred in children. Because most of the serious adverse events reported with lindane products are due to misuse and overuse, especially with the lotion, product package sizes are limited to one and two ounces.

The National Pediculosis Association also discourages the use of lindane products (such as Kwell), because it considers them to be potentially toxic and no more effective than other treatments. Still, no product kills 100 percent of nits, and a fine-toothed comb should be used to remove the remaining nits. Lice medications are not intended to be used on a routine or preventive basis.

All lice-killing medications are pesticides, and therefore should be used with caution. A pharmacist or physician should be consulted before using or applying pesticides when the person is pregnant, nursing, has lice or nits in the eyebrows or eyelashes, or has other health problems (such as allergies). Because the head lice pesticides can be absorbed into the bloodstream, they should not be used on open wounds on the scalp, or on the hands of the person applying the medication. These pesticides should not be used on infants, and should be used with caution on children under age two. In these cases, lice and nits should be removed manually or mechanically.

Pesticides should be used over a sink (not a tub or shower) to minimize pesticide absorption and exposure to the rest of the body. Eyes of the affected individual must be kept covered while administering any pesticide.

All nits must be removed from the hair shaft. Bedding and recently worn clothing should be washed in hot water and dried in a hot dryer. Combs and brushes should be cleaned and then soaked in hot (not boiling) water for 10 minutes. Lice sprays should not be used, according to the National Pediculosis Association. Vacuuming is the best way to remove lice and attached nits from furniture, mattresses, rugs, stuffed toys, and car seats.

Neighborhood parents and the school, camp, or child care providers should be notified of any infestation. Children should be checked once a week for head lice.

Body lice can be killed by placing infested clothing in a hot dryer for five minutes, by washing clothes in very hot water or by burning clothes. *Pubic lice* can be treated with an over-the-counter treatment, including A-200 Pyrinate, RID, or Nix.

lichenification   Thickening of the skin caused by repeated scratching, often by trying to relieve the intense itching of ECZEMA.

lichen myxedematosus   A rare condition of metabolic dysfunction characterized by a variety of skin symptoms.

Symptoms and Diagnostic Path

Symptoms include lichenoid PAPULES of the ears, neck, scrotum, and perianal area. Facial features are exaggerated with deep furrows, which are sometimes very thickened. Other patients have groups of pink wheals and red or flesh-colored small papules. Still others have lichenoid plaques resembling LICHEN PLANUS. Occasionally patients with this condition develop a type of cancer called multiple myeloma.

The condition is a proliferative process related to an abnormal immunoglobulin that stimulates production of mucinous material that deposits in the skin.

Treatment Options and Outlook

Cyclophosphamide, radiotherapy, DERMABRASION, or systemic CORTICOSTEROIDS may eradicate the cells producing the immunoglobulins so that the disease can go into full remission.

See also LICHEN SIMPLEX.

lichenoid drug eruptions   A type of allergic drug reaction causing an itchy eruption of PAPULES most often appearing on the forearms, less often on the lower legs, genitalia, and mucous membranes. While the rash resembles LICHEN PLANUS, the histology and cause is different. Medications most often associated with this condition include antimalarials, thiazides, and tetracyclines.

lichen planus   A common skin disease of unknown origin.

Symptoms and Diagnostic Path

Symptoms include small, flat-topped, itchy pink or purple raised spots on the skin of the wrists, forearms, or lower legs, particularly in middle-aged patients. The inside lining of the cheek may be covered by a lacy white network of spots.

Treatment Options and Outlook

Potent topical steroids and antihistamines are the mainstay of therapy. For extensive cases, PUVA and GRISEOFULVIN or systemic steroids have been used. Most cases resolve spontaneously within two years.

lichen sclerosis et atrophicus (LSEA)   A relatively common benign abnormality of the skin of the vulva characterized by marked thinning of the skin. It occurs in all age groups, but is found most often before puberty and in menopause.

Symptoms and Diagnostic Path

With lichen sclerosis, the vulvar skin often appears white and thin; it is often itchy. Scratching may lead to secondary infections if the skin is broken. As many vulvar conditions have the same symptoms and look similar to the naked eye, doctors often take a biopsy (sample of the skin) to make an accurate diagnosis. There may be an association with autoimmune diseases.

Treatment Options and Outlook

The treatment for lichen sclerosis is either topical testosterone or CORTICOSTEROIDS. High-potency prescription steroid creams are used twice a day for two to three weeks, then once a day, usually at night, for an additional two weeks or until symptoms disappear. Often, the steroid creams will be continued indefinitely once or twice a week. The regimen for testosterone is very similar. Sometimes, simply applying lanolin or vegetable oil provides relief.

Risk Factors and Preventive Measures

It is also important to practice good hygiene, keep the vulva dry, and avoid the use of soaps, lotions and detergents. Over-the-counter antibiotic creams and anti-itch creams should not be used, as they cause more irritation.

lichen simplex A skin disorder characterized by patches of thickened itchy and sometimes discolored skin. It is caused by repeated scratching, usually on neck, wrists, arms, and ankles. It is most prevalent among women and is believed to be caused by extended scratching due to a psychological condition. Patients often rub patches unconsciously when agitated or during stressful situations. This contributes to a cycle of skin thickening and scratching. The skin thickens in reaction to the itching, which in turn causes the skin to thicken even more.

Symptoms and Diagnostic Path

Symptoms include intense, chronic itchy skin that gets worse with scratching or stress. The skin lesions have distinct borders, a flat top, and are typically violet or slightly purple. When scratched repeatedly, the lesions may become leathery, reddened, or darkened. There may be raw areas and scratch marks. The lesions are typically found on the ankle, wrist, neck, anal area, forearms, thighs, lower leg, back of the knee, and inner elbow.

The skin's appearance and a history of chronic ITCHING and scratching is typically used to identify the condition, but a skin lesion biopsy may be needed to confirm the diagnosis.

Treatment Options and Outlook

Dressings to cover and protect the area may be used with or without topical medications, and may be applied for a week or more at a time. The itching and inflammation may be treated with a lotion or steroid cream applied to the affected area. Peeling ointments (such as those containing salicylic acid), may be used on thickened lesions and coal tar soaps or lotions may be recommended. ANTIHISTAMINES (especially those that are a bit sedating) may be needed to reduce itching; steroids may be injected into lesions to reduce itching and inflammation. Psychological counseling to understand the importance of not scratching, plus stress management, may help.

light treatment See PHOTOTHERAPY.

limes and the skin See OIL OF BERGAMOT.

lindane (Trade name: Kwell) A drug (gamma benzene hexachloride), once widely used to treat infestation by SCABIES OR LICE. It is no longer recommended by the U.S. Food and Drug Administration (FDA) or NATIONAL PEDICULOSIS ASSOCIATION (NPA) because of its potential toxicity. Other products, such as permethrin (Elimite), work equally well with less risk.

In 2004 the FDA issued a Public Health Advisory concerning the use of topical formulations of lindane lotion and lindane shampoo for the treatment of SCABIES and head LICE. The warning emphasized that lindane products should be considered as a second-line therapy for the treatment of scabies and lice. While FDA explained that it believed the benefits of lindane outweigh the risks when used as directed, given the potential for neurotoxicity patients should be treated with these medications only if other treatments are not tolerable or other approved therapies have failed. The boxed warning also stated that lindane lotion and shampoo should be used with caution in patients who weight less than about 110 pounds, and that these products are not recommended for infants or premature infants.

These warnings were based on reports to the FDA's voluntary reporting system, which described that about half of reported adverse events occurred in children. Because most of the serious adverse events reported with lindane products are due to misuse and overuse, especially with the lotion, product package sizes are limited to one and two ounces.

Lindane may irritate the scalp and skin, or cause itching. It is thought by some to be toxic to the nervous system. In at least one case, a child allegedly suffered permanent brain damage after being treated with a lindane-based pediculicide.

lipoid proteinosis   See URBACH-WIETHE DISEASE.

lipoma   A common benign tumor composed of mature fat cells that almost never becomes malignant. Women are affected much more often, usually in early-to-middle adult life. The tumors appear on the neck, trunk, abdomen, forearms, buttocks, and thighs.

Symptoms and Diagnostic Path
The tumor may be moveable underneath the skin's surface. Usually painless, it will slowly grow until it becomes several inches across. It can appear at any age and will not spontaneously fade away. They may be confused with other types of tumors.

Treatment Options and Outlook
Most lipoma require no treatment, although LIPOSUCTION or surgical excision are both effective means of removal.

liposuction   The removal of unwanted fat deposits in certain areas of the body, most commonly the thighs, buttocks, abdomen, "handlebar" areas, chin, and knees. It is an excellent method of spot reduction but is not an effective method of weight loss.

It remains the most popular cosmetic surgical procedure in the United States—even more popular than FACE-LIFTS. There are more than 470,000 procedures done annually. The procedure is effective because fat cells do not regenerate after they are destroyed or removed; for example, people who gain weight after liposuction do not regain significant amounts of weight in areas where fat has been removed.

Best candidates for the surgery are those who are healthy, at near-normal weight, who are in their 30s and 40s and whose skin still retains some elasticity and who have isolated pockets of fat in certain areas. These localized fat deposits may be an inherited pattern, and typically cannot be removed via dieting or exercise. Surgical excision but not liposuction is often the only way to eliminate these areas. A recent study has found that injecting a medication that melts fat directly into the lipoma may help shrink it without surgery.

While some surgeons perform liposuction under general anesthesia, it is most frequently done under local anesthesia at a hospital free-standing outpatient facility, or office surgical suite. Sometimes, the removed fat can be transferred into other areas where the fat has wasted away as a way to augment soft tissue.

In traditional liposuction, the surgeon inserts a tube (called a canula) through a small inconspicuous skin incision. The tube is attached to a vacuum pressure unit and is moved through fat, removing the cells. As the canula moves through the fat, it creates tunnels that scar, resulting in a permanent flattening of the area. Unfortunately, in the past this technique sucked out not only fat but blood vessels, tiny nerves, and anything else in the path of the cannula. This tended to cause significant bleeding, bruising, and blood loss, which limited the amount of fat that could be safely removed.

Several years ago, the "tumescent technique" (sometimes also called the super-wet technique) was developed by a DERMATOLOGIST, which allowed removal of significantly more fat during the operation with much less blood loss. With this technique, the fat layer is injected with large amounts of a dilute anesthetic solution of saline and adrenalin before suctioning. The same hollow metal cannulas and high-powered vacuum pumps are then used again to suck out the fat. Most patients are back at work within one or two days. While there is less bleeding than with the traditional technique, patients still frequently require several weeks to recover fully from the bruising, pain, and swelling.

Ultrasonic liposuction Also known as ultrasound assisted lipoplasty (UAL), this is a technical advancement over other liposuction techniques. Introduced in the United States in 1994 and approved by the U.S. Food and Drug Administration in 1996, it is becoming a popular technique for fat removal and body sculpting among plastic surgeons.

In ultrasonic liposuction, a special titanium cannula transmits the ultrasound energy to the fat layer, where it disrupts the fat cells with which it comes in contact. This liquefies the fat, which is then drained or suctioned out through a hollow portion of the cannula under low, gentle vacuum.

Outlook and Lifestyle Modification

Because the technique is more refined and gentle to the tissues, there is less blood loss, less bruising, less pain, and a significantly faster recovery. Studies need to be performed to determine whether UAL offers any advantage over traditional liposuction performed with tumescent anesthesia. An elasticized bandage, sponge, or specially designed garment may be placed over the treated areas. The patient will be able to go home after a few hours, although some patients may stay overnight in the hospital or surgical facility. After several days, the dressings will be temporarily removed so the plastic surgeon can examine the treated areas. There may be swelling, which typically begins to fade within a week or so after surgery; bruising and numbness can last at least three weeks. If stitches need to be removed, this is typically done within 10 days after surgery.

Risks and Complications

Although liposuction is very safe and effective, it is still a surgical procedure and can cause complications such as infection, bleeding, and nerve damage. In addition, aesthetic complications such as skin irregularity or waviness can occur if too much fat has been removed. Fortunately, complications are uncommon and most patients are satisfied with their results.

liquid nitrogen Freezing with liquid nitrogen, otherwise known as cryotherapy, destroys tissue by means of extremely low temperatures of −125° degrees to −130° C (−195° to −200° F). The liquid nitrogen is delivered with either a Q-tip, a spray thermos device, or a contact probe.

It is used for the treatment of lentigines, seborrheic keratoses, actinic keratoses, WARTS, benign tumors, some basal cell and squamous cell carcinomas, and occasionally LENTIGO MALIGNA. Liquid nitrogen on plantar or palmar warts may cause painful blood-filled blisters, however.

See also ACTINIC KERATOSIS; BASAL CELL CARCINOMA; KERATOSIS, SEBORRHEIC; SQUAMOUS CELL CARCINOMA.

livedo reticularis A condition characterized by a reddish blue netlike mottling of the skin, usually on the lower legs. The condition may be intermittent, appearing simply as a normal response to the cold. The permanent form of livedo reticularis may be caused by an underlying systemic disease, such as arteriosclerosis, diseases of COLLAGEN, cerebrovascular disease, and so on. It is caused by enlargement of blood vessels underneath the skin.

Treatment Options and Outlook

Treatment of the underlying condition in secondary livedo will cure this problem. Rewarming the area in cases with no known underlying cause may reverse the problem. However, eventually the blood vessels become permanently dilated and the livedo reticularis will become permanent no matter what the surrounding temperature.

liver spots See LENTIGO, ACTINIC.

van Lohuizen's disease See CUTIS MARMORATA TELANGIECTATICA CONGENITA.

loiasis A form of the tropical parasitic disease FILARIASIS caused by an infestation of the *Loa loa* worm, which travels beneath the skin and causes an inflammation known as a calabar swelling. Swellings tend to be several centimeters in size, and may be preceded by localized pain and itching. The disease may occasionally involve acute allergic symptoms with giant hives, fever, and recurring episodes of angioedema, especially in Caucasian visitors to endemic areas. Evidence of heart or kidney problems may be found in up to 20 percent of such cases.

Loiasis is widely distributed and highly endemic in tropical West Africa. In the Congo River basin up to 90 percent of villagers in some areas are infected. Humans who have microfilariae in the blood are likely the only important reservoir of loiasis, although nonhuman primates can be infected. *Chrysops* flies bite the human and ingest blood containing the microfilariae. These develop into larvae and are returned to man via the bite of the infective fly.

Symptoms and Diagnostic Path

Symptoms of loiasis generally do not appear until several years after the bite of the fly, although they have been known to appear within four months. Repeated infections can occur. The worms move through the skin, causing inflammation. The worms can often be seen migrating across the conjunctiva and cornea of the eye, which is where its nickname "eye worm" comes from. The worm sometimes enters the brain, causing encephalitis. The problem is diagnosed by detecting the microfilariae in the blood.

Treatment Options and Outlook

Diethylcarbamazine or ivermectin has been the primary drug for the past 40 years and has proven very effective in treating loiasis.

Risk Factors and Preventive Measures

Visitors to Africa should take preventive action against insects, including the use of an effective repellent containing Deet or dimethyl phthalate, wearing long pants, and sleeping in well-screened areas.

loofahs A type of natural fibrous sponge harvested from the luffa plant, which grows like a gourd and is then dried and made into sponges, mitts, or woven cloths. Loofahs are a good alternative to a body brush or washcloth, since they help remove dead skin cells. They should not be used on the face, neck, or on broken skin.

Because loofahs are a nutrient source for bacteria and cellular debris from the skin and are usually kept in a damp environment, these products are liable to become contaminated.

To keep a loofah clean, thoroughly wash with mild soap, rinse and then dry after each use. Since this process will not kill some organisms, soak the loofah twice a week in a solution of one part bleach and nine parts water to sterilize.

Loofahs may not *look* contaminated (such as a color change or odor), so consumers should buy new ones regularly—about every two months. A loofah needs to be replaced if it gets soft, or if pieces start to fall off.

Synthetic products are less likely to become contaminated, but they should still be washed and rinsed after each use and replaced after two months of use.

Loofahs, sponges, and brushes should not be shared and if used on an infected part of the skin, they should be thrown away.

Loprox See CYCLOPIROXOLAMINE.

lotion A liquid drug preparation that can be applied to the skin. Lotions have a soothing effect and can be used to cover large areas.

Louis-Bar syndrome A genetic disorder that causes, among many other symptoms, reddish lesions of the skin and mucous membranes in early childhood due to permanent widening of groups of blood vessels (TELANGIECTASIA). The syndrome is inherited as an autosomal recessive trait, which means that the defective gene must be inherited from both parents. The defective gene has been identified as ATM (for "AT mutated") that has been mapped to the long arm of chromosome 11. The ATM gene controls the production of an enzyme that plays a role in regulating cell division after DNA damage.

Symptoms and Diagnostic Path

This syndrome involves a wide range of symptoms. In addition to the telangiectasia, skin symptoms include GRAY HAIR, loss of skin elasticity, and excess subcutaneous fat. Non-skin symptoms include progressively impaired coordination of voluntary movements (ataxia) and impaired functioning of the immune system leading to increased susceptibility to upper and lower respiratory infections. Individuals with ATM also have an increased risk of developing certain cancers, including lymphomas, leukemia, and brain tumors. It affects both sexes equally, typically being diagnosed at about the age of four years.

Treatment Options and Outlook

There is no treatment, other than to ease symptoms. Death usually occurs in adolescence or early adulthood from a lung infection or cancer.

lubricants   Topical preparations containing fats or oils used to help hydrate and protect the skin, making it more pliable by trapping water within the top layer of the EPIDERMIS (stratum corneum).

Lubricants work better if the skin is first soaked for five to ten minutes in water. They may contain animal fats (such as LANOLIN), vegetable oils (such as olive oil), mineral oil, paraffin, petrolatum, or waxes.

Different brands or types of lubricants may have quite different consistency, and choice of preparation should depend on its intended use.

lunula   The white crescent area at the base of the nail.

lupus erythematosus   A chronic autoimmune disease that causes inflammation of connective tissue, which affects the skin and internal organs.

When wolves roamed Europe, it was said that the victim of a wolf (*lupus*) attack bore the sign of the wolf—a red mark on the face. Others who had never been attacked but who bore similar marks were believed to have the "disease of the *lupus*"—lupus erythematosus.

Lupus involves the body's immune system, which launches an attack against itself. In one form (discoid lupus erythematosus, or DLE), the disease affects only the skin; in the second form (systemic lupus erythematosus, or SLE), the disease affects the skin and organs throughout the body. Drug-induced lupus (similar to SLE) occurs after using certain medications, such as the blood pressure drug hydralazine, and procainamide (used to treat irregular heart rhythms). Only a very few people who use these drugs develop drug-induced lupus, and symptoms usually fade when the medications are discontinued.

In about 10 percent of all lupus cases, patients will have symptoms of more than one connective tissue disease, including lupus. This is called "overlap syndrome" or "mixed connective tissue disease."

About 1.5 million Americans have the disease. Lupus strikes nine times as many women as men, usually those of childbearing age. The condition occurs throughout the world, but the incidence is higher among certain ethnic groups (such as African Americans, Hispanics, Asians, and Native Americans). In high-risk groups, the incidence may be as common as one in every 250 women.

An autoimmune disorder, lupus causes the body's immune system to attack its own connective tissue, causing inflammation. Attacks can be triggered by sunlight and by certain drugs such as hydralazine, procainamide, or isoniazid. It is believed that the disease is inherited, and that hormonal factors play a part. Sometimes, a viral infection may trigger symptoms.

About 20 percent of people with lupus have a close relative (a parent or sibling) who already has lupus or may develop lupus. About 5 percent of children born to individuals with lupus will develop the illness.

Symptoms and Diagnostic Path

In both forms of the disease, symptoms wax and wane with varying severity.

In DLE, the rash presents itself as one or more red, circular, thickened areas of skin on the face, behind the ears, and on the scalp. The rash may cause permanent hair loss in affected areas and result in facial scars.

SLE causes a red, blotchy butterfly-shaped rash over the face that does not scar. Most patients feel sick and are tired, experiencing fever, appetite loss, nausea, painful joints, and weight loss. Complications include kidney failure, pleurisy, arthritis seizures, and psychiatric problems.

Less than 5 percent of patients with DLE progress to SLE; patients with SLE may also have skin lesions of DLE.

Treatment Options and Outlook

Although there is no cure, treatment aims at reducing inflammation and alleviating symptoms with nonsteroidal anti-inflammatory drugs, antimalarials, and corticosteroid drugs. Those whose condition is worsened by sunlight should avoid exposure, wear protective clothing, and use sunscreens. Immunosuppressant (or immunomodulating) drugs (chemotherapy) are typically recommended only for patients with the most severe flares of lupus, or to reduce the steroid dose. (A "severe" flare is one that impairs one of the body's organs.) During a severe flair, the function of the organ must be protected. Immunosuppressive or chemotherapy medications suppress the overactivity of the immune system triggered by lupus, which helps limit the damage and preserve the function of the involved organ.

Although this disease may be life threatening if the kidney is involved, the outlook for patients has improved a great deal over the past 20 years.

lupus pernio See SARCOIDOSIS.

lupus vulgaris A type of skin lesion that appears in skin tuberculosis in immune (or partially immune) patients.

Symptoms and Diagnostic Path

Beginning early in life, the condition is characterized by scaly red plaques, which over time will spread, ulcerate, and produce extensive scarring and tissue loss.

Treatment Options and Outlook

Administration of antituberculosis drugs.
See also TUBERCULOSIS, SKIN.

lycopenia A condition characterized by an orange-yellow skin tint caused by eating foods high in lycopene, such as tomatoes or berries. In lycopenia, the skin discoloration may resemble that of hypercarotenemia. High blood levels of lycopene may be raised and mild liver dysfunction may also occur.

Lyme disease A tick-borne illness whose hallmark symptom is a red rash that forms an irregular ring shape surrounding the tick bite. Untreated, Lyme disease in humans can cause a host of problems, including arthritis and disorders of the heart and central nervous system. It is most commonly found in the northeast coastal states from Maine to Maryland, in the upper Midwest, and on the Pacific coast. It is most often contracted in the late spring or early summer when ticks are abundant.

The number of annually reported cases of Lyme disease in the United States has increased about 25-fold since national surveillance began in 1982, with about 22,000 cases annually reported to the Centers for Disease Control and Prevention (CDC) through 2003.

The disease is caused by *Borrelia burgdorferi*, a spirochete form of bacterium transmitted by the bite of deer ticks (*Ixodes scapularis*) and western black-legged ticks (*Ixodes pacificus*). The deer tick, which normally feeds on the white-footed mouse, the white-tailed deer, other mammals, and birds, is responsible for transmitting Lyme disease bacteria to humans in the northeastern and north-central United States. On the Pacific coast, the bacteria are transmitted to humans by the western black-legged tick. *Ixodes* ticks are much smaller than common dog and cattle ticks. In their larval and nymphal stages, they are no bigger than a pinhead (adult ticks are slightly larger).

Most *B. burgdorferi* infections are believed to be caused by exposure to infected ticks during property maintenance, recreation, and leisure activities. People who live or work in residential areas surrounded by woods or overgrown brush are at risk of getting Lyme disease. In addition, those who participate in recreational activities such as hiking, camping, fishing, and hunting, away from home, in tick habitat, and persons who work outdoors, such as landscapers, foresters, and wildlife managers in endemic areas, may also be at risk of getting Lyme disease.

Ticks search for host animals from the tips of grasses and shrubs (not from trees) and transfer to animals or persons that brush against vegetation. Ticks only crawl; they do not fly or jump. Ticks found on the scalp usually have crawled there from lower parts of the body.

There is no evidence that a person can get Lyme disease from the air, food or water, from sexual contact, or directly from wild or domestic animals. There is no convincing evidence that Lyme disease can be transmitted by insects such as mosquitoes, flies, or fleas. The risk of exposure to ticks is greatest in the woods and garden fringe areas of properties, but ticks may also be carried by animals into lawns and gardens.

Symptoms and Diagnostic Path

Lyme disease most often begins with a characteristic "bull's-eye" rash, accompanied by symptoms such as fever, malaise, fatigue, headache, muscle aches, and joint aches. The incubation period from infection to onset of the rash is typically seven to 14 days, but may be as short as three days or as long as 30 days. Some infected individuals have no recognized illness or experience only vague symptoms such as fever, headache, fatigue, and muscle aches.

The signs of early disseminated infection usually occur days to weeks after the appearance of a solitary bull's-eye rash. In addition to multiple red lesions, early disseminated infection may produce disease of the nervous system, the musculoskeletal system, or the heart. Early brain symptoms include lymphocytic meningitis, cranial neuropathy (especially facial nerve palsy), and radiculoneuritis.

There may be joint and muscle pains with or without joint swelling.

If untreated, the infection may progress to disseminated disease weeks to months after infection, with intermittent swelling and pain of one or a few joints—usually large, weight-bearing joints such as the knee. Some patients develop chronic thinking disorders, sleep disturbance, fatigue, and personality changes. Infrequently, Lyme disease may be severe, chronic, and disabling.

An ill-defined post-Lyme disease syndrome occurs in some people after treatment for Lyme disease. However, it is rarely if ever fatal.

The diagnosis of Lyme disease is based primarily on symptoms; patients with early disease may be treated solely on the basis of objective signs and a known exposure. Blood testing may provide valuable supportive diagnostic information in patients with endemic exposure and objective clinical findings that suggest later stage disease.

Treatment Options and Outlook

Antibiotic treatment for three to four weeks with doxycycline, cefuroxime, or amoxicillin is generally effective in early disease. Cefuroxime axetil or ERYTHROMYCIN can be used for persons allergic to penicillin or who cannot take TETRACYCLINES. More advanced disease, particularly with brain symptoms, may require treatment with intravenous ceftriaxone or penicillin for four weeks or more, depending on disease severity. In advanced disease, treatment failures may occur and retreatment may be necessary.

Risk Factors and Preventive Measures

A Lyme disease vaccine (LYMErix) was discontinued in 2002 because of insufficient consumer demand. Protection provided by this vaccine diminishes over time, so consumers who received the Lyme disease vaccine before 2002 are probably no longer protected against Lyme disease.

Whenever possible, people should avoid areas that are likely to be infested with ticks, particularly in spring and summer when young ticks feed. Ticks favor a moist, shaded environment such as leaf litter and low-lying vegetation in wooded, brushy, or overgrown grassy habitat.

Visitors in tick infested areas should wear light-colored clothing so that ticks can be spotted more easily and removed before becoming attached. Wearing long-sleeved shirts and tucking pants into socks or boot tops may help keep ticks from reaching the skin. Ticks are usually located close to the ground, so wearing high rubber boots may provide additional protection.

Applying insect repellents containing DEET (N, N diethyl-*m*-toluamide) to clothes and exposed skin and permethrin (which kills ticks on contact) to clothes should also help reduce the risk of tick attachment. DEET can be used safely on children and adults but should be applied according to Environmental Protection Agency guidelines to reduce the possibility of toxicity.

Since transmission of *B. burgdorferi* from an infected tick is unlikely to occur until after the tick has been attached for at least 36 hours, daily checks for ticks and their prompt removal will help prevent infection. Embedded ticks should be removed using fine-tipped tweezers. PETROLEUM JELLY, a hot match, nail polish, or other products should not be used.

To remove a tick, it should be grasped firmly and pulled away from the skin. It is not a problem if the tick's mouth parts remain in the skin, since the bacteria that cause Lyme disease are contained in the tick's midgut. The tick bite area should be washed with an antiseptic.

In most cases, treating everyone who gets a tick bite with antibiotics is not recommended. Individuals who are bitten by a deer tick should remove the tick and seek medical attention only if there are symptoms of early Lyme disease, ehrlichiosis, or babesiosis.

The number of ticks in residential areas may be reduced by removing leaf litter, brush- and wood-piles around houses and at the edges of yards, and by clearing trees and brush to admit more sunlight and reduce the amount of suitable habitat for deer, rodents, and ticks. A pesticide designed to kill ticks (acaricide) can be very effective in reducing tick populations. If properly timed, a single application at the end of May or beginning of June can reduce tick populations by 68 to 100 percent. The U.S. Environmental Protection Agency and each state determines the availability of pesticides. Consumers interested in applying acaricides should check with local health officials about the best time to apply it, as well as any rules and regulations related to pesticide application on residential properties. Consumers also can contact a professional pesticide company to apply pesticides.

Bait boxes that treat wild rodents with acaricide are now available for home use. Properly used, these boxes have been shown to reduce the number of ticks by more than half. The treatment is similar to products used to control fleas and ticks on pets, and does not harm the rodents. Bait boxes are available from licensed pest control companies in many states.

Other methods for controlling ticks currently under evaluation include vegetation and habitat modification, devices for applying topical acaricides to deer, fungal agents for biological control, and natural extracts that safely repel ticks.

lymphangiosarcoma   See STEWART-TREVES TUMOR.

lymphangitis   Inflammation of the lymphatic vessels that cause tender red streaks to appear on the skin caused by a spread of bacteria (usually streptococci) from an infected wound.

Symptoms and Diagnostic Path

The streaks extend from the site of infection toward the nearest lymph nodes, and is usually accompanied by a fever and a general feeling of illness.

Treatment Options and Outlook

This condition is a clear indication of serious infection, and requires immediate treatment with antibiotics. Antibiotic treatment usually clears up the infection without complication.

lymphocytoma cutis   One of a group of benign inflammatory skin conditions that resemble malignant lymphomas. In most cases, the cause of this disorder is unknown, although it may be induced by bites or stings, injected drugs, vaccinations, or acupuncture. If the lesion persists or spreads, a biopsy must be performed to rule out the possibility that the condition is malignant lymphoma and not a benign condition.

Symptoms and Diagnostic Path

This variant, (also known as cutaneous lymphoid hyperplasia), seen primarily in women, is usually characterized by a single firm, red-brown or purple NODULE or plaque on sun-exposed areas such as the face and extremities.

Treatment Options and Outlook

Although the lesions may be excised, they do respond to injections of CORTICOSTEROIDS directly into the affected area. Superficial, low-dose X-rays may also be administered.

macular amyloidosis See AMYLOIDOSIS.

macule A flat spot on the skin, visible only by differing color that is less than 1 or 2 cm in diameter.

maduromycosis See MYCETOMA.

Maffucci's syndrome A rare syndrome that affects the skin and skeleton, with many large growths with blood-filled spaces due to dilation and thickening of the walls of capillaries (cavernous HEMANGIOMAS), raised masses of capillaries, dilated veins, and bone fractures. Between 25 percent and 30 percent of those afflicted with Maffucci's disease develop cancer.

While no particular pattern of inheritance has been identified, the disease appears early in life, usually around the age of four or five; 25 percent of cases are present at birth. Patients apparently are of average intelligence, with no associated mental problems. More than 100 cases have been reported in the United States.

Symptoms and Diagnostic Path

The syndrome can trigger many superficial and deep hemangiomas that often protrude as soft nodules or tumors, usually on arms or legs (although they can appear anywhere). The hemangiomas in Maffucci's syndrome appear as blue NODULES under the skin. Patients are usually short and may have unequal arm or leg lengths because of bone abnormalities.

The syndrome also can cause benign cartilaginous tumors (enchondromas) that can appear anywhere but are usually found on the bones of the fingers and on the long bones. These bone abnormalities are usually asymmetric and cause secondary fractures. About 30 percent to 37 percent of enchondromas can develop into cancer.

Treatment Options and Outlook

Specific treatment of Maffucci's disease depends on a wide variety of possible symptoms. Surgery may remove or reduce the size of the hemangiomas. No medical care is needed in patients without other symptoms, but careful follow-up is needed to evaluate any changes in the skin and bone lesions, since these lesions can become malignant.

Patients with Maffucci's syndrome usually lead reasonably normal lives with a normal life expectancy if no malignant transformation occurs. Although the skeletal malformations can sometimes be crippling, patients have managed to perform activities of daily living.

magnesium aluminum silicate An oil-absorbing chemical that is included in some skin care products, such as oil-free foundations. It is not considered to be part of an effective treatment for ACNE.

Majocchi's disease A disorder involving inflammation of blood vessels with particular skin symptoms.

Symptoms and Diagnostic Path

Known medically as purpura annularis telangiectodes, this condition is one of a group of diseases called PIGMENTED PURPURIC DERMATOSIS that are all characterized by rust-colored MACULES and PAPULES on the lower legs. In this condition, early lesions may be redder, forming rings, but there is no itching involved.

Treatment Options and Outlook

All forms of these capillary diseases are chronic and tend to resist treatment although topical steroids and UVB PHOTOTHERAPY may help.

Majocchi's granuloma A variant of TINEA COR-PORIS (RINGWORM of the body), in which there is an infection in the hair follicles. This uncommon condition is often found among young women who frequently shave their legs. Occasionally, this problem may be caused by potent topical steroids.

Many species of dermatophytes can cause MG, but it is usually due to *Trichophyton rubrum;* other causes include *T. mentagrophytes* and *Epidermophyton floccosum.* Experts do not know whether these granulomas appear in response to the organism itself, or after the release of follicular contents.

The condition was first described as a "granuloma tricofitico" in 1883 by dermatology professor Domenico Majocchi. (He also described a type of chronic pigmented purpura known as MAJOCCHI'S DISEASE).

Symptoms and Diagnostic Path

Symptoms include patches on any hairy area, such as the scalp, face, forearms, hands, and legs. Majocchi's granuloma may be worsened by shaving legs in an upward direction, which causes the hair follicles to be inoculated with ATHLETE'S FOOT fungus. The lesions may first appear as single or multiple oval patches that evolve into PUSTULES and NODULES with or without background redness and scaling.

If the condition is associated with the use of topical steroids, they may be affected by the complications of topical steroid therapy, including atrophied skin and spidery veins, ROSACEA, or patches of loss of color on the skin that looks like LEPROSY. MG may rarely resemble KAPOSI'S SARCOMA.

Treatment Options and Outlook

Majocchi's granuloma usually responds to topical antifungal or drying powders, such as those that contain miconazole, clotrimazole, or similar ingredients. Severe or chronic infection may require further treatment by a doctor. Stronger, prescription topical antifungal medications, such as KETO-CONAZOLE or sulconazole, may be needed. In some cases, topical CORTICOSTEROIDS may be added to the topical antifungals. Antibiotics may be needed to treat secondary bacterial infections.

makeup A group of COSMETICS including face powder, lipstick, mascara, eyebrow pencil, eye shadow, and eye liner that are used to enhance a person's appearance.

Face powder covers up the outer layer of the skin, creating a velvety finish on the face. This product usually contains titanium dioxide or zinc oxide, with talc, kaolin, ZINC or magnesium stearate, color, and perfume. Powdered silk, sometimes included in face powder, is a powerful marketing tool but contributes very little to the product's function.

Compact powder is compressed face powder with a binding component (such as gum arabic). *Translucent powder* offers an extra opaque quality through the addition of titanium dioxide.

Lipstick is made up of a number of components, including carnauba wax, beeswax, castor oil, LANO-LIN, preservatives, perfumes, and indelible dyes (such as D&C Red #21, D&C Orange #5, and so on).

Mascara is a soap that emulsifies when moistened; liquid mascara is emulsified with alcohol. *Eyebrow pencil* is made with the same pigments as in mascara and is basically a crayon. *Cream eye shadow* is a mixture of a petrolatum and pigment, whereas *stick eye shadow* contains most of the same ingredients as lipstick.

Eyeliner contains pigments in a resin solution that may often be irritating to the eyes. It also contains a small amount of mercury, which has been prohibited in all other cosmetics. However, the amount in eyeliner is not believed to be harmful.

Sensitivity can appear in response to any cosmetic, but the eyes are especially vulnerable. Too frequent or too harsh cleansing of the eyelid can also cause irritation.

malar flush Often a sign of narrowing of a heart valve (mitral stenosis) malar flush is characterized by heightened color and a slight blue tinge over the cheekbones due to a lack of oxygen in the blood. It usually appears after a bout of rheumatic fever.

It is possible, however, to have a malar flush without any heart irregularities: Many people with this high coloring do not have cardiac disease.

mal del pinto See PINTA.

mal de Meleda An extremely rare hereditary skin disease of the EPIDERMIS inherited by autosomal recessive transmission. This means that a defective gene must be inherited from both parents in order to cause the abnormality. Generally, the parents of an affected person are unaffected carriers of the defective gene. Each of the children of such parents has a one in four chance of being affected, and a two in four chance of being a carrier. This disease is progressive and persistent.

The condition was first described in 1826 on the island of Meleda off the coast of Bosnia Herzegovina. Most cases of this disease have been reported in Bosnia, Germany, and France.

Symptoms and Diagnostic Path

During the first few weeks of life, the disease is characterized by yellow-brown, waxy, rough palms and soles of the feet. Other associated abnormalities include poor physical development, short nails and fingers, high palate, and abnormalities of the EEG.

Treatment Options and Outlook

Administration of keratolytics and lactic acid-based creams is the recommended treatment.

malignancy, skin signs of internal There are a range of signs that can appear on the skin in connection with cancer. Some of these signs include multiple SEBACEOUS CYSTS, increased hairiness, dryness, and scaling. Five percent of cancer patients may get metastatic lumps, usually in connection with cancers of the breast, lung, or colon—but usually only after the cancer is well advanced. Up to 25 percent of lymphomas appear first as a skin rash, with small plaques, nodules, or ulcers.

Other examples of cancerous diseases with skin symptoms include ACANTHOSIS NIGRICANS (dark-

ening in body folds, underarms, neck and groin, with velvety brown eruptions), COWDEN'S DISEASE (small oral nodules), dermatomyositis (red, swollen thickened skin especially of the eyelids), GARDNER'S SYNDROME (disfiguring cysts on skin), Paget's disease (weeping, crusting or scaly skin inflammation in anal or groin region, vulva, armpits, or breasts), PEUTZ-JEGHERS SYNDROME (dark pigmented oral spots), PYODERMA GANGRENOSUM (ulcer with bluish borders, covering large areas of skin), BOWEN'S DISEASE, BULLOUS PEMPHIGOID, ERYTHEMA ANNULARE CENTRIFUGUM, ERYTHEMA GYRATUM REPENS, acquired ICHTHYOSIS (Hodgkin's disease or lymphoma), BAZEX SYNDROME, DERMATITIS HERPETIFORMIS, PEMPHIGUS, PORPHYRIA cutanea tarda, and leukocytoclastic vasculitis.

malignant melanoma See MELANOMA, MALIGNANT.

mammoplasty Plastic surgery of the breasts either to increase (breast augmentation) or decrease (breast reduction) their size.

Breast augmentation is the most popular of all operations to reshape soft tissue. In the past, fluids were directly injected into the breast, with some dreadful results. Today, a prosthesis is implanted into a pocket either directly under the breast tissue or underneath the major chest muscle.

In the past, the most common implants were silicone gel. The U.S. Food and Drug Administration (FDA) had asked for a voluntary moratorium on the sale of silicone gel breast implants in 1992 after a number of anecdotal reports linking ruptured implants with immune system disorders. The FDA ruled that silicone implants would be available only if saline-filled implants were not an option (silicone implants were not totally banned). However, the FDA did not conclude that silicone implants posed a health risk, but that implant manufacturers had not provided enough data to confirm their absolute safety. Since then, health risk reports have not been substantiated by controlled clinical trials.

However, critics continue to insist that silicone often leaks from the gel-filled devices, causing cancer and neurological diseases. As a result, more than 90 percent of the U.S. market now uses saline-filled implants, although silicone implants have remained available for women who have undergone mastectomies.

In July 2005, silicone gel-filled breast implants moved a step closer to being reintroduced to the U.S. market after the FDA issued an "approvable with conditions" letter to one manufacturer (Mentor Corp.) for its implants. However, this letter does not mean that the device is approved for marketing in the United States at this time. Federal law prohibits the government from discussing the letter's specific contents, but an approvable letter is one of several intermediate steps in the FDA's review process for new products. Saline inflatables are the implant of choice in the United States. A third type, the double-lumen prosthesis, features a gel-filled inner portion surrounded by a saline inflatable outer jacket.

In breast augmentation, the incision through which the implant is inserted can be made either above the crease under the breast, near the nipple, or high in the armpit. The first method is the most popular: The armpit incision leaves no scar on the breast itself, but it is more risky since the incision is so far from the area on which the surgeon is working.

After the procedure, the breast should look and feel natural: Scars are usually not noticeable.

Risks and Complications

Problems with breast hardness, caused by scar tissue that forms around the implant, may occur in up to 30 percent of patients. This hardness may appear soon after surgery or years after the procedure. Other risks are rare and include loss of nipple sensitivity (5 to 10 percent), infection, or poor healing of scars.

Because breasts that are too large may cause back pain, discomfort during sports, chronic back strain, rashes in the creases, or a psychological burden, some women choose *breast reduction* to solve their health problems. In this surgical technique, excess breast tissue is removed, the nipple position is raised and the skin is trimmed to fit the new shape. The operation usually requires a hospital stay and general anesthesia.

Outlook and Lifestyle Modification

Activities must be restricted for several weeks postsurgery. Some scarring occurs, usually around the nipple, under the breasts and between the nipple and the second scar. It is also possible that the nipple will be less sensitive, and that breast-feeding may become impossible. There is no evidence of an increase in breast cancer. Because breast reduction is not always simply cosmetic, some insurance companies will pay for at least part of the operation.

See also MASTOPEXY; SILICONE IMPLANTS.

manicures   See NAILS, CARE OF.

Mantoux test   See TUBERCULIN TEST.

mask   A type of skin product that can either be rinsed or peeled off that helps the skin to exfoliate (shed its dead outer cells) in order for it to look fresh and vital. Masks also stimulate the skin's circulation, and some help the skin hold moisture better (at least temporarily).

Newer products have been developed for a wide range of tasks such as improving puffy eyes in addition to imparting a healthy glow to the skin and removing dead skin cells. Masks are designed to work quickly—most of them dry in 10 minutes or less and are then removed.

Today's masks are more effective because they include better ingredients designed to clean, tighten, refresh, and moisturize the face. Mixed into these products are substances previously found only in moisturizers such as talc and nylon, to cut down shine; buttermilk (a moisturizing ingredient); caffeine extract; and grapefruit seed to soothe and lessen redness.

Before choosing a mask, consumers should read the label carefully; it's important to know what active ingredients to look for to best treat a specific SKIN TYPE.

Oily skin   The best masks for this skin type are made of kaolin (oil-absorbing clay), bentonite (white clay), aluminum magnesium silicate (talc), witch hazel, alcohol, or zinc oxide. These masks work by cleaning the skin, absorbing excess oil (which cuts down on shine) and preventing bacterial growth. Kaolin and bentonite also cause the skin to perspire, which opens up the pores, allowing the ingredients in the mask to deep-clean the skin. Most oily-skin masks start as a thick paste and dry to a hard crust that is removed by water. Afterward, the skin feels temporarily tightened.

Dry skin The best masks for dry skin include those with collagen, buttermilk, and protein as moisturizers; panthenol (a B vitamin), to help retain moisture; amino acids, to help water penetrate the skin, plumping up skin cells and temporarily filling in fine lines; and oils or lanolin, to help keep moisture close to the skin. Masks for dry skin are usually gel- or cream-based and do not dry and harden on the skin.

Blotchy skin The types of masks to help this skin problem include those made with kaolin, caffeine, grapefruit seed, and plant extracts such as azulene, chamomile, and aloe. All skin types can benefit from products with these ingredients, which can soothe and even out the complexion. Caffeine and grapefruit seeds diminish redness; chamomile extract cuts down inflammation and has a cooling effect on the skin.

Dull skin Masks made of menthol, peppermint, or eucalyptus can help stimulate the skin, leaving it with a tingling feeling. These masks are sometimes made to dry into a stretchy film that is peeled off; others are cream-based and are rinsed off. Both types remove dead skin cells, which create a dull appearance.

mask of pregnancy See CHLOASMA.

mast cell diseases Diseases that involve the mast cell, a large cell in connective tissue with many coarse granules containing the chemicals heparin, histamine, and serotonin, which are released during inflammation and allergic responses. Mast cell diseases (known collectively as MASTOCYTOSIS) include a wide variety of different conditions characterized by tissue invaded by mast cells. These conditions include crops of benign hyperpigmented MACULES or PAPULES (URTICARIA PIGMENTOSA), small nodules common in young children (mastocytoma), and malignant mast cell leukemia. Urticaria pigmentosa is the most common of these diseases. MASTOCYTOMAS represent 10 percent of all cases of mast cell diseases.

Symptoms and Diagnostic Path
Symptoms may include flushing, nausea, vomiting, upper stomach pain, hives, itching, and shock, or "mastocytosis syndrome."

Treatment Options and Outlook
Most patients with mast cell diseases can expect an excellent prognosis with an uncomplicated recovery. In children, the skin lesions often clear up on their own, but in adulthood the lesions don't usually disappear. Occasionally, patients may experience systemic involvement with collections of mast cells in internal organs and a progressively more serious decline into a lymphomalike illness, but this is uncommon. A few cases become malignant.

mastocytomas One of the more common MAST CELL DISEASES that is found almost exclusively in children, characterized by a solitary brown-tan plaque rather like an orange peel (PEAU D'ORANGE) that itches when stroked. Adults do not develop exterior symptoms from mastocytomas.

Symptoms and Diagnostic Path
Mastocytomas usually are diagnosed at birth or within the first few weeks of life. Usually solitary, they may occur in groups of up to four, and they are most often found on the body, neck, and arm (especially near the wrist). The brown/tan plaques may swell or itch, usually the result of gentle rubbing or scratching. BLISTERs also may develop from the plaques. Attacks of flushing (either on the face or all over the body) may occur, sometimes related to bumping the lesion.

Treatment Options and Outlook
While isolated mastocytomas may be removed, it may be best to leave them alone since they almost always spontaneously disappear. Most children

who develop this condition before age five will outgrow it by adolescence or early adulthood. When mastocytosis begins after age five, the abnormal collections of mast cells may sometimes involve the internal organs, and the plaque may not go away.

mastocytosis   The most common variety of MAST CELL DISEASE (also known as urticaria pigmentosa), this unusual condition is characterized by many itchy, yellow or orange-brown MACULES on the skin.

Symptoms and Diagnostic Path

Macules are most often found on the trunk and seldom the face, although they can appear anywhere on the body. The macules range in size from a few millimeters to several centimeters. The skin condition generally worsens after bathing or scratching the skin. Mastocytosis usually appears during the first 12 months of infancy and fades away by adolescence.

Treatment Options and Outlook

There is no satisfactory treatment, although ANTIHISTAMINES such as Benadryl can help control ITCHING, HIVES, and flushing.

Risk Factors and Preventive Measures

Patients should avoid aspirin, codeine, opiates, alcohol, polymyxin B, hot baths, and vigorous rubbing after bathing and showering, since these can release histamine, which can trigger hives, itching, and flushing.

mastopexy   The medical term for reshaping the breasts by trimming excess skin and raising the nipple. Drooping breasts usually follow significant weight loss or frequent childbirth.

In mild cases, the breast appearance can be improved simply by placing an implant underneath the breast tissue in a procedure similar to breast augmentation (see MAMMOPLASTY). In this procedure, the implant fills out the extra skin and raises the nipple, giving the entire breast a more youthful appearance. This process also makes the breast larger; in patients who do not want larger breasts—just more youthful-looking ones—the surgeon can perform a mastopexy. This does leave the same scars as a breast reduction. With this technique, however, nipple sensations are usually left undisturbed and there may be no loss of the ability to breastfeed.

measles   A childhood viral illness causing a widespread blotchy, slightly elevated pink rash, which develops first behind the ears and then elsewhere. The rash lasts from three to five days. Although a commonplace disease, complications (including pneumonia) can lead to death. One attack usually confers lifelong immunity. The patient is infectious while the rash lasts; complete recovery may take two to four weeks.

Once common throughout the world, only about 44 cases of measles were reported in the United States, because of strict vaccination requirements for school-age children. No measles deaths have been reported in the United States in the past few years, but measles still kills more than 1 million victims a year in developing countries—especially among malnourished children with impaired immunity.

The measles virus is very contagious, and is spread by airborne droplets from nasal secretions. Symptoms appear after an incubation period of between nine to 11 days. The patient is infectious from shortly after the beginning of this period until up to a week after symptoms have developed. Infants under eight months of age rarely contract measles, because they still harbor some immunity from their mothers.

Symptoms and Diagnostic Path

The disease begins with a fever, runny nose, sore eyes and cough; the rash appears after three or four days, beginning on the head and neck and spreading down to cover the entire body. The spots may be so numerous that they blend together as a large red area. The rash begins to fade within three days.

Treatment Options and Outlook

Fluids and acetaminophen are given for fever. Antibiotics will not help the virus, but may be needed to treat a secondary infection.

The most common complications include ear and chest infections, usually occurring as the fever returns a few days after the rash appears. There may also be diarrhea, vomiting, and abdominal pain. About one in every 1,000 patients goes on to develop encephalitis (brain inflammation), with headache, drowsiness, and vomiting, beginning seven to 10 days after the rash begins. This may be followed by seizures and coma, sometimes leading to mental retardation or death. (Note: seizures are common with measles and do not necessarily indicate the presence of encephalitis). Very rarely (one in a million cases) a progressive brain disorder called subacute sclerosing panencephalitis develops many years after the illness.

A woman who contracts measles during pregnancy will lose the baby in about one-fifth of cases, but there is no evidence that measles causes birth defects. GERMAN MEASLES during pregnancy can cause birth defects if the mother contracts the disease during early pregnancy. For this reason, girls should be immunized before puberty.

Risk Factors and Preventive Measures

In the United States, children are routinely vaccinated early in the second year by an injection usually combined with mumps and rubella that produces immunity in 97 percent of patients. Side effects of the vaccine are reported to be mild, including low fever, slight cold, and a rash about a week after the shot.

The vaccine should not be given to infants under age one, to those with a history of epilepsy in the family, or to those who have had seizures before. In these cases, simultaneous injection of measles-specific immunoglobulin, which contains antibodies against the virus, should be given.

mechlorethamine A nitrogen mustard used for the past 30 years as a topical treatment for early stages of mycosis fungoides (a disease featuring chronic irritating eruptions). It is administered either as a liquid or ointment, usually over the entire body on a daily basis. Lesions clear up in between 50 and 75 percent of cases within two to six months, although prolonged treatment may be required for more stubborn cases. Some experts recommend daily treatments for six months even after active lesions have disappeared in order to prevent recurrence, but the value of maintenance therapy has not been established.

Mechlorethamine is not effective in those with advanced tumor-stage mycosis fungoides.

Side Effects

This medication is relatively less toxic than other antitumor agents, although more than half of all patients develop an irritant or contact dermatitis. Nitrogen mustard causes fewer problems when applied as an ointment in lower concentrations, gradually increasing the concentration over time. The drug should be stopped if diffuse hyperpigmentation occurs.

See also BASAL CELL CARCINOMA; SQUAMOUS CELL CARCINOMA.

Mees' lines Single or multiple white horizontal bands on the nails that are a sign of arsenic poisoning.

Meissner's touch corpuscles One of three specialized nerve endings found in the skin. Meissner's touch corpuscles are oval structures composed of coiled terminal axons within a basal lamina and collagen fibers. They are primarily found in the palms and soles, and appear to assist in the sensory function of touch.

melanin The pigment that gives skin, hair, and the iris of the eyes their color; the more melanin present, the darker the color. Its level depends on race, heredity, and sun exposure.

Melanin is produced by cells called melanocytes (PIGMENT CELLS), special cells of the EPIDERMIS that are controlled in part by the pituitary gland and by a hormone secreted from the hypothalamus called MELANOCYTE-STIMULATING HORMONE (MSH). Melanocytes produce two types of melanin, eumelanin and phaeomelanin; eumelanin is black or brown, and phaeomelanin is red. The ratio of these two pigments determines hair and skin color.

Exposure to sunlight stimulates a protection reaction by the melanocytes that darkens the skin by increasing melanin. Ultraviolet light B (UVB) increases the production of melanin; UVA oxidizes already-existing melanin to produce immediate darkening. UVB tanning is the slow darkening that develops after several days after sun exposure. Localized excess melanin production causes FRECKLES and lentigines. Many chemical agents stimulate the production of melanin. Other agents that boost melanin production include prostaglandin E2, estrogens and other hormones, and some chemotherapy drugs (such as bleomycin). Ingested metals such as arsenic can darken skin by depositing melanin in the DERMIS.

PSORALENS are organic compounds found in many plants, such as limes and celery, that in combination with UVA stimulate the formation of melanin.

See also DEPIGMENTATION DISORDER; PIGMENTATION; PIGMENTATION, DISORDERS OF.

melanocytes See PIGMENT CELLS.

melanocyte-stimulating hormone (MSH) A hormone that regulates human skin color by stimulating the production of MELANIN. Four different MSH peptides have been identified, all of which are formed in the pituitary gland. Lack of MSH (such as in HYPOPITUITARISM) may cause a decrease of skin color all over the body.

See also PIGMENTATION; PIGMENTATION, DISORDERS OF; PIGMENT CELLS.

melanocyte system, tumors of Tumors that include MOLES, congenital nevus, Spitz nevus (see NEVUS, SPITZ), dysplastic nevus syndrome, halo nevus (see NEVUS, HALO); blue nevus (see NEVUS, BLUE), lentigines (see LENTIGO; LENTIGO MALIGNA), malignant melanoma (see MELANOMA, MALIGNANT).

See also PIGMENT CELLS; PIGMENTATION.

melanoma See MELANOMA, MALIGNANT.

melanoma, acral lentiginous The second least common of four types of malignant melanoma accounting for only 10 percent of all melanomas. It is, however, the most common malignant melanoma in African Americans and Asians. The diagnosis of this form of melanoma is often delayed, which can be fatal.

Symptoms and Diagnostic Path
Lesions are found on the palms, soles, fingers, and toes, or on the mucosal surfaces. The first signs of acral lentiginous melanoma may appear as a darker streak in the nail, sometimes appearing with a brown discolored cuticle (Hutchinson's sign). Not all darker streaks in the nail are the result of malignant lesions. As the lesion develops it may be brown, black, pink, or blue occasionally becoming a nodule, which may ulcerate.

Treatment Options and Outlook
Treatment of acral lentiginous melanoma is described under malignant melanoma.

See also MELANOMA, JUVENILE; MELANOMA, LENTIGO MALIGNA; MELANOMA, MALIGNANT.

melanoma, juvenile Historic name for NEVUS, SPITZ.

melanoma, lentigo maligna A type of malignant lesion that develops from a preexisting lesion of LENTIGO MALIGNA (melanotic Hutchinson's freckle); it makes up about 5 percent of all primary skin melanomas. These lesions, which tend to occur in older women patients, always are found in sun-exposed areas (especially the face).

This type of malignancy tends to grow over a long period of time; the original pigmented lesion appears 10 to 15 years before it becomes malignant. This transformation takes place in up to 5 percent of all patients with lentigo maligna.

Melanoma first appears within the lesion as a slow-growing, deeply colored nodule. Once the malignant cells have invaded the dermis, they may spread as any other type of melanoma.

Treatment Options and Outlook

Treatment for lentigo maligna melanoma is the same as for malignant melanoma.

See also MELANOMA, ACRAL LENTIGINOUS; MELANOMA, MALIGNANT; MELANOSIS.

melanoma, malignant The most deadly form of the three major types of SKIN CANCER, melanomas are brown, black, or multicolored patches, plaques, or NODULES with an irregular outline. Malignant melanoma is much more dangerous than other forms of skin cancer because of its tendency to spread rapidly to vital internal organs such as the lungs, liver, and brain. One in five patients afflicted with malignant melanoma dies of this cancer. It is the most frequently diagnosed cancer among women between 25 and 29, and it ranks second in frequency of occurrence only to breast cancer among those aged 30 to 34.

In 1935 when few people habitually baked at the beach, melanoma was a rare disease, affecting only one in 1,500 Americans. Today, the worldwide incidence of melanoma is increasing at a faster rate than any other type of cancer, with the exception of lung cancer in women. In the United States alone, the incidence has tripled in the last 40 years, nearly doubling in the last decade. An estimated 59,580 Americans will develop melanoma in 2005. Since 1981, the incidence has increased about 3 percent a year.

Those at highest risk have a family history of skin cancer, an abundance of moles (more than 100), fair skin, light hair, and blue-green or gray eyes. A defective gene on chromosome 9 causes an inherited tendency to this type of deadly skin cancer, and that may also play a role in non-inherited melanoma. About 10 percent of melanoma occurs in people with an inherited tendency, and it is unclear what percentage of inherited cases are due to this gene.

Normally, the gene acts as a brake on cancer, but those who inherit a defective version lose part of their protection, making them unusually susceptible to melanoma. The normal gene tells the body how to make a protein called p16, which helps regulate cell division.

Defective versions of the gene also may be involved in many or even most cases of noninherited melanoma, according to research. In those cases, the gene would be inherited in normal form but would mutate following exposure to sunlight or other causes. Researchers hope that studying this gene may someday lead to a screening test for those at risk, and for better treatments for the noninherited disease.

Other risk factors for developing melanoma are severe SUNBURNS in childhood; even one severe burn during childhood or adolescence is a potent precursor of melanoma later in life. Anyone with multiple moles may also suffer from dysplastic nevus syndrome and may be at increased risk for the development of melanoma.

All patients with a history of malignant melanoma have about 5 percent risk of developing another separate, unrelated melanoma of the skin. This process is called multiple primary melanoma formation. If a second melanoma of the skin develops in a patient with a history of melanoma, it is very important to determine whether it is a new skin melanoma (second primary) or a spreading to the skin from the original melanoma. If the lesion has spread, the disease must be classified as Stage III and the likelihood of death in five years rises significantly.

Although melanoma many times begins without the presence of a mole, it most frequently does begin inside a mole. Interestingly, melanoma can arise within all three major categories of moles:

- atypical (dysplastic, unusual) nevus
- congenital (existing at birth) nevus
- plain ordinary moles, which are totally different from seborrheic keratoses

Symptoms and Diagnostic Path

Melanoma usually begins as a pigmented growth on the skin, displaying many shades of color (including brown, black, pink, white, blue, or gray). It often has irregular outlines and may be larger than ordinary moles. The spots may crust, bleed, or itch, and at times they may develop within preexisting MOLES. It is therefore important that any moles that change in any way be examined by a DERMATOLO-GIST. Congenital moles (present at birth) seem to have an increased risk of becoming malignant, and therefore should be examined early in life by a dermatologist. There are four types of melanoma, each with a characteristic growth pattern:

- *Superficial spreading melanoma* This is the most common type, accounting for 70 percent of all cases. This type typically arises from a preexisting nevus and expands in a radial fashion before it enters a vertical growth phase.

- *Nodular melanoma* A more aggressive tumor found more often in men, this accounts for approximately 15 to 30 percent of cases. It begins from normal skin and has no radial growth phase.

- *Lentigo maligna melanoma* This type accounts for less than 10 percent of cases and is found more commonly on the face in females and the elderly. The lesions, typically large and flat, are slow growing and rarely spread.

- *Acral lentiginous melanoma* This type, which occurs on the soles of the feet, accounts for less than 10 percent of lesions but occurs in a higher proportion (35 percent to 60 percent) of nonwhite patients.

Because the skin is so easily seen, malignant melanoma can be easier to spot than internal malignancies. To make sure that people notice skin cancer, dermatologists recommend that everyone examine their skin twice a year, using a full-length and a hand-held mirror. Any suspicious growths should be reported immediately to a dermatologist.

Treatment Options and Outlook

Most skin cancers—even malignant melanomas—can be cured if discovered early enough, which is why attention to symptoms and regular self-examination is highly recommended. When cancers of the skin are discovered early, there are a variety of treatment possibilities, depending on the type of tumor, size, location, and other factors affecting the patient's general health. A biopsy is often needed before a treatment option is selected.

Surgical removal of the tumor and a margin of normal skin is usually required, together with possible surgical removal of nearby lymph nodes. A skin graft may be necessary after the tumor is removed. Tumor removal may be accompanied or followed by radiation, chemotherapy, or medications that stimulate the immune system, such as interferon.

The thickness of the tumor is the single most important factor in determining prognosis. Approximately 77 percent (men) to 88 percent (women) of all malignant melanomas may be cured if treated early. The cure rate approaches 100 percent if the melanoma is found early enough. If deep local spread occurs, the number of people who live for at least five years is about 30 percent. With spread of cancer to distant sites, five-year survival is less than 10 percent.

Scientists have been working on creating a "cancer vaccine" that can prime the immune system to recognize malignant cells and target them for destruction. (The cancer vaccine is a treatment for existing disease; it is called a "vaccine" because it enlists the immune system to kill malignant cells.)

Researchers now report that destroying healthy skin cells can incite the immune system to kill the cancerous versions of these cells, with only mild side effects. The potential treatment targets pigment cells (melanocytes) that, when malignant, become melanoma. In mouse studies, scientists administered a vaccine containing DNA plus an antiviral drug to mice in a series of injections. In response to the treatment, the mice lost not only melanoma cells but also many healthy melanocytes, leaving the black mice with white splotches of hair that lasted for months. The mice remained tumor-free for at least 100 days after receiving the vaccine.

However, when the team implanted new tumors in the mice 100 days after the first tumors had been destroyed, the protection had faded and the mice died of melanoma.

Risk Factors and Preventive Measures

In addition to avoiding excess sun exposure, new research isolating a gene defect that may lead to some cases of malignant melanoma may be used as a screen for people at risk for the disease. These patients could then be counseled to take steps like avoiding too much sun, keeping track of possible precancerous moles, and using SUNSCREEN.

In addition, scientists have found that some foods and nutrients may counteract the development of melanoma: best choices are fish with omega-3 fat and antioxidants (including VITAMINS E and C and beta-carotene). In one Australian study, those who ate a half-ounce of fish daily were less likely to have melanoma than those who ate only one-fifth of an ounce of fish daily.

Melanotan A synthetic hormone that mimics the action of melanocyte-stimulating hormone (MSH), the hormone that induces a tan after sun exposure. It was created and developed at the University of Arizona and the Arizona Cancer Center in 1991. Not yet approved for use by the U.S. Food and Drug Administration, Melanotan may be an effective preventative treatment for people at risk for SKIN CANCER. So far, it is effective only when administered by injection, not orally. Its developers hope it can reduce the risk of skin cancer in high-risk individuals by offering them the protective benefit of a tan without the harm of sun exposure. Its developers believe that Melanotan is effective in promoting skin pigmentation with little or no risk. Its role in actually preventing skin cancer has not yet been determined.

However, it cannot help individuals with ALBINISM or VITILIGO, because these patients do not have skin cells (melanocytes) with receptors for MSH.

The company developing the product claims it will not leave streaks, blotches or, bare spots that are common with other sunless tanning creams and lotions. It is currently undergoing clinical trials.

melanotic freckle of Hutchison See LENTIGO, MALIGNA.

melasma See CHLOASMA.

melioidosis See WHITMORE'S DISEASE.

Mendes da Costa syndrome A disorder of KERATINIZATION also known as erythrokeratodermia variabilis, this is a rare disorder characterized by two types of lesions—fixed plaques and shifting red rings or arcs frequently caused by temperature change. This genetic disorder is carried by only one defective gene (from one parent). Each child of an affected person usually has a one in two chance of inheriting the defective gene and of being affected.

Symptoms and Diagnostic Path

The plaques are most often found on the face, extremities, and buttocks; the red rings may last up to hours or days. It is a form of ICHTHYOSIS, a group of hereditary skin disorders characterized by scaly skin patches.

Treatment Options and Outlook

Treatment with topical and oral retinoids has eased the condition in many patients. Etretinate is often effective, although symptoms rapidly return when treatment stops. Even with treatment, however, this condition is chronic and lasts a lifetime.

meningococcal infections Infections caused by the bacteria *Neisseria meningitidis* that may cause a rash ranging from masses of tiny pinhead-sized red dots to large blue-purple hemorrhagic areas or extensive gangrene. In the few who lack immunity, the meningiococcus bacteria infects the lining of the brain as a form of MENINGITIS, or the bloodstream as either acute or chronic meningococcemia.

The disease is transmitted most often through the air in winter or by nasal droplets in spring. If the infection is introduced to people is closed quarters, it can become epidemic. Spread by a cough, a sneeze, a kiss, or a shared drink, it can kill a healthy teenager within hours.

Symptoms and Diagnostic Path

In addition to the rash, other symptoms include fever, headache, vomiting, delirium, convulsions, stiff neck, and back. Acute meningoccemia is rapidly progressive and often fatal, and needs early and aggressive diagnosis and treatment.

Treatment Options and Outlook

Aqueous penicillin G must be administered every 24 hours for seven to 10 days by IV (or until the patient's fever subsides for five days) to cure the infection. There is a vaccine for group A and group C meningococci. Treatment should also include symptom control, such as reducing fever, maintaining fluid and electrolyte balance, and administering heparin when necessary.

Menkes' kinky-hair syndrome　A hereditary syndrome characterized by twisted, beaded (monilethrix) or fragile (trichorrhexis nodosa) hair shafts, usually associated with mental retardation, seizures and problems in walking or balance.

Symptoms and Diagnostic Path

The syndrome, which is caused by a problem with copper metabolism, causes poor absorption, with low blood and tissue copper levels. Most untreated patients die by the age of four; many survive less than two years.

The condition is an X-linked recessive disorder, which means that it is caused by a defect on the X chromosome, usually leading to problems in boys only. Women can be carriers of the defect, and half of their sons may be affected.

Treatment Options and Outlook

There is no treatment; supplements of intravenous copper are not effective.

menthol　A soothing white substance derived from oil of peppermint that is included in many skin-care products because it feels cool to the touch and may help relieve ITCHING.

Merkel cell cancer　A rare type of malignancy that develops on or just beneath the skin and in hair follicles on the face, head, and neck. Researchers believe that exposure to sunlight may increase a person's risk of this disease. People taking drugs to suppress their immune system after an organ transplant can develop Merkel cell cancer quickly.

The cause of Merkel cell cancer (a type of neuroendocrine cancer of the skin) is not known. However, researchers have learned that it can develop quickly in people who have had an organ transplant and are taking drugs to suppress their immune system. Exposure to arsenic may also increase the risk for Merkel cell cancer. Because this disease occurs so often on the face, head, neck, and extremities, researchers believe that exposure to sunlight may play a role.

Symptoms and Diagnostic Path

This cancer is characterized by firm, painless, red, pink, or blue smooth shiny lumps that vary in size from less than a quarter of an inch to more than two inches. About half of all Merkel cell cancers occur on the sun-exposed areas of the head and neck; another third appear on the arms and legs. Occasionally, tumors also may begin on other parts of the body. This type of cancer occurs mostly often in white men between 60 and 80.

Early detection is important because the disease can spread rapidly, and Merkel cell cancer is difficult to cure once it spreads. However, it is not easy to diagnose this type of cancer because Merkel cells often look like cells found in other types of cancers (especially lung cancer). To diagnose it, a tissue sample is removed from the abnormal area and biopsied. The doctor will also conduct a detailed skin exam, examine lymph nodes for signs of swelling, and may order blood cell counts, a liver functions test, or a CT scan.

Treatment Options and Outlook

Surgery to remove the tumor is the usual treatment for Merkel cell cancer. If the tumor cannot be removed, the patient may require radiation or chemotherapy to try to shrink the tumor. Lymph nodes are often removed because they may contain cancer cells; radiation may be directed at the site of the surgery and at nearby lymph nodes to destroy any remaining cancer cells.

Even fairly small Merkel cell tumors can grow rapidly and often spread to other parts of the body, most often to the regional lymph nodes, or the liver, bones, lungs, and brain. Merkel cell cancer that has spread may respond to chemotherapy, but it is not usually curable by this method.

metabolic disorders, skin signs of Disorders of metabolism often include symptoms of skin abnormalities. In some disorders, skin changes are the first signal of an underlying metabolic problem.

Metabolic diseases with skin symptoms include disorders of amino acid metabolism (phenylketonuria, homocystinuria, ochronosis, HARTNUP DISEASE, arginosuccinic aciduria, and tyrosinemia type II). Diseases of lipid metabolism include xanthomatoses, REFSUM'S DISEASE, XANTHELASMA, GAUCHER'S DISEASE, and FABRY'S DISEASE. Diseases of metal metabolism include problems with the metabolism of ZINC (acrodermatitis enteropathica), iron (HEMOCHROMATOSIS), or copper (WILSON'S DISEASE) and may result in numerous skin signs.

Other metabolic disorders include AMYLOIDOSIS, MUCINOSES, LICHEN MYXEDEMATOSUS, URBACH-WIETHE DISEASE, MUCOPOLYSACCHARIDOSES, FUCOSIDOSIS, gout, and Lesch-Nyhan syndrome.

methotrexate Sometimes used to treat PSORIASIS, this powerful anticancer drug can cause many unpleasant side effects. (It can also make the skin increasingly sensitive to sunlight.) **It should never be given to anyone besides the patient for whom it is prescribed for any purpose, since patients require close medical supervision.**

Side Effects

Possible effects include severe nausea and vomiting, diarrhea and mouth ulcers, black stools, sore throat, fever, chills, unusual bleeding and bruising, abdominal pain, anemia, increased susceptibility to infections, abnormal bleeding, and liver damage with long-term use. Extra fluid intake eases methotrexate toxicity. Infrequently, side effects can include hair loss, dizziness, seizures, shortness of breath, and rash.

Physicians perform routine follow-up medical evaluations in all patients taking methotrexate, including tests to check liver and kidney functions and complete blood counts.

Methotrexate may negatively interact with a range of other drugs. Possible toxicity could occur when taken with anticonvulsants, antigout drugs, diclofenac, nonsteroidal anti-inflammatory drugs, oxyphenbutazone, phenylbutazone, phenytoin, probenecid, pyrimethamine, salicylates (including aspirin), sulfadoxine and pyrimethamine, sulfa drugs, and TETRACYCLINES.

methoxsalen A PSORALEN drug used to treat PSORIASIS, MYCOSIS FUNGOIDES, and VITILIGO that belongs to the class of repigmenting agents. It is taken as a tablet or capsule two to four hours before exposure to sunlight or a sunlamp. In the treatment of vitiligo, it may take between six to nine months before results are apparent; results may be seen in 10 weeks or more for psoriasis.

See also PUVA.

Side Effects

In addition to the above, common side effects include increased skin and eye sensitivity to the sun, and nausea. Other possible side effects include red and sore skin, dizziness, headache, depression, leg cramps, or insomnia.

Precautions

Methoxsalen should not be taken with any other medication that causes skin sensitivity to the sun. Patients should avoid alcohol in any form from 12 hours before taking the drug to at least 24 hours afterward. Combining alcohol with methoxsalen may result in a reaction causing flushed face, severe headache, chest pains, shortness of breath, nausea and vomiting, sweating, and weakness; severe reactions may be fatal.

methyl paraben A preservative used in eyeliners, hair care products, and cold creams that is the frequent cause of allergic reaction to cosmetics.

metronidazole (Trade names: Flagyl, Metryl, Prostat, Satric) An antibiotic particularly useful in fighting infections of the urinary, genital, and digestive systems such as trichomoniasis, amebiasis, and giardiasis, and for the treatment of ROSACEA. It is administered by mouth or by suppository.

Side Effects

Rarely, side effects may include nausea and vomiting, appetite loss, abdominal pain, metallic taste, and dark-colored urine. Drinking alcohol during treatment with this drug can trigger particularly unpleasant reactions, such as nausea, vomiting, hot flashes, headache, and so on.

miconazole   Antifungal agent used for topical treatment of DERMATOPHYTES.

microdermabrasion   An effective skin-freshening technique used to repair the skin, reducing fine lines, sun-induced, age spots, and superficial ACNE scars by removing the very outer layer of skin, and by stimulating the production of skin cells and COLLAGEN. Microdermabrasion is one of the top five nonsurgical cosmetic procedures; more than 1 million microdermabrasions were completed in 2004 (an increase of 28 percent), according to the American Society of Dermatologic Surgery (ASDS). Simple and quick to perform, this painless procedure does not require anesthesia, can be repeated at short intervals, and does not significantly interrupt the patient's life. Microdermabrasion is well suited for patient with mild skin damage as a result of sun exposure and who have busy lifestyles, because the only real down time is during the treatment itself. The procedure does not require an anesthetic and is effective on all skin colors and types.

For thousands of years individuals in search of younger-looking skin have tried to resurface their faces by using a variety of abrasive techniques, using acids, poultices of minerals and plants, and irritants such as fire or rough materials. Microdermabrasion as experts perform it today was developed in Italy in 1985 and quickly spread throughout Europe; eventually, physicians in the United States began to use the procedure as well.

During the procedure, the physician, nurse, or aesthetician uses a sort of sandblasting device to spray the surface of the skin with high-pressure crystals that gently abrades and suctions away the dead outer layer of skin, gently polishing the area as it lessens wrinkles. The handpiece is moved over the treatment area in a single, smooth stroke. Thicker skin on the forehead, chin, and nose can be treated more aggressively.

Each treatment takes between 15 minutes to an hour, and is usually repeated five to six times typically spaced two to four weeks. After the initial series of treatments, monthly to four-times-a-year maintenance treatments are usually recommended, depending on the patient. Microdermabrasion may be combined or alternated with a light chemical peel to increase the effect.

Microdermabrasion is only effective for fine lines and more superficial scars; it is ineffective for deeper wrinkles or scars, or anything but the most superficial pigmentary abnormalities. These are best treated with other methods, such as chemical peels, DERMABRASION, NON-ABLATIVE SKIN REJUVENATION, and LASER RESURFACING.

Risks and Complications

Unlike other skin resurfacing techniques such as dermabrasion, chemical peels, and laser resurfacing, microdermabrasion has fewer significant risks of pigmentary changes or scarring, even though it requires multiple treatments.

Outlook and Lifestyle Modification

After the procedure, the treated area is cleaned with a wet cloth to remove any leftover crystals. After drying, a moisturizer or ointment is applied. Redness usually improves within hours after treatment, allowing a quick return to normal activities. However, the patient may experience a mild sunburnlike sensation for a few days.

The procedure gives the skin an overall fresh, healthy-looking glow without side effects. Normal activities can be resumed immediately. Patients who have good skin tone will show the best results.

After microdermabrasion the skin's appearance can be enhanced even more with topical skin treatments such as TRETINOIN, ALPHA-HYDROXY ACIDS, RETINOIC ACID, and topical VITAMIN C. Patients being treated for HYPERPIGMENTATION (excess skin color) should apply hydroquinone between treatments.

An individualized skin care program, including use of sun blocks and protection from photoaging, is usually recommended for best results. Liberal use of SUNSCREEN and moisturizers can help improve the appearance of the skin by helping to remove skin cells and decrease sensitivity to the sun. The price of a microdermabrasion treatment ranges from $100 to $200.

Scarring has not been documented from microdermabrasion because the procedure barely affects the skin any deeper than the outer layer. This is the reason for both its strong and weak points: Superficial injury results in quick healing and recovery with little risk, but because it is superficial, only fine lines, skin quality, shallow scars, mild sun damage, AGE SPOTS, acne scars, and enlarged pores can be treated. It is not effective for deep wrinkles and scars or ice-pick acne scars because these lesions extend into the deeper layers of the skin. This is also why it does not work for pigment problems such as melasma or post-inflammatory hyperpigmentation, because this treatment does not effectively address the DERMIS, where these problems begin. Instead, patients with these problems should be treated with more traditional resurfacing techniques, such as chemical peels, dermabrasion, NON-ABLATIVE SKIN REJUVENATION, or laser resurfacing.

microlipoinjection   See SKIN FILLERS.

milia   Also known as epidermal cysts, these small, firm white PAPULES are usually found in clusters on upper cheeks and around the eyes. They are commonly (but wrongly) called SEBACEOUS CYSTS. These cysts are extremely common, appearing equally in all races, all ages, and both genders. Milia in newborns are so common that they are considered normal.

Milia are also found in about 40 percent of full-term infants on the forehead, cheeks, and nose.

Symptoms and Diagnostic Path
Milia are superficial, pearly white to yellowish domed lesions that usually appear on the face. About 40 percent of infants have the bumps, which are especially common around the nose, forehead, and cheeks, and also in the mouth. Primary milia in older children and adults also

develop on the face, particularly around the eyes. Secondary milia can be found anywhere on the body at the sites affected by whatever is causing the milia. Eruptive milia occur on the head, neck, and upper body.

Painless and harmless, these bumps may also appear after an injury, chronic ultraviolet light exposure, or BLISTERS, or as a result of blocked PORES.

Treatment Options and Outlook
Epidermal cysts and milia may be removed for cosmetic reasons or to prevent rupture using a fine-gauge needle and a cotton-tipped swab, or a comedone extractor. Inflamed lesions respond well to incision and drainage. Antibiotics are not normally required, unless pathogenic bacteria are present. In infants, no treatment is necessary.

miliaria   A common disorder of the eccrine SWEAT GLANDS that often occurs during hot, humid weather. It is believed to result from blocked sweat ducts, so that eccrine sweat leaks into the epidermis or dermis layers of the skin. The three types of miliaria are classified according to the level at which obstruction of the sweat duct occurs:

- *miliaria crystallina* In this condition, ductal obstruction is least severe, producing tiny, fragile, clear blisters
- *miliaria rubra* (PRICKLY HEAT) In this condition, obstruction occurs deeper within the EPIDERMIS, causing extremely itchy red PAPULES
- *miliaria profunda* This condition obstructs ducts at the junction of the DERMIS and EPIDERMIS, leaking sweat into the dermis and producing subtle flesh-colored papules

Miliaria occurs in individuals of all races, although some studies have shown that Asians, who produce less sweat than Caucasians, are less likely to develop miliaria rubra. Miliaria crystallina and miliaria rubra can occur at any age, but are most common in infancy. Two cases of congenital miliaria crystallina have been reported. Miliaria profunda is more common in adulthood.

High heat and humidity that triggers excess sweating is the primary cause for the development of miliaria. Binding the skin with clothing or bandages can further contribute to pooling of sweat on the skin surface and overhydration of the top layer of the epidermis (stratum corneum). If hot, humid conditions persist, the individual will continue to produce excessive sweat but will be unable to secrete the sweat onto the skin surface due to the blocked ducts. This leads to leakage of sweat en route to the skin surface, either in the dermis or in the epidermis. When the point of leakage is in the stratum corneum or just below (as in miliaria crystallina), there is little inflammation. In miliaria rubra, however, leakage of sweat into the subcorneal layers produces blisters. In miliaria profunda, escape of sweat into the papillary dermis leads to white or red papules that usually do not itch.

Normal skin bacteria, such as *Staphylococcus epidermidis*, are thought to play a role in the development of miliaria. Patients with miliaria have three times as many bacteria as healthy people.

Symptoms and Diagnostic Path

Miliaria crystallina is a common condition in infants, most often at one week of age, and in feverish individuals or those who have recently moved to a hot, humid climate. Miliaria rubra is also common in infants and in adults who have moved to a tropical environment, occurring in up to 30 percent of people exposed to such conditions. Miliaria profunda is more rare, seen only in a minority of those who have had repeated bouts of miliaria rubra.

Miliaria crystallina is usually quite mild and gets better without complications over a period of days, although it may recur if hot, humid conditions persist. Miliaria rubra also tends to improve spontaneously when patients are removed to a cooler environment. Unlike patients with miliaria crystallina, however, those with miliaria rubra tend to have a lot of itching and stinging. They develop a lack of sweat in affected sites that may last weeks and, if generalized, may lead to heat exhaustion. Secondary infection is another possible complication of miliaria rubra, either as IMPETIGO or as multiple discrete ABSCESSes known as periporitis staphylogenes.

Miliaria profunda is itself a complication of repeated episodes of miliaria rubra. The lesions of miliaria profunda do not cause symptoms, but patients may develop compensatory excess facial sweating and a widespread inability to sweat elsewhere, resulting from eccrine duct rupture: This is known as tropical anhidrotic asthenia and predisposes patients to heat exhaustion during exertion in warm climates.

Treatment Options and Outlook

There is no reason to treat miliaria crystallina, as this condition will go away on its own and does not cause unpleasant symptoms. However, miliaria rubra can be very uncomfortable, and miliaria profunda may lead to heat exhaustion, so treatment of these two conditions is necessary.

Topical treatments may include lotions containing CALAMINE, boric acid, or menthol; cool wet-to-dry compresses; frequent showering with soap (although some doctors discourage excess soap); topical CORTICOSTEROIDS, and topical antibiotics. Topical application of anhydrous LANOLIN has resulted in dramatic improvement in patients with miliaria profunda. Anhydrous lanolin is believed to prevent ductal blockage, allowing sweat to flow to the skin surface. Calamine lotion provides cooling relief.

It may be possible to prevent miliaria by using oral antibiotics. Patients have also been treated with oral retinoids, VITAMIN A, and VITAMIN C with variable success. However, there have been no controlled studies to demonstrate the effectiveness of any of these treatments.

Since increased exertion leads to sweating, which greatly worsens miliaria, patients should limit activity (especially in hot weather) until the miliaria is cured. Patients with miliaria profunda are at particularly high risk for heat exhaustion during exertion in hot weather, since they have trouble dissipating heat via evaporation of sweat.

Risk Factors and Preventive Measures

Prevention of miliaria consist primarily of controlling heat and humidity so that the patient is not stimulated to sweat. This may mean treating a fever, reducing tight clothing, limiting activity, providing air-conditioning, or (as a last resort) moving the patient to a cooler climate.

miliaria apocrine   See FOX-FORDYCE DISORDER.

miliaria tuberculosis   See TUBERCULOSIS, SKIN.

milker's nodule   A viral infection by a pox virus that causes tricolored, sometimes-painful, black, red, and white nodules on the fingers of people who milk cows. The poxvirus (paravaccinia) is found widely among cattle and can cause lesions called pseudocowpox in the animals. Cross-species infection can occur when human skin touches these lesions.

Symptoms and Diagnostic Path
Generally, a single red macule appears on the finger (although multiple lesions may occur) between four and seven days after infection. It progresses into a three-colored papule with a crusted center surrounded by a whitish area, in turn surrounded by a red base.

Treatment Options and Outlook
There is no specific treatment, and the lesion usually heals on its own, although it may leave a scar. Topical antibiotics may help to minimize the risk of secondary bacterial infection.

Risk Factors and Preventive Measures
Infected cows should be isolated, and protective gloves should be worn when coming in contact with infected animals.

mineral oil   A clear, odorless oil derived from petroleum that is widely used in cosmetics because it is inexpensive and rarely causes allergic reactions. It can, however, sometimes induce ACNE lesions.

minocycline (Trade name: Minocin)   A tetracycline antibiotic used to treat ACNE.

minoxidil (Rogaine)   A drug that widens blood vessels, used in a topical solution on the scalp to treat androgenetic alopecia (also known as pattern baldness) in men and diffuse hair loss or thinning of the front and top of the scalp in women. It was approved by the Food and Drug Administration in 1988 as a lotion treatment for male pattern baldness, and in 1991 for women with hair loss.

Research has found that after four months, about 25 percent of 2,300 men with male pattern baldness reported moderate to dense hair regrowth, compared with 11 percent using placebo. No regrowth was reported by 41 percent (60 percent using placebo). After one year, 48 percent of those who continued to use minoxidil rated their new hair growth as moderate or better.

Studies have shown that the response to the drug varies a great deal from one person to the next, but patients should not expect to see regrowth before four months of use. Minoxidil is a hair loss treatment, not a cure, and patients must continue to use the drug in order to maintain regrowth. New hair growth is shed after minoxidil use is discontinued.

In general, clinical studies have found that minoxidil works best for those patients who are younger, who have been losing their hair for a short period of time and who have less initial hair loss. The medication's effectiveness appears to be related to the activity level of hair follicles.

Side effects include itching and other skin irritations on the scalp.

mites   Tiny eight-legged parasites belonging to the group (Acarina) that includes ticks. Much like tiny spiders, many of these mites have piercing mouth parts that suck blood from animals and humans. A mite has no antenna or wings. Medically important mites include the many species causing DERMATITIS (*Dermatophogoides*). The SCABIES mite lives in human skin, and CHIGGER BITES can cause a rash. Mites in grain or fruit can cause a variety of skin irritations (commonly called "grocer's itch" or "bakers' itch").

Risk Factors and Preventive Measures
Mites can be avoided by using insect repellents such as dimethyl phthalate when walking through infested areas.

Mohs' microscopically controlled excisions A type of dermatologic treatment in which thin layers of tissue are removed and immediately examined for malignant cells in a specially equipped lab in the doctor's office. Layers are removed until all tissue is cancer-free. The technique is used to remove basal cell and squamous cell carcinomas and a variety of other more rare skin cancers.

Developed by dermatologist Frederic E. Mohs, this method is now used to treat one out of every four or five skin-cancer patients. Mohs' surgery offers the highest cure rate and sacrifices the least amount of healthy tissue because it almost always removes the entire cancer without removing too much surrounding normal skin. In this technique, using local anesthesia the tumor may first be reduced by curettage and then excised; blood flow is usually controlled by electrodesiccation. The excised tissue is then mapped, flattened, frozen, and then cut in horizontal sections and the entire undersurface checked for the presence of tumor. Repeated slices are performed until the margins are clear.

This technique is indicated for patients with recurrent tumors, primary tumors known to have high recurrence rates, and primary lesions where tissue must be preserved (such as on the eyelids, nose, finger, genitalia, and areas around facial nerves).

moisturizer While moisturizing can help dry skin (much like a raisin plumps up in water), no moisturizer can prevent wrinkling. (The only possible exception is a moisturizer containing ALPHA HYDROXY ACID, which may help keep skin young-looking by thinning out dried up cells on the surface.)

The right moisturizer should prevent dryness without causing the skin to break out. Consumers who experience problems with one moisturizer should switch moisturizers rather than discontinue their use. The problems may have resulted from reaction to a specific chemical in that brand.

It is important to test a moisturizer in the store, especially if the consumer has had problems with other moisturizing products. Moisturizer should be applied to an area that will not be washed immediately.

While moisturizers do not have "use by" dates, they can lose effectiveness if stored for too long. Shopping at a store with good turnover will ensure freshness. At most department and chain stores, the cosmetics company automatically changes the stock, but this may not be the case at off-price or discount stores that do not buy directly from a manufacturer.

Some of the newest (and most expensive) products contain humectants (ingredients that help the water stay with the skin longer to keep it supple); some of these substances are expensive. Some experts believe that two humectants—hyaluronic acid and ceramides—are excellent moisturizing ingredients, but they can add significantly to the price of a product. Whether hyaluronic acid is a good moisturizer remains to be proven.

The best humectants include lactic acid and urea, which is not expensive and is very effective. Over-the-counter products containing these compounds are available singly or together.

When shopping for moisturizers, experts suggest that consumers compare ingredients and try the lower-priced product first. While people with dry skin and no ACNE can use oil-based moisturizers, consumers who tend to break out need to be more careful. Those with acne-prone skin should choose water-based products while avoiding products that could aggravate the condition. However, recent information suggests that oil-based products are acceptable as long as they are not comodogenic. Acne-aggravating products include ingredients such as cocoa butter, heavy mineral oil, acetylated lanolin alcohols, isopropyl esters, isopropyl myristate, lanolin, lanolin fatty acid, linseed oil, oleic acid, olive oil, petrolatum, and stearic acid. Moisturizer ingredients that are good for oily skin include beeswax, corn oil, isostearyl neopentate, light mineral oil, octyl palmitate, propylene glycol, safflower oil, sodium lauryl sulfate, and spermacetti.

moles A type of pigmented NEVUS composed of nevus cells. The average young adult has at least

25 moles. However, a change in a mole may be the first sign of an early malignant melanoma.

Malignant melanoma is a serious skin cancer that originates in benign moles about a third of the time. In early stages it can be treated, but in later stages it spreads to other parts of the body and becomes very difficult to treat. See MELANOMA, MALIGNANT.

Regular self-examination is the best way to notice when a mole begins to change shape or size. It is important to realize that common moles and malignant melanoma *do not look alike*. A handy way to remember what features to look for is to remember "A-B-C-D" (asymmetry, border, color, diameter).

A mole that is asymmetrical, that has uneven borders, that changes color or is made up of more than one color, or that has a diameter larger than 6 mm could be a malignant lesion and should be checked immediately by a physician.

molluscum contagiosum　A harmless viral infection that causes clusters of pearly white tiny lumps on the skin's surface. Each PAPULE is a small circle with a central depression that produces a cheesy fluid when squeezed. Infection is easily transmitted by direct skin contact or during sexual contact.

Symptoms and Diagnostic Path

The papules appear primarily in children on the genitals, thighs, and the face and in adults in the genital region and on the lower abdomen. They are also frequently seen in patients with advancing AIDS. Molluscum in patients with AIDS are most frequently seen on the face, in flexural areas, and on the genitals.

Treatment Options and Outlook

The infection may clear up within a few months without treatment, although it usually requires treatment with keratolytics, liquid nitrogen, or by curettage.

Mongolian spot　A congenital blue-black pigmented NEVUS found on the lower back or but-

tocks. The spot, which may appear alone or in a group, may be mistaken for a bruise. It is most common in Asian or African-American children, and is caused by a concentration of pigment-producing cells (MELANOCYTES) deep within the skin. The spots usually disappear by age three or four.

moniliasis　See CANDIDA INFECTION.

monilethrix　A rare condition of the hair shaft featuring multiple constrictions, causing the hairs to look like a string of beads. The disease is caused by a defect in the production of KERATIN. It is an autosomal dominant disorder that is characterized by hair that is normal at birth but which changes in the first months of life. The hair breaks off at the thinned area between the beads.

monobenzone　A permanent depigmenting drug that causes permanent skin bleaching. It is used only in severe cases of VITILIGO to remove residual areas of normal pigmentation.

monochloroacetic acid　Together with di- and trichloroacetic acid, these are caustic treatments used for wart removal, to treat XANTHELASMAM, and to perform moderate-depth facial peels.

morbilli　See MEASLES.

Morgan's lines　A crease often seen on the lower eyelids of patients with inflammation (atopic dermatitis) of the skin.

See also DERMATITIS, ATOPIC.

morphea　A localized form of SCLERODERMA (hardening of the body's connective tissue) in which one or more well-defined, hard, flat, round, or oval patches appear on the skin.

Symptoms and Diagnostic Path

The white or purplish patches may be up to several inches in diameter, usually appearing on the trunk, neck, hands, or feet. There also may be hair loss or ulceration at the affected site. The condition is most often found in middle-aged women, although it can occur at any age.

Treatment Options and Outlook

Treatment includes systemic antibiotics, and potent topical steroids, colchicine, and immunosuppressive drugs may have limited benefit. New treatments being studied include gamma interferon (which may inhibit synthesis of COLLAGEN) and extracorporeal photophoresis (which may alter immune response).

The condition may spontaneously regress over several years.

mosquito bites   Female mosquitoes bite in order to obtain blood to produce their eggs. Because their eggs are laid and hatched in stagnant water, throughout the world they are most commonly found near marshes, ponds, reservoirs, and water tanks.

Mosquitoes are a major health hazard and are responsible for the transmission of West Nile virus, yellow fever, malaria, dengue fever, encephalitis, and many other serious diseases. In parts of the world where mosquito-transmitted diseases are not common, it is the bite itself that presents the greatest difficulty. More infants and children are bitten by mosquitoes than by any other insect.

When the mosquito bites, it injects its saliva that is full of digestive enzymes and anticoagulants. The first time a person is bitten, there is no reaction, but with subsequent bites, the person becomes sensitized to the foreign proteins, and small, itchy, red bumps appear about 24 hours later. This is the most common reaction in young children. After many more bites, a pale, swollen hive begins to appear within minutes, followed by a red bump 24 hours later. This is the most common reaction in older children and teens.

With repeated mosquito bites, some people begin to become insensitive again, much as if they had allergy shots. Some older children and adults get no reaction to mosquito bites unless they go for a long time without being bitten—then the process can start again. Other people become increasingly allergic with repeated stings that can trigger blisters, bruises, and inflammatory reactions. For these people, avoiding being bitten is important.

Symptoms and Diagnostic Path

Mosquito bites may cause swelling and itching for several days; the main problem of these bites is the infections that may be transmitted.

Treatment Options and Outlook

Because mosquitoes can spread disease, the bite area should be washed with soap and water, followed by an antiseptic. To control ITCHING, nonprescription ANTIHISTAMINE, CALAMINE lotion, gels with mild anesthetic, or ice packs can be used.

Risk Factors and Preventive Measures

Mosquitoes are attracted to things that remind them of nectar or mammal flesh. When outdoors, people should wear light clothing that covers most of the body, keeping as much of the skin and hair covered as practical, and avoiding bright, floral colors. Khaki, beige, and olive have no particular attraction for mosquitoes. Mosquitoes are also attracted by some body odors, and for this reason they choose some individuals over others in a crowd. In order to avoid mosquito bites, people should not use fragrances in soaps, shampoos, and lotions.

In general, mosquitoes will choose children as their victims rather than adults; many species prefer biting from dusk until dawn. The problem is worse when the weather is hot or humid. For this reason, children should avoid playing outdoors during the peak biting times. Consumers should use insect repellents, such as

DEET (NN-diethyl-*m*-toluamide): By far the best repellent, it should be applied to all exposed skin. It comes in various strengths, but the more concentrated is more effective; children should use milder versions because there have been a few cases of toxicity involving small children. DEET should not be applied under clothes, or too much of the toxic substance may be absorbed. It should not be applied to portions of the hands that are likely to come in contact with the eyes and mouth. Pediatric insect repellents with only 6 to 10 percent DEET are available. For greater protection, clothing and mosquito nets can be soaked in or sprayed with permethrin, which is an insect repellent licensed for use on clothing. If applied according to the directions, permethrin will repel insects from clothing for several weeks. These specialty items can be purchased in hardware, back-packing, and military surplus stores.

Unless traveling to a high-risk area, gentler insect repellents should be used for children, such as Skedaddle. However, neither these nor the stronger repellents inhibit mosquitoes from landing—only from biting.

chlorine bleach: Bathe in a tubful of warm water with two capfuls of bleach, but do not get the solution near eyes.

bath oil: Although many consumers swear by Avon's Skin-so-Soft, research by the military (and Avon) demonstrate that it is not nearly as effective as DEET.

zinc: Some experts recommend daily doses (at least 60 milligrams) of ZINC, although they warn it can take up to four weeks to become effective; extra supplements should be taken only with approval of a physician.

thiamine chloride: A B vitamin that may repel insects when taken orally; however, it may also cause ITCHING, HIVES, and a rash in sensitive individuals.

Moynahan's syndrome See MULTIPLE LENTIGINES SYNDROME.

mucinoses A group of metabolic disorders involving mucin (the primary component of mucus). These disorders include LICHEN MYXEDEMATOSUS, URBACH-WIETHE DISEASE, and MUCOPOLYSACCHARIDOSES.

mucocutaneous lymph node syndrome See KAWASAKI DISEASE.

mucopolysaccharidoses A group of metabolic disorders including at least seven major types and 14 subtypes, each with an enzyme deficiency in the metabolism of mucopolysaccharides (a group of complex carbohydrates that help make up the connective tissue). None of these disorders can yet be treated, but someday it may be possible to replace the missing enzyme.

HUNTER'S SYNDROME is the only disease in this group with skin symptoms, which include white or flesh-colored PAPULES or NODULES that may merge to form ridges. They may appear before age 10 and may fade away later. In severe forms of this syndrome, patients are mentally retarded and die young. Milder forms may not be fatal, or affect intelligence.

mucormycosis An uncommon invasive fungal infection of the lung and central nervous system usually associated with kidney transplant patients or patients with diabetes or cancers of the lymph or bone marrow. While primary skin infection is rare with this type of fungus, it may be commonly associated with burn wound infections.

Symptoms and Diagnostic Path
Symptoms include a single, painful, hardened area of skin that may exhibit a blackened area in the center. A tissue specimen must be analyzed to diagnose mucormycosis.

Treatment Options and Outlook
Administration of intravenous amphotericin B plus treatment of underlying disease is effective.

multiple lentigines syndrome A genetic syndrome characterized by multiple brown spots similar to FRECKLES (lentigines), heart irregularities, abnormal distance between the eyes, pulmonary stenosis, abnormal genitals, short stature, and deafness. The syndrome is also known as LEOPARD or Moynahan's syndrome; variants include NAME syndrome, centrofacial lentiginosis, or

LAMB syndrome. Multiple lentigines syndrome was originally described as "progressive cardio-myopathic lentiginosis syndrome" by Moynahan. The acronym LEOPARD was applied later to describe the unusual appearance of the numerous lentigines together with the major developmental defects. The acronym stands for the range of developmental symptoms that characterize the disorder:

lentigines
electrocardiographic abnormalities
ocular hypertelorism
pulmonary stenosis
abnormalities of the genitals
retarded growth
deafness

Symptoms and Diagnostic Path

At birth, patients have only a few lentigines, but the number increases rapidly with age until there are hundreds of lesions by adulthood, found on the face palms, soles, lips, and genitalia. Patients with centrofacial lentiginosis have lentigines in a "butterfly" pattern over the nose and cheeks.

While freckles are flat tan or brown spots found only on areas of the skin exposed to the sun that darken with sun exposure, lentigines are medium- to dark-brown spots that appear on all areas of the skin and that do not clear in the absence of sun exposure.

Many patients with multiple lentigines syndrome are also mentally retarded, with abnormal EEGs. The NAME syndrome includes: *n*evi (moles), *a*trial myxoma (tumor in the heart), *m*yxoid neuro-fibromas, and *e*phelides (freckles). The LAMB syndrome includes: *l*entigines (brown flat spots), *a*trial myxoma, *m*ucocutaneous myxomas (tumor of connective tissue), and *b*lue nevi. Both are believed to be a variant of multiple lentigines syndromes.

Generalized lentiginosis (LENTIGINOSIS PROFUSA) is a different genetic disorder characterized by numerous lentigines without other developmental problems.

Treatment Options and Outlook

Most of the symptoms and developmental problems associated with this syndrome are not treatable. Shortly after birth, the infant should be examined by pediatric cardiologists, endocrinologists, and otolaryngologists, aimed at early detecting of atrial myxomas or deafness. It is possible to improve the appearance of the facial skin by superficial DERMABRASION.

The patient's family should understand that all forms of the multiple lentigines syndrome are transmitted as autosomal dominant disorders. This means that the defective gene must be present in only a single parent to cause the syndrome. Each child of an affected person usually has a one in two chance of inheriting the defective gene and of being affected.

mupirocin (Bactroban) A topical antibacterial medication that is very effective in treating superficial streptococcal and staphylococcal infections of the skin. Many doctors use mupirocin instead of systemic antibiotics to treat primary and secondary types of IMPETIGO.

Naftin See NAFTIFINE.

naftifine (Trade name: Naftin) An antifungal agent that, when applied to the skin, is effective against the DERMATOPHYTES and *Candida* species. It is used to treat ATHLETE'S FOOT, JOCK ITCH, and RINGWORM of the body, among other diseases.

Side Effects
Burning or stinging feeling on treated areas is a common side effect. Less common are dry skin, itching, and redness.

nail biting A common habit that is not related to any underlying medical problem. While many children bite their nails in their early school years, most grow out of the habit, although it can continue as a nervous mannerism into adulthood.

Nail biting is one of the causes of recurrent acute inflammation of nail tissues (PARONYCHIA). Warts around the perimeter of bitten nails are not uncommon. Because persistent nail biting can cause pain and bleeding, painting on bitter-tasting preparations may help end the habit.

nail discoloration The most common cause of nail discoloration is nail polish. The deeper the shade of polish, the more likely the pigment will stain the nail. Using a clear base coat before applying color seems to help a bit. Usually, externally induced discoloration involves the whole nail, while discoloration of just a portion usually means there is a problem underneath the nail.

Other causes of externally induced nail discoloration include the use of nail hardeners and synthetic nails, as well as contact with some chemicals (such as photo developer, anti-malarial drugs, or gardening fertilizers), applying HENNA with the bare hands, and smoking.

If the nail continues to be discolored, the patient should see a dermatologist because the problem could be a symptom of an underlying disease. Discoloration can be caused by health problems such as yeast and bacterial infections, inflammatory syndromes (such as PSORIASIS), benign tumors, and even certain cancers (such as melanoma). However, in these cases, stains are located *under* the nail and cannot be removed. Dark-skinned individuals may notice *linear longitudinal* brown streaks in their nails.

Consumers should skip commercial stain-removing products, since many of them do not work well on nails. Instead, for best results in lightening or removing a stain, the nail should be lightly buffed with a white emery block. Buffing will sand off the pigments in the top layers of the nail. (However, this should not be done on a regular basis, since too much buffing thins and weakens the nail.)

nail fungus A hard-to-cure infection (also known as ONYCHOMYCOSIS) that can develop in warm, moist areas of the body and is more common as a person ages.

Symptoms and Diagnostic Path
The fungus can affect the end of the nail on fingers or toes, causing the nail to crumble and turn yellow, thickening and lifting up. Sometimes, white

crumbly patches or white or yellow spots appear on the surface.

Treatment Options and Outlook

For mild infections, cutting the nail back and applying an antifungal medication may help, but recurrence is common. More severe cases may require oral medication. Using conventional antifungals (such as griseofulvin), cure rates are about 30 percent. It takes up to a year for medication to cure a nail infection on smaller toes and up to two years for infections involving the big toe. Newer systemic antifungals are much more effective (cure rate are about 80 percent) in a much shorter period of time.

nail hardeners Fingernail enamels (actually nail polishes) that form a particularly thick coat or that contain nylon fibers to protect or shield the nail. In the past, nail hardeners caused actual physical changes in the keratin through the action of formaldehyde; because these formaldehyde-containing products caused adverse reactions they are limited to concentrations of 5 percent by the U.S. Food and Drug Administration.

See also FINGERNAILS, CARE OF; FORMALDEHYDE, SENSITIVITY TO.

nail-patella syndrome An hereditary disorder characterized by nail abnormalities (especially of the index finger and thumb), kidney problems, mental retardation, and lack of kneecaps. The prognosis is poor for infants whose kidneys are involved.

The condition is an autosomal dominant disorder, which means that only one defective gene (from one parent) is needed to cause the syndrome. Each child of an affected person usually has a one in two chance of inheriting the defective gene and of being affected.

nail polish A lacquer used to apply color to the fingernails to enhance their appearance. Nail polish is composed of solvents, plasticizers (to provide flexibility), resins (for body and adhesiveness), color, and cellulose nitrate (to create a film for the nail).

Resins are responsible for most of the cases of irritation caused by nail polish, but the more severe allergic reactions are often caused by the monomers contained in nail polish extenders.

nails The horny plate at the top of the end of fingers and toes. It is made up of KERATIN (a tough protein that forms the basis of skin and hair), and takes up to six months to grow from base to tip of the finger; toenails take twice as long to grow. Nail growth is also affected by seasonal variations.

While very tough, the nails may still be damaged by crush or pressure injuries. Among the elderly, the nails on the big toes may grow abnormally thick and curved (a condition called ONYCHOGRYPHOSIS).

In addition, the nails can be affected by a variety of bacterial and fungal disorders, especially TINEA (RINGWORM) and candidiasis (THRUSH). The nail folds can also become inflamed or infected (a condition called PARONYCHIA).

Illness in other parts of the body can also include symptoms in the nails, such as the pitting (small indentations in the nail) seen in ALOPECIA AREATA, pitting and separation from the nail bed in PSORIASIS, or scarring and nail bed separation in LICHEN PLANUS.

More generally, some nail symptoms may be indications of a generalized disease. Concave, ridged, and brittle nails can indicate the presence of iron-deficiency anemia, and fibromus nails can be a sign of TUBEROUS SCLEROSIS. Bleeding into the nail beds that causes vertical black lines on the nail bed can be an indication of infection of heart valves.

Unusual nail color can also be an indication of disease: bluish nails may indicate heart or breathing problems; greenish black nails might be caused by a bacterial yeast infection; and hard, curved yellow nails may indicate breathing problems.

nails, care of Despite a wide variety of old wives' tales, there is actually little that can be done—even

Nail

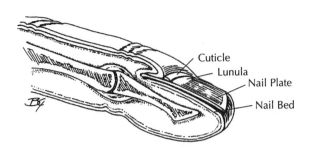

Cuticle
Lunula
Nail Plate
Nail Bed

by consuming calcium or gelatin—to strengthen a healthy fingernail.

Risk Factors and Preventive Measures

Preventive care can include avoiding injuries: Objects should never be pried open with fingernails. Cotton gloves should be worn when doing chores, with heavier gloves for gardening and outside jobs.

Because repeated drenching of nails in detergents and water can make nails brittle, this problem can be prevented by wearing cotton-lined rubber gloves. However, the rubber gloves should be removed before hands begin to sweat. Dry nails that split easily can be treated by applying Vaseline to the nail, cuticle, and fingertips nightly.

Care of the Cuticle

When hands are damp, the cuticle should be gently pushed back with a soft towel or orange stick. Cuticle removers contain substances that dissolve and soften the keratin, and because of the potential hazards of caustic products containing potassium hydroxide, many DERMATOLOGISTS recommend that they be avoided. People with inflamed cuticles should never use cuticle removers to achieve a smooth appearance. Although many manicurists do trim or clip the cuticle, this process can cause inflammation and should be avoided. Constantly immersing hands in water can also lead to inflammation of the cuticle (PARONYCHIA).

Hangnails

These partly detached dried parts of the cuticle should be cut close to the base, and not be picked or torn (which can lead to infection). To head off hangnails, emollients and gloves should be worn in dry, cold weather or while using detergents.

Manicures

Manicures may improve the appearance of fingernails. Carefully done, manicures can be beneficial, but overenthusiastic buffing of nails with abrasive powders may injure the nail matrix. Repeatedly applying and removing nail polish can dry out the nail. Allergic reactions to nail polish usually do not appear on the fingers but instead may appear on the eyelids or neck.

Sculptured Nails

Molded fake nails are created by applying an acrylic monomer on the nail plate. While this procedure is popular because it enhances the length of the nail, it can often induce inflammation and cause a painful separation of the nail plate from the bed.

nails, disorders of Although the fingernails are quite hard, they are susceptible to traumatic damage, usually caused by crushing or pressure. This can cause splitting, ridging, breaking, or bleeding under the nail.

Symptoms and Diagnostic Path

The nails may become abnormally thick and curved (ONYCHOGRYPHOSIS), a condition that usually occurs among the elderly. Fungal or bacterial infection may also damage the nails, especially TINEA and CANDIDA INFECTIONS, or the nails may be affected by skin diseases or more general illnesses. For example, in ALOPECIA AREATA (hair loss) the nails may be pitted. In PSORIASIS, the nails may be pitted and separate from the nail bed (ONYCHOLYSIS). In LICHEN PLANUS, the nails may be scarred and separate from the nail bed. Brittle, ridged, concave nails suggest iron-deficiency anemia. Separation of the nail from its bed is seen in thyrotoxicosis, and fibrous growths on the sides of the nails are a sign of TUBEROUS SCLEROSIS. In endocarditis and bleeding disorders, the nails develop splinterlike black marks.

The color of the nails may indicate possible diseases of the body. Blue nails may be a sign of respiratory or cardiac distress. Hard, curved yellow nails are seen in people with bronchiectasis and lymphedema.

Nail disorders are usually diagnosed by visual inspection.

Treatment Options and Outlook

Treatment of nail disorders is not easy, since creams and lotions do not usually penetrate into the nail deeply enough, and oral medications may take months to be effective.

nails, pitted   Small depressions in the nail plates, typically found in patients with PSORIASIS.

NAME   See MULTIPLE LENTIGINES SYNDROME.

necrobiosis   Gradual process by which cells lose their function and die. Necrobiosis lipoidica causes patchy degeneration of the skin, resulting in white scars. It is most often seen in about one in 300 diabetics, although others can contract this disease.

The lesions usually appear as red papules or plaques, followed by a yellowish depressed plaque. Treatment with steroids injected into the lesions may be effective during early stages.

necrotizing fasciitis   A potentially fatal illness commonly caused by streptococcus bacteria, characterized by an infection with warm, red, tender plaques that become necrotic and spread.

In this condition, commonly called "flesh-eating bacteria," more virulent strains of the strep bacteria destroy the body's protein, affecting the lungs, skin, and bloodstream. The bacteria releases a toxin that can dissolve fat and muscle tissue, causing the skin to die and leading to deadly gangrene. Most often the bacteria enter the body through a very minor cut in the skin (as small as

a paper cut), a bruise, or a scrape. It also can occur after major surgery; in some cases, its origin is a mystery.

The bacteria are usually transferred by respiratory droplets or direct contact with secretions of someone carrying strep A. The bacteria destroy soft tissue beneath the skin, and are often linked with toxic shock syndrome. If muscle also is destroyed, the condition is called necrotizing myositis.

Symptoms and Diagnostic Path

Within 24 hours of infection, the person may feel some pain, which is often far more serious than the original injury. This is quickly followed by flulike symptoms, such as confusion, diarrhea, dizziness, fever, nausea, weakness, and general malaise. As the body becomes dehydrated, the patient begins to feel extremely thirsty. Within three or four days, the wound area begins to swell and the skin may have large, dark marks or a purple rash. These turn into fluid-filled black BLISTERS, although the would itself may appear blue-white, or dark and mottled. The patient's condition typically becomes critical within four to five days, as blood pressure plummets and the body begins to go into shock as a result of toxins from the bacteria. As the body weakens, unconsciousness occurs.

A patient with any of these early symptoms should immediately see a physician to rule out this condition, since the vast majority of these cases are misdiagnosed.

Treatment Options and Outlook

The disease requires aggressive treatment with removal of affected skin and broad-spectrum antibiotics. Other treatments depend on the seriousness of symptoms. Medications to raise blood pressure, blood transfusions, and a new medicine called *intravenous immunoglobulin (IVIG)* are also used. A hyperbaric oxygen chamber is sometimes used in certain cases that involved different types of bacterial infection.

A patient with this condition may experience anything from some mild scars to death. Among those who survive, most patients experience some removal of skin, which often requires skin grafting. Amputation of legs, hands, fingers, toes, or arms also may be required to save the life of the patient. Between 2,000 and 3,000 people die from strep infections each year out of 10,000 to 15,000 cases of serious strep infections in the United States, according to the Centers for Disease Control. Of these 15,000 cases, between 500 to 1,500 involve necrotizing fasciitis; of these, about 100 to 350 people die.

See also BACTERIAL SKIN INFECTIONS.

neomycin (Trade names: Mycifradin; Myciguent) An antibiotic sometimes used to treat skin infections (often together with other drugs). Possible adverse effects include nausea and vomiting, rash, itching, diarrhea, hearing loss, dizziness, and tinnitus (ringing in the ears).

neonatal acne   See ACNE, INFANT.

Netherton's syndrome   A hereditary condition characterized by three primary defects: abnormality in the hair shaft (especially trichorrhexis invaginata, or "bamboo hair"), ICHTHYOSIS linearis circumflexa (a scaling skin disorder), and atopic dermatitis.

This disorder of unknown cause is inherited in an autosomal recessive pattern, which means that a defective gene must be inherited from both parents to cause the abnormality. Generally, both parents of an affected person are unaffected carriers of the defective gene. Each of the affected children has a one in four chance of being affected, and a two in four chance of being a carrier.

See also DERMATITIS, ATOPIC.

neurilemmoma   See NEUROFIBROMA.

neurocutaneous disorders   A group of genetic disorders featuring abnormalities of the skin, nerves, or the nervous system. The diseases are believed to begin in the abnormal development of primitive cells found during the earliest stages of an embryo's development. There are several neurocutaneous syndromes, but the most common ones include NEUROFIBROMATOSIS type 1 and 2, STURGE-WEBER SYNDROME, TUBEROUS SCLEROSIS, ataxia-telangiectasia, and von Hippel-Lindau disease.

Symptoms and Diagnostic Path
The first symptoms most commonly noted in children are skin lesions, including BIRTHMARKS, tumors, and other growths. Symptoms vary considerably from condition to condition and from patient to patient, because neurocutaneous syndromes affect individuals in different ways.

Treatment Options and Outlook
Although there is no cure for these conditions, treatments are available that help to manage symptoms and complications. The conditions are always lifelong, which means that educational, social, and physical problems must be managed throughout a child's life.

neurodermatitis   See LICHEN SIMPLEX.

neurofibroma   A skin tumor that may occur alone or in groups, ranging in color from pale cream to lightly pigmented.

Treatment Options and Outlook
Single neurofibromas may be surgically removed. See also NEUROFIBROMATOSES.

neurofibromatoses   A group of genetic disorders characterized by many soft, fibrous swellings (called NEUROFIBROMAS) growing from nerves in the skin and elsewhere in the body. There also may be CAFÉ-AU-LAIT MACULES (coffee-colored spots) on the skin.

Both forms of NF are autosomal dominant genetic disorders, which may be inherited from a parent who has NF or may be the result of a new or spontaneous mutation in the sperm or egg cell. Each child of a parent with NF has a 50 percent chance of inheriting the gene and developing NF. The type of NF inherited by the child is always the same as that of the affected parent, although the severity and the type of symptoms may differ from person to person within a family. However, up to 50 percent of new cases are spontaneous mutations.

Symptoms and Diagnostic Path

In the past, medical experts classified the disorder into two different types, neurofibromatosis type 1 and type 2 (NF1 and NF2). Today experts know that these are two totally separate disorders caused by two different genes. NF1 occurs far more frequently, accounting for about 90 percent of all cases.

Neurofibromatosis 1 (*NF1*), also known as von Recklinghausen NF or peripheral NF, occurs in one out of 4,000 births and is characterized by multiple café-au-lait spots and neurofibromas on or under the skin. Enlargement and deformation of bones and curvature of the spine (scoliosis) also may occur. Occasionally, tumors may develop in the brain, on cranial nerves, or on the spinal cord. About 50 percent of people with NF also have learning disabilities.

Neurofibromatosis 2 (*NF2*) also known as bilateral acoustic NF (BAN), is much more rare, occurring in one out of 40,000 births. NF2 is characterized by multiple tumors on the cranial and spinal nerves and by other lesions of the brain and spinal cord.

Symptoms and Diagnostic Path

Tumors affecting both of the auditory nerves are the hallmark. Hearing loss beginning in the teens or early twenties is generally the first symptom.

Neurofibromas (the most common tumors in NF), are benign growths that typically develop on or just underneath the surface of the skin but may also occur in deeper areas of the body. They usually develop at puberty, although they may appear at any age. Nodulelike surface tumors are known as dermal neurofibromas; plexiform neurofibromas grow diffusely under the skin surface or in deeper areas of the body.

The presence of multiple neurofibromas is an important symptom of NF, although single neurofibromas may occasionally occur in people who don't have NF. The number of neurofibromas varies widely among affected individuals from only a few to thousands. There is no way to predict how many neurofibromas a person will develop.

Dermal neurofibromas rarely, if ever, become cancerous, but plexiform tumors may very rarely become malignant. Therefore, it is important that patients be in the care of an NF specialist.

Café-au-lait spots, the most common sign of NF, are flat, pigmented spots on the skin that are called by the French term *café-au-lait* (coffee with milk) because of the light tan color. In darker-skinned people, café-au-lait spots appear darker than surrounding skin. People with NF almost always have six or more café-au-lait spots. (Fewer café-au-lait spots may occur in people who don't have NF; in fact, about 10 percent of the general population has one or two café-au-lait spots.) The size of the spots that identify NF varies from one-quarter inch in children to more than several inches in diameter.

Café-au-lait spots are usually present at birth in children who have NF or, generally, appear by two years of age. The number of spots may increase in childhood and occasionally later in life. The spots may be very light in color in infants and usually darken as the child gets older. Smaller pigmented spots, which may be difficult to distinguish from ordinary FRECKLES, may also be present in people with NF. In those who do not have NF, freckling usually occurs in areas of skin exposed to sun. With NF, café-au-lait spots and freckling are present in other areas as well, including the armpit and the groin. Armpit freckling is not seen in every person with NF, but when present it is considered strong evidence of NF. Lisch nodules are common in young children with NF; these brown pigmented areas of the iris resemble little freckles. The nodules increase in number during adolescence, but do not impair vision.

Iris nevi are clumps of pigment in the iris that usually appear around puberty. They can be distinguished from iris freckles by a simple and painless procedure called a slit-lamp examination, which is typically performed by an ophthalmologist. Iris nevi do not cause medical problems and do not affect vision, but their presence can occasionally help confirm the diagnosis of NF.

Children with NF1 are usually checked for height, weight, head circumference, blood pressure, vision and hearing, evidence of normal sexual development, signs of learning disability and hyperactivity, and evidence of scoliosis, in addition to examination of the skin for café-au-lait spots and neurofibromas. Further diagnostic evaluations, including blood tests and X-rays, are usually needed only to investigate suspected problems.

Treatment Options and Outlook

A person with NF should see a physician for evaluation and follow-up care. Specialists from many disciplines may be knowledgeable about specific aspects of NF; those most likely to be familiar with the disorder as a whole include geneticists, neurologists, and pediatric neurologists. NF referral centers that cooperate with the National Neurofibromatosis Foundation have been established in a number of major medical centers in the United States.

Some neurofibromas, depending on their location and size, can be removed surgically if they become painful or infected, or cosmetically embarrassing. However, a new tumor sometimes appears where one has been excised, especially if that tumor was not removed completely, but there is no evidence that removing growths will speed up the appearance of new growths or cause incompletely removed tumors to become cancerous. Healthy children with NF1 are usually examined at six- or 12-month intervals.

Routine checkups for adults with NF1 generally include, in addition to standard physical evaluation, an examination of the skin, blood pressure, vision and hearing, and examination of the spine for scoliosis. Attention is given to any mass that is rapidly enlarging or causing new pain. Other tests can be performed if a medical problem develops. Adults with NF1 who are otherwise healthy usually have periodic checkups at 12-month intervals.

neurotic excoriations A psychogenic skin disease characterized by repeated picking of the skin. This condition should be suspected if the lesions, which are present in all stages of development, are distributed solely in accessible areas, often in parallel lines. There are no primary lesions.

Generally, patients pick at their skin because they feel restless; the root of the tension is sometimes related to a specific cause, such as family problems. Picking their skin is another outlet for these patients' emotional tension.

Symptoms and Diagnostic Path

Lesions are gouged in the skin, leaving white, round papery scars when they heal against a hyperpigmented background. Lesions are noticeable in all stages of healing, and the small ulcers are usually angular, the tip-off that they are self-induced and not primary. They are most often found on the tops of the forearms and over the shoulders.

Treatment Options and Outlook

Usually patients with these neurotic urges to pick at their skin do it compulsively and find it very difficult to stop. Therefore, treatment should center on efforts to identify the source of stress in the patient's life, although psychiatric help is not usually very effective. Attempts to physically prevent the patient from picking may result either in panic or depression.

See also ACNE EXCORIÉE.

nevus (plural: nevi) A BIRTHMARK or skin malformation characterized by too much (or not enough) normal epidermal, connective, adnexal, nervous, or vascular tissue.

Symptoms and Diagnostic Path

There are many different types of nevi, with different appearances: colored or uncolored, with or without hair, lying flat, slightly raised, or on a stalk above the skin. Some nevi may be congenital, but they may develop at any time.

A MOLE is another common type of colored nevus, not usually present at birth. Some nevi have a bluish color, and are known as "blue nevi"; these are often found on the backs of hands in young girls. Most African-American and Asian infants are born with one or more blue-black spots on their lower backs, called MONGO-LIAN SPOTS.

The above examples are all forms of melano-cytic (or pigmented) *nevi,* caused by an overactivity or abnormality of skin cells that produce MELANIN.

The other primary type of nevi are the *vascular nevi* (or HEMANGIOMA), caused by an abnormal collection of blood vessels. They include PORT-WINE STAIN, which does not fade but can be treated with lasers, and STRAWBERRY BIRTHMARK, which usually does disappear in early life.

Nevi are visually diagnosed by a physician.

Treatment Options and Outlook

Most nevi are completely harmless and do not require treatment. Some types of vascular nevi do require treatment for psychological reasons. Any nevus that suddenly appears, grows, bleeds, or changes color should be brought to the attention of a DERMATOLOGIST to rule out the possibility of cancer.

nevus, amelanotic   A nevus that contains no pigment.

nevus, balloon cell   A benign nevus that changes overtime. Under the microscope it consists of balloon cells formed of altered melanosomes. It may be confused with malignant melanoma.

See also MELANOMA, MALIGNANT.

nevus, blue   A type of pigmented BIRTHMARK (NEVUS) caused by an abnormality or overactivity of skin cells producing the pigment MELANIN, which is deep blue in color. The brown melanin pigment is placed in a specific pattern, deep enough in the skin for it to take on a blue color.

See also NEVUS, COMPOUND; NEVUS, CONGENITAL; NEVUS, HALO; NEVUS, SPITZ; NEVUS PIGMENTOSUS; NEVUS SPILUS; NEVUS SYNDROME, DYSPLASTIC.

nevus, compound   One of three main types of benign skin malformation (NEVI), located within the

dermal-epidermal junction and in the underlying DERMIS. Compound nevi are often raised and may have a flat area surrounding the elevated area.

See also NEVUS, BLUE; NEVUS, CONGENITAL; NEVUS, HALO; NEVUS, SPITZ; NEVUS ARANEUS; NEVUS PIGMENTOSUS; NEVUS SPILUS; NEVUS SYNDROME, DYSPLASTIC.

nevus, congenital   Unlike the common acquired nevi (skin malformation) that appears after birth, this type of nevus appears at birth or shortly thereafter, and remains throughout life. Most are small and look very much like acquired nevi. Rarely, congenital nevi may be large (giant congenital nevi), involving major areas of the body. They are usually found on the trunk, upper back, and shoulders. Most have a rough surface and hair.

There is debate over whether small congenital nevi can become cancerous. If there is a risk, it is quite low. The lifetime risk of melanoma developing from giant congenital nevi is higher—approximately 6 percent.

See also BIRTHMARK; MOLE; NEVUS, BLUE; NEVUS, HALO; NEVUS, SPITZ; NEVUS SYNDROME, DYSPLASTIC.

nevus, connective tissue   A BIRTHMARK (also called nevus elasticus of Lewandowsky) involving different parts of the connective tissue that are typically visible at birth but that occasionally do not appear until adolescence. They may be inherited or acquired, and may be associated with other diseases. The nevi may appear alone or in groups of NODULES, PAPULES, or plaques, or in various combinations of these lesions, but individual lesions usually appear as a plaque composed of firm, flat, ivory white or yellow-brown papules, often having a pebbly appearance.

Treatment Options and Outlook

No treatment is necessary for most of these connective tissue nevi, since they are not unsightly. On rare occasions, surgical excision may be performed.

See also BIRTHMARK; MOLE; NEVUS, BLUE; NEVUS, COMPOUND; NEVUS, EPIDERMAL; NEVUS, HALO; NEVUS,

SEBACEOUS; NEVUS, SPITZ; NEVUS ARANEUS; NEVUS DEPIGMENTOSUS; NEVUS PIGMENTOSUS; NEVUS SYNDROME, DYSPLASTIC; PORT-WINE STAIN.

nevus, epidermal An uncommon brown lesion present at birth that may either appear small and singly, or in large groups that are usually either linear or swirled. While this nevus usually is present at birth, it may appear during the first few years of life through puberty, and rarely later in life.

Treatment Options and Outlook
No treatment is normally required, unless the nevus is cosmetically distressing. In that case, small lesions may be excised, but removal of larger epidermal nevi may be difficult or cosmetically unappealing, as the scar may look worse than the nevi. Superficial removal by laser or by chemical destruction are possible treatment options.

See also BIRTHMARK; MOLE; NEVUS, SEBACEOUS; NEVUS DEPIGMENTOSUS; NEVUS PIGMENTOSUS.

nevus, epithelioid See NEVUS, SPITZ.

nevus, halo A skin abnormality in which the skin surrounding the lesion whitens in color, giving a characteristic "halo" appearance.

nevus, sebaceous A skin abnormality present at birth or shortly thereafter that usually appears as a hairless, yellowish orange plaque on the scalp that sometimes may be mistaken for a melanocytic nevus. These lesions should be removed during childhood because they have a tendency to become cancerous, usually at puberty (basal cell carcinoma or other benign or malignant tumor).

See also MOLE; NEVUS, EPIDERMAL; NEVUS DEPIGMENTOSUS; NEVUS PIGMENTOSUS.

nevus, spindle and epithelioid cell Another name for a Spitz nevus (See NEVUS, SPITZ).

nevus, Spitz A solitary pink, purple, or red PAPULE or NODULE that usually appears in childhood. While it resembles malignant melanoma under the microscope, this lesion is benign.

Symptoms and Diagnostic Path
This lesion usually appears on the face in young patients, but among adults is more common on the legs and trunk.

Treatment Options and Outlook
Simple excision will cure this nevus.

See also BIRTHMARK; MOLE; NEVUS; NEVUS, BLUE; NEVUS, COMPOUND; NEVUS, EPIDERMAL; NEVUS, HALO; NEVUS, SEBACEOUS; NEVUS, SPITZ; NEVUS DEPIGMENTOSUS; NEVUS PIGMENTOSUS; NEVUS SYNDROME, DYSPLASTIC; PORT-WINE STAIN.

nevus araneus The medical name for a spider angioma, which looks like a bright red blood vessel with branches radiating out from the center, much like a spider. This condition is common in pregnancy; it is suspected that estrogen plays a role in the development of these lesions which are caused by the expansion of superficial small veins in the skin. They are also often seen in children and in both women and men.

Symptoms and Diagnostic Path
Lesions are found most often over the face, the front of the neck and chest, and the upper arms. They are also often seen in patients with chronic liver disease.

Treatment Options and Outlook
Those lesions associated with pregnancy normally fade after delivery, so generally they do not require treatment. If not, the lesions may be removed by laser surgery with the pulsed dye laser, or they may be electrocoagulated with a fine needle.

See also NEVUS, BLUE; NEVUS, COMPOUND; NEVUS, CONGENITAL; NEVUS, HALO; NEVUS, SPITZ; NEVUS PIGMENTOSUS; NEVUS SPILUS; NEVUS SYNDROME, DYSPLASTIC.

nevus depigmentosus A fairly uncommon disorder of pigmentation that may be either congenital or acquired.

Symptoms and Diagnostic Path

It is characterized by white macules and irregular patches on the trunk or extremities. As the child grows, the macules enlarge.

Treatment Options and Outlook

There is no way to repigment the skin, though cosmetic concealment may be helpful in masking the problem.

See also BIRTHMARK; MOLE; NEVUS, BLUE; NEVUS, COMPOUND; NEVUS, EPIDERMAL; NEVUS, HALO; NEVUS, SEBACEOUS; NEVUS, SPITZ; NEVUS PIGMENTOSUS; NEVUS SYNDROME, DYSPLASTIC; PORT-WINE STAIN.

nevus elasticus of Lewandowsky See NEVUS, CONNECTIVE TISSUE.

nevus flammeus See PORT-WINE STAIN.

nevus of Ito and nevus of Ota Disorders of pigmentation characterized by benign blue-gray-brown pigmented patches of skin located on the face (nevus of Ota) and on the shoulder (nevus of Ito). About 50 percent of these lesions are congenital or appear soon after birth; most of the rest appear at puberty, although a few may not surface until the third decade of life.

Symptoms and Diagnostic Path

The two lesions are similar to a MONGOLIAN SPOT with the pigment found deep in the skin, accounting for the typical blue-gray color.

Nevus of Ota is usually found over the cheek and temple, and is more commonly found in dark-skinned people and Asians; it affects 0.5 percent of all Japanese. Neither type fades with age; while both are benign, they have rarely been associated with melanoma (usually in Caucasians).

Treatment Options and Outlook

Highly effective treatment includes the use of short pulsed lasers, such as the Q-switched ruby laser. This provides excellent results without textural change in most lesions.

See also BIRTHMARK; MOLE; NEVUS, BLUE; NEVUS, COMPOUND; NEVUS, CONNECTIVE TISSUE; NEVUS, EPIDERMAL; NEVUS, HALO; NEVUS, SEBACEOUS; NEVUS, SPITZ; NEVUS ARANEUS; NEVUS DEPIGMENTOSUS; NEVUS PIGMENTOSUS; NEVUS SPILUS; NEVUS SYNDROME, DYSPLASTIC; PORT-WINE STAIN.

nevus pigmentosus A benign tumor composed of MELANOCYTES.

See also BIRTHMARK; MOLE; NEVUS, BLUE; NEVUS, COMPOUND; NEVUS, EPIDERMAL; NEVUS, HALO; NEVUS, SEBACEOUS; NEVUS, SPITZ; NEVUS ARANEUS; NEVUS DEPIGMENTOSUS; NEVUS PIGMENTOSUS; NEVUS SYNDROME, DYSPLASTIC; PORT-WINE STAIN.

nevus spilus A light-brown patch (CAFÉ-AU-LAIT MACULES) sprinkled with dark brown macules that is present at birth or early infancy.

Symptoms and Diagnostic Path

While the overall size of the spot may vary, it is usually several centimeters in diameter and may be found on the trunk or extremities.

Treatment Options and Outlook

No treatment is necessary, although short pulsed lasers such as the Q-switched ruby and O-switched YAG lasers can lighten the lesions.

See also BIRTHMARK; MOLE; NEVUS; NEVUS, BLUE; NEVUS, EPIDERMAL; NEVUS, HALO; NEVUS, SEBACEOUS; NEVUS, SPITZ; NEVUS ARANEUS; NEVUS DEPIGMENTOSUS; NEVUS PIGMENTOSUS; NEVUS SYNDROME, DYSPLASTIC; PORT-WINE STAIN.

nevus syndrome, dysplastic An often-hereditary condition characterized by groups of pigmented skin abnormalities, which in some patients may indicate a predisposition to malignant melanoma. Such cancerous melanomas may grow from the nevi themselves, or elsewhere on the body.

The trait usually has an autosomal dominant mode of transmission, which means that only one defective gene (from one parent) is needed to cause the syndrome. Each child of an affected person usually has a one in two chance of inheriting the defective gene and of being affected. A patient with dysplastic nevi with two or more primary family members with malignant melanoma has a very strong chance—almost 100 percent—of developing the cancer as well.

Symptoms and Diagnostic Path

Dysplastic nevi are different from ordinary nevi in that they are bigger and usually more prevalent (often more than 100). And while ordinary nevi do not usually appear in adulthood, dysplastic nevi continue to develop throughout life. When researchers followed the evolution of dysplastic nevi in 153 patients aged 12 to 73 for seven years, they found new nevi common—even among adults—continuing to appear in 20 percent of adults over age 50. The moles also changed appearance, or disappeared in people of all ages.

Treatment Options and Outlook

Suspect nevi should be seen by a doctor and removed. If a patient's parent has dysplastic nevi *without* melanoma, the chance of the patient developing melanoma is less definite; however, the patient still is at higher risk than the general population.

Patients with dysplastic nevi but no family history of melanoma have "sporadic" dysplastic nevus syndrome. If these patients have high numbers of nevi, they are still at a higher risk for developing malignant melanoma than the general population, but less than for those in the familial dysplastic nevus group.

Risk Factors and Preventive Measures

Patients with multiple dysplastic nevi and a family history of malignant melanoma should avoid the sun and use SUNSCREEN, practice skin self-examination, and see a DERMATOLOGIST every six months. To spot signs of dysplastic nevi that may be turning malignant, check for the "ABCs": the blemish is *asymmetrical,* the *border* is notched or blurred (not smooth and distinct), and the *color* includes mixtures of shades.

See also BIRTHMARK; MELANOMA, MALIGNANT; MOLE; NEVUS; NEVUS, BLUE; NEVUS, COMPOUND; NEVUS, EPIDERMAL; NEVUS, HALO; NEVUS, SEBACEOUS; NEVUS SPITZ; NEVUS ARANEUS; NEVUS DEPIGMENTOSUS; NEVUS PIGMENTOSUS; NEVUS SYNDROME, DYSPLASTIC; PORT-WINE STAIN.

newborn skin   The skin of a newborn usually is smooth and velvety, with a greasy coating that is shed after about a week. At birth, the skin is a reddish purple color, which changes rapidly to pink. The hands and feet may remain purple a little longer, and this coloring may recur later when the child cries, holds its breath, or becomes chilled. There are a variety of disorders that can develop in newborn skin during the first few weeks of life. Most of these are natural phenomena and resolve on their own. Knowing and understanding these disorders is essential if one is to distinguish them from more significant, potentially critical, problems.

See also BIRTHMARKS; CRADLE CAP; DIAPER RASH; INFANT ACNE.

niacin deficiency   See PELLAGRA.

nickel dermatitis   See DERMATITIS, NICKEL.

nifedipine   A drug commonly used to treat angina that is also used in the treatment of circulation disorders such as RAYNAUD'S DISEASE.

Side Effects

Possible effects include fluid retention and swelling, flushing, headache, and dizziness.

Nikolsky's sign   A diagnostic technique in which the skin sloughs off with slight lateral pressure.

Nikolsky's sign is seen in superficial blistering disorders such as in SCALDED SKIN SYNDROME, toxic epidermal necrolysis, and in PEMPHIGUS, but it is not usually seen in deeper blistering diseases such as bullous pemphigoid.

nitrobenzenes Hair dyes used in semipermanent shampoo-in hair color. The color is formulated to last up to a month, but this depends on how often hair is washed.

nits The tiny eggs of a louse that are yellow when newly laid, turning to white once they hatch.

Symptoms and Diagnostic Path
Nits are small, oval-shaped eggs that are "glued" at an angle to the side of the hair shaft. Nits hatch within eight days, and the empty eggshells are carried outward as the hair grows. Both head and pubic LICE lay eggs at the base of hairs growing on the head or pubic area. Nits can be seen anywhere on the hair, especially behind the ears and at the back of the neck.

Nits should not be confused with hair debris, such as fat plugs or hair casts. Fat plugs are bright white irregularly shaped clumps of fat cells stuck to the hair shaft. Hair casts are thin, long, cylinder-shaped segments of dandruff encircling the hair shaft; they are easily dislodged.

Lice infestations are diagnosed by the presence of nits; by calculating the distance from the base of the hair to the farthest nits, it is possible to estimate the duration of the infestation.

Treatment Options and Outlook
All nits must be removed, according to the National Pediculosis Association. Since no lice pesticide kills all nits, thorough nit removal will reduce or eliminate the need for more treatments.

Nits can be removed with a special nit removal comb, with baby safety scissors, or with the fingernails.

nocardiosis An infection by a funguslike bacterium (*Nocardia asteroides*) found throughout the world that starts in the lungs and spreads to tissues under the skin where fistulas develop. This infection is not normally found in healthy patients, and usually occurs in those with a compromised immune system.

Symptoms and Diagnostic Path
Symptoms include fever and cough similar to pneumonia that does not respond to normal short-term antibiotics, with lung damage and brain ABSCESSes.

Treatment Options and Outlook
Sulfonamide drugs (sulfadiazine) or a combination of trimethoprim-sulfamethoxazole (TMP-SMX) are effective. Drainage or resection of abscesses may be necessary. The prognosis is good with early diagnosis, before the infection spreads to the brain.

nodule A solid mass of tissue larger than 1 cm in diameter that may protrude from the skin or occur deep underneath the surface.

non-ablative skin resurfacing A method to refresh the skin using non-wounding lasers and intense pulsed light that work beneath the surface skin layer to stimulate collagen production, tone and tighten skin and improve mild to moderate skin damage.

This noninvasive approach is used to erase fine lines and skin imperfections, buffing the top layers of aged, discolored or irregular skin while avoiding many of the side effects and extended recovery period typical of traditional resurfacing techniques. Non-ablative lasers and intense pulsed light sources work by aiming light energy on the underlying skin, while leaving the surface of the skin untouched. The selective laser erases surface blemishes as the heat effects of treatment stimulate the production of new collagen deep within the skin. Non-ablative therapy also helps correct irregular skin pigmentation and improves skin texture and tone. By directly treating the layers beneath the top layer of skin, the tissue can respond by regenerating skin as if it was repairing a wound. The process seems to stimulate collagen growth and tighten underlying skin, improving skin tone and removing fine lines and mild to moderate skin damage.

The results from non-ablative lasers are more subtle and gradual than a facelift or conventional laser resurfacing, improving the look of the skin after a series of treatment sessions. The advantage to these procedures is that patients can return to work the same day, and because the surface skin is not broken, women can reapply makeup before leaving the doctor's office. Best results usually occur after three to five treatments. Occasional retouch sessions can help maintain the appearance of smooth, healthy skin. The subtle nature of the non-ablative resurfacing make this a favorite approach for younger men and women who want to begin preserving their looks before much damage is done.

Patients seeking nonablative skin rejuvenation are most often treated with lasers (58 percent), according to the American Society for Dermatologic Surgery. An additional 31 percent of patients are treated with intense pulsed light/non-laser sources.

Side Effects

Mild redness may last for a few hours with non-ablative techniques, and makeup may be applied afterward. Four to six treatments are usually necessary because the results from non-ablative techniques are generally less dramatic than those with Er:YAG and CO_2 lasers.

non-Hodgkin's cutaneous lymphomas Slow-growing tumors of the lymphatic system that cause skin symptoms. They may appear in patients with systemic disease or may be the first sign of lymphoma.

Symptoms and Diagnostic Path

The firm smooth skin lesions may be red, blue- or plum-colored and can be found on any part of the body. They may also cause itchiness or dark patches on the skin.

Treatment Options and Outlook

The lesions generally respond to ionizing radiation or to chemotherapy. Because most patients have (or will develop) widespread lymphoma throughout their body, their prognosis is not usually promising.

noninvasive cutaneous infections See TINEA.

Norwegian scabies A type of mild to severe redness and scaling of the skin characterized by thick crusted lesions on hands, nails, and feet associated with a widespread infestation of SCABIES and mites.

Symptoms and Diagnostic Path

Mites are easily seen among the scales. Unlike ordinary scabies, there is little or no ITCHING. The condition may be seen in retarded patients, patients with AIDS, and other individuals suffering from debilitating medical conditions.

Treatment Options and Outlook

Treatment is the same as for scabies.

nose repair An operation (also called rhinoplasty) that alters the nose structure to either correct a deformity caused by injury or disease, or to repair its appearance. In the technique, incisions are made within the nose to avoid visible scars, using a local or general anesthetic. Sometimes, a bone or cartilage graft is used, and the nose is splinted in position for about 10 days.

Risks/Complications

Rarely, complications may include recurrent nosebleeds because of persistent crusting at the site of the incision, or breathing problems because of narrowed nasal passages. These operations usually cause considerable bruising and swelling.

Outlook

Final results may not be noticeable until weeks or months later.

NSAIDS See NONSTEROIDAL ANTI-INFLAMMATORY DRUGS.

nucleic acids The building blocks of protein, these specific chemicals act on the nucleus of cells. They cannot stimulate growth when applied to the skin's surface or to the hair. However, like all proteins, nucleic acids in cosmetics can form a film on the skin or hair shaft to help retain moisture.

nummular dermatitis See DERMATITIS, NUMMULAR.

nutrition and the skin See DIET AND THE SKIN.

Nystatin See MYCOSTATIN.

oatmeal A colloid-containing grain that soothes the skin and can be very helpful for itchy skin conditions. Preparations containing oatmeal can soothe skin irritated by sunburn or allergic reaction. Oatmeal is also included in face masks and soaps because it absorbs oil from the skin's surface and lessens redness of irritating ACNE-prone skin. Nonirritating oatmeal soaps are a good choice for people with sensitive skin.

occupational skin disorders Because the skin has such a large surface area accessible to the environment, it is particularly vulnerable to problems related to occupational trauma and disease. In fact, after traumatic injuries, skin problems represent almost half of all remaining occupational illnesses. As new industrial chemicals and production processes are developed, new skin diseases and problems continue to appear.

Occupational skin diseases include systemic diseases (caused by absorption through the skin), contact dermatitis, PHOTOSENSITIVITY DISORDERS, disorders of pigmentation, SKIN CANCER, connective tissue diseases, hair and nail disorders, occupational infections and infestations, and disorders caused by physical and mechanical agents.

Skin absorption is one way that many toxic substances (such as agricultural pesticides) enter the body. Some of the major industrial chemicals that cause toxic systemic diseases by being absorbed in the skin include aniline dyes, arsenic, benzene, cyanide salts, mercury, methyl-*n*-butyl ketone, polyhalogenated aromatic hydrocarbons, organic solvents, and neuromuscular insecticides.

About 90 percent of all skin diseases acquired via occupations are *contact dermatitis.* Most cases are due to skin irritation, not allergy, through skin contact with an irritating substance. Some common industrial irritants include solvents, acids and alkalies, industrial detergents, cleaning compounds, abrasive soaps, waterless hand cleaners, poison ivy or oak, metallic salts, rubber antioxidants, epoxy resins and hardeners, acrylic resins, biocidal agents, and organic dyes.

Other substances encountered in the workplace that may cause skin problems may include fragrances, cosmetic preservatives, and topical medications included in soaps, hand creams, or first-aid products.

Photosensitivity

Certain industrial chemicals, when present on the skin and exposed to sunlight, can cause an acute SUNBURN or ECZEMA. The resulting photosensitivity may cause redness and swelling, with VESICLES or BLISTERS that later weep, crust, or scale. Chemicals such as creosote and tar may cause burning and stinging after sun exposure. Severe blistering may occur in celery harvesters caused by toxins released by celery fungus, and certain new acrylic resins may produce both phototoxic and photoallergic reactions.

Acne

ACNE may be induced or aggravated by experiences in the workplace as well. Tight-fitting masks may cause ACNE MECHANICA; lubricating oils or grease may irritate the follicles and cause oil acne. Finally, CHLORACNE is caused by exposure to specific aromatic hydrocarbons in the workplace.

Disorders of Pigmentation

The synthesis of MELANIN may be slowed down or speeded up by a variety of occupational substances, leading to disorders of pigmentation. Such changes in skin color may follow any contact dermatitis, and certain photosensitizers (especially tar, pitch, and furocoumarins) may also alter skin pigmentation. Similarly, the loss of pigment may be caused by exposure to a variety of industrial substances, such as phenol. Skin discoloration has been associated with heavy metal contact (especially silver and mercury), and from dyes.

Skin Cancer

Skin cancer was the first type of malignancy to be associated with occupational risks, when in 1775 Percivall Potts discovered that soot caused SQUAMOUS CELL CARCINOMA in the scrotum of London's chimney sweeps.

People who work outdoors in natural sunlight, or who are exposed to ionizing radiation, are at greatest risk for the development of skin cancer. While coal tar and its derivatives (such as pitch and creosote) may contribute to the development of premalignant skin WARTS and keratoses that eventually are transformed into squamous cell carcinoma, researchers have not yet proved that any chemical carcinogen causes malignant melanoma.

Connective Tissue Diseases

Diseases such as SCLERODERMA may be caused by on-the-job exposure to silica in mining operations. Acrosteolysis has been linked to the manufacture of certain polyvinylchloride plastics.

Hair Loss

Hair loss may be caused by a variety of toxic exposures in the workplace or by mechanical accidents. A wide variety of infections may be picked up on the job, often linked to poor hygiene or minor abrasions and lacerations. Finally, heat, electricity, cold, wind, vibration, and radiation may cause a wide variety of skin problems.

Risk Factors and Preventive Measures

Workers should wear protective clothing, use barrier creams, and practice good hygiene. Depending on the job description, gloves, boots, sleeves, aprons, coveralls, and different types of face protection must be worn to keep out toxic substances.

See also DERMATITIS, CONTACT.

oil of bergamot   A type of oil contained in the skin of lemons and limes that, when applied to the skin, can cause burns and BLISTERS after exposure to sunlight.

Although lemons and limes are most notorious for their phototoxic reactions, many other plants and foods also contain the oil in lesser amounts—carrots, celery, figs, parsley, parsnips, coriander, caraway, fennel, and anise. Even perfumes that contain the oil can cause burns when oil-soaked skin is exposed to the sun.

Young children who suck on limes or lemons in the hot sun are particularly prone to skin burns and blisters, since juice of the fruit dribbles onto the face or drops onto the chest, which then causes burns from the ultraviolet rays of the sun.

The chemical in oil of bergamot responsible for the phototoxic reaction is PSORALEN, ironically now used for its therapeutic benefits. Many years ago, a Cairo dermatologist found out that indigenous people along the Nile used plants containing psoralen as a folk remedy to treat VITILIGO, a skin disorder in which the immune system attacks and destroys the skin's pigment. While researchers are not sure why it works, they believe that psoralen, when combined with sunlight, may suppress the immune system and stop the attack on the skin's pigment, or simply that the psoralen augments the sun's ability to produce pigmentation. Psoralen plus sunlight also interferes with the way cells make DNA, thus decreasing cell turnover, so it is also used to treat PSORIASIS (a disease featuring excessive cell turnover).

ointment   A greasy, semi-solid substance that is placed on the skin either to apply drugs or to provide a protective barrier. Most ointments contain petrolatum or wax with an EMOLLIENT for a moisturizing effect.

onychodystrophy   Malformation of a nail.

onychogryphosis   A curved overgrowth and thickening of the nail. The cause is unknown.

onycholysis Separation of part or all of a nail from its bed. It is a common symptom that may be associated with thyroid disorders, an injury to the nail, exposure to chemicals, or use of nail cosmetics combined with a fungi, yeast, or bacterial infection.

Symptoms and Diagnostic Path

A nail that has lifted from its bed at its end can have an irregular border between the pink portion of the nail and the white outside edge. Most of the nail is opaque, either white, yellow, green, or discolored. Depending on the cause of onycholysis, the nail may have collected thickened skin underneath the edge of its nail plate, and the nail plate may have a deformed shape with indentations in the nail surface, a bent nail edge, or coarse thickening of the nail. If the cause is trauma, the lifted area is white or opaque. If it is a yeast, fungal, or bacterial infection, it may be yellow, green, or shades of black. Onycholysis caused by PSORIASIS is usually cream or yellow.

If an infection is suspected as the cause of nail changes, a scraped sample of tissue from beneath the nail plate can be examined under a microscope or sent to the lab to confirm the diagnosis.

Treatment Options and Outlook

Onycholysis is not an urgent problem and can be discussed with a doctor on a routine checkup. However, diabetics should seek treatment quickly to prevent other complications.

Treatment for onycholysis depends on the cause of the problem.

Treatment for hyperthyroidism can permit normal regrowth of the nails. Some oral treatments for psoriasis that are given by mouth may improve nail health. Fungal nail infections can sometimes be treated with prescription medicines. However, the medicines required to treat the nail condition are expensive and potentially toxic.

Regular clipping and application of a topical antifungal such as imidazole derivative is recommended. Patients with *Candida* infection should avoid water. Antibiotics may help if bacteria is present.

Nails are slow to grow and take time to repair themselves. The portion of nail that has separated from the skin surface beneath it will not reattach—onycholysis only clears after new nail has replaced the affected area. It takes four to six months for a fingernail to fully regrow, and twice as long for toenails. Some nail problems are difficult to cure and may permanently affect the nail appearance.

Risk Factors and Preventive Measures

Some things will make onycholysis less likely to occur. Nails should be cut to a comfortable length so that they will be less likely to endure repeated "tapping" trauma in everyday use. Rubber gloves should be worn to avoid repetitive immersion in water. Nails expand after they are exposed to moisture and then shrink while drying, a cycle that over time can make them brittle. Keeping nails dry will also help prevent fungal infections. Frequent exposure to harsh chemicals such as nail polish remover should be avoided.

Because the portion of nail that has lifted away from its bed may catch on edges when moving abruptly, it is a good idea to trim the nail close to its separation.

onychomalacia Softening of the nails.

onychomycosis A fungal disease of the nails that often occurs on the feet, where it may be associated with ATHLETE'S FOOT. It is much less common on the fingernails. The infection is usually caused by *Trichophyton rubrum* or *T. mentagrophytes*.

Symptoms and Diagnostic Path

The infection first causes a discolored nail edge, spreading until the entire plate is discolored, ragged, thickened, and rough. Sometimes, however, there is only a slight infection of the upper surface of the nail, which has a chalky color.

Treatment Options and Outlook

Most topical antifungals are not effective in treating fungal nail infections; fingernail fungal infections usually require systemic treatment. Systemic antifungals such as itraconazole are effective, clearing 70 percent to 80 percent of nail fungus infections. The effectiveness of treatment depends on how faithfully the patient takes the medication. However, if the fungal infection returns, treatment is far less successful because the DERMATOPHYTE may develop resistance to GRISEOFULVIN.

Infections of the toenail are more difficult to treat in part because it can take up to 18 months for a toenail to grow out.

onychotillomania   Pulling, poking, or tearing of the nails that is a manifestation of DELUSIONS OF PARASITOSIS. In this condition, the patient cuts down the nails in search of parasites. It may also occur as a nervous habit.

open wet dressings   A type of topical preparation useful in conditions characterized by VESICLES, PUSTULES, exudates, and crusts, such as in a poison ivy rash. These dressings cool and dry the skin by evaporation; as they are removed, they help remove the crusts and exudate from the surface. Appropriate use of open wet dressings can control exudation and inflammation.

The solutions usually consist of room-temperature water or saline. Other agents include silver nitrate, BUROW'S SOLUTION, potassium permanganate, 5 percent acetic acid, and sodium hypochlorite.

orf   A viral infection with skin symptoms caused by a subgroup of poxviruses found around the world in sheep and goats. Human infection is usually caused by direct contact with infected material from animals or animal products. Veterinarians, farmers, shepherds, and butchers are especially at risk.

The infection is characterized by large crusting purple PUSTULES with a white center and a red edge appearing on the hands.

Symptoms and Diagnostic Path
Following an incubation period of up to a week, a firm red PAPULE appears and enlarges into a large crusted hemorrhagic pustule. The lesions usually appear alone on the fingers, hands, forearms, or (occasionally) the face. There is sometimes an accompanying low fever.

Treatment Options and Outlook
No treatment (other than prevention of secondary infection) is required. The infection will heal spontaneously within three to six weeks; primary infection confers lifelong immunity.

Risk Factors and Preventive Measures
Those working with animals should watch for lesions around the mouths of sheep or goats. There have been no reports of infection spreading from one human to another.

orthokeratosis   Normal production of keratin (KERATINIZATION).

Osler-Weber-Rendu disease   A genetic disorder of the blood vessels in which small vessels are dilated in the skin and mucous membranes. The condition affects about one in 10,000 people, both men and women from all racial and ethnic groups.

The disorder is named after several doctors who studied the condition between 50 and 100 years ago. In 1896, Dr. Rendu first described this condition as a hereditary disorder involving nosebleeds and characteristic red spots that was distinctly different from hemophilia. Drs. Weber and Osler reported on additional features of the disease in the early 1900s. Still, a century later it is often misdiagnosed in affected individuals, and many doctors do not understand all of its manifestations.

A patient with this condition has a tendency to form blood vessels that lack the capillaries connecting an artery and vein. This means that arterial blood under high pressure flows directly into a vein without first having to squeeze through the very small capillaries. This place where an artery is connected directly to a vein tends to be a fragile site that can rupture and bleed. This type of abnormal blood vessel in which a small artery is attached to a small vein is called a TELANGIECTASIA. Telangiectasia tend to occur at the surface of the body, such as the skin and the mucous membrane that lines the nose.

In the mid-1990s scientists discovered two genes (one on chromosome 9, one on 12) that are responsible for most cases. There may be one or more other genes that can cause this condition, but if so they are quite rare. Any individual will have only one of these two abnormal genes. Normally, these genes tell the body to produce a substance that is involved in the formation of blood vessels; patients make less of one of these substances. This in turn can interfere with normal formation of a blood vessel. The abnormal gene is usually inherited from one parent who has the condition, which is a "dominant" disorder, meaning it only takes one abnormal copy of the gene, from only one parent, to cause the problem. Each child of a parent with the gene has a 50 percent chance of inheriting it. If a given child does not inherit the gene from a parent, they will not pass the gene to their children or grandchildren. However, it is possible for an individual with the gene to have such mild symptoms that they are not recognized, or that symptoms are recognized but not attributed to the disease. Very rarely, a new mutation occurs in a sperm or egg cell of an unaffected parent and causes the disease in the child. But in most cases, the abnormal gene has been in the family for generations.

Currently, scientists are trying to understand better exactly how it is that the abnormal gene can interfere with normal blood vessel formation.

In a normal person, arteries carry blood under high pressure to all areas of the body after being pumped by the heart. Veins carry blood under low pressure on its way back to the heart. An artery does not usually connect directly to a vein; instead, very small blood vessels called capillaries link an artery to a vein.

Symptoms and Diagnostic Path

The telangiectasias occur primarily in the nose; skin of the face, hands, and mouth; and the lining of the stomach and intestines (GI tract), lungs, and brain. It is not currently known why they tend to occur in certain parts of the body and not others. Its location in the body determines what problem a telangiectasia might cause. In most locations, and at any size, a telangiectasia is more likely to rupture and bleed.

The lesions in this disorder may be present at birth, but more often they appear after puberty and progress with age. Hemorrhage is common and often serious. Telangiectasia of the skin of the hands, face, and mouth are found in about 95 percent of all people with the disease. These often do not become apparent until the 30s or 40s, when they appear as small red-to-purplish spots or distinct areas of delicate, lacy red vessels. In some individuals, they become quite prominent by late adulthood; in others they are subtle. These telangiectasia on the skin and in the mouth can bleed also, but they are less likely to than those in the nose. Both telangiectasia of the skin and nosebleeds have a tendency to become more numerous with increasing age. But with this, too, there are many exceptions.

Symptoms may vary considerably, even within a family. A parent may have horrible nosebleeds, but no problems in an internal organ, while their child may rarely have a nosebleed but have more problems with internal organs. It is not possible to predict how likely someone is to have one of the hidden, internal telangiectasias based on how many nosebleeds or skin lesions they have. About 95 percent of patients have recurring nosebleeds by the time they reach middle age. The average age at which nosebleeds begin is 12, but they can begin as early as infancy or as late as adulthood. The nosebleeds can be rare or can occur daily. When a nosebleed occurs it can last only seconds, or occasionally hours. The amount of blood lost may be one or two drops, or enough to require a blood transfusion. Most patients are in between the two extremes. About 25 percent of those will develop bleeding in the gastrointestinal tract that may range from mild to severe.

There is currently no test that can be done to determine if someone has HHT, although soon genetic testing of a blood sample will be able to reveal the condition. Until then, a physician must decide whether someone has the disease based on symptoms and family history. Since it is so variable, and since in many individuals the symptoms are so few, it can be difficult to be certain about the diagnosis.

The diagnosis is considered definite if three or more of the following four criteria are present and "suspected" if two of the following four criteria are present:

- Nosebleeds: spontaneous and recurrent
- Telangiectasia: multiple, at characteristic sites, including lips, mouth, fingers, and nose.
- Internal telangiectasia: lung, brain, GI, liver, or spinal
- Family history: parent, sibling, or child with the disease.

Treatment Options and Outlook

Although there is not yet a way to prevent the telangiectasia from occurring, most can be treated once they occur. They should be treated if they are causing a significant problem, such as frequent nosebleeds.

Telangiectasia of the skin can be treated with laser therapy if they bleed to an extent that is bothersome or are a cosmetic concern. Lesions of the skin are usually best treated by a dermatologist who has expertise in the use of lasers.

osteopoikilosis with connective tissue nevus   See BUSCHKE-OLLENDORFF SYNDROME.

otitis externa   An inflammation of the outer ear caused by infection or the result of an inflammatory skin disorder (such as atopic ECZEMA or seborrheic DERMATITIS). The condition is also known as "swimmer's ear" because it can occur after swimming in dirty or heavily chlorinated water. The risk of getting swimmer's ear rises with the frequency of swimming, the longer the person stays in the water, and the longer the head is submerged.

Symptoms and Diagnostic Path

Swimmer's ear usually causes redness and swelling in the ear canal, a discharge, and sometimes eczema around the ear opening. ITCHING may become painful and deafness can occur if pus blocks the ear.

Swimmer's ear also can be caused by excessive washing, perspiration, irritation of the ear canal after removing a foreign object, allergies, or a generalized skin disease.

Malignant otitis externa is a rare (and sometimes fatal) form of the disease caused by the bacterium *Pseudomonas aeruginosa*. This type of otitis sometimes spreads into surrounding bones and soft tissue, and usually affects elderly diabetics with a lowered resistance to disease.

Treatment Options and Outlook

Usually the only required treatment is a thorough cleaning and drying of the ear together with antibiotic, antifungal, or anti-inflammatory drugs. A wick should be used to instill drops into the ear in ear canals that are badly swollen. Patients should avoid getting the ear wet until the condition is completely healed.

otoplasty   A cosmetic operation to correct oversized or malformed ears. By the age of six, most children's ears have reached adult size and an operation to repair them may be considered. In the operation, an incision is made behind the ear, and excess skin is removed; at this time, the ear itself can be reshaped or recurled. The day after surgery, bandages are removed, and smaller, lighter bandages are applied until the sixth day, when stitches are removed. A ski headband can be worn at night for a month after the operation to prevent distortions of the ear as it heals.

oxytetracycline   A TETRACYCLINE antibiotic used to treat a wide variety of infections, including chlamydia, SYPHILIS, ROCKY MOUNTAIN SPOTTED FEVER, cholera, and the PLAGUE.

Side Effects

Possible side effects include rash, increased skin sensitivity to the sun, nausea, and vomiting. Because oxytetracycline may discolor developing teeth and bones, it is not prescribed during pregnancy or for youngsters under the age of 12.

PABA The abbreviation for the active ingredient in SUNSCREEN—PARA-AMINOBENZOIC ACID—which is very effective in blocking ultraviolet B (UVB) rays of the sun.

Some people are allergic to PABA and its esters, especially if they are allergic to the "-caine" group of anesthetics (lidocaine, benzocaine, and so on) or to certain hair dyes. Allergic reactions to PABA resemble SUNBURN.

pachydermoperiostosis A rare hereditary disease characterized by thickened furrows on the face (especially on the forehead), with large, active sebaceous glands and oily skin. In addition, there is often a marked folding of the scalp skin (cutis verticis gyrata) and excessive sweating.

It is an autosomal dominant disease, which means that only one defective gene (from one parent) is needed to cause the syndrome. Each child of an affected person usually has a one in two chance of inheriting the defective gene and of being affected, and a one in two chance of being unaffected.

pachyonychia Thickened nails that may occur as an inherited disease.

padimate O A derivative of PABA that can block the damaging effects of the sun. See PABA.

pallor Abnormally pale skin (especially of the face) that may be a symptom of a disease or a simple deficiency of the skin pigment MELANIN or a constriction of blood vessels in the skin.

Melanin deficiency can be caused by a lack of exposure to the sun, or it can be the result of the hereditary condition known as ALBINISM.

Constriction of blood flow to the skin is a reaction of the body in an effort to shunt blood to the vital organs and the brain. Constricted blood vessels in the skin may be caused by severe pain, injury, fainting, extreme cold, or excessive blood loss, leading to shock. Pallor may also be a symptom of anemia, caused by the lack of hemoglobin pigment in blood vessels in the skin.

Pallor as a symptom of disease may be caused by kidney disorders such as pyelonephritis or renal failure, or from hypothyroidism. Other diseases that might cause pallor include lead poisoning or scurvy.

palmar-plantar keratosis A descriptive term for the thickening of the horny layer of palms and soles as seen in a wide variety of acquired and hereditary disorders. These include CORNS, CALLUSES, WARTS, hand ECZEMA, HOWEL-EVANS SYNDROME, MAL DE MELEDA, and so on.

panniculitis A general term for a group of conditions involving inflammation of fat tissue just beneath the skin, caused by a wide variety of diseases. Different types of panniculitis can be divided into two main types: mostly septal or mostly lobular, depending on where the inflammation is found.

Symptoms and Diagnostic Path
Although there are many different causes, most types of panniculitis have the same symptoms: pain, tenderness, raised NODULEs, and sometimes large flat areas of thickened skin. As the skin hardens,

it forms lumps, patches, and lesions. There may be a discoloration of the skin (either red or dark brown). After the inflammation subsides, there may be a slight skin depression, either temporary or permanent.

Panniculitis is diagnosed by a skin biopsy to distinguish the different microscopic features of individual types of panniculitis.

Treatment Options and Outlook

The underlying cause of the panniculitis should be treated (if known). The affected area should be elevated and compression hosiery should be worn, if possible. Anti-inflammatory medications such as aspirin or ibuprofen may be administered for the pain; oral or injected systematic steroids may treat the inflammation. Other medications may include potassium iodine or antibiotics (such as TETRACYCLINE or hydroxychloroquine). Persistent lesions may need to be surgically removed.

panthenol A VITAMIN B complex that can add strength and body to hair by filling in cracks on the shaft, thereby firming up the fiber.

panthothenic acid A B vitamin found in liver, eggs, and dried brewer's yeast (and the ROYAL JELLY of bees) that some people erroneously believe can prevent gray hair.

papilloma A generic term usually referring to a nonmalignant tumor resembling a WART with a broad base, that arises from the EPITHELIUM (cell layer that forms the skin and mucous membranes)—most commonly on the skin, tongue, or larynx and in the urinary tract, digestive tract, or breasts.

papilloma virus, human (HPV) A very common and extremely contagious virus that can cause abnormal warty tissue growth on the feet, hands, vocal cords, mouth, and genitals. More than 100 types of HPV have been identified; each type infects certain parts of the body and produces a specific type of wart. Some cause WARTS, including PLANTAR WARTS on the feet, common hand warts, juvenile warts, and GENITAL WARTS. The most common type of HPV is the basic wart on hands or feet. These are not associated with cancer, but are very stubborn to treat. A wide variety of benign and cancerous growths also may be associated with HPVs, some of which has been demonstrated to cause vulvar or cervical cancer in some women.

HPV is one of the most common causes of sexually transmitted diseases in the world. About 30 of the more than 100 different type of HPV are spread through sexual contact. Some types of HPV cause genital warts—single or multiple bumps that appear in the genital areas of men and women, including the vagina, cervix, vulva, penis, and rectum.

About 20 million people are currently infected with HPV, and at least half of all sexually active men and women acquire a genital HPV infection at some point in their lives. By age 50, at least 80 percent of women will have acquired genital HPV infection. About 6.2 million Americans get a new genital HPV infection each year. There are high-risk and low-risk types of HPV. High-risk HPV may cause abnormal Pap smear results, and could lead to cancers of the cervix, vulva, vagina, anus, or penis. Low-risk HPV also may cause abnormal Pap results or genital warts.

Symptoms and Diagnostic Path

Many people infected with HPV have no symptoms. A health care provider usually diagnoses warts by visual inspection. Any woman with genital warts should be examined for possible HPV infection of the cervix. If a woman has an abnormal Pap smear, it may indicate the possible presence of cervical HPV infection. A laboratory worker will examine cells scraped from the cervix to see if they are cancerous.

Treatment Options and Outlook

There is no known cure for HPV. There are treatments to remove warts, but they often disappear even without treatment. There is no way to predict whether the warts will grow or disappear. Anyone who suspects genital warts should be examined and treated, if necessary. A recently-developed vaccine that appears to prevent HPV infection has not yet been approved by the U.S. Food and Drug Administration.

papovaviruses One of a group of viruses producing nonmalignant tumors in humans. Papovaviruses are divided into two types: polyomaviruses and PAPILLOMA VIRUS. Polyomaviruses induce tumors in rodents; at least three polyomaviruses are believed to cause disease in humans; BKV, JCV, and SV40. Papilloma viruses induce benign tumors of the head and neck and several varieties of skin WARTS on hands, feet, mouth, and genitals.

papular acrodermatitis See GIANOTTI-CROSTI SYNDROME.

papular dermatitis of pregnancy Also known as Spangler's dermatitis of pregnancy, this condition is a rare, severely itchy disease that can occur at any time during pregnancy. Abnormal hormone levels are linked to this disorder, especially high levels of gonadotrophins and low cortisol and estrogen levels.

Symptoms and Diagnostic Path
The condition is characterized by uniform crusted, excoriated red PAPULES that appear in groups of wheals. As the lesions fade, the skin may become hyperpigmented, but this will fade after pregnancy.

Treatment Options and Outlook
Administration of systemic CORTICOSTEROIDS is recommended. Associated with 30 percent of stillbirth or spontaneous abortion cases, this condition recurs with subsequent pregnancies.

papular mucinosis See LICHEN MYXEDEMATOSUS.

papular urticaria A condition caused by a hypersensitive reaction to insect bites (especially fleas, bedbugs, mosquitoes, and dog lice). The condition appears primarily in children aged two to seven; the disease is rare in infancy and uncommon in adulthood.

Symptoms and Diagnostic Path
The lesions appear solid instead of as a swelling, and are sometimes indistinguishable from an insect bite. They are generally found on exposed areas of the skin, especially the face and arms and legs. In some cases, they represent an overreaction to INSECT BITES, while in others the lesions appear faraway from the insect bite site as an allergic reaction to the bite.

The lesions transform into an inflammatory, firm, red-brown persistent PAPULE. Extremely sensitive people may also experience vesicles and blisters. Bacterial infection and excoriations may appear.

In the eastern United States, the problem appears almost exclusively in the summer when fleas are numerous; on the West Coast the problem is found throughout the year.

Treatment Options and Outlook
A topical steroid cream should be applied as soon as the itchy spots appear; antihistamine tablets at night may be useful for severe ITCHING. Antibiotic cream should be applied if the spots get infected.

papules Small, solid slightly raised areas of the skin less than half an inch in diameter. They may have a varied appearance: either rounded, smooth or rough, skin-colored or red, pink, or brown. The characteristic lesion in skin conditions such as ACNE or LICHEN PLANUS is a papule.

papulosquamous diseases Conditions characterized by scaling papules or plaques, with sharply defined margins. Crusts, excoriation, or weeping are rarely seen. PSORIASIS is the most typical of the papulosquamous diseases; others include PARAPSORIASIS, LICHEN PLANUS, seborrheic dermatitis, FUNGAL INFECTIONS and SYPHILIS. See DERMATITIS, SEBORRHEIC.

para-aminobenzoic acid See PABA.

parabens, sensitivity to A group of preservatives used in foods, drugs, and cosmetics that can cause a severe redness, swelling, ITCHING, and pain in the skin. They also can cause anaphylactic shock in susceptible individuals.

Foods commonly preserved with parabens include mayonnaise, salad dressings, mustard, processed vegetables, ice cream, some baked goods, jellies and jams, soda, fruit juices, syrups, and candy. Medications, with parabens include creams; SUNSCREENS; eye, ear, and nose drops; deodorants; rectal and vaginal medications; cleansers; bandages; and local anesthetics. Cosmetics containing parabens include foundations, powders, cover-up sticks, bronzers, makeup removers, blushes, highlighters, lipsticks, quick-dry nail products, mascaras, eye shadows, and eye liners.

However, considering how widespread parabens, sensitivity to this preservative is not common. The most commonly used parabens are methylparaben, ethylparaben, p-hydroxybenzoic acid, propylparaben, and butylparaben.

Symptoms and Diagostic Path

Allergic reactions to parabens can cause severe redness, swelling, ITCHING, and pain; severe allergic reaction in sensitive consumers may lead to anaphylactic shock.

Treatment Options and Outlook

Anyone diagnosed with a parabens allergy should avoid products containing this substance. Once a sensitive person has been exposed and the reaction appears on the skin, treatment is the same as for any acute skin rash: topical corticosteroids free of paraben preservatives, emollients, and treatment of any bacterial infection.

See also ALLERGIES AND THE SKIN; PABA.

parapsoriasis A hard-to-treat group of diseases characterized by different-sized superficial scaling plaques. Resembling PSORIASIS, parapsoriasis is not related at all to that disease.

There are three main types of parapsoriasis: parapsoriasis guttata (small plaque parapsoriasis), parapsoriasis lichenoides chronica, and parapsoriasis en plaques (large-plaque parapsoriasis).

PARAPSORIASIS VARIOLIFORMIS ACUTA is a completely different condition, and should not be classified among these diseases.

Symptoms and Diagnostic Path

The first two forms of parapsoriasis are chronic and cause no serious complications, but parapsoriasis en plaques is serious and may progress to MYCOSIS FUNGOIDES. All forms of the disease usually begin with one lesion covered with a fine spreading scale, appearing first on the trunk, arms, or legs.

Parapsoriasis guttata is characterized by fine macules and papules resembling guttate psoriasis, dusted with a fine silvery scale. This condition does not respond to antipsoriasis treatment. The lesions appear on the trunk at any age in both men and women, and may persist for years. ITCHING does not usually occur.

Parapsoriasis lichenoides (or retiform parapsoriasis) is characterized by raised, dull red, scaly papules that appear on the neck, trunk, arms, and legs. The patient's general health is not affected, and itching is not a problem.

In *parapsoriasis en plaques,* lesions are larger than those of either lichenoides or guttata, and they are flatter than lesions in psoriasis. Plaques range from yellow-red to brown with a fine scale, found primarily on the trunk, thighs, and buttocks. Unlike the other two types of parapsoriasis, these lesions may itch and in many cases this type of parapsoriasis may progress to mycosis fungoides.

Treatment Options and Outlook

Treatment for both parapsoriasis guttata and lichenoides may not be necessary, since the lesions cause no problems, although sunlight (UVB and PUVA) or topical CORTICOSTEROIDS may be helpful in clearing them up. Parapsoriasis en plaques may respond to topical steroids, sunlight (ultraviolet B) or PUVA. Patients with parapsoriasis en plaques should be carefully followed by a dermatologist.

parapsoriasis varioliformis acuta A disease that features a papular, scaly rash unrelated to other forms of PARAPSORIASIS. It is also known as acute parapsoriasis, pityriasis lichenoides et varioliformis acuta, or Mucha-Habermann syndrome.

Symptoms and Diagnostic Path

Acute onset appears much like CHICKEN POX with groups of papules, vesicles, and pustular crusted lesions that progress to a necrotic stage, leaving chicken pox–like scars. They typically form on the insides of the forearms and back of the legs.

Treatment Options and Outlook

Large doses of tetracycline, penicillin G, or ERYTH-ROMYCIN are administered for a month; for chronic cases this treatment may not help. While small doses of oral METHOTREXATE will control the disease, when the drug is stopped the lesions return. This condition primarily occurs in patients in their 20s and 30s and lasts from a few weeks to years. Often, it simply disappears without treatment.

parasitic infestations   A wide range of skin symptoms may occur with parasitic infestations, which are endemic in many developing countries throughout the world where poverty, poor hygiene, and poor sanitary facilities are common. Infestation from parasites are divided into those caused by protozoa (single-celled animals), by helminths (worms), and by arthropods (mites or ticks).

Protozoal infestations that cause skin symptoms include LEISHMANIASIS, African and South American trypanosomiasis, amebiasis, trichomoniasis, and TOXOPLASMOSIS.

Parasitic worm infestations with skin symptoms are divided into roundworms (class Nematoda) and flatworms (class Trematoda, or flukes, and Cestoidea, or tapeworms).

Arthropod infestations include mites, ticks, and insects.

Symptoms and Diagnostic Path

Symptoms of parasitic infections vary depending on the type of parasite involved, but ITCHING and skin irritation are common.

Treatment Options and Outlook

Treatment for parasitic infestations depends on the particular parasite involved.

paresthesia   See PINS AND NEEDLES SENSATION.

paronychia   Swelling and inflammation of infected skin at the base of the nail usually caused by the yeast *Candida albicans*. Acute paronychia is the result of bacteria.

Symptoms and Diagnostic Path

The condition begins with a tender red area that may draw pus, and is most often found among women with poor circulation or those who must wash their hands often.

Treatment Options and Outlook

Antifungal or antibiotic drugs will cure this problem. The hands must be kept dry. Any ABSCESSes must be surgically drained.

patch   A flat area of skin larger than one cm in diameter that differs in color from the skin around it.

patch test   A test to discover the cause of an allergic reaction by reproducing allergic contact dermatitis. In the test, the physician places a suspected ALLERGEN in contact with the patient's unbroken skin under occlusion for 48 hours. Positive reactions show redness, swelling, and/or BLISTERS.

The physician can select suspended allergens from a screening tray of chemicals often found in commercial products or with the products that are suspected. The chemical is placed on an adhesive-backed gauze pad, taped in place on the back or inner arm for 48 hours. The reaction is influenced by the skin condition, the concentration and the volume of the testing substance and the vehicle used, the length of time of the test, and the number of readings. The standard tray of allergens is frequently updated by the International Contact Dermatitis Research Group and the North American Contact Dermatitis Research Group.

The standard patch test covers the most common skin allergies, which make up about 80 percent of contact sensitivities. To test for other allergies, supplementary patch testing must be carried out. The type of patch test is determined by the kind of dermatitis, the history of exposure, and the experience of the dermatologist.

If a reaction occurs, the physician can then describe the substance, what common products contain that substance, and what substitutions are available.

Pautrier's micro abscess A characteristic small collection of leukocytes (or white blood cells—lymphocytes) found in the top layer of skin in patients with MYCOSIS FUNGOIDES.

See also DERMATITIS, CONTACT.

pearly penile papules See ANGIOFIBROMA.

peau d'orange French for "skin of an orange," this is a skin symptom caused by fluid retention in nearby lymph glands, dimpling the skin like an orange peel. The fluid retention may be caused by breast cancer in the area around the nipple, in LICHEN MYXEDEMATOSUS, or in some types of skin lymphoma.

pediculi See LICE.

pediculosis Any type of louse infestation.
See also LICE.

pellagra A nutritional disorder affecting the skin caused by a deficiency of niacin (found in meat, yeast extracts, and some cereals). Pellagra is found primarily in parts of India and southern Africa where people live mostly on corn.

While corn has as much niacin as other cereals, the niacin in corn is not absorbed by the body unless first treated with an alkali such as lime water. Corn is also low in tryptophan, an amino acid that the body converts to niacin. This is why other diseases that increase the breakdown of tryptophan, such as inflammatory bowel disease, can also cause pellagra.

Symptoms and Diagnostic Path
First signs of pellagra include ITCHING and inflammation, especially in sun-exposed sites; weak-ness; weight loss; lethargy; depression; and irritability. Severe attacks include bright red weeping BLISTERS, a swollen tongue, DERMATITIS, diarrhea, and, in severe cases, dementia and memory loss.

Treatment Options and Outlook
Several weeks' supplementation with niacin and a varied diet rich in protein and calories will reverse pellagra.

pemphigoid A very rare group of autoimmune blistering diseases in which the body's immune system mistakenly perceives as foreign one or more proteins that naturally occur in the skin or mucous membranes. The immune system responds by producing antibodies against itself that attack these proteins. Because these proteins are responsible for keeping the skin intact, when they are damaged, it results in BLISTERS that do not heal easily. In some cases, these blisters can cover a significant portion of the body. Experts believe some people inherit a tendency to develop this disease, and some groups are at higher risk, but pemphigoid seems to affect different races or genders equally.

Symptoms and Diagnostic Path
There are two major types of pemphigoid—bullous pemphigoid (BP) and cicatricial pemphigoid (CP). The type of autoantibodies produced determines which version of pemphigoid a person develops and in which layer of the skin the blister occurs.

Bullous pemphigoid This type of pemphigoid is characterized by itchy large, tense blisters on the skin. It usually begins with itchy red plaques, followed by intense blisters over several weeks or months. The condition spreads across the body with oozing erosions that may be either painful or itchy.

Cicatricial pemphigoid Primarily a disease of the elderly (between 60 and 80 years) it is rarely seen in young adults. Lesions appear in mucous membranes including the nose, mouth, eyes, esophagus, larynx, urethra, and anus. The gums are often involved, which can cause gingivitis. Temporary small blisters on the head and neck occur in more than 20 percent of patients.

Pemphigoid can be diagnosed after a visual examination of the skin lesions, a biopsy of the lesions, and treatment of the biopsied skin sample to reveal antibodies in the skin (direct immunoflourescence) and in the blood (indirect immunoflourescence).

Treatment Options and Outlook

Prompt doses of steroids (usually prednisone or predinisolone) are needed to control pemphigoid, which is easier to manage than PEMPHIGUS. Patients with small areas of blisters can be treated with topical or intralesional steroids, but patients with more severe or widespread disease are prescribed systemic CORTICOSTEROIDS such as prednisone. Once the disease is under control, the medications are reduced slowly to minimize the risk of side effects. Several other drugs are often used in combination with prednisone, such as antibiotics, immunosuppressants, and METHOTREXATE.

Up to 70 percent of patients with BP will experience a remission within five years of diagnosis, although some patients may experience a relapse. BP lesions should heal without scarring unless secondary infection occurs. Appropriate wound care is important to promote healing and prevent infection and scarring. Spontaneous remissions of CP are rare; this disease is progressive and often does not respond to steroids.

pemphigus An uncommon skin disorder featuring skin BLISTERs most often found in patients between ages 40 and 60. Pemphigus is a more serious disorder than another similar condition, bullous PEMPHIGOID, which features itchy blisters that are not normally fatal. Pemphigus appears more often among Jews and other ethnic groups of Mediterranean and Indian descent.

Pemphigus may be associated with other autoimmune diseases, such as myasthenia gravis and LUPUS ERYTHEMATOSUS. Various forms of pemphigus include pemphigus vulgaris, pemphigus vegetans, pemphigus foliaceus, pemphigus erythematosus, and fogo selvagem.

In pemphigus, antibodies circulate in the blood that react against the intercellular substance of the outer skin layer. These antibodies lead to the formation of blisters.

Symptoms and Diagnostic Path

Blisters first break out in the mouth and nose, then on the skin; the precise location and type of lesions vary depending on the variety of pemphigus. The easily ruptured skin lesions often form raw, painful areas that may become infected and then form a crust.

Treatment Options and Outlook

CORTICOSTEROID drugs given over a long period of time together with immunosuppressant drugs can control the disease. Antibiotics may be given for any resulting skin infections. If the blisters appear over a large area, the condition can lead to secondary skin infections that may be fatal.

pemphigus, familial benign chronic See HAILEY-HAILEY DISEASE.

pemphigus v. pemphigoid There are two types of blistering disorders caused by autoimmune problems in which a patient's own antibodies attack the skin cells. The attack may occur at various layers of the skin. PEMPHIGUS causes a cleavage within the top layer of the skin, with flaccid blisters that break easily. PEMPHIGOID produces a split below the top layer of the skin, causing deeper, tense BLISTERs. Pemphigoid is seen most often in the elderly.

Both are treated with similar medications. Severe cases may require more intensive treatment. Either may recur.

penicillin and derivatives The first group of antibiotic drugs to be discovered (the sulfas are considered to be antibacterials); natural penicillins are derived from the *Penicillium* mold, but can also be produced synthetically. Penicillins are used to treat a wide variety of infections, and include amoxicillin, ampicillin, penicillin G, penicillin V, and penicillin.

Side Effects

Allergic reactions include skin rash, HIVES, and anaphylaxis. Any patient allergic to one type of penicillin should not be given any other. Side effects include vomiting and diarrhea.

See also PENICILLIN RASH.

penicillin rash An allergic skin rash in response to the administration of PENICILLIN and derivatives. The red rash usually appears as HIVES or as a fine macular or papular rash; it can be widespread. These allergic reactions are not uncommon and range from immediate hypersensitivity (including potentially fatal anaphylaxis) to SERUM SICKNESS reactions. Hypersensitivity of one type or another to penicillin is believed to occur in about 1 or 2 percent of the general population.

Anyone who develops such a rash should immediately stop taking the medication and contact a physician. Anaphylaxis should be handled as a medical emergency.

penile warts See WARTS.

peptides A combination of two or more AMINO ACIDS that are used in shampoos, conditioners, and moisturizers because of their ability to retain moisture and strengthen the hair shaft. Peptides form a film on the hair shaft, making the hair seem thicker—they can also fill in cracks on the shaft and make hair shinier. On the skin, peptides form a film that retains moisture.

Physiologically, peptides are found throughout the body's endocrine and nervous systems. Many hormones are peptides; in the nervous system peptides are found in nerve cells throughout the brain and spinal cord.

percutaneous A medical term meaning "performed through the skin." Percutaneous procedures include injections into veins, muscles, or other body tissues, and biopsies in which tissue or fluid is removed with a needle.

perforating disorders A family of several disorders characterized by perforation of elements of the DERMIS through the overlying EPIDERMIS. The perforating disorders include ELASTOSIS PERFORANS SERPIGINOSA, perforating collagenosis, perforating FOLLICULITIS, and KYRLE'S DISEASE. Perforation has also been reported to occur in dermal diseases, including GRANULOMA ANNULARE, necrobiosis lipoidica diabeticorum, and PSEUDOXANTHOMA ELASTICUM.

perfume sensitivity See FRAGRANCE, SENSITIVITY TO.

periarteritis nodosa An uncommon disease of small and medium-sized arteries that causes the arterial wall to become inflamed and weakened, tending to form aneurysms. Many different groups of blood vessels may be involved, including the coronary arteries supplying blood to the heart, and the arteries of the kidneys, intestine, skeletal muscles, and nervous system.

This disorder has been linked to a poorly functioning immune system triggered by exposure to the hepatitis B virus. While it may develop at any age, it is most common among adult men.

Symptoms and Diagnostic Path

Initial symptoms include fever and aching muscles, with a general malaise, appetite and weight loss, and sometimes nerve pain. High blood pressure, muscle weakness, skin ulcers, and gangrene are often associated with the disease.

Treatment Options and Outlook

Large doses of CORTICOSTEROID drugs are given together with immunosuppressant drugs. Without treatment, the condition is almost always fatal within five years by heart attack, kidney failure, intestinal bleeding, or complications of high blood pressure. With treatment, about half of all patients survive for five years.

periderm The outer two layers of fetal epithelium (tissue that covers the external surface of the body) that generally disappear before birth, persisting only as the cuticle.

perifollicular fibromas Small lesions on the face made up of fibrous tissue around hair follicles.

See also ANGIOFIBROMA.

periodic acid-Schiff (PAS) stain One of the most common tests for the presence of fungi and certain microorganisms in tissue sections.

perioral dermatitis See DERMATITIS, PERIORAL.

perleche Inflammation, dryness, and cracking of the corners of the mouth. Perleche is associated with the collection of moisture at the corners of the mouth, which encourages invasion by yeasts and bacteria, especially *Candida albicans,* and streptococci. In children, this is often caused by lip licking, drooling, thumb sucking, and mouth breathing. Adults may be troubled by age-related changes in their mouth and poorly fitting dentures. Rarely, vitamin B deficiency can be the cause.

Treatment Options and Outlook

An antifungal cream followed by a CORTICOSTEROID in a nongreasy base is usually effective.

permanent makeup Also known as "dermapigmentation," this is a technique in which pigment is implanted in the skin to simulate the lines drawn with makeup pencils on eyelids, brows, or lips. Like TATTOOING, dermapigmentation involves dipping a needle into pigment that is injected into the bottom layer of the skin. Each injection leaves behind a tiny dot of pigment. The dots when placed closely enough together look like an unbroken line.

While the procedure is fairly straightforward, it is painful, it carries some risks, and it is permanent.

The technique is most frequently performed by an aesthetician working in a skin-care salon. While a medical professional is better qualified to handle complications, many physicians do not perform the procedure.

Dermapigmentation (like tattooing) is not well regulated: Anyone may perform the procedure, and any state or local ordinances are usually not well enforced. Consumers interested in the procedure should find out how the practitioner was trained; ask to see before-and-after photos; and call past clients to see how pleased they were with the work. Clients must also understand what the end result will look like; dermapigmentation does *not* look like real eyebrow hairs, for example—it looks like makeup. Consumers should realize that once placed in the skin, the pigment cannot be removed.

To some people, dermapigmentation on the sensitive eye or lip area is extremely painful, while others dismiss it as merely uncomfortable. Physicians may use injectable anesthetics (such as those used by dentists) to numb the area, but these may cause swelling and bruising that would otherwise not occur.

It is very important that the procedure be performed in a sterilized environment. In a skincare salon, the dermapigmentation area should be separate from other rooms to protect against contamination from fumes or hair. All parts of the machine that come in contact with the skin and the pigment must be disposable or removable for sterilization *after each use.*

Autoclave sterilization (steam under pressure) is acceptable; dry heat sterilization is not. Because blood is drawn during the procedure, the technician should wear goggles, a face shield, and double gloves.

Pigments should be gamma-irradiated for sterility and approved by the U.S. Food and Drug Administration. Common tattooing dyes, India ink, and vegetable dyes should never be used. Pigment used around the eyes must be an ophthalmologist-tested blend of iron oxide suspended in glycerine and alcohol.

While there have been no irritating reactions to eye pigments, lip lining requires an allergy test before the operation because the ingredients used to produce reddish tones often cause an allergic reaction.

To help decide on colors, the consumer should bring in eye pencils and lipsticks. The pigment shades would not match the pencils exactly because the colors change in contact with skin tone. Custom-mixing colors is not a good idea, because if they are improperly blended they can separate and result in the absence of one of the desired hues.

Placement of the pigment is critical; if placed only on the top layer of skin it will soon be sloughed off. Special needle guns used in the procedure are designed to penetrate skin only as deep as is necessary. This is particularly important around the eyes, where contact must never be made with the eyeball. Occasionally eyebrow pigment is placed too high or with too much of a curve, but once applied, the color cannot be changed.

For more information or for a recommendation of local dermatologists, contact the American Academy of Dermatology, Box 681069, Schaumburg, IL 60168; for a trained anesthetician, call the Aestheticians International Association at (504) 469-1016.

permethrin A synthetic substance that in a 5 percent cream is approved by the U.S. Food and Drug Administration for the treatment of SCABIES. Because of its low toxicity, it is widely prescribed, especially for children. In treating scabies, a single application of permethrin is applied to the entire skin surface and washed off eight to 14 hours later.

pernio See CHILBLAIN.

pet-borne illnesses A wide range of pet-borne illnesses can cause skin symptoms in humans. These include allergies to pet dandruff (see PET DANDER ALLERGY), HOOKWORM, infections from bites, CAT-SCRATCH FEVER, MITES, fleas, RINGWORM, and TOXOPLASMOSIS.

pet dander allergy Allergies to pet dander can cause itching and skin rash in sensitive people. In the case of an allergy, the immune system identifies a normally harmless substance (called an "allergen") as dangerous, and produces antibodies to fight it. The allergen stems from substances in the pet's oil-producing glands, in its skin, or from its saliva. Some experts also believe that cat dander also may contribute to the problem.

Symptoms and Diagnostic Path

Those allergic to cats experience an allergic reaction, which can cause itching, puffy eyes, wheezing, rash, or shortness of breath.

Treatment Options and Outlook

Antihistamines are the primary treatment for most allergies. Repeated allergy shots may allow a patient to build up immunity over a period of several months. However, because people may react adversely to the shots, and because repeated shots are inconvenient, a severe cat or dog allergy is best managed by removing the pet.

Risk Factors and Preventive Measures

Not surprisingly, the best way to handle pet allergies is to avoid pets. But even after removing pets, it may take weeks or months for the allergens to be completely removed from carpeting and furniture. Washing the pet once a week for several weeks will reduce the amount of the airborne allergens by 90 percent. Removing carpeting and upholstered furniture, mopping floors often and vacuuming with a high-efficiency filter will help. An effective air cleaner can remove up to 99 percent of the dust, including pet allergens. Pets should be kept outside as much as possible. Because super-insulated homes have higher allergen levels, good fresh-air circulation will help.

See also PET-BORNE ILLNESSES.

petechiae Flat pinhead-sized spots of red or purple appearing in the skin or mucous membranes caused by a localized hemorrhage from small blood vessels. Petechiae are seen in individuals with bleeding disorders and sometimes appear with bacterial endocarditis (inflammation of the heart's lining).

petroleum jelly An inexpensive oily substance also known as petrolatum used in products to treat chapped, dry, or raw skin. Derived from petroleum, it is commonly used as an ointment base, a protective dressing or an emollient to soften the skin. An excellent protectant against water evaporation, it is very mild and has not been associated with allergies or irritation. It can, however, trigger ACNE in people with oily or acne-prone skin.

Peutz-Jeghers syndrome An inherited autosomal dominant disorder featuring small brown or blue-brown spots on the lips and in the mouth. It is associated with many polyps in the small intestine; while there are often no other symptoms, the polyps may occasionally produce pain or bleeding.

Lesions appear early in childhood and may fade during adolescence. About one-third of affected individuals exhibit symptoms in the first 10 years of life.

Symptoms and Diagnostic Path

In addition to skin lesions, symptoms include abdominal pain, vomiting, and gastrointestinal bleeding. There appears to be a 2 to 3 percent chance for the eventual development of gastrointestinal cancer. Because the polyps are usually numerous and widespread, removal is not often possible.

Treatment Options and Outlook

Bleeding polyps may be removed, but generally treatment aims at symptom management.

phenytoin hypersensitivity syndrome A type of drug reaction causing skin symptoms in response to the anticonvulsant drug used to treat epilepsy. While fairly rare, the reaction can be severe; it usually occurs during the first week of phenytoin use. Phenytoin (Dilantin) is also used occasionally to treat migraines and to control certain types of arrhythmia (irregular heart beat). Cross reaction with other anticonvulsants is common; therefore, physicians should treat with caution.

Symptoms and Diagnostic Path

The syndrome is characterized by fever, a widespread eruption consisting of red PAPULES and plaques with facial swelling, generalized tender swollen lymph nodes, leukocytosis, and liver dysfunction.

Treatment Options and Outlook

The syndrome is reversed when medication is stopped.

phlegmon Intense inflammation of connective tissue, often causing ulcers or abscesses.

photoallergy A condition that occurs after a person experiences an adverse reaction after ingesting or applying a substance (called a photosensitizer) and subsequently exposing the skin to sunlight. Photosensitizers can be applied to the skin or taken internally. Some photosensitizers occur within the body; excessive porphyrin molecules cause PORPHYRIA.

Topical photosensitizers are common ingredients of cosmetics, face creams, perfumes, after-shave lotions, and soaps. Others include medications such as coal tars and PSORALENS that are deliberately used to induce photosensitivity to help treat various skin disorders, or phenothiazines and sulfonamides, which may produce unintended photosensitivity when applied to the skin. Antibacterial agents (such as the halogenated salicylanilides and related compounds) were once used in deodorant soaps; first-aid creams were responsible for an epidemic of photosensitivity reactions in the 1960s.

Plants such as celery, wild carrots, gas plant, limes, and meadow grass contain photosensitizing psoralens. Industrial contaminants and air pollutants such as tars and polycyclic aromatic hydrocarbons are also potent photosensitizers.

Commonly used photosensitizers include sulfonamides, thiazide diuretics, sulfonylureas, phenothiazines, and certain tetracycline derivatives (such as doxycycline). While some of these are more potent, thiazide diuretics produce the most reactions because they are used most frequently.

Symptoms and Diagnostic Path

The reaction is characterized by itchy papular lesions resembling POISON IVY or blistering that may extend beyond the area of exposure. Immediate HIVES occur rarely.

Treatment Options and Outlook

Prevention is the best option; patients using a known photosensitizer should avoid exposure to sunlight. Those who develop a reaction should avoid the photosensitizer. Treatment of lesions depends on the type extent and severity of response. Cool tap water compresses can be applied continually or intermittently; topical application of CORTICOSTEROID cream or lotion can reduce inflammation. Systemic antihistamines may lessen the itch. If the process is severe and extensive, systemic corticosteroids (such as those used in extensive poison ivy cases) may be needed.

photochemotherapy Treatments involving the interaction between chemicals and the sun, also called PUVA therapy (psoralens molecules combined with UVA energy). The PSORALENS (a group of photosensitizing chemical compounds) are taken either orally or topically followed by irradiation with long-wave ultraviolet light A (UVA) rays one to two hours later, for five to 10 minutes two or three times per week until remission. The most common psoralen used in the United States is 8-methoxy psoralen.

Photochemotherapy in the treatment of VITILIGO has been practiced since 1400 B.C. in India, using plant-derived psoralens. Today, physicians use synthetic psoralens that become activated after they absorb UVA radiation.

This treatment has been successful in the treatment of a variety of conditions including PSORIASIS, vitiligo, and MYCOSIS FUNGOIDES; other diseases such as solar HIVES may also respond.

Side Effects

Patients who receive too much drug or UV light can develop severe SUNBURN with BLISTERS and swelling. The psoralen may produce nausea, vomiting, or light-headedness. Prolonged use of PUVA may cause cataracts, solar keratoses, and skin cancer.

photodermatitis Skin inflammation caused by light or ULTRAVIOLET RADIATION.

photophytodermatitis Skin inflammation caused by plant products on the skin, activated by light or ULTRAVIOLET RADIATION.

See also OIL OF BERGAMOT.

photosensitivity Also known as sun sensitivity, this is a toxic skin reaction to the sun that can be triggered by a variety of substances, such as some prescription medications and consumer products—as well as some physical disorders. It often occurs because a substance (called a photosensitizer) has been ingested or applied to the skin. Examples of photosensitizers include certain drugs, dyes, chemicals in perfumes and soaps; plants such as buttercups, parsnips, and mustard; and fruits such as limes and lemons.

Drugs are the primary cause of photosensitivity; those that are known to cause sun sensitivity include TETRACYCLINES, furosemide (Lasix), GRISEOFULVIN, sulfonamides and nalidixic acid, phenothiazine, piroxicam and naproxen, tretinoin (Retin-A), diphendramine, and birth control pills. Other medications that may cause a problem include anticancer and photochemotherapy drugs, antidepressants and antipsychotics, antihistamines, antiparasitic drugs, diuretics, and hypoglycemics.

Sun sensitivity can also be triggered by the coal tars in some medicated soaps and shampoos, or the OIL OF BERGAMOT in certain perfumes or toilet soaps.

Photosensitivity also can be caused by some disorders, including LUPUS ERYTHEMATOSUS and the PORPHYRIA group of blood disorders.

Fortunately, relatively few people ever become photosensitive; the risk is higher for those who only have intermittent exposure to sunlight and those who have light skin and who tend to burn instead of tan.

About 10 percent of individuals have an adverse reaction to sunlight without any photosensitizing medications. These individuals suffer from POLYMORPHIC (or polymorphous) LIGHT ERUPTION, an itchy eruption characterized by red papules 24 to 72 hours after sun exposure that last several days after the affected person avoids the sun. Frequently known as "sun poisoning," this reaction often develops on the first sunny outing in the spring or during a winter holiday to a sunny destination. It is usually mild, but the itch, swelling, and rash can be so severe that it can ruin a holiday. It can be prevented by getting small amounts of sun before going on holiday, or with pretreatment (PUVA or PUVB).

Symptoms and and Diagnostic Path

Any abnormal reaction to the sun causing exaggerated SUNBURN, painful swelling, HIVES, or blistering should be considered to be a sign of photosensitivity. A photosensitive reaction can occur in less than half an hour or it can take until 48 to 72 hours after exposure.

Treatment Options and Outlook

Known photosensitizers should be avoided; susceptible people who report skin reactions without using any photosensitizing agents should also avoid exposure to the sun and should use a SUNSCREEN. Polymorphic (-ous) eruptions may be treated with systemic CORTICOSTEROIDS or antihistamines.

phototherapy Treatment with light, including sunlight, nonvisible ultraviolet light (UVA or UVB), or visible blue light. Moderate exposure to sunlight is the most common form of phototherapy and is effective in treating up to 75 percent of PSORIASIS patients.

The most recent form of phototherapy is called PUVA, which combines long-wave ultraviolet light (UVA) with a PSORALEN drug (such as METHOXSALEN) to sensitize the skin to UVA. It is especially effective in the treatment of psoriasis and some other skin diseases, such as VITILIGO and MYCOSIS FUNGOIDES.

Short-wave ultraviolet light (UVB) is effective in the treatment of psoriasis.

Visible blue light is the treatment of choice for infant JAUNDICE, caused by the accumulation of bilirubin (bile pigment) as the result of a poorly developed liver. Experts believe the light breaks down the bilirubin in the skin, allowing it to be excreted.

COMMON PHOTOSENSITIZING DRUGS

Antibiotics
aureomycin (Chlortetracycline)
griseofulvin (Fulvicin)
minocycline (Minocin, Dynacin)
quinolone (Aprofloxacin, naladoxic acid)
sulfa drugs
tetracycline (Tetracycline)
Antiarrythmics
quinidine (Cin-Quin, Duraquin, etc.)
Antidepressants
amitriptyline (Elavil)
desipramine (Norpramin)
Tranquilizers
chlordiazepoxide (Librium)
chlorpromazine (Thorazine)
Diuretics
hydrochlorothiazide (Esidrix)
chlorothiazide (Diuril)
chlorathalidone (Hygroton)
furosemide (Lasix)
triamterene (Dyrenium)

phototoxic Pertaining to injury by ultraviolet radiation or light.

phrynoderma Also called "toad skin," this is an eruption of solid, elevated palpable lesions seen in patients with severe VITAMIN A deficiency.

pian See YAWS.

piebald skin A condition of two-toned skin, either white and black, or white and brown. It is an inherited autosomal dominant condition, which means that only one defective gene must be inherited from a parent to cause the disease. Each child has a 50 percent chance of inheriting the affected gene and developing the disease.

Symptoms and Diagnostic Path

It is characterized by a white forlock and stable white flat discolorations with hyperpigmented centers; discolorations are usually found on the trunk, face, forearms, and mid-leg (hands and feet are not affected).

Some patients with the condition are also deaf (WAARDENBURG'S SYNDROME).

Treatment Options and Outlook

It is difficult to repigment white areas, and the lack of MELANIN-producing cells in hair follicles next to affected skin means that PSORALEN and UVA (PUVA) therapy will not be very effective. Full thickness grafts of normal skin may result in successful repigmentation.

piedra See TRICHOSPOROSIS.

pigmentation Color of skin, hair, and eyes determined by MELANIN (pigment) produced by special cells called melanocytes (PIGMENT CELLS). The more melanin in the body, the darker the color. The amount of melanin any person produces is the result of heredity and exposure to sunlight. Three other pigments that contribute to normal skin color are oxygenated hemoglobin, reduced hemoglobin, and carotenoids.

Skin color can range from a pale white to deep black, and hair color ranges from white, blond, light to dark brown, black, red, or gray. Eyes can be any shade from the bluest sky blue to the very blackest black.

In humans, pigmented skin and hair protects against the harmful effects of sunlight; in other animals, color may provide camouflage against predators (as in chameleons) or act as a sexual attractant (as in peacocks). Some experts believe that the human pigmentation system may have developed as a skin protectant for animals with very little hair covering.

All pigment cells are produced from the neural crest (except those of the retina, which come from the primitive forebrain). A person's neural crest is formed by the sixth week of gestation, although the precursors of pigment cells probably begin their migration to the skin, ears, eyes and other organs before the neural crest is completely formed. By the eighth week of gestation, pigment cells can be identified in the DERMIS.

See also PIGMENTATION, DISORDERS OF.

pigmentation, disorders of Skin color is determined by the MELANIN—its amount, its distribution, its character, and its chemistry—which together determine the color and hue of the skin's pigmentation.

Lightened Skin

Pigment cells that are absent from an area of skin, produce too few melanosomes, or are unable to produce enough melanin, result in skin that is very light in color. An absence of pigment cells may cause PIEBALD SKIN, WAARDENBURG'S SYNDROME, or VITILIGO. Lack of skin color may also be caused by trauma, exposure to cold, or chemicals. Hypopigmentation (too little pigmentation), due to abnormal formation of melanosomes, may indicate TUBEROUS SCLEROSIS, HYPOMELANOSIS OF ITO, NEVUS DEPIGMENTOSUS, or CHEDIAK-HIGASHI SYNDROME. Loss of pigment due to a drop in the production of melanin may be caused by ALBINISM and TINEA VERSICOLOR. PITYRIASIS ALBA is caused by a decrease in the transfer of melanosomes.

Finally, there are many infections and inflammatory skin disorders that leave behind hypopigmented skin, including drug reactions, LEUKONYCHIA, and post-inflammatory hypopigmentation. Patches of pale skin are also a symptom of a range of disorders, including PSORIASIS and PHENYLKETONURIA.

Darker Skin

Hyperpigmentation is a common problem, especially among patients with dark skin. Among those with darker skin, most skin irritations cause heightened skin color. Hyperpigmentation may also be a sign of a serious metabolic or nutritional problem. Most lesions that are hyperpigmented are benign, although some (such as MELANOMAS) are cancerous.

Patients may notice patches of dark and light skin after an episode of ECZEMA, psoriasis, or tinea versicolor. Those with CHLOASMA experience dark areas on the face caused by hormonal changes while taking birth control pills, or during pregnancy or menopause. Dark skin patches on the face may also be caused by some perfumes or cosmetics, especially when they contain photosensitizing chemicals. These chemically induced patches usually fade with time. Other types of skin darkening unrelated to sun exposure may occur with ADDISON'S DISEASE or Cushing's syndrome.

Permanent areas of dark pigmented skin are usually caused by an abnormality in the melanocytes, such as with a FRECKLE or MOLE. The disease ACANTHOSIS NIGRICANS is characterized by dark patches of velvety thick skin usually found in the skin creases.

Other disorders involving hyperpigmentation include LENTIGO SIMPLEX, MULTIPLE LENTIGINES SYNDROME, NEVUS SPILUS, Mongolian spot, NEVUS OF ITO AND NEVUS OF OTA, NEUROFIBROMATOSIS, hereditary cases of hyperpigmentation and Addison's disease.

Other Changes

Still other pigment changes occur with an excess of bilirubin, which turns the skin yellow, or too much iron, HEMOCHROMATOSIS, which turns the skin bronze.

pigment cells Also called melanocytes, these pigment-producing cells are located in the BASAL CELL layer of the EPIDERMIS (top skin layer). They are controlled by a hormone secreted by the pituitary gland in the brain and produce MELANIN (pigment color) by oxidizing tyrosine. Pigment cells are also found in the hair bulb and are a normal part of cells in the mucous membranes. In dark-skinned people, these pigment cells normally produce large amounts of melanin, and oral mucous membranes are very dark. In Caucasians, pigmentation may not be normally visible in mucous membranes.

Large amounts of melanin indicate an efficient effective protection against many chemical and physical toxins. Short wave ultraviolet light, chemical carcinogens, and phenols produce free oxygen radicals within the epidermis and dermis. It may be that a primary function of melanocytes is to remove FREE RADICALS formed in the skin during inflammatory conditions. Melanocytes protect other cells of the epidermis from damage by release of radical oxygens.

Human pigment cells produce two types of melanin: eumelanin (black and brown) and phaeomelanin (red). The ratio between the two types determines a person's skin and hair color.

See also PIGMENTATION; PIGMENTATION, DISORDERS OF.

pigmented nevi   See NEVUS.

pigmented purpuric dermatosis A group of disorders characterized by reddish brown spots or patches caused by the leakage of blood through the tiny capillaries the skin. Exactly why the capillaries should become leaky is not known for certain, but a hypersensitivity reaction to viral infection, food additives, and medications has been cited. Types of pigmented purpuric dermatosis include:

Gougerot-Blum syndrome (pigmented purpuric lichenoid dermatosis): Itchy red brown spots and bumps that join together to form a thickened patch

Schamberg's disease (progressive pigmented purpura): Nonitchy, flat brown patches with rust-colored spots that look like cayenne pepper

MAJOCCHI'S DISEASE (purpura annularis telangietoides): Similar to Schamberg's disease, but with dilated capillaries arranged in rings

Lichen aureus: Patches have a yellowish hue and usually occur over VARICOSE VEINS.

pilar Pertaining to the hair.

pilosebaceous Relating to the hair follicles and their sebaceous glands.

pimples The common name for a small PUSTULE or PAPULE, pimples are usually found on the face, neck, and back, especially in adolescents with ACNE.

See also ACNE, ADULT; ACNE, TREATMENT FOR; ACNE MYTHS; ACNE PRODUCTS, OVER-THE-COUNTER.

pinch graft A small type of SKIN GRAFT used to cover leg ulcers. Only 4 to 10 mm thick, this graft is taken from anesthetized skin from the upper thigh by picking up a small amount of skin with the tip of a small needle and slicing with a scalpel or razor blade. The grafts are kept in sterile saline and transferred to the wound area, leaving a 2-mm space between grafts. An adhesive spray is then applied, followed by a semipermeable dressing with edges extended beyond the margin of the ulcer. Gauze and an elastic dressing are used to cover the wound, which is left untouched for up to four days. Strict bed rest is required. The wound can be checked through the semipermeable dressing and accumulating fluid can be drained. Dressings are removed in five to six days. Wiping the wound with alcohol allows it to form a scab that will come off in two or three weeks. As the grafts take, the grafted sites grow together and cover the entire wound site.

See also ALLOGRAFT; ARTIFICIAL SKIN; AUTOGRAFT; HETEROGRAFT; SKIN GRAFT.

pins and needles sensation The common term for paresthesia, a tingly or prickly sensation in the skin that is usually associated with numbness or loss of sensation and sometimes with a burning feeling.

A temporary pins and needles feeling is caused by a disturbance in the nerve impulses along the pathway from skin to brain, such as when an arm is bent under the body during sleep. Persistent pins and needles sensations may be caused by a group of nerve disorders called neuropathy. This condition is frequently seen in patients with diabetes.

pinta A skin infection found in some remote tropical American villages caused by the microorganism *Treponema carateum,* a close relative of the bacterium that causes SYPHILIS. It seems to affect only dark-skinned people and is thought to be transmitted either by direct contact or by flies that carry the infective spirochetes.

Symptoms and Diagnostic Path

Symptoms include thickening and loss of pigment of the skin, particularly on the face, neck, buttocks, hands, or feet. Up to a year after infection, red skin patches appear that subsequently turn blue, brown, and then white.

Treatment Options and Outlook

Rarely disabling or fatal, PENICILLIN or TETRACYCLINE will cure the disease, but patients may be permanently disfigured.

pitted nails See NAILS, PITTED.

pityriasis alba A common childhood skin condition featuring irregular, fine, pale scalp patches on the cheeks caused by a mild ECZEMA. Up to a third of children have this disorder. The skin condition often worsens after exposure to the sun because inflamed skin in the patches does not tan well. The disease may persist into adulthood.

Symptoms and Diagnostic Path

Symptoms include small white round or oval patches that are lighter than surrounding skin; the borders of the rash are not clearly visible. The lesions may be flat or slightly elevated, with very small fine scales on the face, outer upper arms, neck, and upper trunk. The lesions may get red in the sun, but they will not tan.

The rash seems to worsen when the skin is dry and may be flakier during the winter months. However, the rash is most obvious during the summer, when the surrounding skin gets tan and the patches of rash do not.

Treatment Options and Outlook

The condition usually responds well to EMOLLIENTS or mild topical steroids. Patches clear but return; the lesions usually fade by adulthood.

pityriasis rosea A common mild skin disorder of childhood and young adulthood characterized by a single large round spot (called a herald patch) on the trunk, followed days to a week later by slightly raised, scaly-edged, round or oval pink-to-copper colored spots on the trunk and upper arms. The condition is not believed to be contagious.

The cause of the disease is unknown, although many speculate that it is due to a virus.

Symptoms and Diagnostic Path

In addition to the above symptoms that last for about six to eight weeks, pityriasis rosea may cause itching.

Treatment Options and Outlook

Mild ITCHING may be relieved by applying CALAMINE LOTION or ZINC OXIDE shake lotion; more severe itching may be treated with ANTIHISTAMINE DRUGS, topical steroids, or PHOTOTHERAPY. The rash usually clears up without treatment, but a physician should rule out other conditions that may cause a similar rash.

pityriasis rubra pilaris A chronic disease of KERATINIZATION that can be inherited or acquired and is characterized by papules with greasy plugs, generalized skin redness, and yellow thickening of the palms and soles.

In the inherited form, the lesions resemble PSORIASIS, and may begin in infancy and last throughout life with occasional periods of remission. The acquired type of pityriasis rubra pilaris usually appears in adulthood. The lesions disappear within three years in 80 percent of cases. Treatment may shorten that time.

Symptoms and Diagnostic Path

Firm, pink, red, or orange follicular PAPULES may form groups of lesions that either remain localized to the extensor surfaces of the skin or eventually cover the entire body. There may be scaling on the scalp. When the lesions spread over the entire body, a few small clear areas of normal skin ("skip areas") may be seen on the trunk.

Treatment Options and Outlook

Etretinate, ISOTRETINOIN (Accutane), and METHOTREXATE are the most effective treatments. Etretinate and isotretinoin produce remission within several months. Combining the retinoids with ultraviolet B (UVB) phototherapy also may help. Topical creams are not usually effective.

plague A serious infectious disease transmitted by the bites of rats or fleas that was the scourge of early history. Nicknamed the Black Death during the pandemic of the 14th century, its primary symptom is the black patches on the skin caused by bleeding around swollen lymph glands. Recent outbreaks among humans have occurred in Africa, South America, and Southeast Asia. Plague is also found among ground squirrels, prairie dogs, and marmots in parts of Arizona, New Mexico, California, Colorado, and Nevada. Between one and 40 Americans contract plague during the spring and summer months each year. Worldwide, more than 2800 cases are reported yearly.

Fleas found on rodents throughout the world carry the bacterium *Yersinia pestis* that causes plague. The great pandemics of the past occurred when wild rodents spread the disease to rats in cities, and then to humans when the fleas jumped off dying rats. A bite from an infected flea leads to bubonic plague, a form of the disease characterized by BUBOES (swollen lymph glands). Pneumonic plague affects the lungs, and is a complication of bubonic plague; it is also spread via infected droplets during coughing. Bubonic plague causes enlarged, tender lymph nodes, fever, chills and prostration. Septicemic plague is characterized by fever, chills, prostration, abdominal pain, shock, and bleeding into skin and other organs. Pneumonic plague causes fever, chills, cough, and difficulty breathing, followed by rapid shock and death if not treated early.

Symptoms and Diagnostic Path

Two to five days after infection, patients experience fever, shivering, seizures, and severe headaches followed by buboes—smooth, oval, reddened, and very painful swellings in the armpits, groin, or neck.

Treatment Options and Outlook

Administration of streptomycin, chloramphenicol, or TETRACYCLINE reduces the risk of death to less than 5 percent. Those in contact with anyone who has pneumonic plague are given antibiotics as a preventive measure at the first sign of disease.

Left untreated, half of plague patients will die. If blood poisoning occurs as an early complication, a patient may die before the buboes appear.

plantar wart A firm, rough-surfaced WART found on the sole of the foot that may appear alone or in clusters. The plantar wart is caused by an infection with human PAPILLOMAVIRUS (HPV) often contracted by walking barefoot on surfaces where the virus is lurking. This virus thrives in warm, moist environments, making infection a common occurrence in swimming pools and public showers.

Symptoms and Diagnostic Path

Plantar warts tend to be hard and flat, with a rough surface and well-defined boundaries; warts are generally raised and fleshier when they appear on the top of the foot or on the toes. Plantar warts are often gray or brown, although the color may vary, with a center that appears as one or more pinpoints of black.

If left untreated, warts can grow to an inch or more in circumference and can spread into clusters of several warts; these are often called mosaic warts. Like any other infectious lesion, plantar warts are spread by touching, scratching, or even by contact with skin shed from another wart. The wart may also bleed, which can help to spread the virus.

Occasionally, warts can spontaneously disappear after a short time, and, just as frequently, they can recur in the same location.

When plantar warts develop on the weight-bearing areas of the foot—the ball of the foot, or the heel, for example—they can be the source of sharp, burning pain. Pain occurs when weight is brought to bear directly on the wart, although pressure on the side of a wart can create equally intense pain.

Treatment Options and Outlook

Warts can be very resistant to treatment and have a tendency to recur. Self-treatment is advisable at first, since over-the-counter preparations containing acids or chemicals are readily available. Self-treatment with such medications should be avoided by people with diabetes and those with cardiovascular or circulatory disorders.

Most effective treatments damage the tissue where the wart virus lives; the most effective is liquid nitrogen, a very cold liquid that is sprayed onto the wart. After treatments at least every three weeks, the wart will clear slowly.

Topical treatments with acids such as trichloroacetic acid, salicylic acid, or lactic acid are painted on or applied in a medicated bandage. When liquid nitrogen cryotherapy is combined with one of these medications, warts clear more quickly.

Plantar warts are very stubborn. It is far better to see a physician for specialized treatment by a simple surgical procedure, performed under local anesthetic. Lasers have become a common and effective treatment, using CO_2 laser cautery performed under local anesthesia either in a podiatrist's office or an outpatient surgery facility. The laser reduces post-treatment scarring and is a safe form for eliminating wart lesions.

Preventive Measures

To avoid getting plantar warts;

- avoid walking barefoot, except on sandy beaches
- change shoes and socks daily
- keep feet clean and dry
- avoid direct contact with warts from other people or from other parts of the body

plastic and reconstructive surgery The specialty of plastic surgery includes two branches: reconstructive surgery and cosmetic surgery. Plastic and reconstructive surgeons use special techniques to repair visible skin defects and problems in underlying tissue, caused by heredity, burns, injuries, operations, aging, or disease.

The word *plastic,* from the Greek *plastikos,* means "to fit for molding" or "to give form"—it does not refer to the synthetic materials that are sometimes used in plastic surgery.

Reconstructive surgery is performed on abnormal structures of the body, caused by congenital defects, developmental abnormalities, trauma, infection, tumors, or disease. It is generally performed to improve function, but also may be done to approximate a normal appearance. This includes procedures done to repair birth defects, such as cleft lip and palate repair, and deformities caused by accidents or disease, such as facial reconstruction following cancer surgery, burn care, reattachment of limbs, and breast reconstruction following mastectomy. The average plastic surgeon spends 60 percent of the time performing reconstructive surgery.

Cosmetic surgery is performed to reshape normal structures of the body in order to improve the patient's appearance. This includes procedures such as FACE-LIFTS, nose reshaping, and other procedures done to improve appearance and enhance the patients' quality of life.

A variety of techniques are used to provide skin cover for damaged areas, including SKIN GRAFTS, skin and muscle flaps, Z-plasty, and TISSUE EXPANSION. These techniques may be performed in addition to grafts or implants.

Since the early 1990s, the practice of plastic surgery has become more complex through the use of microsurgical techniques to join blood vessels, allowing the transfer of blocks of skin and muscle from one part of the body to the other.

More than 1 million plastic and reconstructive surgeries are performed in hospitals each year, according to the National Center for Health Statistics.

See also COSMETIC SURGERY; Z-PLASTY.

plethora A florid, bright red flushed complexion that may be caused by dilation of blood vessels near the skin's surface due to alcohol, heat, spicy food, and so on. More rarely, it can be caused by an excess number of red blood cells, as in polycythema rubra vera.

pockmark A term referring to the deep, pitted scars of ACNE lesions. The appearance of pockmarks can be improved by a variety of techniques, including DERMABRASION, chemical peels, or LASER RESURFACING.

poikiloderma Pigment changes of the skin, causing a dappled or mottled appearance with areas of both increased and decreased color. *Poikiloderma* is a word that means "varied, multicolored skin" from the Greek *poikilos* (mottled) and *-derma* (skin). The exact cause is unknown, but it is clear that the sun is the major factor causing this condition. In some cases, a substance in cosmetics sensitizes the skin to the Sun's ultraviolet light. In others, it is simply caused by excess sun exposure. The neck area under chin that is usually shaded from the sun is spared. Contributing factors include fair skin, accumulated sun exposure, and in women, hormonal factors.

Symptoms and and Diagnostic Path
Symptoms include mottled changes that have brown hyperpigmentation, a netlike proliferation of fine red vessels, intermingled with white skin. It is commonly known as "red neck," from which the derogatory term *redneck* derives. Fair-skinned farmers and outdoor workers who spend hours a day outside over many years develop diffuse redness of the neck, which is sometimes combined with brown discoloration of a permanent tan.

Treatment Options and Outlook
The results of treatment are encouraging. Patients should protect themselves from the sun, use a daily broad spectrum SPF 30+ SUNSCREEN, and avoid all perfumes on the affected area, including those in soap. Hydroquinone-containing preparations may help fade the pigmentation. Pulse-dye LASER TREATMENT (and some other vascular lasers) are very effective at decreasing the overall red

color and sometimes even the brown color after a series of treatments. A combination of sun avoidance, lightening agents, and laser treatments can dramatically improve poikiloderma.

See also ROTHMUND-THOMSON SYNDROME.

poison ivy (*Toxicodendron radicans; Rhus toxicodendron*) Sensitivity to this plant's oil (urushiol) is the most common allergy in the country, affecting almost half of all Americans at one time or another. In a few cases, it can be quite serious; if symptoms such as swelling appear within four to 12 hours, patients should seek immediate medical treatment.

One of the most common poisonous plants in the United States, its leaves may be notched or smooth, and almost always grow in groups of three—two leaves opposite each other and one at the end of the stalk. However, according to some experts there are exceptions, and leaves may sometimes appear in groups of five, seven, or even nine. In early fall, the leaves sometimes turn bright red. While it usually grows as a long, hairy vine (often wrapping itself around trees), it can also be found as a low shrub growing along fences or stone walls. Poison ivy has waxy yellow-green flowers and greenish berries, which can help identify the plant in late fall, winter, and early spring before the leaves appear. Poison ivy is found throughout the United States, although it is most common in the eastern and central states.

The ITCHING and blistering is caused by the reaction of the body's blood vessels to the plant's urushiol oil. Sensitivity to this oil ranges from nonexistent to severe, and an allergy can spring up in previously immune people at any time. The urushiol oil that causes the rash is a colorless or slightly yellow resin, whose name comes from a Japanese word meaning lacquer. The entire plant contains this oil, and is therefore poisonous: leaves, berries, stalk, and roots.

Urushiol is easily transferred from an object to a person, so anything that touches poison ivy (clothing, gardening tools, a pet's fur, athletic equipment) can be contaminated with urushiol and cause poison ivy in anyone who then touches the object. Urushiol remains active for up to one year, so any equipment that touches poison ivy must be washed. Even the smoke from burning poison ivy is toxic and can irritate the lungs, since urushiol can be carried in smoke. Therefore, individuals should never burn poison ivy plants as a way to get rid of them; the smoke given off by these burning plants is particularly dangerous and can enter the nasal passages, throat, and lungs of anyone who breathes it.

As the leaves die in the fall, the plant draws certain nutrients and substances (including the oil) into the stem. But the oil remains active, so even in winter if broken stems are used as firewood kindling or as vines on a Christmas wreath they may cause a rash.

Symptoms and Diagnostic Path

While not every person is allergic to poison ivy, about seven out of 10 people are sensitive to urushiol and will develop contact dermatitis if exposed to a large enough dose.

Children rarely have allergic reactions to urushiol, primarily because it usually takes several exposures to develop a sensitivity to the resin. Symptoms vary from one person to the next; some people exhibit only mild itching while others experience severe reactions, which may include terrible burning and itching with watery BLISTERS. The skin irritation, swelling, blisters, and itching may appear within hours or days, usually developing within 24 to 48 hours in a sensitized person. The skin becomes reddened, followed by watery blisters, peaking about five days after contamination and gradually improving over a week or two, even without treatment. Eventually, the blisters break and the oozing sores crust over and then disappear.

Despite a common misconception, poison ivy is *not* spread by scratching open blisters or by skin-to-skin contact, but by the oil (urushiol) found in the plant. Anything that brushes against this oil is contaminated and can cause poison ivy if it contacts the skin.

However, doctors recommend not scratching blisters, since any remaining urushiol that has not been washed off can be transmitted to another part of the body. In addition, scratching the blisters may cause a skin infection from bacteria present on the fingernails.

Animals can also transmit poison ivy from their fur to their owners' skin. Any animal suspected of coming in contact with poison ivy should be given a bath.

Allergy to poison ivy may also indicate that a person is also sensitive to related plants, including cashews, pistachios, mangos, and Chinese or Japanese lacquer trees.

A small percentage of sensitive individuals are seriously allergic, and will begin to develop a rash and swelling in only four to 12 hours after contact (as opposed to the normal 24 to 48). One of the few real emergencies in dermatology, such an extreme sensitivity should be immediately treated at the hospital as soon as possible; a shot of CORTICOSTEROIDS will lessen swelling.

Treatment Options and Outlook

If it is not possible to wash off the oil before the allergic reaction begins, the best nonprescription treatment is generally considered to be CALAMINE lotion, a soothing skin protector that cools the skin and absorbs the oozing, forming a protective crust that keeps the skin from sticking to clothes.

Because the cooling effect of calamine shrinks the blood vessels, this also helps stop the blister formation. Patients should stop using calamine once the oozing stops, so as not to dry the skin too much and worsen itching again.

Itching also can be treated with compresses soaked in cold water. Products containing local anesthetics (such as benzocaine) should be avoided because they themselves cause a contact dermatitis. Some experts recommend cooling counterirritants such as phenol or menthol, which may be effective, although they may sting and may not be strong enough to stop the discomfort.

Nonprescription oral antihistamines (such as Chlor-Trimeton or Benadryl) also may be effective; systemic antihistamines do not work against the rash, although their sedative action may help the patient sleep. Nonprescription cortisone creams, however, are too weak to be very effective, although they may provide minor relief for minimal itching.

Colloidal oatmeal (such as Aveeno, available at drugstores) will dry up oozing blisters, and can be applied with a cloth or used in the bath, which also eases itching.

Widespread, severe poison ivy is treated by dermatologists with topical steroids; if quite severe, systemic steroids may be administered.

Risk Factors and Preventive Measures

Most important is proper protection—gloves, long sleeves, heavy socks, and pants tucked into boots. Before going out and working in a poison ivy-infested area, consumers should spray deodorant or antiperspirant on arms, legs, clothes, and pets. Deodorant sprays contain activated clay known as organoclay, and antiperspirants contain the clay and aluminum chlorohydrate, both of which have been found to neutralize urushiol oil. Antiperspirant contains both oil-fighting ingredients, but it is also irritating and should not be sprayed on the face or in body folds.

Short of avoiding the plant, the best method for preventing a rash from exposure to poison ivy before the allergic reaction takes hold is to *immediately* wash off the oil—first with alcohol, followed by water (soap is not necessary). Or, wash the affected area immediately after contact (within 10 minutes, if possible) with yellow laundry soap (such as Castile) and *cold* water, lathering several times and rinsing the area in running water after each sudsing. Do not scrub with a brush.

Any clothing that might have come in contact with urushiol must be washed several times. If the urushiol is washed off, there is little or no further treatment of mild cases of the rash.

Anyone who comes in contact with poison ivy out in the wild should wash in a cold running stream. If no water is available, there are a host of other possibilities, including rinsing with paint thinner, acetone, horse urine, ammonia, and meat tenderizer. Organic solvents (paint thinner or acetone) work very well in washing off the urushiol oil, but they should not be used on a regular basis. (Regular skin contact with solvents can cause a rash). Solvents *are* recommended for eliminating the poison ivy on garden tools, car upholstery, and so on.

Other products designed to prevent poison ivy and poison oak are presently being investigated by the Food and Drug Administration.

Extremely sensitive individuals may be desensitized to the effects of poison ivy with allergen extracts, although results have been disappointing sometimes and often do not last longer than one season. The vaccine is given by mouth or injection. The procedure requires a great deal of time (three to six months). Adverse reactions to the desensitization include swelling, dermatitis, gastroenteric disturbances, fever, and inflammation at the injection site. Because of these problems, immunization is only recommended for those sensitive people who live or work near the ivy. Convulsions have occurred in children following oral administration of the plant's extract. No cream, lotion, or spray has been proven effective as protection against the allergen, although studies are continuing.

Alternatively, recent research suggests a different vaccine may be available for millions of Americans tormented each summer with the itchy rash. Researchers at the University of Mississippi have developed an experimental vaccine that seems to prevent an allergic reaction and may lessen the painful symptoms after the rash appears. Researchers explain the vaccine works best as an injection, and probably would be most helpful for those who are highly sensitive to the plants. The agent has been tested on animals, but has not yet been tested on humans. Researchers at the university have been studying the oily compounds of the plants that make the skin blister and itch to create less-toxic forms of the oil, which allow the body to tolerate the plants in the laboratory.

polyarteritis nodosa   See SYSTEMIC NECROTIZING VASCULITIDES.

polychondritis, relapsing   See RELAPSING POLYCHONDRITIS.

polycystic ovary syndrome   See STEIN-LEVENTHAL SYNDROME.

polymorphic light eruption   An allergic reaction to certain wavelengths of the Sun that affects 10 percent of the population, causing bumpy, scaling, blistering, itchy, or red patches hours or days after exposure to the sun. More women than men are affected by this condition, which usually appears between adolescence and the 30s.

Symptoms and Diagnostic Path

The eruption is characterized by red MACULES, PAPULES, plaques, and BLISTERS, and begins anywhere between an hour and 24 to 36 hours after exposure to the sun, and lasts three to five days. The itch can be quite severe.

Treatment Options and Outlook

Patients should avoid the sun and always use a SUNSCREEN of at least SPF 15; patients tend to improve as the summer progresses. Slow exposure to the sun can increase tolerance. Nonprescription topical steroids or prescription steroids and ANTIHISTAMINES also may be effective.

See also SOLAR URTICARIA; PHOTOSENSITIZING DISORDERS.

polymyositis-dermatomyositis   A rare systemic connective tissue disease characterized by inflamed, weak muscles that may cause a rash. The disorder may affect children under age 10 and adults between ages 40 and 60. There have been reports of cases associated with cancer in up to 40 percent of adult cases.

The course of this disease varies and is unpredictable, lasting for many years or sometimes leading to death within 12 months.

Symptoms and Diagnostic Path

Reddish purple discolored swollen eyelids, scaly red flush over the cheeks and forehead, red PAPULES over the surfaces of finger joints, and a dusky red rash on the arms and upper back, plus pigment changes of the skin (POIKILODERMA).

Treatment Options and Outlook

CORTICOSTEROIDS may be given in the early stages; the disease may be chronic, requiring therapy for years. In those who fail to respond to steroids, immunosuppressive drugs (such as METHOTREXATE, cyclophosphamide, azathioprine, and chlorambucil) may be effective. A combination of CORTICOSTEROIDS and methotrexate is probably most effective, especially in childhood dermatomyositis.

polymyxins A group of antibiotics derived from the bacterium *Bacillus polymyxa* used to treat infections of the skin. These drugs, which include colistin and polymyxin B, are often given as drops or in ointment form and are often used in antibiotic eye drops or skin ointments. Taken orally, colistin is associated with pseudomembranous enterocolitis—a severe, life-threatening type of diarrhea sometimes caused by antibiotics.

pompholyx The appearance of BLISTERS on the hands or feet without known cause. Once called dyshidrotic pompholyx, this term is no longer used since the SWEAT GLANDS play no part in the disease's cause. *Pompholyx* means "bubble" in Greek and the words simply denote a blistering ECZEMA of the palms and soles, respectively.

Symptoms and Diagnostic Path

In general the blisters are found on the sides of the fingers, spreading to the central palms and the soles of the feet that may merge into large blisters. Itching is intense and secondary infection is common (especially on the feet).

Treatment Options and Outlook

Low- or mid-potency steroids are often not very effective; high potency steroids are required. Soaking the hands in a potassium permanganate solution, normal saline, or BUROW'S SOLUTION for 10 or 15 minutes followed by wet dressings (0.05 percent silver nitrate solution or shake lotions) gives rapid relief. However, the silver nitrate or potassium permanganate may stain the hands.

pore The tiny opening of the oil or SWEAT GLANDS at the skin's surface. The size of a pore is regulated by heredity, and contrary to popular opinion, it is not possible to shrink large pores. In addition, hot water does not open pores, and cold water does not close them.

It is possible to make pores *appear* smaller by using an alcohol-base astringent that contains aluminum chloride or aluminum hydroxide. This will temporarily reduce oiliness and minimize light reflection, which can magnify pore size. In addition, Retin-A and prescription strength GLYCOLIC ACID can refine the skin's texture, which may also help pores *look* smaller.

Women can also use a water-based foundation and powder to make pores look smoother and more even.

porokeratosis A disorder of KERATINIZATION that includes three separate autosomal dominant syndromes, all featuring a lesion with a raised border and central furrow or depression; the center may be scaly or atrophic. "Autosomal dominant" means that only one defective gene must be inherited from a parent to cause the disease. Each child has a 50 percent chance of inheriting the affected gene and developing the disease.

Symptoms and Diagnostic Path

In *porokeratosis of Mibelli,* the lesions—craterlike patches with a raised border that enlarge to form lesions—may appear anywhere on the body, either alone or in groups arranged in a line or in segments. This rare, chronic progressive skin disorder is seen usually in males and first appears in early childhood (usually before age 10). Lesions slowly enlarge as the child grows older.

Disseminated superficial actinic porokeratosis is an autosomal dominant skin disorder occurring on sun-exposed areas in fair-skinned individuals (usually women) over age 16. It is characterized by many brownish red MACULES with depressed centers and sharply-ridged borders. The palms and soles are spared. Unlike the Mibelli form, the border of the lesion is less distinct, the centers of the lesions are not as atrophied and they are often itchy. Number of lesions will increase with time.

The lesions of *porokeratosis plantaris, palmaris et disseminata* are most similar to those of disseminated superficial actinic porokeratosis, although they occur at an earlier age (in the second decade) and lesions first appear on palms and soles. The number of lesions will increase with time.

Treatment Options and Outlook

Because of the small danger of the development of SQUAMOUS CELL CARCINOMA (especially in the Mibelli type), physicians should follow this disease closely. FLUOROURACIL 2 percent or 5 percent cream applied twice daily for three weeks may be useful in some patients.

In the Mibelli form, surgical removal of small lesions (especially on arms and legs) may be effective.

Patients with the disseminated superficial actinic form should avoid sunlight and use SUNSCREENS. Lesions (if not too numerous) may be treated with LIQUID NITROGEN.

porphyria A group of rare inherited disorders that cause a rash or skin blistering that in some instances is brought on by sunlight, as a result of abnormalities of the metabolism of chemicals in the body called porphyrins. The diseases result in the increased production and excretion of porphyrins; each type has distinct clinical, biochemical, and genetic features.

Porphyrins are involved in the manufacture of heme, a component of hemoglobin (the oxygen-carrying pigment in the blood). When blocks occur in the chemical process that produces heme, porphyrins build up.

Porphyria includes the more common types of acute intermittent porphyria, variegate porphyria, and porphyria cutanea tarda, and rare varieties, including hereditary coproporphyria, protoporphyria, and congenital erythropoietic porphyria.

Estimates of the combined prevalence of the disease in the United States are about one per 10,000 to 50,000.

Symptoms and Diagnostic Path

Porphyrias with skin symptoms include variegate porphyria and hereditary coproporphyria, both of which cause blistering of sun-exposed skin, together with abdominal pain, cramps in the arms and legs, muscle weakness, psychiatric disturbances, and so on. Attacks also may be brought

on by a variety of drugs, including barbiturates, phenytoin, birth control pills, and TETRACYCLINES. Porphyria cutanea tarda causes blistering skin, but there are no abdominal or nervous system problems. In this variety, wounds are slow to heal and the urine may be pink or brown. Protoporphyria often causes mild skin symptoms after exposure to sunlight, such as burning and stinging without blister formation.

Treatment Options and Outlook

Specific treatment depends on the variety of porphyria. For porphyria cutanea tarda, avoiding causative agents such as alcohol and estrogen and treatment with phlebotomy and/or antimalarials such as hydroxychloroquine is recommended.

Portuguese man-of-war sting See JELLYFISH STINGS.

port-wine stain The common name for nevus flammeus, a permanent large purple-red BIRTHMARK.

Symptoms and Diagnostic Path

Present at birth, port-wine stains are usually sharply outlined and flat, although the surface may sometimes have a pebbly feel. Most commonly appearing on the face, they can range in size from a few millimeters in diameter to half the body's surface. They do not enlarge, but they do increase in size proportionally as the child grows, becoming darker over time. Three out of every 1,000 people will be born with a port-wine stain.

Port-wine stains may appear alone or as part of a multisystem disorder, such as STURGE-WEBER SYNDROME, which also features seizures and eye abnormalities such as glaucoma. There are a normal number of vessels that are larger than normal.

Blood vessels in port-wine stains have an abnormal nerve supply, which may account for the vessels' enlargement over time.

Treatment Options and Outlook

A simple port-wine stain, when it does not occur as part of another syndrome, is more than a cosmetic problem. If treated early in childhood, the psychological burden on the child may be relieved.

The most successful method of removal is the PULSED DYE LASER, popular because it has a low rate of scarring and its effectiveness is not as dependent on an operator's experience. Total clearing with pulsed dye laser treatment is uncommon, but dramatic lightening after a series of treatments is not unusual. Pulsed dye laser treatment decreases the solid color mass, thins thickened lesions, and lightens all types of port-wine stains. By treating patients early in their lives, the psychological burden is eased, the risk of darkening and thickening is reduced, and the risk of bleeding and infection eliminated.

Pulsed dye laser treatment has become the gold standard of treatment. Since it was introduced, the pulsed dye laser has been modified several times to lengthen the wavelength and the pulse duration, two changes that have enhanced results significantly.

Until the late 1980s, the ARGON LASER was the treatment of choice for these birthmarks. The laser works by emitting light that is absorbed by the hemoglobin in the dilated blood vessels that make up the birthmark. However, this therapy is limited because of its substantial rate of scarring—the continually delivered laser energy dissipates into the surrounding dermis, causing thermal damage. Less-than-optimum treatment can result in pale, immature port-wine stains. In addition, the extent of clearing and the rate of scarring is highly dependent on the skill and experience of the operator.

Choosing a wavelength that is more selectively absorbed by hemoglobin and delivering it in a pulse shorter than the cooling time of the abnormal vessel produces better results.

Excision and grafting for smaller lesions, or tattooing for larger ones, are best avoided, considering how effective laser treatment is. CAMOUFLAGE COSMETICS also may be used to mask lesions.

post-herpetic neuralgia A chronic pain syndrome experienced by between 9 percent and 34 percent of patients following an attack of SHINGLES that is often difficult to treat and can persist for years.

Typically, the onset of shingles is heralded by an attack of skin pain, followed by the development of a painful skin rash within several days. The rash usually fades away within two to four weeks, but the nature, severity, and duration of the continuing pain vary considerably among individuals.

Because the nerves have been damaged after a shingles attack, they can produce strong pain impulses that may last for months or years after the shingles blisters heal. Not everyone with shingles will develop post-herpetic neuralgia, but the older the patient and the more severe the shingles, the more likely that post-herpetic neuralgia may occur. As many as 75 percent of patients aged over 70 years have pain a month after the rash heals, and 50 percent are still having pain a year later.

Four additional risk factors have been identified for the development of post-herpetic neuralgia

- greater acute pain severity
- greater rash severity
- abnormal sensitivity in the affected skin during the acute phase
- the presence of a painful feeling before the rash occurs (prodome)

Symptoms and Diagnostic Path

Post-herpetic neuralgia pain usually occurs only in the area affected by the rash, and may come and go with a burning, throbbing, or sharp and shooting nature. Allodynia (pain provoked by normally harmless stimuli) is common. Some patients experience marked allodynia without numbness, while others have marked sensory loss in the affected area with minimal allodynia. There also may be areas of scarring or loss of skin pigmentation.

Use of antiviral drugs such as ACYCLOVIR, famcyclovir, or valacyclovir to treat the acute shingles seems to reduce the risk of developing post-herpetic neuralgia and the overall duration of pain. Thus, with widespread use of these antiviral drugs, it is likely that less than 22 percent of patients with acute shingles will experience pain for three months or more after the beginning of the rash.

Researchers are studying whether the use of drugs such as TCAs, gabapentin, oxycodone, and tramadol or nerve block during acute shingles may reduce the risk of developing post-herpetic neuralgia. Administration of the chicken pox vaccine is also being studied as a way to prevent shingles in the first place.

Treatment Options and Outlook

Simple measures such as use of cold packs for short-term pain relief or occlusion with cling film may be sufficient in some instances, but many patients require drug treatment. Research suggests that starting treatment as soon as possible after the beginning of the rash may be a key in preventing post-herpetic neuralgia.

Tricyclic antidepressants have been regarded as first-line treatments for some time; recent research has shown nortriptyline to be the preferred drug of this class. The anticonvulsant gabapentin, sustained-release oxycodone, and topical lidocaine patches are also used as first-line treatments for post-herpetic neuralgia Lidocaine patches may be preferred for patients with significant pain from normally nonpainful sources (allodynia), or occasional intermittent pain, whereas nortriptyline is a suitable option for those patients with depressive symptoms in addition to pain. Trial and error may be required to find the most suitable treatment for each individual patient.

Cognitive-behavioral therapies, including relaxation training, biofeedback, and hypnosis, can help manage chronic pain. Pain management centers offer a multidisciplinary approach that usually incorporates such measures, with the aim of improving function and improving quality of life, as well as reducing pain.

For patients who do not respond to any of the first-line treatments, alternative treatment approaches that may be considered include tramadol, selective serotonin reuptake inhibitors (particularly paroxetine or citalopram), anticonvulsants other than gabapentin (such as sodium valproate or carbamazepine), transcutaneous electrical nerve stimulation (TENS), topical capsaicin, lidocaine infusion followed by oral mexiletine, and nerve blocks.

post-inflammatory pigmentation A discoloration left on the skin after an underlying trauma, skin infection, ECZEMA, or a drug reaction has healed.

Symptoms and Diagnostic Path

In people with dark skin, the color tends to be more intense and last for a longer period.

Treatment Options and Outlook

Bleaching agents such as those containing hydroquinone may be used, and a mild steroid may help. The pigmentation tends to clear with time, and normal skin color should return slowly within a few months. Further trauma to the area (and sun exposure) should be avoided.

potassium iodide A simple chemical that has been used for a century to effectively treat lymphatic SPOROTRICHOSIS (chronic fungal skin infection). In saturated solution, it is prescribed on a slowly increasing dose until adverse effects appear, or until a response is noted. Potassium iodide is not effective against any other fungal infection.

Side Effects

Common side effects include ACNE-like lesions, nausea and vomiting, and hypothyroidism.

potassium para-aminobenzoate A chemical once used to treat LICHEN SCLEROSIS ET ATROPHICUS and SCLERODERMA. However, there is little scientific evidence that it works.

potassium permanganate An antiseptic drug with an astringent effect on the skin useful in treating inflammation (DERMATITIS). It is applied directly to the skin as a dressing or dissolved in water for a soak.

Once a popular remedy for dermatitis, its tendency to stain skin, nails, and clothing purple has caused this drug to lose favor among physicians. Moreover, if not fully dissolved, potassium permanganate can cause a chemical burn on contact with skin.

poultice   A warm pack made of a soft, moist substance such as kaolin (white clay) spread between layers of soft fabric as a way of providing moist heat to the skin. In the past, poultices were widely used to reduce pain or inflammation and improve circulation in a particular area, or to soften the skin to allow matter to be expressed from a boil. Poultices containing kaolin retain heat for a long period of time.

precancerous conditions   Conditions in which cancer has a tendency to develop. Precancerous conditions of the skin include ACTINIC KERATOSES, DYSPLASTIC (or atypical) NEVI, LENTIGO MALIGNA, BOWEN'S DISEASE, and SQUAMOUS CELL CARCINOMA in-situ.

pregnancy and the skin   A wide variety of skin changes can be brought about by pregnancy. While it is true that many women notice an improvement in the condition of their skin during pregnancy, some annoying skin problems also can occur. Changes during pregnancy may also be associated with preexisting skin conditions such as ACNE, ATOPIC DERMATITIS, and PSORIASIS.

Some of the many skin changes that arise during pregnancy include itchiness, stretch marks, blood vessel overgrowth and broken blood vessels, mole growth or darkening, and skin darkening in patches or all over the body.

Normal Skin Changes

A certain number of physiological changes occur in the skin because of hormonal changes that take place during pregnancy. While they do not affect health, they may be psychologically distressing. About 90 percent of pregnant women experience an increase in pigmentation, usually a mild darkening of areas of the body that are already darkly pigmented (such as the underarms, the nipple and areolae, vulva, anus, and inner thighs). A dark line often appears in the middle of the abdomen from the pubic bone to the belly button. (This line is already present on the skin, but does not really become visible until pregnancy).

Ordinary FRECKLES, some scars, and many MOLES may also darken. These are harmless, but since malignant melanomas and premalignant DYSPLASTIC NEVI are sensitive to hormonal change, any suspicious-looking moles should be brought to the attention of a physician. HYPERPIGMENTATION is usually most pronounced among dark-haired, dark-skinned women and usually begins in the first trimester, continuing throughout the nine months and usually fading after the birth. Generally, however, the sites that became darkened never return to their exact pre-pregnancy color.

Melasma

Called the "mask of pregnancy," or chloasma, this is a special type of hyperpigmentation affecting the face that may appear in up to 75 percent of all pregnancies. It is more common in dark-skinned women, is often worsened by sun exposure, and also occurs in up to one-third of women on birth control pills. It has been suggested that this condition may be hereditary.

Pruritus Gravidarum

This common disorder is characterized by ITCHING, which in some is mild and in others is generalized and severe. It occurs in the third trimester and disappears after the birth, but tends to recur with subsequent pregnancies or with the administration of birth control pills. Symptoms include itching over the entire body, loss of appetite, nausea, and vomiting.

PUPPP

Another common disorder is PRURITIC URTICARIAL PAPULES AND PLAQUES OF PREGNANCY (PUPPP), which appears during the third trimester only in first pregnancies and is characterized by itching and red papules that resemble HIVES. They usually begin on the abdomen and later spread onto the thighs, buttocks, and arms. There is no increase in fetal problems or death associated with this syndrome. Patients usually respond to antihistamines and topical CORTICOSTEROIDS, although some women need a brief course of oral corticosteroids to control the itching. The disease does not reappear after birth, nor is there a recurrence with birth control pills or subsequent pregnancies.

Papular Dermatitis

Spangler's dermatitis of pregnancy is a rare, severely itchy disorder that may begin at any time during the nine months. It is associated with a 30 percent chance of stillbirth or spontaneous abortion. The disorder, which can recur during subsequent pregnancies, may be characterized by red papules that become crusted and excoriated, followed by a darkening of skin after the lesions fade. The disorder is treated with oral corticosteroids.

Immune Progesterone Dermatitis of Pregnancy

This rare disorder of the first three months of pregnancy is characterized by PAPULES and PUSTULES on the arms, legs, and buttocks that may resemble acne or psoriasis. The problem may recur with subsequent pregnancies. Administration of estrogens can suppress the lesions, which may be brought on by the administration of birth control pills with progesterone.

Herpes Gestationis

This unusual autoimmune blistering disorder is similar to bullous pemphigoid. It appears in one in 50,000 pregnancies, can occur at any time during pregnancy and is characterized by blistering and itching. It is treated with topical and sometimes systemic steroids. There is no conclusive proof that it is associated with an increased risk for fetal injury and death. There is a tendency for the condition to recur, with increased severity, in subsequent pregnancies.

Prurigo Gestationis of Besnier

This third-trimester disorder is characterized by small papules that are crusted and excoriated on the arms, backs of hands, tops of feet, thighs, legs, and trunk. It is not associated with any fetal or maternal problems.

Impetigo Herpetiformis

This type of pustular psoriasis occurs primarily during the third trimester and may occur during subsequent pregnancies. It is thought to be associated with a significant increase in death rates for mother or child. Associated with hypoparathyroidism, it is characterized by symptoms such as fever, chills, prostration, vomiting, diarrhea, convulsions, and weight loss. Skin symptoms include red macules followed by sterile pustules, especially in body folds and mucous membranes. The individual lesions may itch and burn. Treatment is the same as for pustular psoriasis, except that antimetabolites or ETRETINATE are avoided.

Jaundice

This yellowing of the skin may appear during the last trimester, caused by obstruction of liver ducts. It is not usually a serious problem and resolves quickly after delivery.

Blood Vessel Lesions

Vascular spider angiomas caused by circulating estrogens appear in the first or second trimester, but most (75 percent) have already faded seven weeks after the birth. Spider veins and varicose veins may also occur.

pressure injuries Continuous pressure on the skin can cause several different problems, including CORNS, CALLUSES, and BEDSORES (pressure sores).

A corn appears when there is focal pressure over a bony prominence or a bone spur. Although they are most common on the foot, calluses, which are larger and less focal than corns, can form on any surface where there is recurrent pressure or friction (such as the soles of runners' feet, the fingers of guitar players, or the middle finger of people frequently holding a pencil or pen).

The initial thickening of the STRATUM CORNEUM is an attempt by the skin to protect itself; pain and fissures may develop if the pressure continues. Eliminating this pressure or friction usually produces a permanent cure, but sometimes surgical removal may be necessary. Special inserts in shoes, wearing two pairs of socks, and wearing well-fit shoes may help to prevent the cause of sores.

Pressure sores may form over any bony prominence (especially on the heels, base of the spine, and elbows) and are caused by continual pressure on the skin, which interferes with blood flow in patients who are unconscious, bedridden, or who have abnormal sensations. The process is affected by a person's age, nutrition, and general physical shape.

Risk Factors and Preventive Measures

Skilled, vigilant nursing care can prevent most of these ulcers from forming; any reddened area should receive special attention. Bedridden patients should be turned every two hours to distribute their weight, and the skin should be kept clean and dry. Urine and feces should be promptly removed before they irritate the skin; dusting powder may also help. Other preventive aids include sheepskins, water and air mattresses, and foam rings.

pressure sores See BEDSORES; PRESSURE INJURIES.

pretibial fever See LEPTOSPIROSIS.

prickle cell layer See STRATUM SPINOSUM.

prickly heat An irritating skin rash also known as heat rash that is associated with obstruction of the SWEAT GLANDS and accompanied by aggravating prickly feelings. The medical term for prickly heat, miliaria rubra ("red millet seeds") refers to the appearance of the rash. A milder form of the condition, miliaria crystallina, sometimes appears first as clear, shiny, fluid-filled BLISTERs that dry up without treatment.

While physicians are not completely sure of the mechanism behind the development of prickly heat, it is thought to be associated with sweat that is trapped in the skin.

Symptoms and Diagnostic Path

Numerous tiny, red itchy spots occur, covering mildly inflamed parts of the skin where the sweat collects (especially the waist, upper trunk, armpits, and insides of the elbows). With prickly heat it is comfortable to sleep only in cool surroundings, and lack of sleep and intense skin irritation can make the patient irritable.

Treatment Options and Outlook

Slow acclimation to hot weather will reduce the chance of prickly heat. Avoiding heavy activities in the heat will also help prevent the problem. Frequent cool showers and sponging the area will relieve the itching. CALAMINE lotion and dusting powder may also ease the discomfort. Clothing should be clean, dry, starch-free, and loose to help sweat evaporate. Sweating from fever can be reduced with drugs such as acetaminophen.

procarbazine (Trade name: Matulane) A chemotherapy drug used to treat certain cancers of the skin, among other conditions. It inhibits growth of cancer cells by preventing cell division.

Side Effects

In addition to typical anticancer drug side effects, which include nausea and vomiting, procarbazine may cause a sudden rise in blood pressure if taken with certain foods or drinks (such as cheese or red wine), which can be fatal.

progeria A rare autosomal recessive disorder characterized by premature old age, including excessive wrinkling of the skin. The condition is usually diagnosed at six to 12 months of age. Cells taken from affected patients show only a few generations of cell division before they stop reproducing, instead of the 50 generations that occur in cells from healthy youngsters.

Symptoms and Diagnostic Path

There are two forms of the disease, both of which are rare. In Hutchinson-Gilford syndrome, aging starts around age four; within eight years the affected child has all the external features of old age, including sagging skin on the face and body, baldness, loss of fat, and internal degenerative changes. In WERNER'S SYNDROME (or adult progeria), the condition begins in early adult life and follows the same rapid progression.

Treatment Options and Outlook

There is no treatment, and the outlook is not good for either type of this condition. Patients with Hutchinson-Gilford syndrome typically die at puberty. Patients with Werner's syndrome die in early adulthood.

progressive systemic sclerosis   See SCLERODERMA.

prolidase deficiency   A rare inherited disease in which the enzyme prolidase is absent. Skin symptoms include chronic recurrent ulcers of the lower legs, diffuse spider veins (TELANGIECTASIA), and shallow scarring with darkened skin color over face and buttocks. Other skin symptoms include fragile skin; purple papules (PURPURA); gray hair; reddened fissures of hands and feet; papular lesions on face, arms, and legs; and dry crusted areas on face and buttocks.

Other symptoms associated with this enzyme deficiency include nose abnormalities, jaw problems, multiple dental cavities, mental retardation, joint problems, and recurrent ear and sinus infections.

There is no treatment.

promethazine   An ANTIHISTAMINE drug used to relieve itching in a variety of skin conditions, including HIVES and ECZEMA. The drug is also used to relieve nausea and vomiting, and as a premedication sedative.

Side Effects
Dry mouth, blurred vision, and drowsiness.

Propionibacterium acnes   A type of bacterium that is one of the more important factors in the development of ACNE. *P. acnes* is found deep in the sebaceous follicle. While it is important in the development of inflammatory acne, acne is not a bacterial infection; instead, inflammation probably stems from the effect of the byproducts of this bacterium within the cell.

propylene glycol   A substance used to improve spreadability of a topical cosmetic product which can worsen ACNE.

protozal infections   Infection caused by single-celled animals account for a number of skin conditions, including LEISHMANIASIS, trypanosomiasis, amebiasis, TRICHOMONIASIS, and toxoplasmosis.

See also PARASITIC INFECTIONS.

prurigo   The general term for several itchy skin eruptions consisting of dome-shaped PAPULES and nodules.

See also PRURIGO NODULARIS.

prurigo nodularis   A skin condition characterized by intense ITCHING. Experts believe that the disease may represent some problem with skin sensory nerves. It primarily affects middle-aged women and drives affected individuals to pick and dig at their skin. Repeated picking produces nodular lesions.

Symptoms and Diagnostic Path
Lesions, which are found most often on the upper back, back of the neck, arms, and shins, are skin-colored with a warty, rounded surface topped by a crust.

Treatment Options and Outlook
There is no one specific treatment for this condition but picking must be stopped. Topical or intralesional steroids are often administered, while some patients respond slowly to a modified GOECKERMAN REGIMEN of tar ointments and daily exposure to ultraviolet-B light (UVB). CRYOTHERAPY also may be helpful in treating the lesions.

pruritic urticarial papules and plaques of pregnancy (PUPPP)   A common disorder that appears during the third trimester of pregnancy characterized by ITCHING and red papules resembling HIVES.

The disorder, which appears in one out of every 300 first-time pregnancies, does not occur in repeat pregnancies.

The cause of PUPPP is not known, but studies show that between 4 percent and 10 percent of patients with the condition are pregnant with twins, which suggests a relationship between skin distension and the development of PUPPP.

Most studies also have found patients with higher weight gain developed PUPPP when compared to normal pregnancies, further supporting the role of increased skin distension. One large series of cases revealed an infant male/female ratio of 2-to-1. Investigators have recently identified fetal DNA in the skin of mothers with PUPPP.

Symptoms and Diagnostic Path

Lesions may first appear in the abdominal area, and spread to the thighs, buttocks, and arms. The lesions usually fade away within one or two weeks after the birth. There is no evidence of death of either the fetus or the mother.

Treatment Options and Outlook

ANTIHISTAMINES (for ITCHING) and topical CORTICO-STEROIDS are effective, although initial control may require a brief course of oral corticosteroids. The condition fades away within a week of delivery. The disorder does not reappear after birth, nor does it recur with subsequent pregnancies or with the use of birth control pills.

See also PREGNANCY AND THE SKIN.

pruritis gravidarum This common itchy condition, also known as intrahepatic cholestasis of pregnancy, appears in up to 2.4 percent of pregnancies during the last trimester and disappears after birth. This reversible condition, which appears to have a genetic component, causes itching without producing primary skin lesions. It tends to recur with subsequent pregnancies or with birth control pill use.

While the health of the mother is not affected by this condition, its effect on the fetus is more controversial. Some experts report premature births and intrauterine asphyxia among infants whose mothers have the condition, but most argue that there is no fetal risk.

Cause is unknown, but lab studies reveal elevated bilirubin (a bile pigment); the itchiness is proportional to the concentration of bile acid in the skin. Placental estrogens and progestins are believed to interfere with the liver's excretion of bile acids.

Symptoms and Diagnostic Path

ITCHING that is localized at first and then spreads over the entire body may be associated with anorexia, nausea, and vomiting and, rarely, JAUNDICE. The liver may be enlarged and tender; stools are clay-colored and urine dark.

Treatment Options and Outlook

While the itching can be severe, it virtually always stops after the birth. OATMEAL baths and ANTIHISTAMINES are effective, although more aggressive treatment may be necessary, involving cholestyramine and vitamin K. Phenobarbital can help promote bile excretion.

See also PREGNANCY AND THE SKIN.

pruritus Itching.

pseudoacanthosis nigricans See ACANTHOSIS NIGRICANS.

pseudofolliculitis barbae A condition of ingrown hairs in the beard area that is very common among African-American patients, occurring in either sex on any shaved part of the body. Shaving increases the chances of this problem by sharpening the free hair end. Short, curly hairs are more likely to penetrate the skin than long straight ones.

Symptoms and Diagnostic Path

Numerous inflammatory papules and pustules (ranging from just a few to hundreds) in any hairy area together with darker skin color. The disease disappears if the beard or other hair is allowed to grow. While early lesions include reddened papules with pustules, those who have had the problem for a long time have firm, hyperpigmented PAPULES.

Treatment Options and Outlook

The best treatment is to discontinue shaving, which will slow the appearance of new lesions, ultimately allowing some of the embedded hairs to be released from the skin. As the beard grows, warm-water compresses should be applied for 10 minutes, three times daily to smooth lesions and remove crusts. The beard may be trimmed during this time, but not shorter than half an inch. Ingrown hairs should be released each day with a clean toothpick or sterile needle; *they should not be plucked, since this may cause more irritation when the hair breaks through the hair follicle.* After releasing the hair, a topical CORTICOSTEROID lotion should be applied. If there is infection, systemic antibiotics may be prescribed.

If the beard must be shaved, a close shave should be avoided to stop the immediate penetration by sharpened hairs.

Before shaving, the face should be washed with an abrasive soap and rough washcloth to loosen embedded hairs. Then, areas of ingrown hairs should be massaged with a toothbrush. Warm-water compresses should be applied for several minutes. A single-blade razor (not a double blade) should be used with the grain, in one direction, using short, even strokes. Some people find relief with special razors designed to prevent a close shave, and some electric shavers are also designed to prevent close shaving. The skin should not be pulled tight, since the released skin falls on the stubble and causes more shaving bumps. Any ingrown hairs should be released after shaving, followed by a nonirritating aftershave. If the lotion causes any itching or burning, a prescribed topical corticosteroid lotion should be applied.

Alternatively, chemical hair-removers may be effective. For some people, topical Retin-A (tretinoin) or glycolic acid is effective over the long term, although heightened irritation may occur at first.

Laser hair removal has revolutionized the treatment of pseudofolliculitis barbae. A series of treatments permanently decreases hair growth and converts remaining dark, thick hairs into finer, lighter-colored ones. By doing so, the cause of pseudofolliculitis is removed. With no terminal thick hairs to cause inflammation, the disease ends. All skin types, even very dark skinned individuals, can be treated with long-pulse diode and Nd:YAG lasers.

pseudoxanthoma elasticum A chronic hereditary disease involving abnormalities in connective tissue, causing the elastic fibers of the skin to fragment and calcify. There are four different forms of pseudoxanthoma elasticum: two caused by autosomal recessive inheritance (the most common) and two caused by autosomal dominant inheritance. A genetic autosomal dominant trait means that only one defective gene (from one parent) is needed to cause the syndrome.

One of any of the four types of this condition can appear in one out of every 40,000 live births.

Symptoms and Diagnostic Path

Skin symptoms include stiff, thickened, yellow-tan skin in mucous membranes of the mouth, cheek, and inner lips, in the armpits, groin, the navel, and the neck. Other general characteristics of the disorder include vision problems caused by hemorrhages in the retina, persistent high blood pressure, severe chest pain, and dizzy spells. There are also speech problems and brief, minor strokes, with abdominal pain and severe pain in the calf muscle.

Lesions are usually distributed equally on the left and right sides of the body, and may group together to affect a larger area of skin. Some people have described these areas as having a "chicken skin" or "cobblestone" appearance or have described the neck as appearing unwashed.

The areas of lesions tend to progress downward from the neck, affecting the underarm, the inside of the elbow, the groin, and the back of the knee. Sometimes the navel and inner lip are affected. Generally, the progression of skin lesions is slow. In late stages of the disease, the skin may develop loose and saggy folds.

A skin biopsy by a dermatologist can reveal elastic fibers of the skin that are clumped and fragmented, and include small amounts of calcium. Both the age of onset and the age of detection vary greatly from one individual to another, as does the extent of skin involvement. In some individuals, there is no apparent skin involvement, whereas in others, skin involvement may be extensive.

Once PXE is diagnosed, the affected individual should consider all the ramifications of this disease. A detailed history should be taken by the dermatologist and the patient should obtain a referral to an ophthalmologist and a cardiologist. PXE can cause difficulties in the eyes, cardiac, vascular, and gastrointestinal systems. There may be special issues for women and pediatric patients.

Treatment Options and Outlook

There is not yet a treatment for the disease, but there are several treatments for complications. Cosmetic surgery may be used to tighten the skin if this effect is considered unsightly. The outcome of the cosmetic surgery is usually good, although stretched scars have been reported in some cases.

Aerobic exercise and good diet low in fat and cholesterol may help. All exercise should be safe from the risk of head trauma or increasing pressure in the eye (this would exclude football, soccer, weight lifting, and so on). Patients should avoid smoking or becoming overweight and should try to lose weight if obese. Patients with mitral valve prolapse should take prophylactic antibiotics before dental work and avoid nonsteroidal anti-inflammatory drugs (such as aspirin or ibuprofen) since they may cause gastric irritation or encourage bleeding.

Patients should visit a doctor on a regular basis in order to monitor pulses in the extremities, blood pressure, and cholesterol. In addition, an ophthalmologist should monitor any retinal changes.

The life expectancy of people affected by PXE is the same as the general population. However, life-threatening complications can occur as a result of involvement of major arteries.

There is no way to predict the rate of progression or the extent of skin involvement, nor is there any evidence regarding the effect of environment or diet on the progression or the extent of skin involvement.

psoralens Organic compounds found in many plants such as limes, lemons, celery, and parsnips that stimulate the formation of MELANIN in combination with ultraviolet light (UVA). Capable of inducing phototoxic reactions in the skin when exposed to sunlight, this substance is now being studied for its therapeutic benefits.

Many years ago, a Cairo dermatologist found out that indigenous people along the Nile used plants containing OIL OF BERGAMOT as a folk remedy to treat VITILIGO, a skin disorder in which the immune system attacks and destroys the skin's pigment. While researchers are not sure why it works, they believe that psoralens, when combined with sunlight, may suppress the immune system and stop the attack on the skin's pigment while stimulating melanin production. Psoralens also stops cells from making DNA, eventually killing them, which may explain why it helps those with disorders characterized by rapid cell replication, such as PSORIASIS.

Psoralens, together with ultraviolet light-A (UVA), is the most commonly used form of photochemotherapy. Called psoralen-UVA (or PUVA), it became available in the mid-1970s. PUVA therapy consists of oral or topical administration of a psoralen and irradiation of the skin with UVA light. The most widely used psoralen in the United States is 8-methoxypsoralen, administered orally followed by a one-hour exposure to UVA. PUVA may interfere with the migration of inflammatory cells to the skin, and is effective in managing psoriasis (it alleviates the problem in almost 90 percent of cases). It may also be used in the treatment of other forms of psoriasis, for cutaneous T-cell lymphomas, atopic dermatitis, LICHEN PLANUS, and vitiligo.

Psoralen alone may produce ITCHING and nausea in a small number of patients, and the risks of PUVA can be either acute or chronic. SUNBURN-like redness may occur together with BLISTERS. These effects can be prevented by carefully assessing dose. However, the chronic long-term toxicity is not yet determined. PUVA is carcinogenic in experimental situations. Hyperpigmentation occurs in most patients, and some experience lentigines and mottling of skin color. There is also a risk of premature aging of the skin, ACTINIC KERATOSES, BOWEN'S DISEASE, and SQUAMOUS CELL CARCINOMA. Prior skin cancer, previous exposure to ionizing radiation, arsenic ingestion, and (perhaps) the previous use of tar preparations may increase the chance of abnormal growths in those patients. The formation of cataracts is another risk, although there have been few reports of premature cataracts in those patients treated with PUVA without eye protection.

psoriasiform A medical term meaning "like PSO-RIASIS." It refers to any sharply-marginated plaque with thick scales.

psoriasis A chronic skin disorder affecting more than 4.5 million men and women, producing silvery, scaly plaques on the skin. The most common type of psoriasis is called plaque psoriasis (or psoriasis vulgaris), characterized by raised, inflamed lesions covered with silver-white scales. Other, far less common forms include pustular, guttate, inverse, and erythrodermic psoriasis. In erythrodermic psoriasis, red scaly involvement of the entire skin makes temperature and fluid control difficult, placing a significant strain on internal organs such as the heart and kidneys, that may require hospitalization.

Psoriasis usually begins between 15 and 35, affecting 2.1 percent of the population but it can begin at any age. Rarely, even some infants develop the condition. The condition is considered mild if less than 10 percent of the body is affected; more than 10 percent indicates a severe problem. About 30 percent of patients have moderate to severe cases.

The *location* of the symptoms, more than the extent, influences how disabling the condition may be. Psoriasis only on the palms and soles of the feet can be physically disabling, while psoriasis on the face can be emotionally disabling.

Normally, a person with psoriasis experiences cycles of improvement and flare-ups; the disease can go into remission for a periods ranging from one to 60 years.

The cause of psoriasis is unknown, although researchers believe that some type of biochemical stimulus triggers the abnormal cell growth in the epidermis. While normal skin cells take a month to mature, patients with psoriasis have skin cells that overmultiply, forcing the cells to move up to the top of the skin in only seven days. As the number of cells builds up, the epidermis thickens and the extra cells pile up in raised, red and scaly lesions. The white scales covering the red lesions is made up of dead cells that are continually shed; the inflammation is caused by the buildup of blood needed to feed the rapidly dividing cells.

While anyone can develop psoriasis, there also seems to be a hereditary link, and a family association, in one out of three cases. If one parent has psoriasis, each child has a 10 to 25 percent chance of developing the condition. If both parents have psoriasis, each child has a 50 percent chance. It is not known whether just one gene, or a collection of genes, predisposes a person to the condition. Experts do believe that one gene modified by others in combination with certain environmental factors produce the condition.

Skin trauma, emotional stress, and some kinds of infection may trigger the development of psoriasis. The condition sometimes forms at the site of a surgical incision or after a drug reaction. Psoriasis that appears after trauma is known as the "Koebner phenomenon." Alcohol abuse makes psoriasis more aggressive and more difficult to treat and control.

Symptoms and Diagnostic Path

The first lesions of plaque psoriasis appear as red, dots that can be very small; these eruptions slowly get larger, producing a silvery white surface scale that is shed easily. When forcibly removed, the scales may leave tiny bleeding points known as the AUSPITZ'S SIGN. The plaques, which often appear in the same place on the right and left sides of the body, often cover large areas of skin, merging into one another. The most common sites are elbows, scalp, and genitals. Lesions vary in size and shape from one person to another.

Certain races seem more susceptible to developing psoriasis. Caucasians have the highest percentage, although East Africans are also at risk; African Americans have a low incidence of the disease, probably because their origins are primarily West African.

The most common places to find the scaly patches are on the scalp, elbow, knees, and trunk, although they can be found anywhere on the body. Patches spread over wide expanses of skin can lead to intense itching, skin pain, dry or cracking skin, and swelling; body movement and flexibility may also be affected.

Potentially more disabling than the physical discomfort of psoriasis is the emotional impact of a disfiguring disease. Psoriasis can be unsightly and erode self-confidence, inducing depression, guilt, or anger.

Between 10 and 30 percent of patients develop psoriatic arthritis. Mild cases are milder than rheumatoid arthritis but in several cases can be very disabling. Psoriatic arthritis causes inflammation and stiffness, often affecting the fingers and toes.

About 1 million Americans have psoriatic arthritis (about 0.5 percent of the country). Psoriatic arthritis usually develops between the ages of 30 and 50, but it can develop at any time. Although psoriasis typically appears before psoriatic arthritis, arthritis can develop even without the characteristic skin lesions.

Psoriasis is usually diagnosed by observation. There are no blood tests for the disease, although physicians sometimes examine a skin biopsy under the microscope to confirm the diagnosis. Sometimes small pits in the fingernails, yellow discoloration of the nail, or collections of scaly skin under the nail can help to diagnose the condition.

Treatment Options and Outlook

There is no cure for psoriasis, but there are treatments that can clear plaques or significantly improve the skin's appearance. Treatment is aimed at slowing the excessive cell division, resulting in remissions lasting up to a year or more. Once the treatment is effective, it is discontinued until the psoriasis returns. Type of treatment depends on the type of psoriasis, its location and severity, patient age, and medical history. Experts suspect that psoriasis is caused by a malfunctioning immune system that allows skin cells to grow too fast, resulting in dry, red, scaly patches. Topical medications slow down the excessive cell reproduction and ease inflammation associated with psoriasis. There are many effective topical treatments. While many can be purchased over the counter, others are available by prescription only.

Topical medications (EMOLLIENTS, steroids, VITAMIN D or A derivatives, ANTHRALIN, salicylic acid, and COAL TAR preparations) are used for mild to moderate psoriasis. These may be used alone or in combination with each other or with ultraviolet light (UVB). Regular sunbathing may help clear up a case of psoriasis for some patients because of the exposure to natural UVB.

For more severe cases, the topical treatments above will be combined with psoralen plus UVA, chemotherapy (METHOTREXATE), and oral retinoid medications (such as Tegison). Treatments for severe psoriasis are toxic and must be weighed against their potential risks.

A new treatment for localized psoriasis involves using a laser to target small psoriatic plaques. The laser produces high-intensity UVB light at the wavelengths most effective for clearing psoriasis. Because the light is so intense and the laser can be aimed just at the spot of psoriasis, clearing can occur in just six to eight treatments. Cleared areas may remain clear for six to eight months.

DERMATOLOGISTS usually begin with the mildest therapy and work up to the one that is most effective in clearing up the skin problem. No single treatment works for everyone, and each patient reacts differently to the drugs. Systemic medications are prescription medications that affect the entire body. They are usually used only for patients with moderate to severe psoriasis who do not respond to or who are not eligible for topical medications or ultraviolet (UV) light treatments.

"Biologics" are medications developed from cells rather than combinations of chemicals like traditional drugs. They block or eliminate immune system cells involved in psoriasis and psoriatic arthritis. Biologics that have been approved include Amevive, the first approved biologic medication; Enbrel; and Raptiva. Remicade has been approved to treat psoriatic arthritis and is being studied for treating psoriasis.

Other systemic medications for these diseases can also affect the immune system in a more general way. Cyclosporine is a prescription systemic medication used to treat psoriasis; it has been available since 1995 to help prevent organ rejection in transplant patients. In 1997 Neoral (one brand name of cyclosporine) was approved as a psoriasis treatment.

Methotrexate is a systemic medication, usually sold as a generic, that was first used to treat cancer; researchers discovered in the 1950s that it could clear psoriasis, and it was eventually approved for this use in the 1970s.

Soriatane (acitretin) is a prescription oral RETINOID (a synthetic form of vitamin A). Synthetic retinoids were introduced as experimental drugs in the mid-1970s and were approved in the United States in the 1980s. Soriatane is currently the only oral retinoid approved specifically to treat psoriasis.

Other systemic medications sometimes used to treat psoriasis include Hydrea, mycophenolate mofetil, sulfasalazine, and 6-Thioguanine.

pulsed dye laser   A type of laser tuned to a specific light wavelength that uses flashes of light that are only a few millionths of a second long. Its bright light is well absorbed by blood vessels, which are then destroyed without harming surrounding skin.

In use with blood vessels, only yellow light is used to target hemoglobin—the substance that gives blood its red color. As a result, when used to treat birth defects of blood vessels, only the abnormal blood vessels are destroyed; surrounding tissue is left undamaged by the laser light. In treating pigment disorders such as liver spots and CAFÉ-AU-LAIT MACULES, green light is chosen to target the melanin.

This type of laser is particularly effective in removing BIRTHMARKS such as PORT-WINE STAINS at a very low risk of side effects. It is also effective in treating facial redness, ROSACEA, broken blood vessels in the face, STRETCH MARKS, and SCARS, as well as a variety of blood vessel tumors. The pulsed dye laser has revolutionized treatment of many of these conditions. Until the 1980s, port-wine stains could be treated but the risk of scarring was great. With the pulsed dye lasers, port-wine stains can be lightened drastically with a risk of scarring significantly less than 1 percent. Other blood vessel problems can all be treated with the pulsed dye laser.

During the treatment, the physician holds a handpiece against the skin and pulses the laser; patients say the light feels like a rubber band snapping and stinging against the skin. Although most adults tolerate the procedure without anesthesia, some children may need an anesthetic or medication to relax during treatment. Some lesions (such as a spider angiomas or dilated blood vessels) may require only one to three treatments, while larger, darker, thicker lesions such as port-wine stains may need six to 12 or more sessions.

Risks and Complications

There are few significant risks with this procedure. Patients may notice a tingling or burning sensation for a few hours after treatment.

Two types of treatment settings are used. If purpura (bruising settings) are selected, immediately after the treatment, a purple discoloration appears at the treatment site, which lasts for five to 10 days. As this color fades, the treated area may still look red, but will slowly fade to normal skin color over the next few weeks. Crusting may develop in the first several days and last up to two weeks. Some patients may experience a temporary brown discoloration of the skin for several months.

If non-bruising settings are used, the treated area gets red and a bit swollen for a few hours to a few days, but bruising does not develop. Application of ice for 10 minutes every hour on the day of treatment reduces the amount and duration of swelling.

Outlook and Lifestyle Modification

A soothing ointment (such as Aquaphor Healing Ointment) may be applied immediately after treatment. Patients should limit sun exposure before the treatment, because tanned skin will absorb the laser light and make the treatment less effective, and it also will increase the risk for temporary brown discoloration to occur after treatment. Treated skin also may be sensitive to the sun and should not be exposed for several weeks. A SUNSCREEN of SPF 30 is suggested.

PUPPP   See PRURITIC URTICARIAL PAPULES AND PLAQUES OF PREGNANCY.

purpura   A group of disorders characterized by purplish or reddish brown areas of discoloration, visible through the skin and caused by bleeding within underlying tissue. "Purpura" also refers to the discolored purple areas themselves, which range from the size of a pinhead to an inch in diameter. Smaller bleeding points are called

PETECHIAE; larger areas of discoloration are called BRUISES or ecchymoses.

Symptoms and Diagnostic Path

Common purpura (or senile purpura) is the most common of all bleeding disorders. It affects mostly middle-aged or elderly women, causing large discolored areas on the thighs but especially on backs of the hands and forearms, the result of thinning of the tissues supporting blood vessels beneath the skin. Bleeding may also be seen in the membrane lining the mouth.

Purpura caused by a lack of platelets in the blood, called thrombocytopenia, is usually the result of a disease of the bone marrow such as leukemia or aplastic anemia, or a side effect of drugs or excessive radiation.

Henoch-Schonlein purpura (or anaphylactoid purpura) is caused by inflammation of blood vessels in the skin, and is associated with inflammation of blood vessels in the gut, joints, and kidney as well.

Other types of purpura can be found in SCURVY, resulting from a VITAMIN C deficiency, and in certain infections, autoimmune disorders, blood poisoning, or blood chemical disturbances.

Treatment Options and Outlook

Common purpura is difficult to treat. Avoidance of systemic and topical steroids are advised as they thin the skin even further. Avoiding trauma (even a slap on the wrist) is essential. Henoch-Schonlein purpura responds only to immunosuppressant drugs and systemic CORTICOSTEROIDS. In severe cases, plasmapheresis (removal of blood, replacement of plasma and retransfusion) can be effective. Platelet deficiency is treated by curing the underlying cause. Autoimmune thrombocytopenia purpura is usually treated with corticosteroid drugs or a splenectomy.

pus The product of inflammation, this is a pale yellow or green creamy fluid composed of millions of dead white blood cells, fluid, partly digested tissue, bacteria, and other substances found at the site of a bacterial infection. A collection of pus in solid tissue is an ABSCESS.

The main organisms that form pus include staphylococci, streptococci, pneumococci and *Escherichia coli*. Some bacteria (*pseudomonas aeruginosa*) produce blue-tinged pus.

pustule A small pus-containing skin blister found on skin that may or may not be caused by infection. They are often found at the opening of hair follicles (folliculitis). *Staphylococcus aureus* is a frequent cause of bacterial FOLLICULITIS, while the pustules in ACNE are not infectious.

PUVA The combination of the oral or topical photosensitizing chemical PSORALEN (either trioxsalen or methoxsalen) plus long-wave ultraviolet light-A (UVA), the most commonly used form of photochemotherapy helpful in treating PSORIASIS, VITILIGO, MYCOSIS FUNGOIDES, and several other skin disorders. Only becoming clinically useful in the mid-1970s, PUVA therapy consists of oral or topical administration of a psoralen and irradiation of the skin with UVA light. Treatments (which last five to 10 minutes) are given two or three times a week until remission, when the therapy is reduced to once a week or every other week. The most widely used psoralen in the United States is 8-methoxsoralen, administered orally followed by a one-hour exposure to UVA.

The exact reason why PUVA works is not known, but it leads to a decrease in the rate of DNA synthesis, which may explain why it helps those with disorders characterized by rapid cell replication (such as psoriasis). PUVA also may interfere with the migration of inflammatory cells to the skin. PUVA is highly effective in the management of psoriasis (it clears the problem in almost 90 percent of the time). It also may be used in the treatment of other forms of psoriasis, for cutaneous T-cell lymphomas, atopic dermatitis, LICHEN PLANUS, and vitiligo.

Side Effects

Patients who receive too much drug or ultraviolet light can develop severe SUNBURNS. Psoralens alone may produce itching and nausea in a small number of patients, and the risks of PUVA can be either acute or chronic. Sunburnlike redness may occur together with BLISTERS; these effects usually can be prevented by carefully assessing doses. However, the chronic long-term toxicity is not yet determined; PUVA is known to be carcinogenic in experimental situations. HYPERPIGMENTATION occurs in most patients, and some experience lentigines and mottling of skin color. There is a risk of premature aging of the skin, ACTINIC KERATOSES, BOWEN'S DISEASE, and SQUAMOUS CELL CARCINOMA. Prior skin cancer, previous exposure to ionizing radiation, arsenic ingestion, and (perhaps) the previous use of tar preparations may increase the chance of abnormal growths in those patients. The formation of cataracts is another risk, although there have been few reports of premature cataracts in those patients treated with PUVA without eye protection.

pyoderma A purulent (containing or characterized by pus) condition of the skin.

pyoderma gangrenosum A rare ulcerative condition characterized by ulcers that are surrounded by bluish gray discolored skin; it is found in about 5 percent of patients with underlying disease such as inflammatory bowel diseases (ulcerative colitis and Crohn's disease), rheumatoid arthritis, chronic active hepatitis, and Wegener's granulomatosis.

Symptoms and Diagnostic Path

Lesions begin as pustules that quickly progress to a necrotic (composed of dead tissue) ulcer; lesions often enlarge several centimeters each day. In about a third of cases, injury to the skin precedes the onset of the lesion. The blue-gray necrotic edge of the ulcer is characteristic of this disease.

Treatment Options and Outlook

Pyoderma gangrenosum can be very difficult to treat, and the underlying disease must be identified. Treatment of such underlying disease often helps to heal and prevent new ulcers.

Treatment may involve topical and systemic CORTICOSTEROIDS, DAPSONE, SULFAPYRIDINE, anticancer drugs, MINOCYCLINE, and CLOFAZIMINE. The lesions should be protected from injury and any underlying disease should be treated.

pyogenic granuloma A non infectious capillary tumor, that may appear anywhere on the skin but is frequently seen on the lips, gums, digits, arms, legs, or trunk (often after trauma).

Symptoms and Diagnostic Path

The solitary lesion usually begins as a small red PAPULE that quickly grows; as it develops, it becomes friable and bleeds easily. The condition is common in pregnant women (granuloma gravidarum), especially in the gums.

Treatment Options and Outlook

Surgical excision by electrosurgery or CURETTAGE AND ELECTRODESICCATION, or laser (argon, CO_2 and dye lasers have all been successful.) Some pyogenic granulomas recur after surgery and may require treatment.

pyridoxine deficiency See VITAMIN B_6 DEFICIENCY.

pyrilamine An ANTIHISTAMINE drug used to treat HIVES. Unlike other antihistamines, this drug rarely causes drowsiness.

quartz lamp A vacuum lamp of melted quartz glass used as a source of ULTRAVIOLET RADIATION.

Queensland tick typhus A disease in the spotted fever group caused by ticks infected with the *Rickettsia australis* organisms.

Symptoms and Diagnostic Path

The first sign of this disease is usually a lesion at the site of the tick bite that becomes an ulcer of deadened skin up to 5 mm across with a red areola, also called the *tache noir* ("black spot").

Treatment Options and Outlook

Specific antibiotics and administration of fluids and electrolytes are recommended, as well as prompt treatment of the associated high fever. TETRACYCLINE and chloramphenicol are effective, responding within 24 hours. Therapy should be continued for two weeks after the onset of fever. Treatment with CORTICOSTEROIDS has been effective for neurological complications of this infection.

quick-tanning lotions See SELF-TANNING PRODUCTS.

racket nail One of the most common congenital nail deformities. It is caused by a problem with the thumb, which is shorter than normal, producing a nail that is very short and wide. This is an autosomal dominant trait, which means that only one defective gene (from one parent) is needed to cause the syndrome. Each child of an affected person usually has a one in two chance of inheriting the defective gene and of being affected. The condition, which occurs most often in women, can affect either one or both thumbs.

radiation dermatitis See DERMATITIS, RADIATION.

radiation and the skin In the first half of this century, an X-ray machine was commonly found in every dermatologist's office. With the dawn of other treatments, including antibacterials, antifungals, CORTICOSTEROIDS, chemotherapy, and improved surgical treatment, and as the long-term consequences of radiation therapy became better known, radiotherapy became less frequently used. Today, it is confined largely to the treatment of malignant tumors.

The penetration of X-ray radiation varies. The shorter the wavelength, the deeper it can penetrate tissue. X-rays must be chosen to match tissue penetration. Superficial X-ray radiation is primarily used to treat BASAL CELL and SQUAMOUS CELL CARCINOMA of the face. While most of these cancers are treated by surgical excision, in some patients radiation is the treatment of choice (it is nontraumatic and better preserves cosmetic appearance). X-ray radiation is also used to treat eyelid cancers.

Other skin tumors (KAPOSI'S SARCOMA and MYCOSIS FUNGOIDES) may also be treated with superficial radiation.

Electromagnetic radiation includes a spectrum of wavelengths, beginning with the shortest (X-rays and gamma rays), followed by ultraviolet (UV), visible light, infrared, microwave, and radio waves.

Ionizing radiation (as produced by X-rays) produces FREE RADICALS in tissue, which lead to damage and structural changes in cells, delaying the growth and eventually killing the cells.

See also BASAL CELL CARCINOMA; DERMATITIS, RADIATION; RADIATION ERYTHEMA; RADIATION THERAPY FOR SKIN CANCER; RADIODERMATITIS.

radiation erythema Also known as Roentgen erythema, this is a brief reddening of the skin with varying amounts of swelling following exposure to radiation of between 300–400 cGy. The transient redness lasts between 24 and 72 hours; a longer-lasting reddening follows in a week, and may last for another week. It appears to be an early response to injury to the EPIDERMIS and DERMIS (first and second layer of skin). Darkening of the skin caused by the excess production of MELANIN follows. There is usually no significant pain associated with this level of radiation exposure.

See also DERMATITIS, RADIATION; RADIATION AND THE SKIN; RADIATION THERAPY FOR SKIN CANCER; RADIODERMATITIS.

radiation therapy for skin cancer Treatment of BASAL CELL or SQUAMOUS CELL CARCINOMA by X-rays that produce ionizing radiation. As the radiation passes through disease tissue, it destroys the abnormal cells. If the correct dosage of radiation is given, normal cells suffer little or no damage. Radiation, which is usually passed through diseased tissues by X-rays (or electrons) produced by a linear accelerator, cures most SKIN CANCERS.

Side Effects

Radiation for the treatment of skin cancer may produce fatigue, nausea and vomiting, and hair loss from the affected area. Skin reddening and blistering after treatment are common and may be alleviated with CORTICOSTEROID drugs. Long-term side effects may include skin cancer in areas of chronic RADIODERMATITIS (atrophy of the skin and loss of hair and/or sweat glands).

radioallergosorbent test   See RAST TEST.

radiodermatitis   A mottled increase and decrease in skin pigment caused by exposure to ionizing radiation. The area usually has no hair and is covered with dilated blood vessels over the thin surface of the patch. Radiodermatitis is considered to be a precancerous condition that may eventually progress to a malignant skin tumor.

The skin may have been exposed to ionizing radiation either by accident, or deliberately during radiation therapy; in either case, the radiation energy either injures or kills the individual cells, or causes a DNA mutation. The degree of radiation that reaches the cells depends on the type of radiation (X-rays, gamma rays, or neutrons); high-energy radiation used to treat deep tumors may actually cause less total energy to the skin than lower-energy radiation of X-rays. Temporary hair loss may follow 300–400 cGy of superficial radiation to the skin; hair loss may be permanent following larger doses.

Symptoms and Diagnostic Path

Radiation erythema causes a temporary reddening of the skin that lasts up to 72 hours, followed by a longer-lasting redness that appears in about a week and may take another week to fade. Hyperpigmentation due to excess MELANIN production follows. There is no discomfort associated with this type of radiodermatitis.

Acute radiodermatitis can be expected following radiation therapy for cancer; it may also occur following accidental exposure to radiation. In this acute form, the skin reddening does not disappear after a week, but instead progresses to an inflammatory reaction by the second week, characterized by blistering, crusting, and pain. As the inflammation begins to heal over the ensuing months, a nonpigmented scar and TELANGIECTASIAS appear; hair and sweat glands may be permanently destroyed.

Chronic radiodermatitis can appear years after extensive radiation exposure, characterized by atrophy of the skin, with telangiectasias and mottling. The skin becomes dry and easily injured, healing slowly. There is no hair on the exposed area, and sweat and sebaceous glands may be destroyed. There is an increased risk of SKIN CANCER (most commonly BASAL CELL CARCONIMA). When SQUAMOUS CELL CARCINOMA develops, it is often more aggressive than this type of cancer induced by sun exposure.

Treatment Options and Outlook

Acute radiodermatitis should be treated with cool tap water and protective dressings; ITCHING can be relieved with emollients, shake lotions, or witch hazel. Mild analgesics may relieve pain; the area should not be rubbed. Secondary infection is treated with antibiotics. Topical steroids are not effective with this type of skin condition.

There is no treatment for *chronic radiodermatitis,* other than protecting the area from injury or exposure to the sun and watching carefully for early signs of skin cancer.

See also RADIATION AND THE SKIN; RADIATION ERYTHEMA; RADIATION THERAPY FOR SKIN CANCER.

rash   The popular term for a group of spots or red, inflamed skin that is usually temporary and is only rarely a sign of a serious underlying problem. It may be inflammatory, infectious, cancerous, or it may represent an underlying disease.

RAST test   The abbreviation for radioallergosorbent test, used to diagnose allergies. The principle behind these tests is that there is a specific antigen for every antibody. Any antibody will bind only to its own antigen. This test detects antibodies to antigens.

rat-bite fever   A condition following the bite of a rat that causes two similar type diseases—*sodoku*, caused by *Spirillum minus*, and *septicemia* caused by *Streptobacillus moniliformis*. *Spirillus minus* causes skin ulcers and recurrent fever; *Streptobacillus moniliformis* causes skin inflammation, muscular pain, and vomiting. Following the rat bite, the wound heals but after one to three weeks, it becomes tender and swollen. Skin lesions appear, together with enlarged lymph nodes, general malaise, loss of appetite, and joint pain.

Treatment Options and Outlook

Intravenous administration of PENICILLIN G is effective in both cases.

Raynaud's phenomenon   A disorder of blood vessels that causes the skin of the fingers to turn white in the cold; in rare cases, the blood flow is permanently decreased, leading to ulceration or gangrene at the tips of affected fingers and toes.

On exposure to cold, the blood vessels of people with Raynaud's phenomenon suddenly contract, cutting off blood flow. Fingers of young women are most often affected.

Possible causes of Raynaud's phenomenon include arterial diseases (Buerger's disease, atherosclerosis, embolism, and thrombosis), connective tissue disease (rheumatoid arthritis, SCLERODERMA, and systemic LUPUS ERYTHEMATOSUS), and medications (ergotamine, methysergide, and beta blockers).

Raynaud's phenomenon is also a recognized occupational disorder in some people who use pneumatic drills, chain saws, or other vibrating machines; it is also sometimes seen in typists, pianists, and those whose fingers suffer repeated trauma.

Symptoms and Diagnostic Path

During exposure to cold, the skin of the digits turns white. As blood flow returns, the skin turns blue; upon being reheated, the skin turns red. Feelings of tingling, numbness, or burning may occur during an attack.

Treatment Options and Outlook

Hands and feet of affected individuals should be kept as warm as possible. Cigarette smoking further constricts the blood vessels and can worsen the condition, and thus should be avoided. Vasodilator drugs may be administered to relax the blood vessel walls and help prevent vasoconstriction. In severe cases, sympathectomy (cutting of the nerves controlling the caliber of arteries) may be effective.

Patients with Raynaud's phenomenon should wear the proper clothes for the temperature. Perspiration is more responsible for cold hands and feet than cold temperatures, so it is important to wear fabrics that soak up excess sweat and keep it from contacting the body. Hands and feet are especially prone to getting cold because they are natural areas of perspiration, which is why woolen socks and fleece boots make a person sweat and feel cold instead of warm.

This condition can occur in any season and is related to changes in temperature, so that grocery shopping or going to an air-conditioned theater in summer can provoke Raynaud's phenomenon.

razor bumps   The common name for PSEUDOFOLLICULITIS BARBAE.

reactive perforating collagenosis   A rare skin disease characterized by small papules with a central plug of oily material. They are caused by seeping of abnormal COLLAGEN through the overlying EPIDERMIS (top layer of skin). This hereditary condition usually appears in childhood. The lesions are usually found on the backs of the hands, forearms, elbows, and knees.

Treatment Options and Outlook

No treatment is needed, since the lesions usually disappear on their own, but removing the lesions by freezing with LIQUID NITROGEN or ELECTRODESICCATION may be effective.

von Recklinghausen's disease See NEUROFIBRO-MATOSIS.

reconstructive surgery See PLASTIC SURGERY.

reduction mammoplasty See MAMMOPLASTY.

Refsum's disease A rare genetic metabolic disease caused by a lack of the enzyme phytanic acid oxidase that causes mild scaling of the skin on the trunk, arms, and legs similar to ICHTHYOSIS. This results in a buildup in many organs of phytanic acid, a compound chiefly of dietary origin.

The disorder is an autosomal recessive trait, which means that a defective gene must be inherited in a double dose to cause the abnormality. Generally, both parents of an affected person are unaffected carriers of the defective gene. Each of the children has a one in four chance of being affected, and a two in four chance of being a carrier.

Symptoms and Diagnostic Path
In addition to the skin symptoms, the disease is characterized by night blindness, cataracts and other eye problems, skeletal abnormalities, kidney or heart problems, and hearing problems.

Treatment Options and Outlook
Eating a low-phytanic acid diet is recommended. Some patients find relief with plasma exchange (a procedure that reduces the concentration of unwanted substances in the blood).

relapsing polychondritis A rare chronic autoimmune inflammatory disease in which cartilage in the ear, nose, joints, eyes, blood vessels, trachea, and bronchial tubes may be destroyed.

Symptoms and Diagnostic Path
Skin signs are characterized by abnormal cartilage in the outer ear, which is large, swollen, tender, and red, lasting for one or two weeks before it fades and then recurs. Recurrent attacks will eventually destroy the cartilage, and result in "cauliflower ear." There are a number of other symptoms affecting other areas of the body; death can occur from aneurysms and cardiac valve disease.

Treatment Options and Outlook
Topical steroids do not work, but high doses of systemic CORTICOSTEROIDS can control or ease inflammation. Because of the frequent spontaneous remissions and recurrences, it is hard to evaluate response to therapy. DAPSONE, which may be safer than steroids, has been effective for some patients, but it also can cause serious side effects.

About 30 percent of patients usually die within four years, usually as a result of obstruction or collapse of the airway. Even if heart and bronchial tube defects do not occur, the disorder can cause deformities of the ears and nose.

renal failure and skin symptoms See KIDNEY DISEASE AND SKIN SYMPTOMS.

Renova See TRETINOIN.

reportable skin diseases Skin conditions (CHICKEN POX, MEASLES, SYPHILIS, TUBERCULOSIS, and RUBELLA) that must be reported to local health authorities by the physician responsible for care of the affected person. In turn, local health authorities must report some of these diseases to the national Centers for Disease Control.

Notification of certain potentially harmful infections is important because it enables public health officials to take the necessary steps to control the spread of infection. Reporting also provides valuable statistics on the incidence and prevalence of the disease, which can be used to formulate health policies such as immunization programs and improvements in sanitation.

resorcinol (Trade name: Rezamid) An ointment that causes the skin to peel, which is used to treat ACNE, DERMATITIS, and fungal infections, and contained in hair lotions for DANDRUFF. Its mechanism of action is unknown.

It is available in concentrations of 2 percent or less. In preparations of 3 percent and higher, local swelling, dermatitis, ITCHING, and peeling may occur. More seriously, there is also the possibility of systemic toxicity; if the drug is absorbed into the body, it can cause a decrease in activity of the thyroid gland, and convulsions. For this reason, products containing resorcinol should not be applied to broken skin or to large areas of the body. In addition, resorcinol may discolor dark or black skin.

Resorcinol is usually added to sulfur as an acne treatment; although resorcinol by itself is not considered to be effective against acne, it appears to enhance the action of sulfur. The U.S. Food and Drug Administration allows a combination of 8 percent sulfur with 2 percent resorcinol, or 8 percent sulfur with 3 percent resorcinol monacetate.

Resorcinol is considered to be a rather old-fashioned agent and is no longer commonly used.

Restylane   See HYALURONIC ACID GEL.

retinoic acid   See TRETINOIN.

retinoids   Synthetic or naturally occurring derivatives of VITAMIN A that have a range of effects on the skin, including wound repair, inhibiting tumor promotion, and so on. Today, retinoids are widely used in the treatment of stubborn cases of ACNE, PSORIASIS, prevention of SKIN CANCER, reversal of aging, and disorders of KERATINIZATION (the depositing of KERATIN within the cell).

Primary dietary sources of vitamin A are the beta-carotenes in the yellow and green leafy vegetables and also in some animal fats and fish oils. Vitamin A (RETINOL) is sent to the liver, where more than 90 percent of the body's stores are stockpiled.

They may be used topically as in retinoic acid or systemically as in ISOTRETINOIN, the generic form of Accutane, or ETRETINATE, the generic term for Tegison.

retinol   The principal form of VITAMIN A found in the body. It is essential for growth, vision in dim light, and maintenance of soft mucous tissue. Retinol (the alcohol of retinoic acid) and refined palmitate are both often found in skin-rejuvenating creams. While less effective than retinoic acid (Retin A), these two substances likely do help to slow the skin aging process and do reverse at least some of the changes caused by sun damage. Their greatest benefit is that they are less irritating than retinoic acid and are available without a prescription.

retinyl palmitate   A form of VITAMIN A that some studies suggest may be transformed into retinoic acid in the skin. Retinyl palmitate is less irritating than retinoic acid, but many experts believe that commercial skin care products do not contain enough of this substance to prevent or reduce aging.

See also RETINOIDS.

rhinophyma   Bulbous deformity and redness of the nose found almost exclusively in men over age 40, usually as a complication of severe ROSACEA (a skin disorder of the cheeks and nose). As nose tissue thickens, small blood vessels enlarge and the sebaceous glands become overactive, making the nose excessively oily.

Symptoms and Diagnostic Path

This condition causes the nose to thicken and become reddened and bulbous, with a waxy, yellowish appearance.

Physicians can usually diagnose this condition by visual inspection alone, although a skin biopsy may be needed to confirm the diagnosis in unusual cases.

Treatment Options and Outlook

Rhinophyma can be treated with a variety of surgical procedures, with a laser, scalpel, or dermabrasion. Skin grafting is not necessary, since the remaining tissue rapidly regenerates. Some physicians have found that the ACNE medication ISOTRETINOIN (Accutane) offers good results. Although the condition can be corrected surgically, the problem may recur.

rhinoplasty See NOSE REPAIR.

rhinoscleroma A chronic bacterial infection caused by *Klebsiella rhinoscleromatis* that is common in rural areas throughout the third world.

Symptoms and Diagnostic Path

The disease begins with increased nasal secretion and crusting, followed by an enlargement of the nose, upper lip, palate, or neighboring areas. If the infection spreads to the respiratory tract, breathing may become difficult and a tracheotomy may be necessary.

Treatment Options and Outlook

This progressive disease is difficult to treat, but systemic antibiotics such as gentamicin and tobramycin have been effective. Alternatively, oral administration of ciprofloxacin may help, although this drug has not been widely studied as a therapy for this condition. The condition may be fatal due to breathing obstructions or continuing infection.

rhytidectomy See FACE-LIFT.

Richner-Hanhart syndrome The common name for tyrosinemia type II, a hereditary metabolic disease caused by the absence of the enzyme tyrosine aminotransferase.

The condition is an autosomal recessive trait, which means that a defective gene must be inherited from both parents to cause the abnormality. Generally, both parents of an affected person are unaffected carriers of the defective gene. Each child of parents who both carry the defective gene has a one in four chance of being affected, and a two in four chance of being a carrier.

Symptoms and Diagnostic Path

The skin erodes on fingers, palms, and soles of the feet in symmetric lines, becoming crusted and wasted. The lesions may be so painful that they interfere with movement. Other signs of the condition include mental retardation, excess tearing, and eye problems.

Treatment Options and Outlook

A diet low in tyrosine and phenylalanine is advised. If diagnosed early enough, it is possible to prevent some of the problems (including mental retardation) associated with the disease.

rickettsial infections Diseases caused by the bite or feces of parasites called rickettsiae. The infections can be grouped as the spotted fevers (ROCKY MOUNTAIN SPOTTED FEVER, RICKETTSIAL POX, other tickborne fevers); the TYPHUS group (epidemic or louseborne typhus, endemic or murine typhus, and scrub typhus); Q fever; and trench fever.

Rickettsiae are microorganisms that share features of both bacteria and viruses. Like bacteria, rickettsiae have enzymes and cell walls, use oxygen, and can be controlled or destroyed by antibiotics. Like viruses, rickettsiae can live and multiply only inside cells. Rickettsiae normally live in ticks, mites, fleas, and lice, and they can be spread to humans by the bites of these bloodsucking insects. In people, rickettsiae usually live inside the cells lining small blood vessels, causing the blood vessels to become inflamed or blocked or to bleed into the surrounding tissue.

Symptoms and Diagnostic Path

A rickettsial infection may cause a fever, a skin rash, and a feeling of illness. Because the characteristic rash often does not appear for several days, an early diagnosis is difficult. Flea or lice infestation or a prior tick bite, particularly in a geographic area where a rickettsial disease is common, is a helpful clue in making the diagnosis.

The diagnosis of a rickettsial infection can be confirmed by identifying the organism in special cultures of blood or tissue specimens, by identifying the organism under a microscope using certain stains, or by identifying antibodies to the organism in a blood sample.

Treatment Options and Outlook

A rickettsial infection responds promptly to early treatment with the antibiotics chloramphenicol or TETRACYCLINE, both of which are taken by mouth. Improvement usually takes 24 to 36 hours, and fever usually disappears in two to three days.

When treatment is not so prompt, improvement is slower and the fever lasts longer. Antibiotics should be continued for at least 24 hours after the fever disappears, and may be given intravenously to people who are too ill to take them orally. If a person is severely ill and in a late stage of disease, a CORTICOSTEROID may be taken for a few days in addition to the antibiotic to relieve serious toxic symptoms and help relieve the inflammation of blood vessels.

See also *RICKETTSIA RICKETTSII.*

rickettsial pox   An urban disease transmitted by mites on common house mice that has been reported in cities since 1946. The responsible microorganism is *Rickettsia akari,* which belongs to the spotted fever group of these parasites.

Symptoms and Diagnostic Path

A local lesion develops between one and three weeks after a mite bite, beginning as a red papule that breaks down into an area of dead crusted skin, at which time it may be associated with local swelling of lymph nodes. Within a week after the lesion appears, fever, chills, headache, and myalgias occur, followed in a few more days by a rash over the body. This rash develops into an eruption similar to CHICKEN POX.

Treatment Options and Outlook

Treatment involves antibiotics (TETRACYCLINES or chloramphenicol), fluid and electrolytes, and prompt treatment of complications. The lesions may not be very severe, and the disease itself is mild and self-limiting.

See also RICKETTSIAL INFECTIONS.

Rickettsia rickettsii   A type of intracellular parasitic microorganism that looks like a small bacterium but that can reproduce only by invading cells of another life form. These parasites live primarily off insects and insectlike animals such as lice, fleas, ticks, and mites. In turn, these insects can transmit the parasite to rodents, dogs, or humans through saliva or feces. Human diseases spread by different types of these microorganisms include ROCKY MOUNTAIN SPOTTED FEVER and various forms of TYPHUS.

See also RICKETTSIAL INFECTIONS; RICKETISIAL POX.

rifampin   An antibacterial drug used to treat LEPROSY that is usually prescribed with other antibacterials because some strains of bacteria quickly develop resistance to rifampin alone. It is also used to eradicate *Staphylococcus aureus* from nasal cavities. Because it is so expensive, it is typically used as an adjunct treatment.

Side Effects

Harmless, orange-red discoloration of urine, saliva, and other body secretions; muscle pain; nausea and vomiting; diarrhea; JAUNDICE; flulike symptoms; rash and ITCHING.

ringworm   The popular term for TINEA, a superficial fungal infection of the skin.

Ritter's disease   The former name for staphlococcal SCALDED SKIN SYNDROME.

Rocky Mountain spotted fever   A rare infectious disease caused by the *Rickettsia* parasite (similar to a bacteria), characterized by a spotted rash. Transmitted to rabbits and other small mammals primarily by tick bites, it is found most often in wooded areas along the Atlantic coast, but it gets its name from its original occurrence in the Rocky Mountain states. The incidence of the disease has been rising steadily since 1980; there are more than 1,000 cases reported each year. Diagnosis may be difficult because the disease has symptoms resembling several other infections. Lab tests on blood and tissues are needed to confirm the diagnosis. Rocky Mountain spotted fever has been a reportable disease in the United States since the 1920s. In the last 50 years, between 250 and 1,200 cases have been reported each year, although it is likely that many more cases go unreported.

Symptoms and Diagnostic Path

Mild fever, muscle pain loss of appetite, nausea and vomiting, and slight headache may develop slowly about a week after a tick bite. Sometimes, however, symptoms appear suddenly with high fever and prostration. Two to five days after symptoms appear, small pink itchy spots appear on wrists and ankles, spreading centrally over the rest of the body. The illness subsides after about two weeks. The typical red, spotted rash occurs in only 35 to 60 percent of patients with Rocky Mountain spotted fever. In those who have a rash it may also appear later in the course of the disease on the palms or soles in up to 80 percent of patients. On the other hand, up to 15 percent of patients never develop a rash.

Rocky Mountain spotted fever can be tough to diagnose in its early stages, even by experienced physicians familiar with the disease because the symptoms are so common to many other infectious and noninfectious diseases.

Treatment Options and Outlook

Antibiotic drugs TETRACYCLINE or chloramphenicol usually cure the disease. Untreated cases with very high fever may end in death from pneumonia or heart failure.

Risk Factors and Preventive Measures

People in tick-infested areas should use insect repellent and examine themselves daily for ticks.

See also RICKETTSIAL INFECTIONS; *RICKETTSIA RICKETTSII*.

rodent ulcer The popular term for BASAL CELL epithelioma (tumor of the covering of the internal and external surfaces of the body) that has become large and eroded.

Rogaine See MINOXIDIL.

rosacea A chronic disorder affecting facial skin of the nose, cheeks, chin, or forehead that may include redness, pimples, PUSTULES, solid raised lesions, dilated blood vessels (TELANGIECTASES), and, less commonly, disfigurement and enlargement of the nose.

Rosacea affects about 14 million Americans (about one in 20), typically between ages 30 and 60. While it is sometimes called "adult acne" because the pimples usually appear during the 30s and 40s, rosacea is actually a different condition, and the pimples are not usually associated with BLACKHEADS and WHITEHEADS.

The condition affects fair-skinned patients more often than those with dark complexions, although it can affect all skin types. Most rosacea patients have a history of blushing more often and easily. Rosacea also may affect members of the same family because of similar skin conditions or genetic predisposition. Rosacea occurs at a particularly high rate among Irish Americans, although other nationalities—English, Scots, or Eastern Europeans—also may develop this conspicuous condition.

While women are more likely to develop rosacea, men are more likely to develop RHINOPHYMA (the large, bulbous nose associated with the condition). Rosacea is not linked with alcoholism, although alcohol may worsen the condition; teetotalers may also develop rosacea.

Doctors do not know exactly what causes rosacea, but most suspect that some people inherit a tendency to develop the disorder. People who blush frequently also may be more likely to develop rosacea. Some researchers believe that people who have rosacea have blood vessels that dilate too easily, triggering flushing and redness. Other theories suggest that the condition may be triggered by bacteria, mites, or fungal infection, but no link has been proven between rosacea and bacteria or other organisms on the skin, in the hair follicles, or elsewhere in the body.

Different people experience flare-ups caused by different triggers, which may include any of the following: alcoholic beverages, emotional stress, heat (including hot baths), menopause, spicy foods and drinks, strenuous exercise, sunlight, wind, very cold temperatures, and long-term use of topical steroids on the face.

Symptoms and Diagnostic Path

Rosacea develops slowly and usually gets worse unless treated. In most patients, the condition waxes and wanes repeatedly for no apparent reason. Earliest signs include a red face (especially on cheeks and nose) that may come and go. This redness is caused by enlarged blood vessels under the skin that looks like a blush or SUNBURN. Gradually, the redness becomes permanent and more noticeable; facial skin also becomes very dry. As the redness gets worse, pimples may appear. Thin red lines (called telangiectases), which are really enlarged blood vessels, may appear on the surface of the skin. In the most advanced stages (especially in men) the nose may become lumpy and swollen from excess tissue.

Rosacea is aggravated by sun, hot liquids, spicy foods, alcohol, vigorous exercise, heat, cold and wind, fluorinated steroids, menopause, endocrine disturbances, and emotional stress.

It can be diagnosed visually by a dermatologists.

Treatment Options and Outlook

There is no cure for rosacea, but treatment can control the condition and improve the skin's appearance. The treatment of choice for the diffuse redness and dilated blood vessels is laser surgery, which may improve the skin's appearance with very low risk.

Topical and oral medications can control redness and reduce papules and pustules; a combination of topical and oral forms of prescription drugs may be recommended. The most widely prescribed therapy for rosacea is topical metronidazole, which has been proven effective in clinical studies. Oral antibiotics such as TETRACYCLINE, minocycline, ERYTHROMYCIN, or doxycycline are also commonly used; they tend to produce better results and work more quickly than topical medications. Still, it usually takes several weeks for drugs to take effect, and they may have to be taken regularly to keep rosacea under control. Up to 80 percent of patients can expect significant improvement from oral or topical therapy, or a combination of both.

Prescription and nonprescription mild topical steroids are occasionally used on a short-term basis to help control redness; long-term use of topical steroids is not recommended.

Surgery may be used to correct the nose enlargement in RHINOPHYMA. A fine electric needle or a laser may also be used to eliminate enlarged blood vessels, and also decrease the overall redness, thus improving appearance.

In addition, a DERMATOLOGIST may recommend specific moisturizers, soaps, sunscreens, or other products as needed to improve the condition of the skin. Only very mild soaps or cleansers should be used; alcohol or irritating ingredients and excessive cleaning of the skin should be avoided. High-quality moisturizers should be applied only after the topical medication has dried. Sunscreens of SPF 15 or higher are often recommended when prolonged sun exposure is expected.

roseola infantum   A common infectious disease of early childhood also known as *exanthema subitum* (Latin for "sudden rash") that can affect youngsters aged six months to six years. The disease, is caused by the human herpes virus 6 and 7.

Symptoms and Diagnostic Path

The disease is characterized by the abrupt onset of irritability and a fever, which may climb as high as 105° F. By the fourth or fifth day, the fever breaks, suddenly returning to normal. At about the same time, a rash appears on the trunk, often spreading quickly to the face, neck, and limbs, fading within hours and disappearing within two days. Other symptoms may include sore throat, enlarged lymph nodes, and, occasionally, a febrile seizure.

Treatment Options and Outlook

There are no serious complications, and there is no specific treatment other than acetaminophen for the fever. A single attack appears to confer permanent immunity.

Rothmund-Thomson syndrome (RTS)   An extremely rare inherited multisystem disorder that is usually apparent during early infancy, typically characterized by distinctive abnormalities of the skin, defects of the hair, clouding of the lenses of the eyes, short stature and other skeletal abnormalities, malformations of the head and face, and other physical problems. In rare cases, mental retardation may be present. The range and severity of symptoms may vary from case to case. RTS is also known as POIKILODERMA congenita and poikiloderma atrophicans.

Symptoms and Diagnostic Path

During early infancy, individuals with Rothmund-Thomson syndrome develop abnormally red, inflamed patches on the skin accompanied by abnormal accumulations of fluid between layers of tissue under the skin. The patches typically first appear on the cheeks. In most cases, additional areas of the skin may then become involved to a lesser degree, such as the skin of the ears, forehead, chin, hands, forearms, lower legs.

Inflammation eventually tends to recede, and the skin of affected areas develops a condition known as poikiloderma, characterized by abnormal widening of groups of small blood vessels (telangiectasia); skin tissue degeneration; and patchy areas of abnormally decreased pigmentation (DEPIGMENTATION) and/or unusually increased pigmentation (HYPERPIGMENTATION). In many cases, additional skin abnormalities also may occur. Patients are usually short, with either baldness or abnormal hair growth. There is an early onset of cataracts and an abnormally low bridge of the nose ("saddle nose"). Teeth tend to be underdeveloped and the jaw protrudes.

There may be bone defects from birth and contractures of soft tissue involving the limbs. The bone defects may include abnormally small hands and feet, and underdevelopment or absence of the thumbs or bones in the forearm. Underactivity of the ovaries in females or testes in males can lead to irregular menstruation and delayed sexual development in boys and girls. There is a tendency to anemia and an increased risk of bone cancer.

Rothmund-Thomson syndrome is inherited genetically as an autosomal recessive trait. This means that both parents have one RTS gene but do not have the disease. Each of their children stands a 25 percent chance of not having either RTS gene, a 50 percent chance of having one RTS gene (and, as the parents, being normal) and a 25 percent risk of having both RTS genes and the disease. The RTS gene has been mapped and is found on chromosome 8.

The disease gets its name from Dr. August von Rothmund, a German ophthalmologist (1830–1906), who in 1868 reported having seen a familial disorder with cataracts, saddle nose, and skin atrophy in an isolated inbred Alpine village. Matthew S. Thomson was a British dermatologist (1894–1960) who in 1923 and 1936 described "A hitherto undescribed familial disease" and termed it *poikiloderma congenita*. Today, it is generally thought that Thomson's finding was the same disease that was seen in the Alps long before by Rothmund.

Treatment Options and Outlook

Patients should use broad-spectrum SUNSCREENS. TELANGIECTASES can be treated with pulsed-dye laser therapy. Keratolytics and RETINOIDS have been somewhat successful in treating the skin lesions.

Ophthalmology evaluation in early years for detection and management of cataracts is necessary, together with dental, orthopedic, endocrine, and hematology referrals for care depending on related symptoms.

The prognosis for survival, barring such complications as bone cancer, is fairly good.

royal jelly A substance secreted from the digestive system of worker bees that some people mistakenly believe improves skin condition. Royal jelly is fed to male bees and worker bees for a few days after they are born. Because the queen bee eats royal jelly throughout her life, royal jelly became associated with health and long life.

Studies have shown that royal jelly does not prevent aging in humans.

rubella See GERMAN MEASLES.

rubber sensitivity See ALLERGIES AND THE SKIN; LATEX ALLERGY.

rubeola Another name for MEASLES.

rubor Redness.

Rud's syndrome A rare congenital syndrome characterized by mild to fairly severe ICHTHYOSIS (rough, scaly skin), dark, warty growths (ACANTHOSIS NIGRICANS), excess sweating of palms and soles, epilepsy, hair loss, deformed teeth, mental retardation, seizures, and hypogonadism.

St. Anthony's fire The common name for ERY-SIPELAS, a potentially fatal streptococcal infection of the skin characterized by deep swellings on the face, with severe headache and blistering. Severe cases require hospitalization and intravenous antibiotics.

salicylic acid A drug used to treat a variety of skin disorders, including DERMATITIS, ECZEMA (topically), PSORIASIS, ICHTHYOSIS, ACNE, and WARTS. The drug is also sometimes used for fungal infections.

Salicylic acid pads or solutions can be very effective for the treatment of warts. It is important to avoid treating normal surrounding skin to prevent its irritation. This can be avoided by coating the rim of the wart with zinc oxide paste or PETROLEUM JELLY.

Side Effects

This drug may cause inflammation and even skin ulceration if used for a long period of time or if applied to a large area of skin. It is poisonous and should never be ingested.

salmon patch See STORK BITE NEVUS.

salve A healing, soothing (often medicated) ointment for the skin.

sarcoidosis A rare disease characterized by inflammation in the skin and other tissues throughout the body (especially the lungs) that occurs primarily in young adults. Often appearing abruptly, its incidence is highest among widely disparate ethnic groups—primarily African Americans, but also Scandinavians, Irish, and Puerto Ricans.

Despite decades of research, scientists still know very little about the disorder, and its cause remains unknown.

An unusual form of the disease, called Lofgren's disease, is characterized by a very rapid onset, with a HIVE-like skin rash and acute lung problems, enlarged lymph nodes and fever. This condition usually disappears as quickly as it came.

Symptoms and Diagnostic Path

The typical symptom of the disease is the sarcoidal granuloma. Its most common symptom involves lung disease, but in the acute form of the disease purplish swellings on the legs may occur with fever, generalized aches, and lymph node enlargement.

Chronic sarcoidosis may cause a variety of symptoms, including a purple facial rash, painful joints, bloodshot eyes, and numbness. However, about a third of affected people have no symptoms at all; in these people, X-rays reveal enlarged lymph nodes in the center of the chest.

Finally, about one patient in 20 will experience scarring and thickening of the lungs, abnormally high blood levels of calcium, and kidney damage.

Sarcoidosis initially may be confused with tuberculosis or a deep fungal infection. The condition is often diagnosed by first ruling out these other problems.

Treatment Options and Outlook

About 90 percent of patients recover completely within two years with or without treatment. However, the remainder develop a chronic form of the disease. Oral CORTICOSTEROID drugs (such as prednisone) may relieve ERYTHEMA NODOSUM, fever, and lung or eye problems. Steroids are given because their anti-inflammatory effects suppress the sarcoid granulomas often found in the disease. This treatment usually produces a rapid reduction of symptoms within weeks, although it still takes about a year for the disease to disappear. Hydroxychloroquine is sometimes prescribed to treat skin abnormalities.

For the very seriously ill patient with life-threatening complications, more potent anti-inflammatory drugs (such as the anticancer drug METHOTREXATE) may be administered.

In symptom-free patients, the disorder will fade away with or without treatment in about two years. In another third, the condition responds to drug therapy, but these patients may require treatment for many years.

sarcoma Cancer of the connective tissue, blood vessels, or the tissue surrounding and supporting organs. Examples of sarcoma include KAPOSI'S SARCOMA (mainly affecting the skin, and common in AIDS patients), and osteosarcoma and chondrosarcoma (both affecting bones).

Sarcoptes scabiei The mite responsible for the skin infestation of SCABIES.

scab A crust that forms on a healing superficial skin wound or infected area, composed of dried fibrin and serum leaked from the wound, along with pus, skin scales, and other skin debris. Another name for a scab associated with burns is ESCHAR.

scabicides Insecticides (such as LINDANE) designed to treat SCABIES by killing the mites that cause the infestation. These lotions usually kill the mites, but itching may continue for up to two weeks.

scabies A highly infectious skin infestation caused by the mite *SARCOPTES SCABIEI*, which burrows into the skin and lays its eggs. Mites are usually passed during close body contact.

The mite is transmitted by direct, prolonged, skin-to-skin contact with a person already infested with scabies. Contact must be prolonged (a quick handshake or hug is not enough). Infestation is easily spread to sexual partners and household members, and by sharing clothing, towels, and bedding. People with weakened immune systems and the elderly are at risk for a more severe form of scabies, called Norwegian or crusted scabies.

Deprived of the human body, mites do not survive more than 48–72 hours, but on a human an adult female mite can live up to a month.

Pet scabies Humans cannot become infested by catching the mites from pets, because animals have a different kind of scabies mite. If a pet is infested with scabies (also called mange), and they are in close contact with a human, the pet's mites may infest human skin and cause ITCHING and skin irritation. However, the mite will die in a few days and cannot reproduce. The mites may cause itching for several days, but the human does not need to be treated with special medication to kill the mites. However, until the pet is successfully treated, mites can continue to burrow into the skin and cause symptoms.

Symptoms and Diagnostic Path

A person who has never been infested with scabies may develop symptoms within four to six weeks. A person who has had scabies before may develop symptoms within several days. It is not possible to become immune to a scabies infestation. Symptoms include tiny red scaly PAPULES on the skin between the fingers, on wrists and genitals, and in armpits that cause intense itching (especially at night). Reddish lumps may appear later on arms, legs, and trunks.

The infestation can be diagnosed by a physician by visual inspection of the skin. In addition, a doctor may take a skin scraping to look for mites, eggs, or fecal matter. However, a false negative from a skin scraping is possible, because there are often fewer than 10 mites on the entire body of an infested person, which makes it easy for an infestation to be missed.

Treatment Options and Outlook

Insecticide lotion (such as LINDANE, gamma benzene hexachloride, or permethrin) should be applied to all skin, which kills the mites (although itching may continue for up to two weeks later). The insecticide is usually left on overnight for eight hours, and occasionally treatment is repeated the following night. Bedclothes and intimate apparel should be washed twice to prevent reinfection. All members of a family and close friends should be treated at the same time.

Itching may persist for two or three weeks after treatment, which does not mean that mites are still alive. Alternative medication can relieve severe itching. No new burrows or rashes should appear after one or two days of treatment.

scald A burn on the skin caused by steam or hot liquid.

scalded skin syndrome, staphylococcal (SSSS) A syndrome of acute exfoliation of the skin following a reddened skin infection (CELLULITIS) most common in children and neonates, and rare in adults. SSSS is caused by an exotoxin from a staphylococcal infection.

First recognized as a distinct condition in the mid-1800s, this disease has been incorrectly called by many different names, including Ritter's disease, toxic epidermal necrolysis, and PEMPHIGUS neonatorum. Only recently was its cause discovered to be a toxin-producing strain of *Staphylococcus aureus.*

Epidemics have occurred in contaminated nurseries, and the strain of bacteria may be transmitted by a carrier who has no symptoms. The condition has also been reported among adults, most of whom had poorly functioning immune systems.

Symptoms and Diagnostic Path

Symptoms usually begin with evidence of a primary staph infection, of the nose, throat, skin, or GI tract, including IMPETIGO, conjunctivitis, ear infection, or sore throat with fever, malaise, or irritability. The center of the face becomes tender, and the skin around the mouth becomes reddened, weeping, and crusting in a way that resembles potato-chip scales. The trunk may also become involved. In some patients, the rash stabilizes, while in other cases flaccid blisters begin to develop all over the skin within 24 to 48 hours. Large areas of skin slough off, and hair or nails may be lost.

Treatment Options and Outlook

Prompt administration of antibiotics and fluids are generally given in the hospital. Patients often appear very ill, with low fluid levels and risk of secondary infection. The skin is treated with wet dressings for crusted sites and antibiotic ointments such as bacitracin. Patients usually heal without scarring within a week.

The death rate in children is very low (between 1 and 5 percent) unless the child has a blood infection or a serious underlying medical condition. The death rate in adults is higher (between 20 to 30 percent).

scaling disorders of infancy It is completely normal for newborns to shed their skin, and it is particularly noticeable in babies who have gone beyond full term. However, excessive scaling may indicate one of the ichthyoses, a group of disorders featuring dry, rough, and scaly skin caused by a defect in KERATINIZATION (the process by which skin cells become horny as they move upward toward the outer layer of skin).

There are four major types of ICHTHYOSIS, three of which occur during the neonatal period: X-linked ichthyosis, lamellar ichthyosis (nonbullous congenital ichthyosiform erythroderma), and epidermolytic hyperkeratosis. The fourth type of scaling disorder, ichthyosis vulgaris, rarely develops before age three months and most commonly occurs in older children. In addition, COLLODION BABY and HARLEQUIN FETUS describes the skin condition of some of these affected infants.

Symptoms and Diagnostic Path

In *X-linked ichthyosis*, up to a third of the affected male infants are born scaly, and the rest begin to show the signs by three months of age. This condition is characterized by dirty brown scales that usually cover the entire body, except for the face, palms, and soles of the feet. Female carriers may have certain eye abnormalities, but they show no skin symptoms.

Babies with *lamellar ichthyosis* are born with red, scaly skin over their body, including the palms, soles, and flexible surfaces. As the baby ages, the redness fades and yellow-to-brown thick scales appear over the body, especially in areas of the body that are flexed. These infants may suffer with secondary infections due to the large areas of moist broken skin. The disorder is usually inherited in an autosomal recessive way, which means that a defective gene must be inherited in a double dose to cause the abnormality. Generally, both parents of an affected person are unaffected carriers of the defective gene. Each of their children has a one in four chance of being affected, and a two in four chance of being a carrier.

In *epidermolytic hyperkeratosis* (bullous congenital ichthyosiform erythroderma), affected infants develop crops of blisters over large areas of their body during the neonatal period. This causes dry, eroding, reddened skin, together with frequent secondary infection. Sepsis (blood poisoning) may follow, especially in young infants. In this condition, the scales are wartlike and flake off easily in great numbers. Palms of the hands and soles of the feet are usually unaffected.

Other scaling conditions found in infancy include atopic eczema, seborrheic dermatitis (see DERMATITIS, SEBORRHEIC), and PSORIASIS.

scar An area of fibrous tissue left behind on the skin after damaged tissue has healed. When tissue is damaged, the body repairs the wound by increasing production of the tough protein COLLAGEN at the wound site. The collagen helps construct new connective tissue to repair the defect. If the edges of the wound are brought together during healing (such as after the surgical excision), the scar is narrow and pale; if the edges remain wide apart (such as after a BURN), the scar is more extensive.

A KELOID is a large, irregular scar that grows beyond the site of initial surgery. This type of scar is most common among African Americans and Asians, and tends to run in families.

A HYPERTROPHIC SCAR is an overgrown scar that remains within the confines of the initial injury or cut. The tendency toward the development of hypertrophic scars may be inherited. Hypertrophic scars are usually pink and relatively firm.

There is not always a clear-cut difference between keloids and hypertrophic scars, since both are characterized by the same type of fibrous connective tissue. However, keloids tend to keep growing, whereas hypertrophic scars tend to reach a certain size, level off, and spontaneously regress.

Treatment Options and Outlook

Surgical excision of both types of scars is generally not very effective. They tend to recur and they can become larger and more unattractive than before the operation. Prolonged application of pressure by special appliances after surgical removal may prevent recurrence, but it is frequently impractical. Newer treatments, however, have improved the ability to deal with raised scars. Intralesional injections of CORTICOSTEROIDS, silicone gel dressings, or laser therapy are effective treatments for at least some scars.

Risk Factors and Preventive Measures

Because wounds that heal quickly and neatly are less likely to scar, all wounds should be cleaned and kept slightly moist during healing. Scabs should not be picked, which would increase the likelihood of scarring.

To minimize scarring without stitching, a butterfly bandage (available at most drugstores) can be applied. This helps keep the wound closed. Eating a balanced diet, especially rich in the mineral ZINC, also can help heal wounds quickly.

To help prevent keloids, earlobe piercing and excision of nevi and other lesions on keloid-prone areas should be done with caution in young people (especially those with dark skin). To help prevent hypertrophic scars, injury to the skin (especially in early adulthood) should be avoided.

scarlet fever An infectious bacterial childhood disease characterized by a skin rash, sore throat, and fever, that is much less common and dangerous than it used to be. No longer a reportable disease, experts do not know exactly how many cases occur today in the United States, although it is believed that the disease has been on the increase for the past several years. Once a very serious childhood disease, scarlet fever now is easily treatable.

Scarlet fever is caused by infection with *Group A streptococcus*. Scarlet fever strains of group A strep produce toxins that are released in the skin, causing a bright red rash the consistency of sandpaper.

In the past, the disease was associated with poor living conditions. In 1737, a scarlet fever epidemic in Boston killed 900 people; another epidemic in New York City in the late 1800s killed 35 percent of children who contracted the disease; that same year, 19 percent of Chicago children who got the disease perished.

Inexplicably, by the 1920s the death rate of the disease dropped to 5 percent for reasons that are still not completely understood. It is believed that the scarlet fever bacteria underwent a natural mutation that made it less virulent. The introduction of PENICILLIN reduced the death rate even more.

Today, most cases occur in middle-class suburbs, not in inner cities. Because it is possible to get a streptococcal infection and scarlet fever more than once, and because the incidence of all strep infections is rising, prompt medical attention when streptococcus infection is suspected is important. A child with a sore throat or skin rash should be brought in for medical evaluation. Anyone can develop scarlet fever, but most cases are found among children aged four to eight.

Scarlet fever bacteria are spread in droplets during coughing or breathing, or by sharing food and drink. When bacterial particles are released into the air, they can be picked up by others close by. For this reason, some experts advise children to avoid drinking fountains. The hallmark rash is caused by a toxin released by the bacteria.

Symptoms and Diagnostic Path

After an incubation period of two to four days, the first signs of illness is usually a fever of 103° to 104°F, accompanied by a severe sore throat. The face is flushed and the tongue develops a white coating with red spots, rather like a white strawberry. The patient may seem tired and flushed. Twelve to 18 hours after the fever, a rash appears as a mass of rapidly-spreading tiny red spots on the neck and upper trunk. The scarlet fever rash is unique in that it feels rough, like fine sandpaper, and is quite distinctive.

Other common symptoms include headache, chills, and vomiting, and tiny white lines around the mouth, as well as fine red striations in the creases of the elbows and groin. After a few days, the tongue coating peels off, followed by a drop in fever and a fading rash. Skin on the hands and feet often peel.

Treatment Options and Outlook

A 10-day course of antibiotics (usually penicillin or ERYTHROMYCIN), with rest, liquids, and acetaminophen is effective.

Children are contagious for a day or two after they begin treatment, but after that they can return to school. Alternatively a shot of long-acting penicillin that slowly releases the antibiotic over several weeks may be effective.

As with other types of sore throat caused by the streptococci bacteria, untreated infection carries the risk of rheumatic fever or glomerulonephritis (inflammation of the kidneys).

scarlatina Another name for SCARLET FEVER.

scarlatiniform Resembling SCARLATINA, the delicate red rash of SCARLET FEVER.

Schamberg's disease The common name for progressive pigmented PURPURA, one of several subtypes of PIGMENTED PURPURIC DERMATOSIS that share the symptom of rust-colored MACULES and PAPULES (especially on the lower legs). The red pigment changes are caused by the leaking of blood into tissues.

Symptoms and Diagnostic Path

In this subtype, there is no ITCHING; the small macular spots and brown pinhead-sized macules are found on the lower part of the leg. The red color and tiny size give these lesions their common name—CAYENNE PEPPER SPOT.

Treatment Options and Outlook

There is no really satisfactory treatment, but the condition is more of a cosmetic problem than a medical one, since internal organs are not involved and the lesions do not itch. Patients may find support stockings helpful. While systemic CORTICOSTEROIDS are usually effective, their risk is usually greater than any benefit that would accrue from their use. Topical CORTICOSTEROIDS (especially under wet dressings) may help.

schistosomiasis, visceral A parasitic disease (also called bilharziasis) that causes an itchy rash where flukes (flatworms) have penetrated the skin. The disease, found in most tropical countries, affects more than 200 million people around the world.

The disease is caused by one of three types of flukes (schistosomes) acquired from bathing in infested lakes and rivers in the Far East, West Indies, Africa, South and Central America, and the Middle East. The flukes penetrate the skin, where they develop within their host into adults. Their eggs provoke inflammatory reactions.

Symptoms and Diagnostic Path

While it also causes problems in other organs, the skin symptoms of this condition include DERMATITIS, HIVES, and skin lesions, due to the deposits of eggs in the skin. The relatively minor skin symptoms of this form of schistosomiasis is quite different than the marked skin inflammation in SWIMMER'S ITCH (the second form of schistosomiasis).

About one to two months after the penetration of the skin, hives again appear. Skin lesions caused by the egg deposits may appear in the genital and perineal (the region of the body between the anus and the urethral opening) areas.

Treatment Options and Outlook

The drug praziquantel has revolutionized the treatment of this form of schistosomiasis since the 1980s; one dose can kill the flukes and prevent further damage. Alternative drugs are oxamniquine and metriphonate.

Risk Factors and Preventive Measures

There is no vaccine to prevent the disease, and visitors to the tropics should assume that all lakes and rivers are unsafe for swimming.

scleroderma A general term for several chronic autoimmune conditions (also called systemic sclerosis) that involve the abnormal growth of connective tissue. In some forms of scleroderma, patients experience only hardened, tight skin, but in other forms, the problem goes much deeper, affecting blood vessels and the heart, lungs, and kidneys. Scleroderma is considered to be both a rheumatic and a connective tissue disease. Rheumatic diseases are characterized by inflammation and pain in the muscles, joints, or fibrous tissue. A connective tissue disease affects the major substances in the skin, tendons, and bones. It is twice as common in women, especially between the ages of 40 and 60.

Scleroderma's cause is unknown, but it is not infectious or transmittable. Studies of twins also suggest it is not inherited. Instead, scientists suspect that scleroderma may be the result of inflammatory activity, a type of noninherited genetic activity, environment, or hormones.

Abnormal immune or inflammatory activity Scientists believe scleroderma is an autoimmune disease, which occurs when a patient's own immune system for some reason attacks its own cells. The immune system of scleroderma patients may stimulate certain cells to produce too much COLLAGEN, which then forms thick connective tissue around the cells of the skin and internal organs. In milder forms, this buildup is limited to the skin and blood vessels, but in more serious forms it also interferes with normal function of skin, blood vessels, joints, and internal organs.

Genetic makeup While genes may put certain people at risk for scleroderma, the disease is not passed from parent to child as some genetic diseases are. However, some research suggests that having children may increase a woman's risk of scleroderma. When a woman is pregnant, cells from her baby can enter her bloodstream and remain in her body for many years. Recently, scientists have detected fetal cells from former pregnancies in the skin lesions of some women with scleroderma. Experts suspect that these fetal cells may either trigger an immune reaction to the woman's own tissues or set off a response by the woman's immune system to remove those cells. Either way, the woman's healthy tissues may be damaged in the process. Further studies are needed to find out if fetal cells play a role in the disease.

Environmental triggers Research suggests that exposure to some environmental factors such as viral infections, adhesive and coating materials, and organic solvents such as vinyl chloride or trichloroethylene may trigger the disease in people genetically predisposed to it.

Hormones By the end of the childbearing years (ages 30 to 55), women develop scleroderma at a rate seven to 12 times higher than men, which leads scientists to suspect that there must be something unique to women (such as the hormone estrogen) that is linked to the disease. However, the role of female hormones has not yet been proven.

Symptoms and Diagnostic Path

There are two basic groups of scleroderma diseases— localized and systemic. It is the localized type of scleroderma that primarily affects the skin and related tissues and, in some cases, the muscle below. Internal organs are not affected by localized scleroderma as they are in the systematic variety, and will never progress to the systemic form.

Localized scleroderma Often the skin lesions in localized scleroderma improve or go away on their own over time, although the skin damage that occurs when the disease is active can be permanent. However, for some people, localized scleroderma is serious and disabling. There are two generally recognized types of localized scleroderma—morphea and linear scleroderma (and some people have both types of localized scleroderma).

Morphea is characterized by reddish patches of skin that thicken into firm, oval-shaped areas, with a center of ivory with violet borders. These patches

sweat very little and have little hair growth. Patches appear most often on the chest, stomach, and back, although they also may appear on the face, arms, and legs.

Morphea can be either localized or generalized, but both types of morphea generally fade out in the three to five years, although people are often left with darkened skin patches and, in rare cases, muscle weakness. Localized morphea typically involves only one or a few reddish patches from about a half-inch to 12 inches in diameter. The condition sometimes appears on areas treated by radiation therapy. Generalized morphea spreads over the entire body with darker, harder patches.

Linear scleroderma is characterized by a single line or a band of thickened or abnormally colored skin that appears down an arm or leg, or down the forehead.

Systemic scleroderma This type of scleroderma affects the skin, but also penetrates into the tissues beneath, affecting the blood vessels and major organs. Systemic sclerosis is typically broken down into **diffuse** and **limited** disease. People with systemic sclerosis often have all or some of the symptoms that some doctors call CREST, which stands for Calcinosis, RAYNAUD'S PHENOMENON, Esophageal dysfunction, Sclerodactyly, and Telangiectasias.

The formation of calcium deposits in the connective tissues is called *calcinosis*, which can be detected by X-ray. These deposits are often found on the fingers, hands, face, and trunk and on the skin above elbows and knees; they can break through the skin, causing painful ulcers. Raynaud's phenomenon is a condition in which the small blood vessels of the hands and/or feet contract in response to cold or anxiety, so that hands or feet turn white and cold, and then blue. As blood flow returns, they become red. Fingertip tissues may suffer damage, leading to ulcers, scars, or gangrene. Esophageal dysfunction impairs the function of the esophagus so that swallowing is difficult, causing chronic heartburn or inflammation. Sclerodactyly results in thick, tight, shiny, darkened skin on the fingers because of excess collagen deposits within skin layers. The condition makes it difficult to bend or straighten the fingers. TELANGIECTASIAS are small dilated blood vessels on the hands and feet.

Limited scleroderma Limited scleroderma typically begins slowly, affecting the skin only on the fingers, hands, face, lower arms, and legs. Many people with limited disease have Raynaud's phenomenon for years before skin thickening starts, while others experience initial skin problems covering the body, which then slowly improves, leaving only the face and hands with tight, thickened skin. This is typically followed by the development of telangiectasias and calcinosis.

Diffuse scleroderma This type of scleroderma begins abruptly, as skin suddenly thickens and tightens over much of the body, symmetrically affecting the hands, face, upper arms, upper legs, chest, and stomach. Internally, the disease can damage the heart, lungs, and kidneys. People with diffuse disease often feel tired, lose appetite and weight, and have painful joint swelling.

After the first three to five years, the disease often stabilizes, and skin thickness and appearance remain about the same, while little internal damage occurs and symptoms subside. Gradually, the skin starts to change again, so that the last areas to thicken become the first to begin softening. Some patients' skin returns to almost normal, while others have thin, fragile skin and neither hair nor sweat glands. More serious damage to heart, lungs, or kidneys is unlikely to occur.

People with diffuse scleroderma face a serious long-term outlook if they develop severe kidney, lung, digestive, or heart problems, but less than a third of patients with diffuse disease develop these problems.

Treatment Options and Outlook

There is no effective treatment. Symptoms may be controlled with antihypertensives, physical therapy, dialysis, and CORTICOSTEROID drugs.

scorpion stings The sting of most species of scorpion cause pain similar to a bee sting, but the more toxic varieties can cause sweating, restlessness, diarrhea, and vomiting—and can be fatal to children.

Symptoms and Diagnostic Path

Symptoms that appear within two to four hours after a toxic scorpion sting indicate a serious medical problems. A scorpion sting produces severe pain and swelling at the site of the sting; a nontoxic scorpion sting will swell and become discolored, forming a BLISTER. These symptoms may last for eight to 12 hours. If the sting was from *C. exilicauda*, the sting will be followed by a PINS AND NEEDLES SENSATION at the sting site. The area of the sting would not get swollen or discolored, but within one to three hours may trigger itching eyes, nose, and throat; tightness of the jaw muscles, speech problems, extreme restlessness, numbness, frothing at the mouth, nausea and vomiting, incontinence, drowsiness, muscle twitching and painful spasms, irregular heartbeat, breathing problems (including respiratory paralysis), and sometimes convulsions. Death is rare because toxicity is dose related, but the smaller the victim, the higher the risk of a fatal sting.

Treatment Options and Outlook

Medical attention is usually necessary only for infants and the elderly, or if the person is having trouble breathing. An antivenin is available for severe reactions. Local anesthetics and powerful painkillers may be administered.

Fatalities have occurred as long as four days after a sting, but it is not true that *any* scorpion will be fatal. In fact, only one out of a thousand stings is fatal.

Risk Factors and Preventive Measures

Scorpions would not run after a human and attack, but they will sting if they are picked up or stepped on. They prefer moist, dark places and often hide in clothing or shoes. Residents in endemic areas should always shake out all shoes, bedding, and clothing before using and should modify the area surrounding a house, moving trash, logs, boards, stones, bricks, and any other objects, mowing the grass, and pruning overhanging bushes and tree branches. Garbage cans should be stored off the ground, and firewood should never be brought inside the house unless it is placed immediately onto a fire. Homeowners also should add weatherstripping inside and out around doors, baseboards, and windows, and plug any holes in the walls with steel wool, pieces of nylon scouring pad, or small squares of screen.

scratch A skin mark caused by the stroking of the skin with fingernails or a sharp instrument.

scrofuloderma See TUBERCULOSIS SKIN.

scurvy A disease caused by inadequate intake of VITAMIN C that results in skin hemorrhages, causing widespread bruising. It is rare today in developed countries because of widespread consumption of fresh fruit and vegetables; body stores of the vitamin can protect against scurvy for about three months. However, it is still seen in developed countries among the elderly who have poor diets. It has primarily been associated with sailors, who used to suffer from scurvy because of a lack of fresh fruit during long sea voyages.

The body's normal production of COLLAGEN is disrupted by inadequate supplies of VITAMIN C; as the collagen production becomes unstable, it weakens small blood vessels and slows wound healing. Hemorrhages and widespread bruising occur, together with bleeding gums and loosening of teeth. Pain results from bleeding into muscles and joints. Follicular purpura of the skin is classical.

The disease is especially serious in children, since bleeding into the membranes around the long bones may interfere with growth. Fatal hemorrhages in and around the brain may also occur.

Treatment Options and Outlook
Large doses of vitamin C will stop bleeding within 24 hours, quickly easing bone and muscle pain.

Risk Factors and Preventive Measures
The body can obtain enough vitamin C through modest consumption of fruit (especially citrus fruit) and vegetables; other sources of vitamin C include milk, liver, kidneys, and fish.

sea bather's eruption A rash of red bumps that appear on the skin creases covered by a bathing suit after swimming in salt water. The symptoms usually become noticeable within several hours of swimming, and last for several days before clearing up.

Sea bather's eruption was first described in 1949 as an itchy rash occurring in bathers off the eastern coast of Florida.

Sea bather's eruption is a hypersensitivity skin reaction to the larval form of the thimble jellyfish, *L. unguiculata*. The rash typically occurs underneath a bathing suit, which is believed to trap the jellyfish larvae against the skin. It remains uncertain whether the discharge of venom by the trapped larvae may play an important role in the appearance of the rash.

Factors that promote the discharge of venom by the larvae include wearing bathing suits for long periods after swimming, exposure to freshwater through showering, and mechanical stimulation.

Due to seasonal variation in the concentrations of thimble jellyfish larvae in endemic areas, there is an increased incidence of sea bather's eruption during May through August, with a peak in May/June. This coincides with the warm Gulf streams running along the Atlantic coastline of Florida and the corresponding spawn of thimble jellyfish larvae, which results in the high seasonal concentration of the jellyfish. The occurrence of sea bather's eruption in Palm Beach saltwater swimmers in May has been estimated to be 16 percent.

Similar rashes have been reportedly linked to the larvae of the sea anemone *Edwardstella lineata* in an outbreak of sea bather's eruption on Long Island. Various types of larvae in other waters likely can produce similar rashes.

Symptoms and Diagnostic Path
Apparently, some people are more susceptible to the condition than others, since in any group of swimmers only certain people will experience sea bather's eruption. Relatively rare signs and symptoms of sea bather's eruption include nausea, headache, sore throat, cough, diarrhea, and abdominal pain.

Children more commonly demonstrate body-wide symptoms, including fever, nausea, abdominal pain, and diarrhea. These symptoms may be mistaken for viral gastritis.

Diagnosis of sea bather's eruption is made based on history of exposure and physical examination.

Laboratory studies and skin biopsy are unnecessary.

Treatment Options and Outlook

Patients with sea bather's eruption require only symptomatic or supportive therapy. High-potency topical steroids in combination with oral ANTIHISTAMINES are typically used to treat the rash. Systemic CORTICOSTEROIDS should be reserved for patients with severe rash or pronounced associated systemic symptoms.

Alternative remedies made with vinegar, rubbing alcohol, sodium bicarbonate, sugar, urine, olive oil, and meat tenderizer may help.

Risk Factors and Preventive Measures

Studies suggest that the risk of developing sea bather's eruption in patients exposed to high seasonal concentrations of larvae while swimming in salt water can be reduced if bathers shower with the bathing suit off, regardless of length of time in the water or timing of showers.

sea urchins   The spines of sea urchins can break off in or underneath the skin, causing an immediate burning, swelling or ITCHING, and redness or a delayed reaction featuring a flesh-colored nodule appearing several months after being stung.

Treatment Options and Outlook

For an immediate reaction, the wound should be placed in extremely hot water for at least a half hour to relieve pain; spines must be surgically removed in an emergency room to eliminate the risk of infection.

Even so, some spines will remain lodged and will take several months to be ejected by the body's defenses.

seaweed   A plant whose gelatin-like substance is used as the main ingredient in peel-off masks. Seaweed is also used in face creams and lotions to help provide body to the products.

seaweed dermatitis   See DERMATITIS, SEAWEED.

sebaceous cyst   A nonspecific term for a harmless large, smooth nodule under the skin, usually found on the face, ear, scalp, trunk, or genitals (a CYST on the scalp is called a wen). These cysts may grow very large and may become red and inflamed either spontaneously or after trauma. The inflammation is usually the result of disruption of the cyst wall, causing the contents (usually a mixture of KERATIN) to leak out. These cysts are often wrongly thought to be infected because of their appearance, and antibiotics are incorrectly administered.

Treatment Options and Outlook

Incision and drainage is recommended. Large or bothersome cysts should be removed surgically under local anesthetic; if the entire cyst wall is removed, recurrence is rare. Inflamed cysts should not be excised until the inflammation has subsided.

sebaceous glands   Tiny glands that secrete a lubricating substance called SEBUM either into hair follicles or directly onto the skin's surface. Most of these glands are located on the scalp, face, and around the anus; none are found on the hands or soles of the feet. The production of sebum is partly controlled by male sex hormones. Problems with

Cross Section of Skin Revealing Sebaceous Gland

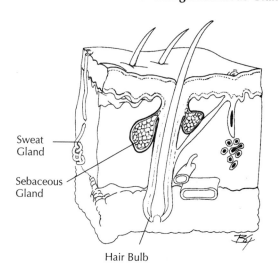

Sweat Gland

Sebaceous Gland

Hair Bulb

the sebaceous glands may lead to excessively oily skin (SEBORRHEA), ACNE, RHINOPHYMA, or sebaceous hyperplasia.

seborrhea Excess SEBUM secretion, causing increased facial oiliness and a greasy scalp. While the exact cause of this excess production is not understood, male sex hormones (androgen hormones) do play a role in the problem. Not surprisingly, therefore, the problem is most common in adolescent boys and men.

Symptoms and Diagnostic Path
Symptoms include excessive oiliness of the skin, especially of the scalp and face, without redness or scaling. Patients with seborrhea may later develop seborrheic dermatitis, which is characterized by both redness and scaling.

Treatment Options and Outlook
Seborrhea usually disappears by adulthood without treatment, but people with seborrhea are also more likely to have other skin problems such as ACNE vulgaris and seborrheic DERMATITIS. Seborrhea is very difficult to treat. Washing the face frequently and the use of acne products reduce skin oiliness only temporarily. The only medication known to reduce sebaceous gland activity is ISOTRETINOIN (Accutane), which reduces the size of the glands during treatment and for several months afterwards. The side effects of Accutane usually preclude its use for seborrhea.

seborrheic dermatitis See DERMATITIS, SEBORRHEIC.

seborrheic keratoses See KERATOSES, SEBORRHEIC.

sebum An oily substance produced by the SEBACEOUS GLANDS in the skin. Composed of fat and wax, sebum lubricates the skin and protects it from becoming soggy when wet, or cracked when exposed to hot, dry temperatures. Sebum also helps protect the skin from bacteria and fungi. Oversecretion of sebum causes SEBORRHEA (oily skin and scalp) and may lead to seborrheic DERMATITIS or ACNE.

sebum-suppressive agents The only medication known to suppress SEBUM production is ISOTRETINOIN (Accutane), which works by suppressing the sebaceous glands. Topical agents may be used to defat the skin, but sebum activity is *not* affected and within minutes, the skin's oiliness returns.

self-tanning products A cosmetic product designed to produce an "artificial" tan without requiring exposure of the skin to the sun. The main ingredient in most topical products is DIHYDROXYACETONE (DHA), a chemical that acts only on the skin's superficial cell layers. When the DHA combines with certain amino acids and KERATIN in the skin's outer layer, it produces a natural golden color. However, as the skin sheds its dead cells, the tan fades—usually within a few days of application.

Some self-tanning products also include a SUNSCREEN up to 15 SPF; others contain no sunscreens at all. Topical self-tanning products should be applied at least several hours before going out in the sun, and preferably the night before. Sunscreen should then be applied at least an hour before going outside.

For best results, users should exfoliate before application because the DHA may be absorbed unevenly in areas where there is a thick layer of dead cells—especially hands, elbows, and knees. The depth of color is determined by how often the product is reapplied, not by how much is applied at one time. It can take between three to five hours for a self-tanner to develop fully.

Most self-tanning formulations have a short shelf-life once opened because DHA degrades quickly, and should be used up within three months of opening.

Tanning pills are another self-tanning product, but these drugs are available only outside the United States and are not recommended by DERMATOLOGISTS. There are two types; one type of drugs contain canthaxidine, a chemical that colors the skin but can damage the eyes and liver.

The second contains PSORALEN, also available as a psoralen-containing cream. Neither is available in the United States, and both are considered dangerous by dermatologists because of the potential for severe SUNBURNS.

Several self-tanning synthetic hormones that color the skin and also seem to protect against sun damage are currently under investigation.

Senear-Usher syndrome   The common name for the blistering disease PEMPHIGUS erythematosus.

Symptoms and Diagnostic Path

Symptoms are usually limited to the face, where it appears as a butterfly rash over the nose and cheeks. Its severe scales and crusts may also appear on the scalp and the upper areas of the chest and back.

Treatment Options and Outlook

Topical medications including cleansing baths using BUROW'S SOLUTION or silver sulfadiazine cream, and application of topical CORTICOSTEROIDS may ease symptoms. Systemic corticosteroids are the primary method of treatment, beginning with doses high enough to completely stop the formation of new BLISTERS. Immunosuppressive therapy together with corticosteroids improves control of the disease.

Most patients on long-term systemic corticosteroids develop side effects, such as high blood pressure, weight gain, infection, potassium loss, gastrointestinal bleeding, osteoporosis, and cataracts.

senile keratoses   See KERATOSES, SENILE.

sensitive skin   Some people appear to have skin that is extraordinarily sensitive, easily ITCHING, burning, chafing, stinging. This type of skin is also called problem-sensitive skin. Individuals with sensitive skin often develop difficulties while using cosmetics. While popular myth holds that fair or thin-skinned women have the most sensitive skin, in fact any type of skin in men or women can be highly reactive to a variety of irritants.

Some of the most common irritants are cold air, dry air, water, and ultraviolet light. Other non-environmental irritants that can induce contact dermatitis include primary and secondary irritants. Primary irritants can cause the skin to react the very first time they contact the EPIDERMIS. (This group includes strong acids or alkalies that burn the skin.) Secondary irritants are milder, and produce an irritation only after the skin has become sensitized to the substance over time. For example, these could include soaps, detergents, moisturizers, SUNSCREENS, and so on.

"Hypoallergenic" cosmetics and products are designed for the consumer with sensitive skin. This may indicate that a product has no added fragrance or that the manufacturer has avoided certain compounds known to be irritating. Unfortunately, when a person has become sensitive to a range of ingredients, it can become harder and harder to find products that do not trigger an allergic response. This group of patients is not necessarily allergic to agents, but they may more easily develop irritant reactions.

See also DERMATITIS, IRRITANT; DERMATITIS, CONTACT; DERMATITIS, ALLERGIC.

serum sickness   A brief illness featuring a skin rash that develops about 10 days after an injection with an antiserum derived from animals (such as anti-rabies serum obtained from horses). Antisera can be obtained from either human or animal blood that contains specific antibodies (substances that play a role in immunity), and may be given to protect against dangerous infections.

When an antiserum is prepared from animal blood, a protein in the serum may be identified by the body's immune system as a potentially harmful foreign substance (called an antigen). In serum sickness, the person's immune system produces antibodies that combine with the antigen to form particles called immune complexes. They are deposited in various tissues, stimulating more immune reactions and leading to inflammation and other symptoms. Serum sickness is different from anaphylactic shock, another type of hypersensitivity reaction in response to antiserums.

Anyone who has ever had serum sickness should remember the injection to which they are sensitive and warn medical personnel against its future use.

Symptoms and Diagnostic Path

About a week after exposure to the antiserum, an itchy rash may appear, followed by enlarged lymph nodes, painful joints, and fever. In severe cases, a state similar to shock develops. Symptoms usually fade within a few days.

Treatment Options and Outlook

Soothing lotions may help with the itching; nonsteroidal anti-inflammatory drugs may relieve joint pain and an antihistamine may curtail the illness period. In severe cases, systemic CORTICOSTEROIDS may be prescribed.

Sezary syndrome   A rare T-cell lymphoma causing total body redness (with scaling), because of an abnormal overgrowth of lymphoid cells in the skin, liver, spleen, and lymph nodes. Sezary syndrome primarily affects middle-aged and elderly patients.

Symptoms and Diagnostic Path

The patchy redness appears first, followed by hair loss, thickening of the palms and soles, and distorted nail growth. Malignant T-cells also accumulate in the bloodstream.

Treatment Options and Outlook

Treatments include topical and systemic anticancer drugs, electron beam radiation, and PUVA therapy. Low doses of METHOTREXATE also has been reported to help a group of patients, and does not cause secondary leukemia. Also beneficial may be photopheresis—giving the PSORALEN methoxsalen followed by irradiation of the blood with UVA.

shagreen patch   A sign of TUBEROUS SCLEROSIS that involves large area of protruding skin on the lower back.

shake lotion   A suspension of powder in a liquid, such as water or oil.

shampoo   Liquid hair cleaner designed to wash away dirt and oil. All shampoos clean hair by removing oil (produced from the oil glands in the scalp) and debris the oil attracts to the hair shaft. Inexpensive shampoos may be about 90 percent water with added detergent cleansing agents—usually either SODIUM LAURETH SULPHATE, SODIUM LAURYL SULFATE, ammonium laureth sulfate, and ammonium lauryl sulfate. More expensive products vary from 30 to 50 percent solids. Other shampoo ingredients include slip agents or oils such as dimethicone, lecithin, cyclomethicone, and mineral oil, with thickeners and ingredients to add lubrication and texture, such as stearyl alcohol, cetyl alcohol, or protein; detangling agents such as tricetylmonium chloride, benzalkonium chloride, or quaternium 1 through 80; foaming agents (linoleic DEA or cocamide DEA); preservatives, coloring agents, and/or fragrances. Many manufacturers add other ingredients, including aloe vera, amino acids, COLLAGEN, vitamins, herb or fruit extracts, and a variety of unusual oils.

The formulation of shampoos for various types of hair is very complex; even the addition of .1 percent of an active ingredient can change the formula. Therefore, it is difficult to judge any product's performance based on the label ingredients alone, since performance is determined by the *concentration* of ingredients and how they function when mixed with other ingredients. Even expert cosmetic chemists cannot judge the performance of a product based on reading label ingredients alone.

Some manufacturers have begun to add SUNSCREENS in shampoo, but they are not given an SPF rating, because rating is based on the ability of a sunscreen to allow greater sun exposure to an individual without producing a sunburn. Since a sunburn is evaluated by skin redness, the test is impossible to do on hair. Instead, manufacturers have proposed establishing measures of "hair protective factors" as a way of measuring a product's ability to protect hair. Hair is very susceptible to damage from ultraviolet light, especially if it has been colored or permed. Sunscreen for hair is most effective when included in conditioners or finishing sprays.

How to Use

Shampoo should be applied to the scalp, especially if the user has long or chemically treated hair. Hair near the scalp will be oilier, and looks flat and sticky with oil buildup; hair at the ends does not get nearly the lubrication. Those with seriously damaged or dry hair should never apply shampoo to the ends of the hair shaft; enough shampoo will reach this area as the hair is rinsed.

Shampoo *must* be thoroughly rinsed out of the hair, or it will make the shafts look dull and flaky with residue.

Anyone with coarse, permed, color-treated, or damaged hair should not use a combination shampoo and conditioner. A shampoo and conditioner's uses are actually opposite; the shampoo is designed to clean oil off the hair, while the conditioner coats the hair.

Those with oily hair should not use conditioner unless the hair is colored or permed, since conditioners add lubricants and coatings to the hair, which is already struggling with excess oil.

For those with chemically treated hair, conditioners designed for oily hair (these products use little or no oils and lighter weight lubricants) should be applied only to the ends of the hair, avoiding the scalp.

After washing, hair should not be scrubbed dry with a rough towel; it should be dried gently by a blotting or gentle squeezing motion. Rough treatment on wet hair can damage the cuticle.

shaving and the skin Daily shaving exfoliates the skin. The best way to get a nondamaging shave is to first soften the hair with warm water; hot water can inflame the skin. Shaving soap or cream helps hold moisture, softening and lifting the hairs. Gel and cream-containing moisturizing shaving creams help individuals with dry or easily irritated skin.

Shaving creams that contain OIL OF BERGAMOT (found in some lime scents), should be avoided because they can cause a photosensitivity reaction in the sun.

Blades should be changed after three to six shaves. A light touch with smooth, even, long strokes along the grain produces the closest, least-irritating shave. In the case of nicks, a styptic pencil (aluminum chloride) can help.

After shaving, cool water or a mild after-shave lotion should be used to tighten pores and smooth skin. Talcum powder after shaving does not really provide much benefit, but applying a mild moisturizer after shaving may be helpful.

shingles A viral infection caused by the VARICELLA-ZOSTER VIRUS, a virus of the herpes family that causes a painful, red blistering of the nerves that supply certain areas of the skin. The problem begins during a CHICKEN POX attack (usually in childhood); after the spots fade, the virus lies dormant in sensory nerves for many years. For reasons that aren't entirely clear, the virus may reemerge and cause an episode of shingles. This is found most often in those over age 50.

Although rarely fatal, shingles has been the scourge of the elderly and the immunocompromised because it causes such terrible pain; each year, the condition affects 500,000 people each year in the United States about one in 544. Researchers believe that current population trends will bring more cases of shingles as the numbers of elderly and those with failing immune systems increases.

Symptoms and Diagnostic Path

The first sign of shingles is an excessive sensitivity in an area of skin, followed by pain. After about five days a rash appears, turning first into tense BLISTERS, and then yellow lesions within three more days. The blisters then dry out and crust over, gradually dropping off, leaving small pitted scars behind. Because the nerves have been damaged after the shingles attack, once the blisters heal the nerves constantly produce strong pain impulses that may last for months or years. The older the patient and more severe the rash, the more likely the pain (called POST-HERPETIC NEURALGIA) will persist.

Shingles often affects a belt of skin over the ribs on one side, which is where herpes zoster gets its name (*zoster* is the Greek word for belt). Sometimes the disease affects the lower part of the body or the upper half of the face on one side. The common name for the disease—shingles—comes from the Latin word for belt—*cingulus*.

Treatment Options and Outlook

Prompt use of antiviral drugs—such as ACYCLOVIR (Zovirax), famciclovir (Famvir), and valacyclovir (Valtrex) can shorten the rash and lessen the chance of pain later. These drugs are most effective if used within 72 hours after the rash appears; patients should seek medical help at the first sign of shingles. Both drugs slow reproduction of the virus and shorten the course of the infection. There is some evidence that the drugs may also decrease the chances for nerve pain following an attack.

Doctors often prescribe various pain medications for people with shingles. Because the pain of shingles can be so intense, some researchers have looked for other ways to block the pain.

When the herpes zoster virus inflames nerves, they pump out a chemical messenger called glutamate. Glutamate then travels to receptors on nearby cells, which transmit pain signals to the brain. Shingles triggers such a flood of glutamate that some cells stop functioning, while others become hypersensitive. This probably explains why shingles patients can feel great pain even when skin is touched only lightly.

There are drugs that can block the receptor sites where glutamate lands, and researchers are studying whether these drugs will help relieve shingles pain. In 1999, the U.S. Food and Drug Administration approved a patch form of the anesthetic lidocaine. The patch, called Lidoderm, provides pain relief for some people with shingles. Because Lidoderm is applied to the skin, it has less risk of side affects than pain medications taken in pill form.

A cold, wet compress applied to the blisters and avoiding direct heat on the lesions may help. The medication Zostrix (active ingredient: CAPSAICIN, a red pepper derivative) may help relieve the postherpetic neuralgia, once all the blisters have disappeared. Experts believe the capsaicin blocks the production of a chemical necessary for pain impulse transmission between nerve cells. It should not be applied to active shingles blisters; as a counterirritant, Zostrix is designed to be used on unbroken, healed skin that hurts, not for open, oozing infections.

For severe pain from shingles, some experts recommend injecting a sympathetic nerve block in the appropriate place to block the nerves supplying the area of pain. This block typically relieves pain in up to 80 percent of patients. In some cases, it can permanently end shingles pain. Prompt intervention by a pain specialist can sometimes head off post-herpetic neuralgia.

Risk Factors and Preventive Measures

Recent studies have found that a stronger version of the chicken pox vaccine was able to cut the incidence of shingles in half. In April 2005 the U.S. Food and Drug Administration received a license application from the manufacturer for the zoster vaccine. If approved for use, the vaccine has the potential to prevent hundreds of thousands of cases of shingles in the United States each year. It works by boosting the type of immunity necessary to hold the virus in check.

shock, electrical See ELECTRICAL BURN; ELECTRICAL INJURY.

sickle-cell ulcers Skin symptoms occur in about half of patients with sickle-cell anemia, a hereditary disease that affects African Americans characterized by the production of an abnormal type of hemoglobin. The skin ulcers associated with this condition usually appear between ages 10 and 20 and appear on the lower legs, with recurrent attacks of fever and pain in the anus, legs, and abdomen. They are caused by partial obstruction in the blood vessels and decreased oxygen in certain areas caused by abnormal hemoglobin.

Symptoms and Diagnostic Path

The sickle-cell lesions look like well-defined punched-out skin defects that are painful and heal slowly; they may be complicated by infection.

Treatment Options and Outlook

Affected limbs should be elevated and immobilized. The ulcers should be cleaned with antibacterial solutions; the wounds also should be debrided in order to promote healing. Blood transfusions may be necessary.

silica A mineral included in face and body powders and paste-type masks. Silica is soothing and forms a moisture-retaining film on the skin.

silicone implant A synthetic implant once widely used in cosmetic surgery because it was resistant to body fluids, permeable to oxygen, and not rejected by the body. The implants have been used in breast reconstruction or breast enlargement for several million American women. Medical-grade silicone is included in more than 500 products, including a range of over-the-counter medications, and in hair spray, processed foods, skin creams, and cosmetics.

History

Silicone gel-filled breast implants have been available since 1963 and were originally made out of a thick, smooth envelope of silicone rubber filled with a silicone gel. In the early 1980s, the shell was reformulated to minimize the amount of certain types of silicone that "bled" through the envelope.

Among the more than 2 million women who have had breast implants containing a soft polymer called polydimethylsiloxane (PDMS), reported illnesses from reactions to the implants include autoimmune disorders such as LUPUS ERYTHEMATOSUS, rheumatoid arthritis, and chronic fatigue. In some cases, silicone invaded the surrounding tissue or implant capsule.

In 1992, based on complaints that the implants ruptured or caused systemic disease, the U.S. Food and Drug Administration (FDA) called for a voluntary moratorium on the use and distribution of silicone gel-filled breast implants. This call followed a 1991 advisory panel ruling that found "no evidence that these implants are unsafe" but noted that "there is also insufficient evidence to prove safety."

Today, while the FDA has not formally approved silicone gel-filled breast implants, they have allowed their continued use under certain guidelines. The FDA also concluded that the implants were of significant benefit for reconstructive patients, and ruled that the implants should be available to those who want them. However, only a small number of women who want the gel-filled implants for cosmetic augmentation are allowed to have them; these women must be part of a research study and their names must be recorded in a registry. The FDA also requires manufacturers to conduct more studies to prove the device's safety and effectiveness.

Women who have an "urgent need" for an implant have immediate access to the device; these include women who have expanders, whose implants have ruptured, or who are facing mastectomy and who want reconstruction with silicone.

However, critics continue to insist that silicone often leaks from the gel-filled devices, causing cancer and neurological diseases despite a lack of supporting scientific data. As a result, more than 90 percent of the U.S. market now uses saline-filled implants, although silicone implants have remained available for women who have undergone mastectomies.

In July 2005 silicone gel-filled breast implants moved a step closer to being reintroduced to the general U.S. market after the FDA issued an "approvable with conditions" letter to one manufacturer (Mentor Corp.) for its implants. However, this letter does not mean that the device is approved for marketing in the United States at this time. Federal law prohibit the government from discussing the letter's specific contents, but an approvable letter is one of several intermediate steps in the FDA's review process for new products.

Procedure

Surgical insertion of the device can be performed under local or general anesthesia, and is usually an outpatient procedure. It can be placed either directly beneath the breast tissue or under the muscles. For reconstructive surgery after mastectomy, the existing surgical incision is usually used, and the implant can be placed at the time of mastectomy or at a later date.

Side Effects

There have been a variety of different problems that women have experienced, which has led the FDA to crack down on silicone implants.

Hardening of the implant The most common side effect is called "capsular contraction." Normally a surgical pocket is created for the implant that is larger than the device itself. A membrane called a capsule forms around the implant, and under the best circumstances, it maintains its original dimensions, allowing the implant to rest inside it. However, for reasons that seem to be related to a person's individual characteristics, the scar capsule shrinks in some women and squeezes the implant, causing the implant to become hard. These levels of contracture are measured on a scale of one to four (one so soft as to be undetectable, and four to be as hard as a grapefruit). The contraction may occur right after surgery, or only many years later, in one or both breasts. Some researchers believe that a low-grade bacterial contamination may trigger this process.

This hardening is not hazardous to the health, but it can interfere with the cosmetic result and cause discomfort or pain. If it becomes troublesome, a physician may recommend surgically scoring the tight capsule of scar tissue or surgically removing it. However, hardening can recur.

For some women who have developed hardened implants, a "closed capsulotomy" can provide dramatic immediate relief. In this procedure, a forceful squeeze of the breast can tear the scar capsule, allowing additional space for the implant and restoring softness. This simple procedure causes very little pain and—when it works—the relief is immediate, eliminating the necessity for surgery.

However, in some women excessive force is required to tear the capsule, which can be painful and sometimes ruptures the implant. The FDA states that a closed capsulotomy should not be performed, although some physicians feel the procedure is appropriate for some patients. If the implant does break, a closed capsulotomy can push the loose gel into nearby tissues.

Rupture Sometimes the implants break on their own. This could happen in the wake of a car accident or normal breast movement and compression. This type of "silent rupture" may be detected on a mammography or by physical examination, although neither method is 100 percent successful. If this should happen, the free gel will usually be kept within the scar-tissue capsule around the implant.

A rupture should be suspected if the breast changes in appearance or texture. Rarely, an accident can tear the scar envelope itself, and push the gel into subcutaneous areas such as the chest wall, down into the abdomen, the arm, or the breast tissue.

Within two to six weeks, gel that has escaped is surrounded by new scar tissue and can form granulomas, which can either mask or mimic a tumor. This is one reason why direct injection of silicone into the breast is not recommended.

Cancer An FDA advisory panel in 1991 concluded that the potential risk from cancer from polyurethane-coated implants is probably less than one in 1 million. Studies of women who have had implants for 10 or 20 years have found no higher incidence of breast cancer in this group than in those women without implants.

Other experts are concerned that the implants may block the detection of breast tumors via mammography. The American College of Radiology, the American Cancer Society, and the American Society of Plastic and Reconstructive Surgeons agree that a woman with breast implants should have routine mammography at the same rate as a woman without implants but that she should be referred to mammographic facilities accredited by the American College of Radiology who are familiar with the special "Eklund" views required for adequate evaluation of the breast. If possible, these women should return to the same place for all future mammograms. This type of mammography is more expensive, since a minimum of four X-rays is required to adequately evaluate the breast; thus, the amount of radiation is also higher.

Rheumatic disorders Some experts have speculated that there may be an association between silicone and autoimmune or rheumatic disorders, especially SCLERODERMA and LUPUS ERYTHEMATOSUS. Since scleroderma, lupus, and similar diseases are not commonly found in the population, it is difficult to research and compare the link between them and implants.

Silvadene   See SILVER SULFADIAZINE.

silver nitrate   A salt of silver that is applied in creams or solutions to destroy WARTS and treat wounds and BURNS. It is also used in eyedrops to prevent a serious form of conjunctivitis in all newborns.

Side Effects

Silver nitrate may cause irritation or pain and if used for a long time, it may cause permanent blue-black skin discoloration. It is extremely poisonous when ingested.

silver sulfadiazine   An antibacterial cream used to prevent infections in skin grafts or second- and third-degree burns. It is especially helpful in keeping burn sites sterile, thereby reducing the chance of secondary infection.

Side Effects

Possible side effects include allergic reactions (with RASH, ITCHING, or burning). Although rare, long-term use may produce serious blood disorders or kidney damage. It is not recommended for patients who are sensitive to sulfonamide drugs, nor should it be used for newborns or premature infants.

skin   The outermost covering of body tissue that weighs twice as much as the brain—about six to nine pounds, stretching over 18 square feet. It is also a sensory organ, and contains many cells sensitive to touch, temperature, pain, pressure, and itching. The skin protects the internal organs and keeps the body at the correct temperature—not too warm and not too cold.

When the body is hot, the SWEAT GLANDS in the skin perspire, cooling the body, and helping the blood vessels in the dermis to dilate, dissipating the heat. If the body gets cold, the blood vessels in the skin constrict, conserving the body's heat. The skin also takes in oxygen and secretes waste, and manufactures hair, nails, and VITAMIN D.

The skin completely renews itself every 30 days; as older cells are sloughed off on the surface, new cells are produced in lower layers of skin. After these new cells have grown and divided, they begin to migrate over a two-week period up to the surface, where they replace older cells.

The hair and nails are extensions of the skin and are primarily made up of KERATIN, the main constituent of the top layer of the skin.

There are two layers of skin—the EPIDERMIS and DERMIS. The *epidermis* is the top skin layer, whose thickness varies from about a ½ inch on soles of feet and palms to 1/25 inch over the eyelids; most of the epidermis is no thicker than a page in this book, made up of about 20 overlapping layers near the skin surface. The epidermis is good at holding water, which helps make the skin elastic and maintains the body's balance of fluid and electrolytes.

A small proportion of epidermal cells are called Langerhans cells, and are located in the mid-zone of the stratum spinosum, the middle layer of the epidermis. They are also found in the dermis, lymph nodes, and thymus, and they are important in recognizing and presenting antigens to keratinocytes and to lymphocytes. They serve as the early warning system of the body's immune system, picking up antigens in the skin and circulating to the draining lymph areas via the dermal lymphatics in order to elicit an immune reaction.

The epidermis is also divided into three layers—the basal layer (named because its cells form the *base* of the epidermis)—is also referred to as the *Stratum germinativum* because this layer of cells is always producing—or germinating—new cells. The second subdivision of epidermis is called the prickle cell layer (or *Stratum spinosum*), composed of squamous cells. The topmost layer is called the "horny layer" (*Stratum corneum*). The basal layer is also home to the class of cells called MELANOCYTES, the pigment-producing cells that give birth to MELANIN (responsible for giving color to the skin). One out of every six cells in the basal layer is a melanocyte. Production of the melanin is under the control of a hormone secreted from the hypothalamus of the brain called melanocyte-stimulating hormone (MSH). It is believed that melanin is capable of absorbing ultraviolet light and thus protecting against the harmful effects of the ultraviolet rays that occur with suntanning.

Cross Section of Skin

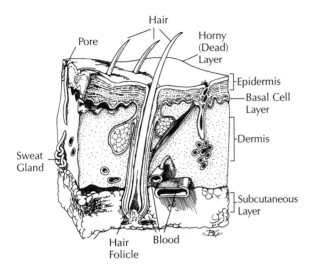

Differences in skin color are due to genetically determined differences in how much melanin there is, and where it is found in the body. In general, the darker the skin the more melanin in the epidermal cells, and the more densely arranged. Sunlight stimulates this melanin production, and a suntan simply means that more melanin has been produced as a way of protecting the skin against the harmful effects of the sun. While the culture may consider a suntan to be a characteristic of attractiveness, to the body it means a protective response to injury.

The epidermis is modified in different areas of the body; it is thick over the palms of the hands and soles of the feet, and contains more keratin. This contrasts with the thin epidermis over most of the rest of the body. The epidermis can get even thicker with use, and can result in a callus on hands or feet.

The junction where epidermis and dermis meet is an area of many furrows called rete ridges, which anchors the epidermis with the dermis and allows the exchange of nutrients between the two.

The *dermis* is the second layer of skin, made up of connective tissue and various specialized structures like HAIR FOLLICLES, sweat glands, and SEBACEOUS GLANDS that produce oily SEBUM. It is the

sebum that makes the skin waterproof, allowing a person to sit in a tub without soaking up water like a sponge. Blood vessels, lymph vessels, and nerves are also found throughout the dermis. Hair and sweat glands are actually epidermal appendages that migrate into the dermis during fetal development.

skin, cleansing Skin should be cleansed daily to remove dirt and grease, bacteria, and odor. Soaps are the products used for these purposes. There are differences in the types of soaps that may be used on the skin, and they differ in outward appearance, fragrance, cost, and composition.

For example, superfatted soaps, which are designed to improve mildness, contain excess fatty material and leave an oily residue on the skin. Transparent soaps contain glycerin and varied amounts of vegetable fats. Other soaps may be produced for specific purposes, such as oatmeal soap for skin that tends to break out. The choice of a proper soap depends on a person's age, skin texture, skin problems, and personal needs. All soaps are good at cleansing, but because of age, heredity, climate, and skin texture, there are many different methods of proper skin cleansing.

Infancy

In infancy, the skin's oil glands are not very active, although the SWEAT GLANDS are quite active. Tepid water is recommended for bathing, and a mild soap may be used sparingly to remove skin oil. The diaper area requires special attention: Soiled diapers should be changed frequently to avoid the harsh irritant potential of urine and feces. Removal of fecal material may require gentle rubbing with a cotton ball soaked in warm water. Soap should not be used if an irritating rash appears—in fact, a great deal of soap is not required at this early age. It is not necessary to wash the skin after removing a diaper soaked in urine only, since an infant's urine is sterile.

Childhood

As the child gets older, the need for soap increases, but if a rash appears, then the soap should be discontinued. It may be particularly difficult to use soap on a child who has ATOPIC DERMATITIS, an inherited dry, scaly condition of the skin. Preteens have a greater need for daily soap and bathing, as the sweat and oil glands are now functioning with more efficiency and can withstand repeated use of soap.

Teenagers

During puberty (13 to 19 years) the oil glands function at peak capacity—especially on the scalp, forehead, face, and upper chest. Some degree of ACNE and an oily complexion are quite common, and routine showering or bathing should become a habit. While frequent washing may appear to decrease oiliness, it will not alleviate acne by itself.

Adulthood

As the skin continues to age, the oil glands secrete much less oil, and soap may begin to cause drying. While some people may continue to cleanse with soap for a long time without any adverse effects, others will experience excess dryness. Seasonal variations affect the skin, too, and must be taken into consideration. Cold, wind, sunlight, and other environmental factors play a role in skin dryness.

If soap is used too often in later life, skin disease may develop; it may be better to cut down on the use of soap, especially on the lower extremities—especially during the colder months. Cleansing creams or lotions may be good substitutes, although certain areas of the body may continue to require soap. It's especially important to cleanse the body folds with soap.

skin, congenital absence of   See APLASIA CUTIS.

skin, nerves of   The skin is filled with a vast web of nerves that have considerable functional overlap, producing sensitivity to temperature, touch, pressure, itch, and pain. The nerve endings are found within the papillary and reticular dermis—some extend into the lower portion of the EPIDERMIS (outer layer of the skin). Great collections of sensory nerves also surround hair follicles and hair bulbs, which enable fine body hairs to act as a sort of sensing antenna.

There are three types of special nerve endings found in the skin—Meissner's touch corpuscles, pacinian corpuscles, and hederiform endings. Meissner's touch corpuscles are composed of oval coils of terminal axons within COLLAGEN fibers, found mostly on the palms and soles of the feet and thought to be associated with touch. Pacinian corpuscles are composed of an axon core inside a capsule found in the deep protein of the feet and palms; they may be especially tuned to detect vibration.

Hederiform ("ivy-shaped") endings include the Merkel cells, found alone or in groups in the basal epidermis, which may function as touch receptors, although their exact function is not clear.

skin, newborn   At birth, the skin of an infant may be covered by a soft, cheesy, white material called vernix that serves to protect young skin; in the past this was almost always immediately removed, but lately more physicians assume it may have a protective benefit.

Many babies are born with skin marks, splotches, or rashes that are quite normal and temporary. Some newborns have ACNE, as a result of the mother's hormones still in the baby's system; these fade away in a few months. There may be scratch marks, superficial bruises, or a purplish mottling of the skin due to a temporary instability of the blood vessels. Such blisters on the lips, feet, or hands are normal, and will fade away.

More than half of all babies and up to 80 percent of premature infants experience JAUNDICE, a yellow discoloration of the skin due to a buildup of bilirubin (a product released normally when blood cells are broken down). It may be that an infant's liver is not ready to handle the job, but there is not usually cause for concern. Bilirubin levels may normalize on their own, or the baby may need to rest under special blue lights for a few days or refrain from nursing until the levels drop.

BIRTHMARKS are often apparent, and in most cases should be left alone. However, some experts believe that a MOLE (or congenital nevus) present at birth should be removed to forestall the potential later transmutation into a malignant melanoma. A STORK BITE NEVUS (a type of HEMANGIOMA) is a harmless small, flat, pink skin blemish found in up to half of all infants, usually around the eyes, that disappears within the first year of life. Those around the nape of the neck may persist indefinitely.

See also NEVUS, CONGENITAL.

skin biopsy   The most common procedure in dermatology that involves cutting a small piece of skin for analysis and requires only a local anesthetic. It is used to establish a diagnosis by providing specific, reliable information about the problem. The biopsy will include all of the skin and some subcutaneous tissue that is large enough to contain hair complexes and sweat glands.

Most commonly, the sample will be taken for histopathologic examination by routine light microscopy, but special studies (immunofluorescence microscopy or electron microscopy) may be performed. It may also be processed for a bacterial, fungal, or viral culture.

DERMATOLOGISTS commonly use four different techniques—punch, shave, excisional, or wedge (incisional) biopsy. The punch (trephine) biopsy is most commonly used by dermatologists for a routine diagnostic biopsy. It is used to remove a portion of a larger lesion, to remove small lesions completely, or to sample a representative area involved in widespread disease.

Shave biopsy is a simple technique used to remove lesions (or parts of them) protruding above the skin's surface. This technique is quick and easy and provides good cosmetic results afterward. However, it does not allow for the sampling of the DERMIS underlying the lesion. This type of biopsy is often used to rule out cancer in SEBORRHEIC KERATOSES and cutaneous horns. It is rarely used to diagnose an inflammatory skin disease.

Excisional biopsy is occasionally used to excise an entire lesion, especially in the case of malignant melanoma and DYSPLASTIC NEVI, since the appearance of the cells may differ widely within one lesion in these conditions. Excision also allows for a much bigger chunk of tissue than a punch biopsy. However, this type of biopsy carries greater risk of significant scars, bleeding, and infection.

The *wedge* (*incisional*) *biopsy* involves a narrow incision that extends deep into a nodule or subcutaneous tissue that is used when it is important to assess the subcutis. This type of biopsy may be used to diagnose panniculitis, large vessel vasculitis, or a deep fungal infection. While the technique is similar to an excisional biopsy, the incision is usually narrower and extends more deeply.

skin cancer   Skin cancer is the most common of all cancers; basal cell and squamous cell cancers affect more than one million Americans each year—a number that is rising rapidly. Another 59,580 people will be diagnosed with malignant melanoma in 2005. But it is also the easiest cancer to cure if diagnosed and treated early. Prolonged exposure or intermittent overexposure to sunlight is the primary cause of skin cancers. In fact, about 90 percent of all skin cancer is related to sun exposure, and most skin cancers are found on parts of the body exposed to sunlight.

Because ultraviolet light can damage DNA, exposing the skin to sunlight increases the risk that an individual will develop skin cancer.

Skin type is also a very important factor in the development of skin cancer, since fair-skinned individuals who tend to burn easily and tan poorly are at greatest risk and dark skinned people are at a reduced risk.

French scientists have discovered they can determine a person's skin cancer risk by measuring a specific mutation in a tumor-suppressor gene called p53. They found specific changes in the building blocks for this gene in three-quarters of samples taken from sun-exposed skin of cancer patients, according to scientists at the International Agency for Research on Cancer in Lyon. Almost no DNA from nonexposed skin of these patients—or the skin of those who spend less time outdoors—had this mutation.

Symptoms and Diagnostic Path

There are three basic types of skin cancer: basal cell, squamous cell, and melanoma. BASAL CELL CARCINOMA usually appears as a small, shiny bump on sun-exposed areas, such as the face, neck, chest, upper back, and hands, primarily in fair-skinned people (especially those who burn easily). The lesions gradually grow and may crust, bleed, or ulcerate, although they usually do not spread. Local destruction of the skin and underlying tissues may be considerable if this type of cancer is left untreated.

SQUAMOUS CELL CARCINOMA usually appears as a red, scaly patch. It grows slowly, occasionally becoming a nodule and frequently becoming crusted and eroded. Bleeding is common. Basal cell and squamous cell cancers are almost certainly related to cumulative sun exposure, occurring mostly on exposed places. Unlike basal cell carcinoma, squamous cell cancers grow and may spread (metastasize).

Basal and squamous cell cancers account for about 1 million new cases each year; cure rates are excellent if these lesions are discovered and effectively treated early.

Malignant melanoma is the third type of cancer, the most deadly of the three. Melanoma is the most common cancer among people aged 25 to 29. Melanomas are usually small brown, black, or multicolored patches, plaques, or NODULES with an irregular outline. They may crust on the surface or bleed, and many of them appear in preexisting moles. Melanoma is much more dangerous than other forms of skin cancer because of its tendency to spread rapidly to vital internal organs as the lungs, liver, and brain.

SKIN CANCER WARNING SIGNS

Any spot (or sore or growth) that:

- changes color
- increases in size or thickness
- changes in texture
- is irregular in outline
- is bigger than 6mm (the size of a pencil eraser)
- appears after age 21
- continually itches, hurts, crusts, scabs, erodes, or bleeds
- does not heal
- increases in size and appears pearl-colored, translucent, tan, brown, black, or multicolored

---

Because the skin is so easily visualized, skin cancer can be easier to spot than internal malignancies. To make sure that skin cancer is rec-ognized early, DERMATOLOGISTs recommend that individuals examine the skin twice yearly, using a full-length and a hand-held mirror. When doing a self-exam, examiners should look for the early warning signs (see box) but also look for any *changes* in the skin. Coupled with yearly skin exams by a physician, self-exams are the best way to ensure early detection and treatment of skin cancer.

Treatment Options and Outlook

Most skin cancers (even malignant melanoma) can be cured if discovered early enough, which is why attention to symptoms and regular self-examination is highly recommended. When cancers of the skin are discovered early, there are a variety of treatment possibilities, depending on the type of tumor, size, location, and other factors affecting the patient's general health. A biopsy is often studied before a definitive therapy is selected.

Malignant melanoma causes 75 percent of all deaths from skin cancer.

Risk Factors and Preventive Measures

Because exposure to the sun seems to be the most important environmental factor in causing skin cancer, avoiding the sun or protecting against it can help prevent skin cancer. Ultraviolet (UV) radiation is also a factor in the development of lip cancer, so protecting the lips against the sun is also important.

Consumers also should realize that UV rays from artificial sources of light, such as tanning beds and sun lamps, are just as dangerous as those rays from the sun, and should also be avoided.

In addition to avoiding excess sun exposure, scientists have found that some foods and nutrients *may* counteract the development of melanoma: best choices are fish with omega-3 fatty acids, and antioxidants (including VITAMIN E, VITAMIN C, and beta carotene).

See also MELANOMA, MALIGNANT.

skin care for infants When babies are born, their pigment production is not complete; even children who will go on to have dark eyes and hair are fairly light at birth. Slowly, as the child gets older the skin color changes and begins to correspond more closely to that of the parents. While young skin heals faster than older skin, it is also less able to protect itself from injury (including injury from the sun).

A child's skin should be examined regularly, while diapering, bathing, and dressing. Any change (MOLE, growth, spot, or sore) should be pointed out to the pediatrician or DERMATOLOGIST. While it is normal for toddlers to develop new moles and other brown spots, ones that continue to change should be checked by a doctor.

Some medications make skin ultra-sensitive—when prescribed, ask the physician if the sun should be avoided.

Preventing Sunburn in Infants

It may take several years until an infant's MELANIN production is fully developed; until then, the skin is especially vulnerable to the sun—even darker skin.

Because a baby's skin constitutes a larger percentage of total body mass than an adult's, they are especially vulnerable to anything affecting the skin. A bad SUNBURN can cause serious fluid and electrolyte loss, fever, faintness, delirium, shock, low blood pressure, and irregular heart beat.

Under six months As SUNSCREENS have not been approved for their age group, infants under six months of age should be kept out of the sun entirely, under carriage hoods, canopies, and tightly woven umbrellas. Since sand, concrete, snow, and water reflect ULTRAVIOLET RADIATION, it is better to park a baby carriage on grass instead of a patio; even on overcast days, as much as 80 percent of the sun's harmful radiation can still penetrate the clouds.

Over six months Babies over age six months should avoid the hours from 10 A.M. to 3 P.M. when the sun is most intense. A broad-brimmed hat will shade ears, nose, and lips, and may reduce a baby's chance of cataracts in later life. The sun can penetrate some fabric (even cotton undershirts, which only have an SPF of about 8)—so clothes alone won't provide protection. Limit time spent in the sun, regardless of hour or season.

After a baby reaches six months of age, experts agree on the importance of using sunscreen.

Unscented sunscreens are a better choice because they do not attract insects. The sun protection factor (SPF) should be at least 15, manufactured by a major drug company, and purchased at a store with a large turnover. Some sunscreens are available without PABA, which can cause skin irritation in some people.

No matter how safe and effective the product seems, it is a good idea to test it on a child's skin before regular use. Normally, creamy products work best on youngsters because they don't dry the skin and can be easily seen.

The sunscreen should be applied on all exposed areas, and under thin clothing, 15 to 30 minutes before exposure (it takes that long for the ingredients to penetrate the skin).

For a baby under one year, sunburn should be treated as a medical emergency. If the child is over age one, the doctor should be called if there is pain, blistering, decreased urine output, lethargy, or fever above 101°F.

Treatment Options and Outlook

In case of sunburn, water or juice can replace fluids, especially if the child is not urinating; acetaminophen is given for fever over 101°F. The skin should be soaked in tepid, clear water, followed by a light moisturizing lotion. Dabbing plain CALAMINE lotion may help.

Alcohol should not be used, and no medicated cream (such as hydrocortisone or benzocaine) should be used unless a baby's pediatrician prescribes it. The child should be kept completely out of the sun until the burn is healed.

Sunscreen Recommendations

A sunscreen for children should have an SPF of 15 or higher, and SPF 15 lip balm for face and hands—the waxy form stays on and does not sting or taste bad. Toddlers can even apply it themselves.

The child's skin should be coated well, rubbing on hands, ears, nose, lips, and areas around the eyes. Contact with eyes or eyelids should be avoided.

Sunscreen should be applied before going into the sun, and every two hours thereafter, or more often if the child plays in water or is perspiring. Children should be taught to use sunscreen early, so they will be more likely to use it regularly as adults.

Zinc oxide on the nose and lips may give more protection. Baby oil should never be placed on the child before going outdoors—it makes the skin translucent, letting the sun's rays pass through more easily.

skin care product allergy Allergic reactions to skin care products are rare (only 210 for every 1 million applications), but they can develop after years of trouble-free use. The perfuming agents in creams, soaps, and cosmetics are often the cause (even some products called "unscented" contain tiny amounts of fragrance to hide chemical odors).

See also COSMETIC ALLERGY.

skin characteristics A description of a person's skin (oily, dry, or in-between) often referred to as "skin type" among consumers and cosmetician.

Oily skin People with this type of skin usually have enlarged pores, a shiny nose, and a tendency to have breakouts, ACNE, or BLACKHEADS. People with an oil problem should keep their skin clean, while not scrubbing too hard, which can stimulate the overproduction of oil.

Only products formulated for oily skin should be used; in the oiliest areas, an astringent or toner with a high alcohol content is a good idea. Oil-free moisturizers may be used, and women with oily skin should use only water-based makeup.

On the positive side, people with oily skin are less likely to experience premature aging lines, although eventually even the oiliest skin becomes drier, causing WRINKLES and lines.

Dry skin People with this type of skin usually have invisible pores and a tendency to itch, flake, get chapped, and develop tiny premature wrinkle lines around mouth or eyes.

This type of skin should be cleaned with soaps that moisturize; transparent soaps are a good choice, but their added alcohol may leave skin dry, so be sure to follow with a moisturizer. Lips may need special protection against chapping in win-

ter. One suggestion is to use a humidifier or pan of water indoors during winter to keep indoor air moisturized.

Combination skin Most people with this type of skin have basically trouble-free complexions with a supple, flexible smooth texture. Some areas of the skin may be dry (such as forehead and eyes) and other parts may be oily (such as the nose). People with this type should use products designed for normal skin, but use specially designed products on spots that are oily or dry.

skin color There are three pigments that give skin its color—MELANIN, which provides brown tones; carotene, which produces yellow tones; and hemoglobin, the red pigment in blood that provides red and pink color. A person's skin is actually a blend of the various pigmentations, and the healthy "rosy glow" comes primarily from hemoglobin. In some people, lack of this healthy rosy color is caused by low hemoglobin levels or impaired circulation of the blood in the skin.

See also BLEACHING CREAMS; PIGMENTATION; PIGMENTATION, DISORDERS OF; PIGMENT CELLS.

skin cream Lotions designed to retain moisture and keep skin smooth and soft. These products usually include at least one of the following: LANOLIN, petrolatum, COLLAGEN, mineral oil, and squalene.

Many products also include preservatives that keep the product stable and fresh. The most common preservatives include PARABENS (ethyl-, methyl-, and butyl-), quaternium-15, and imidazolidinyl urea. In addition, because many fragrances can cause allergies, many skin creams and other products also offer fragrance-free products.

skin disorders Despite its surprising resiliency, any number of things can go wrong with the skin: it can become irritated and inflamed; it can be burned. The skin is also prey to production problems—too little or too much oil, MELANIN, or skin cells.

In fact, skin-related complaints account for up to 10 percent of all ambulatory patient visits in this country. Since the skin mirrors the general condition of the patient, many systemic conditions may be accompanied by dermatologic manifestations. And because disorders of the skin are so readily visible, dermatologic complaints are often the primary reason for patient visits.

Congenital Skin Conditions
BIRTHMARKS are pigmented skin blemishes present at birth that include MOLES, MONGOLIAN SPOTS, and HEMANGIOMAS.

Infection/Infestations
The skin can be infected with either viruses, bacteria, or fungi. Viral infections include CHICKEN POX, WARTS, HERPES SIMPLEX, MOLLUSCUM CONTAGIOSUM, and HERPES ZOSTER. Bacterial infections include BOILS, CELLULITIS, ERYSIPELAS, and IMPETIGO. Fungal infections include ATHLETE'S FOOT, JOCK ITCH, and RINGWORM. Parasites include SCABIES, worms, FLEAS, TICKS, and LICE.

Tumors (Neoplastic Disorders)
Noncancerous tumors are very common skin problems, and include seborrheic keratoses and most types of NEVI. Types of skin cancer are BASAL CELL CARCINOMA, SQUAMOUS CELL CARCINOMA, MALIGNANT MELANOMA, PAGET'S DISEASE OF THE NIPPLE, MYCOSIS FUNGOIDES, and KAPOSI'S SARCOMA.

Autoimmune Disorders
Caused when the body attacks its own tissues, these skin disorders include LUPUS ERYTHEMATOSUS, VITILIGO, DERMATOMYOSITIS, MORPHEA, SCLERODERMA, PEMPHIGOID, and PEMPHIGUS.

Disorders of Hypersensitivity
A wide range of skin symptoms can occur because of hypersensitivity. These include contact dermatitis, HIVES and anaphylaxis, reactive erythemas, drug reactions, vasculitis, and photosensitivity diseases.

Scaling and Bullous Disorders
Although uncommon, the bullous diseases are a dramatic and serious group of skin diseases. They include pemphigus, BULLOUS PEMPHIGOID, HERPES GESTATIONIS, EPIDERMOLYSIS BULLOSA, DERMATITIS HERPETIFORMIS, and HAILEY-HAILEY DISEASE.

Trauma
The skin's role as protector of vital underlying organs means that it is vulnerable to injury itself. Injuries may be due to cold (CHILBLAINS, IMMERSION FOOT, or FROSTBITE), to heat (BURNS or erythromelalgia), or to pressure (CALLUSES, CORNS, or BEDSORES).

Occupational Skin Conditions
Injuries excluded, dermatoses account for nearly half of all remaining occupational illnesses. They can include systemic disease due to skin absorption, contact dermatitis, PHOTOSENSITIVITY DISORDERS, ACNE, PIGMENT disorders, tumors; connective tissue disease, granulomatous reactions, and disorders of the hair or nails.

Disorders of Structure/Function
These can include inherited skin diseases, disorders of keratinization (ICHTHYOSIS, REFSUM'S DISEASE, FOLLICULAR HYPERKERATOSES, ACANTHOSIS NIGRICANS, and so on), disorders of pigmentation (LENTIGO SIMPLEX, NEVUS SPILUS, NEUROFIBROMATOSIS, FRECKLES, MELASMA), diseases of the dermis (CUTIS LAXA or PROGERIA), disorders of the subcutaneous tissue (such as POLYARTERITIS NODOSA), ACNE or ROSACEA, disorders of hair (such as ALOPECIA), disorders of the nails (such as PACHYONYCHIA), MAST CELL DISEASES (such as URTICARIA PIGMENTOSA), and diseases of nutrition and metabolism (such as VITAMIN A DEFICIENCY or PHENYLKETONURIA).

skin fillers Substances that replace components of the skin to erase WRINKLES and other imperfections. The top fillers are HYALURONIC ACID GEL (Restylane and Hylaform), human collagen, bovine collagen, and Sculptra. Wrinkles are caused by the loss of three skin components—collagen, ELASTIN, and HYALURONIC ACID. DERMATOLOGISTS can replace collagen and hyaluronic acid that are lost as the skin ages and one day may be able to replace elastin, as well. Although doctors cannot reverse aging, they can erase its effects by using injectable soft tissue fillers, which are designed to produce a smoother, more youthful appearance with minimal recovery time and maximum safety.

Injectable soft tissue fillers are used to improve the appearance of fine lines and wrinkles, fill out hollow cheeks, lighten scars, lessen deep folds, and repair other facial flaws. Results are often immediate, however, it may take more than one treatment to achieve the desired effect. The length of time and results will vary. In the past, doctors have used bovine (cattle) collagen and the patient's own body fat to safely diminish wrinkles and give the face a more youthful appearance. Today, human collagen and hyaluronic acid promise to be a better solution.

Bovine collagen

The oldest and best-known filler is purified bovine collagen, which dermatologists use to fill in fine lines around the eyes and deep lines from the nose to the corners of the lips, as well as enlarge lips and erase acne scars. Typically, a series of injections will help fill out the imperfections and give almost immediate results, each session lasting about 10 to 30 minutes. However, while these methods are effective, the fillers are not a long-term solution; they require frequent office visits to maintain the youthful look. The procedure must be done again within three or four months, depending on the size of the area treated, how much collagen was injected, and how healthy the filled skin was. The procedure often causes some redness, swelling, or bruising around the injection site, which usually disappears in a few days. Patients risk possible allergic reactions.

Body Fat

Dermatologists have been successfully injecting the patient's own body fat into wrinkles for years, which eliminates potential allergic reactions and avoids the need for allergy testing.

In this procedure, the dermatologist transfers the patient's own fat from a part of the patient's body with excess fat to an area that has lost fat as a result of aging. Typically, the fat is used to plump up deep creases around the nose and mouth, to fill

scars, or to replace fat pads in the cheeks. This technique may require follow-up visits to achieve the desired effects. Results last longer than with bovine collagen—typically over one year.

Potential side effects with this method are unlikely, although sometimes lumps can develop around the lips or the eyes, where body fat does not naturally occur.

Human-based collagen

Two products containing human-based collagen (CosmoDerm and CosmoPlast) were approved in March 2003 for the correction of facial wrinkles, acne scars, restoration of the lip border, and other soft-tissue contour problems. Allergy testing is not required with this method. Side effects are usually limited to temporary redness and swelling around the injection site. As with bovine collagen, results are noticeable almost right away, and last about four to eight months. Multiple treatments may be needed to achieve the desired effects.

AlloDerm is another soft tissue filler made of human tissue donated in much the same way as other transplantable organs and approved by the U.S. Food and Drug Administration for cosmetic use. It may be used to enhance the lips or to fill in lines and creases that develop with aging.

AlloDerm is processed from donated human cadaver tissue prepared in such a way that it retains its underlying structure. It has been used for a variety of surgical reconstructive procedures to replace lost, damaged, or diseased tissues, and is now used to fill in facial wrinkles, where it is considered stable and may last from one to two years.

A micronized form of AlloDerm, called Cymetra, is also available. This material is rehydrated with lidocaine in the physician's office before injection so the procedure is much less painful.

Because it is human derived, no skin test is required. Studies so far have found no evidence of allergic reactions, although temporary bruising, redness, and swelling occurs in a few patients.

AlloDerm is obtained from tissue banks, which surgically remove a thin layer of skin from deceased donors, using sterile operating room techniques. The skin is placed into a antibiotic solution and processed to remove the top layer of skin cells and all of the cells in the deepest layer. The remaining material—the AlloDerm—is a collagen framework that provides strength to the skin, but without any components left to cause the rejection or inflammation. Therefore, when transplanted to a patient, the AlloDerm graft gradually becomes a natural part of the patient's own tissue.

AlloDerm was first used in 1992 to treat burn patients and in 1994 for periodontal and plastic surgery. Currently, more than 50,000 patients have received AlloDerm grafts.

AlloDerm is the only available product capable of regenerating normal soft tissue. Since it is human tissue, it does not trigger an inflammatory or allergic reaction, and the pretreatment skin testing required with bovine collagen is not needed. In addition, patients report that the graft does not feel hard the way other synthetic materials do. When AlloDerm is used as an implant, it completely eliminates any need to transplant donor fat or skin from one part of the body to another area.

Although AlloDerm appears to be long lasting, there have been reports of a small number of patients completely absorbing the AlloDerm within six months. AlloDerm lip enhancement is irreversible after a period of seven to eight weeks.

Hyaluronic acid gels

Although human collagen was an improvement over bovine collagen because it did not trigger allergies, dermatologists still needed a filler that could safely and effectively replace hyaluronic acid, the other primary component lost in aging skin. Several new fillers have been approved by the FDA that can replace the skin's hyaluronic acid lost during aging. These products work by filling as well as by pulling water into the skin, plumping up the skin, and adding volume.

Dermatologists have known for a long time that wrinkles are caused by the loss of three skin components—collagen, elastin, and hyaluronic acid. Today, doctors can replace two of these components (collagen and hyaluronic acid). Hyaluronic acid holds together collagen and elastin, providing a framework for the skin. When injected into the skin in gel form, hyaluronic acid binds to water and adds volume to easily fill in larger folds of skin around the mouth and cheeks. Patients notice an immediate plumping of the skin in the treated areas.

Approved in 2005, hyaluronic acid gels (Restylane and Hylaform), are injected into facial tissue to smooth wrinkles and folds, especially in the folds around the nose and mouth. Hyaluronic acid is a protective, lubricating, and binding gel substance that is produced naturally by the body. Restylane and Hylaform work by temporarily adding volume to facial tissue and restoring a smoother appearance to the face for an effect that lasts for about six months.

They are injected by a doctor into areas of facial tissue where moderate to severe facial wrinkles and folds occur. The gels temporarily add volume to the skin and can give the appearance of a smoother surface. They will help smooth moderate to severe facial wrinkles and folds. In one study, most patients needed just one injection to smooth out the wrinkles; about one-third of patients needed more than one injection to get a satisfactory result.

One of the main advantages of hyaluronic acid gels are that they do not trigger allergic reactions, nor is there a risk of transmitting animal diseases by injection as there is with bovine collagen. Since a skin check for allergies is not required with hyaluronic acid gel, patients can be treated on their first visit to the dermatologist. In addition, hyaluronic acid treatments last about four to six months and require less volume to fill wrinkles and hard-to-treat skin folds compared to collagen.

These gels do have side effects, and pain is a problem. Since hyaluronic acid get does not contain the anesthetic lidocaine, injections can be painful. In addition, there is usually temporary inflammation that produces swelling and redness following injection with hyaluronic acid gel—especially in the lip area.

Some dermatologists combine hyaluronic acid and collagen for the most benefits with each filler. Injecting collagen first numbs and supports the area, stabilizing the skin to prevent bruising. Then hyaluronic acid gel is injected painlessly. Using these fillers together replaces two of the skin components that are lost with skin aging.

Silicone

Until it was banned by the FDA in 1992, injectable silicone was used in the United States for many years to successfully treat wrinkles and acne scars as well as enhance lips, cheekbones, and the chin. However, problems emerged when medical-grade silicone was diluted with foreign substances, such as mineral oil, and when it was injected in large volumes.

What makes silicone unique is that the results are permanent. Studies are showing that once the desired results are achieved, there is no need for future treatments unless it becomes necessary as the patient ages or disease processes continue.

Unfortunately, side effects may include delayed reactions that trigger redness and lumpiness as the body rejects the silicone. In the past, more problems were reported with silicone breast implants. However, side effects are rare when silicone is injected by a dermatologic surgeon skilled in the microdroplet technique, in which tiny amounts of silicone are injected at four- to eight-week intervals until the desired effects is achieved.

Fibroblasts

Harvesting the patient's own collagen-producing cells (FIBROBLASTS) holds promise for filling fine facial lines, enhancing lips and correcting scars. Results reportedly last a bit longer than bovine collagen, and side effects are minimal. However, the procedure is time-consuming. First, a dermatologist must remove a small amount of skin tissue and close the area with adhesive or sutures; the tissue is shipped to a company that cultures the fibroblasts, using its patented process. In six weeks, the harvested cells are delivered to the dermatologist's office; the patient must return for skin testing because the substance in which the cells are grown can cause an allergic reaction. If the patient does not develop an allergic reaction within two weeks, treatment can begin.

New fillers

Polymethylmethacrylate One of the newest permanent injectable skin fillers awaiting FDA approval, this is mixture of micronized plastic spheres and bovine collagen. When injected into the skin, the collagen holds the synthetic spheres

in place until it disperses after injection, leaving the spheres behind to plump up the wrinkles. These spheres stimulate the body's own production of collagen, which then forms around the spheres.

The primary benefit of polymethylmethacrylate is that it is a permanent solution, which also can be a problem if it is not injected properly. Other side effects include temporary swelling and redness (especially in the lips) and permanent or long-term lumps.

Hydroxylapatite with a methylcellulose vehicle Patients interested in a more permanent solution than collagen but who want to avoid the permanent results of polymethylmethacrylate may someday soon be able to choose hydroxylapatite with a methylcellulose vehicle, which is currently approved for other purposes. It is now being studied as an injectable skin filler. This filler contains calcium hydroxylapatite beads (a substance now used to replace missing bones). Hydroxylapatite with a methylcellulose vehicle temporarily corrects wrinkles and may last about a year, although its exact length of improvement has not yet been fully studied. However, if not injected properly, the calcium beads might cling together and could exhibit a lumpy treated area.

skin graft A technique used by both dermatologists and plastic surgeons to repair areas of lost or damaged skin in which the healthy skin is removed from one part of the body and reattached to the damaged area. If successful, new cells grow from the graft and cover the damaged area with fresh, new skin.

Skin used for a graft may be removed from another part of the patient's body, or taken from an identical twin; otherwise, skin from anyone else is rejected as foreign by the recipient's body. (Skin from an unrelated donor may provide temporary cover, however). Although all skin grafts leave scars, a skin graft is performed when the damaged area is too large to be stitched together or because an ungrafted area would result in unsightly or restrictive scarring.

There are two types of skin grafts—split thickness and full thickness grafts. A *split-thickness graft* is used when large areas (such as burns) must be covered; the area that has been "harvested" will regenerate in a few days to weeks and can provide more donor skin. *Full-thickness grafts* include a deeper, thicker section of the skin, and are often used for facial grafts because the transferred skin looks more normal. They have a more natural color and texture, and contrast less than split-thickness grafts. However, full-thickness grafts are less likely to successfully attach themselves. In addition, donor sites cannot be reharvested, and must be stitched closed after the graft section has been removed. Split-thickness grafts are usually cut from the abdomen or thigh; full-thickness grafts are often taken from behind or in the crease in front of the ear.

Pinch grafts may be used in an attempt to treat leg ulcers when there is good granulation tissue. In this procedure, grafts are taken from anesthetized skin (usually the upper thigh) by pinching a small amount of skin with a needle and slicing it with a scalpel or razor blade. The grafts are transferred to the ulcer bed with a small space between grafts, sprayed with an adhesive and covered with a semi-permeable dressing with edges extending beyond the margin of the ulcer. Gauze and an elastic dressing cover the wound, which is left in place for three or four days. Strict bed rest is required. The physician can examine the pinch graft through the semi-permeable dressing, draining accumulated fluid when necessary. Dressings may be removed in five or six days, or left in place if there is no infection. Cleansing with alcohol helps the wound to form a firm crust that will fall off in two or three weeks. The grafts will extend to the skin of the adjacent graft and fill up the ulcer.

skin infections Because the skin represents the outer barrier to the world, it is responsible for defending the interior of the body against a wide range of attackers, including bacteria, viruses, insect venom, and fungi. Skin infections can range from a local superficial problem (such as IMPETIGO) to a wide-spread and possibly fatal infection.

Examples of bacterial skin infections include IMPETIGO, ECTHYMA, FOLLICULITIS, BOILS, CARBUNCLES, ERYSIPELAS, SCARLET FEVER, CELLULITIS, and so on. Viral infections with skin symptoms include HERPES SIMPLEX, CHICKEN POX and SHINGLES, WARTS,

MEASLES, GERMAN MEASLES, RUBEOLA, FIFTH DISEASE, AIDS, and so on.

Fungal infections can be noninvasive, invasive and systemic. They include RINGWORM (tinea), CANDIDA infection, CHROMOMYCOSIS, CRYPTOCOCCOSIS, and so on.

Rickettsial infections are conveniently grouped as the spotted fevers (ROCKY MOUNTAIN SPOTTED FEVER, RICKETTSIAL POX, and so on), the typhus group (TYPHUS), Q FEVER, and TRENCH FEVER.

Parasitic infections are endemic in many developing countries, where poverty, poor hygiene and inadequate sanitary facilities create favorable conditions for infection. The infections enter the United States with the immigration of foreign students, diplomats, and immigrants. Protozoal infections include LEISHMANIASIS and AMEBIASIS; helminthic infections (worms) include PINWORMS, HOOKWORMS, STRONGYLOIDIASIS, CUTANEOUS LARVA MIGRANS, FILARIASIS, and so on. Ectoparasite (a parasite that lives on the outside of the host) infections include SCABIES and LICE.

See also SKIN DISORDERS.

skin patch Also called a transdermal patch, this is multilayered disk ranges in size from that of a small coin to several square inches. It introduces a controlled release of a medication into the system through the skin. The patches are painless and usually do not irritate the skin. The patch works by maintaining a reservoir of the drug and releasing it through the skin via an adhesive-coated polymer membrane. Effective drug levels can be maintained this way for some time.

Patches have been used to deliver scopolamine; nitroglycerin and other nitrates to treat heart disease; hormones for birth control in women; and nicotine to people trying to stop smoking. Researchers have found ways to introduce estradiol to postmenopausal women who need estrogen replacement, and to administer timolol and clonidine hydrochloride to treat high blood pressure.

skin scams Many beauty products promise to "reverse the tracks of time" by removing wrinkles. Unfortunately, this is something no skin cream can do. Terms like *antiaging, rejuvenation,* and *cellular renewal* sound wonderful, but they do not permanently alter the characteristics of aging skin. In truth, these skin products simply moisturize the skin, plumping it up so lines and creases are less noticeable. Experts say the special wrinkle-fighting ingredients in the supercream formulas are of limited value.

COLLAGEN, for example, is commercially manufactured from animal protein with the idea that, applied topically, it will enhance the production of a person's own collagen. But collagen molecules are just too large to be absorbed into the skin. Other anti-aging skin formulas include RNA and DNA, super-oxide dismutase, and glycosphingolipid, which some claim can "rejuvenate" cells. None of them has been shown to have any effect on internal body chemistry, experts say.

According to the U.S. Food and Drug Administration, if skin products alter the structure or function of the skin, they are regarded as drugs, not cosmetics. Manufacturers would have to submit data to demonstrate that these products were safe and performed their intended function—something not now required of cosmetics.

Other products with little value include quail egg omelettes for the face, seaweed cleansers, moisturizers with bee jelly, and oils squeezed from turtles, sharks, and minks.

skin tags Known medically as *acrochordons,* these common lesions are small brown or flesh-colored flaps of skin that usually occur spontaneously and tend to run in families.

They are found most often in middle-aged women, on the neck, under the arm, under the breasts, and on the eyelids.

Skin tags do not usually cause problems, although they may be irritated by rubbing clothing or jewelry. Anal tags often occur as a complication of anal fissures or hemorrhoids. Skin tags appear to be more common in overweight individuals.

Treatment Options and Outlook
Skin tags can usually be removed with electrosurgery or by cryosurgery. Larger lesions may be removed with scissors or a scalpel, followed by electrodesiccation or cauterization.

skin tuberculosis See TUBERCULOSIS, SKIN.

skin tumor, benign A group of skin tumors that are not cancerous. These include Cutaneous SKIN TAGS, SEBORRHEIC KERATOSES, ACTINIC KERATOSES, BIRTHMARKS, LIVER SPOTS, MOLES, KELOIDS, and WARTS.

skin tumor, malignant See SKIN CANCER.

skin type While the phrase "skin type" has come to mean the skin's *characteristics* (whether the skin is oily, dry, or in-between), dermatologists use the term "skin type" to indicate a person's relative sensitivity to sun exposure. Because a person's skin characteristics can vary from one part to another, dermatologists prefer to treat specific areas and conditions of each area of the skin. Skin characteristics tend to become more oily in summer, under stress, during adolescence and in hot, humid climates.

Skin type, according to DERMATOLOGISTS, is classified into six groups, according to the skin's tendency to sunburn.

SUNBURN TYPE

TYPE I: Always burns, never tans. Very fair with red or blond hair and FRECKLES.

TYPE II: Burns easily, tans minimally. Usually fair-skinned.

TYPE III: Sometimes burns, gradually tans.

TYPE IV: Minimum burning, always tans. Usually white with medium pigmentation.

TYPE V: Very seldom burns, always tans. Medium to heavy pigmentation.

TYPE VI: Never burns but tans darkly. Blacks as well as others with heavy pigmentation.

SLE See SYSTEMIC LUPUS ERYTHEMATOSUS.

smallpox A highly infectious viral disease causing skin rash and flulike symptoms that has been totally eradicated since 1980.

A medical scourge of the 19th century, smallpox was characterized by a rash that spread over the body, turning into PUS-filled BLISTERS that crusted and sometimes left deeply pitted scars. Complications included blindness, pneumonia, and kidney damage, and there was no effective treatment for the disease, which killed up to 40 percent of affected individuals.

Smallpox was eradicated through a cooperative international vaccination program that was successful because the disease affected only humans. Patients were easily recognized and infectious only for a short time. As a result of the eradication program, smallpox vaccination certificates are no longer required for international travel. Most countries have stopped vaccinating because the vaccine itself is now more dangerous than the disease, since the vaccine can cause encephalitis and there is now no chance of contracting smallpox.

However, after the events of September and October 2001, the U.S. government took precautions to deal with a possible bioterrorist attack using smallpox as a weapon. The risk for smallpox occurring as a result of a deliberate release by terrorists is not known, but the government considers it very low. Still, by the end of 2002, the government had stockpiled about 286 million doses of smallpox vaccine—enough to vaccinate every person in the United States.

The virus responsible for smallpox is still maintained at laboratories at the Centers for Disease Control in Atlanta and at a research institute in Moscow. A recent suggestion to destroy the virus was met by such criticism among the scientific community, who value the virus for scientific purposes, that any attempt to do so has been postponed.

soap and the skin Soap is an emulsifier that attaches to water molecules and to oil and dirt molecules, pulling them together. This is why soap is better at washing away oily dirt than water alone.

Many people choose to clean their skin with soap (in fact, Americans take more than 60 billion showers and baths each year) and the choices of soap are almost limitless—from 100 percent pure, hard-milled, and scented to translucent bars or liquids. Soap has been around for quite some time

(scented bars of soap were excavated from Pompeii, and Phoenicians were milling soap 700 years before that), and the majority of Americans still turn to a bar of soap to clean their skin.

The downside of soap is that some skins are irritated by heavily perfumed products, and deodorant soaps may be troublesome to others. Moreover, some people with very dry skin or with ECZEMA may find that soap's fatty acids are too irritating; for them, a soapless cleanser or detergent (acid rather than alkaline) is a good choice. (Soaps are made from natural animal fat, while detergents are synthetic).

Antibacterial Soap

Dermatologists note that there is a place for the antibacterial cleanser such as Dial, Safeguard, or Liquid Lever 2000, a mild product that contains moisturizer in addition to deodorant and antibacterial agents and that is safe for children over the age of 18 months. Antibacterial soap is ideal for cleaning the fingers before inserting contact lenses, after handling suspicious things, or after being around people with coughs and colds. However, these cleansers are no better at killing bacteria than plain soap and hot water.

Old-Fashioned Soap

Soap used to be made by combining an alkali with fat (such as vegetable oil) and water. Soaps such as Ivory come under this heading, but many other products that seem like soap are really detergents.

Detergent Soap

While many consumers assume that "detergent" is synonymous with "household cleaner" and is therefore too harsh for the skin, in fact many companies add extra emollients to detergent formulas to make their products milder. Still, detergents do tend to be harsher than soap. Dove is an example of a soap that is really a detergent.

Superfatted Soap

A cleansing product with extra oils or fats (such as coconut or mineral oil, LANOLIN, or COLD CREAM) included in the formula. In addition, excess fatty acids are added to ensure that the pH is not too alkaline. These products tend to leave an oily film.

Glycerin Soap

Usually transparent, these soaps contain the humectant GLYCERIN as an ingredient. Examples include Basis and Neutrogena.

Castile Soap

Often advertised as being especially pure, the real difference between castile and other soaps is that castile products are made with olive oil instead of other fats.

Medicated Soap

This cleansing product, which includes antibacterial ingredients, is considered to be a drug and is therefore subject to drug regulations. In fact, some medicated soaps, such as soaps containing salicylic acid or benzoyl peroxide, are sold only by prescription.

Deodorant Soap

These cleansing products contain ingredients that fight body odor by killing bacteria. They are not recommended as facial cleansers.

Whatever kind of soap is used, it must be completely rinsed off the skin or the resulting residue can dry the skin and attract dirt.

Old beauty advice held that any type of soap was bad for the skin. The reasoning was that no matter how mild or pure, soap was still too drying. Formerly, people were advised to use a nonsoapy cosmetic cleanser containing no alcohol or grains, followed by a toner or astringent.

Today many skin care experts note that there are plenty of mild, non-drying soaps available that are fine for everyone, such as glycerin or superfatted soaps. A consumer should select the mildest product that is effective.

Despite the plethora of fancy "beauty bars," featuring exotic ingredients such as milk and honey, essence of eucalyptus, pear nectar, and freesia, all soaps still contain sodium or potassium salts. It may not be glamorous, but soap works by emulsifying surface oils, carrying dirt away in the foam.

All soaps by definition are alkaline, and strip the skin of its outside oily layer. Some soaps have a neutral or slightly acid pH, until they come in contact with water, whereupon they become alkaline. Therefore, no matter what a particular company may claim, a soap cannot truly be pH-balanced.

How to Use Soap

It is important not to *over-clean* the skin; even those with oily or problem skin should wash with soap just twice a day (or once in the evening if skin is very dry). Experts recommend 10 rinses to ensure that the skin is free of residue. If the skin has a tight, drawn feeling after washing, most likely the skin has been overcleansed or too strong a soap has been used.

A person's skin condition may change drastically with the seasons. In cold, harsh weather the skin is prone to dryness and chapping. Hot, humid weather may lead to more washing, which could irritate the skin.

See also CLEANSING PRODUCTS.

sodium laureth sulfate Cosmetic detergents that exert liquefying action, removing oil and soil from the hair and skin. This ingredient produces eye and skin irritation in experimental animals and in some human test subjects; irritation may occur in some users of cosmetic formulations containing the ingredient. The irritant effects are similar to those produced by other detergents, and the severity of the irritation appears to increase directly with concentration.

Sodium laureth sulfate may induce eye and skin irritation, but it is considered safe as presently used in cosmetic products.

sodium lauryl sulfate (SLS) A detergent cleanser and emulsifier in creams and lotions that may cause allergic reactions in some people.

The longer this ingredient stays in contact with the skin, the greater the likelihood of irritation, which may or may not be evident to the consumer. Sodium lauryl sulfate appears to be safe in formulations designed for brief use followed by thorough rinsing from the surface of the skin. In products intended for prolonged contact with skin, concentrations should not exceed 1 percent.

soft tissue augmentation   See SKIN FILLERS.

solar keratoses   See ACTINIC KERATOSES.

solar lentigo   A condition in which the skin darkens because of an excess of MELANOCYTES (MELANIN-producing cells). Solar lentigo appears in patients with fair skin who have a history of chronic sun exposure; the lesions usually appear after age 40.

Symptoms and Diagnostic Path

Symptoms include moderately dark brown, large spots (called "age spots" or "liver spots") with irregular borders. The outer skin layer is atrophied with fine, paperlike wrinkles. Like LENTIGO SIMPLEX, solar lentigo does not fade in the winter or darken in the summer.

Treatment Options and Outlook

The most important part of treatment is to avoid any further skin darkening by avoiding the sun, and applying SUNSCREENS or sunblocks before going outside. Bleaching creams applied every day for up to a year may be effective. More aggressive treatment includes LIQUID NITROGEN cryotherapy or short pulsed laser treatment such as Q-switched ruby lasers.

solar urticaria   The medical term for sun-induced HIVES, this is an allergic reaction to certain wavelengths of the sun that appears immediately after exposure.

Treatment Options and Outlook

The treatment of choice is a nonsedating antihistamine such as terfenadine.

See also POLYMORPHIC LIGHT ERUPTION.

solar UV index   A daily warning index forecasting the ultraviolet (UV) light radiation exposure for the United States designed to help people avoid SKIN CANCER. The index is issued daily by the National Weather Service to predict the amount of dangerous ultraviolet light that will reach the Earth's surface at noon the next day. The scale is generally from 1 to 11+. The higher the number, the greater the level of radiation from the sun.

The goal of the warnings, is to remind people of the danger of the sun to their skin so they will use SUNSCREENS, sunglasses, and reduce exposure to themselves and their children. Damage from sun exposure accumulates over time, and much of the injury is done when people are youngsters.

THE GENERAL CATEGORIES OF HAZARD ARE:

Minimal (index of 0–2): Fair-skinned people may burn in 30 minutes; those with darker skin may be safe up to two hours.

Low (3–4) Fair-skinned people may burn in 15 to 20 minutes; others may be safe from 75 to 90 minutes.

Moderate (5–6) Fair people may burn in 10 to 12 minutes; others may be safe for 50 to 60 minutes.

High (7–9): Fair people may burn in 7 to 8½ minutes; others may be safe for 33 to 40 minutes.

Very high (10 and up): Fair people may burn in 4 to 6 minutes; others may be safe for 20 to 30 minutes.

The Environmental Protection Agency prepared the index in collaboration with the National Oceanic and Atmospheric Administration and the Centers for Disease Control and Prevention. The index is available online at: http://www.epa.gov/sunwise/uvindex.html.

Solumbra   A type of 30+ SPF sun-protective clothing that can provide medically accepted sun protection. The Solumbra products are regulated as medical devices and have been evaluated in medical research. Solumbra material is soft and lightweight and offers head-to-toe sun protection. It is available in hats, shirts, pants, and accessories for adults and children.

A typical 30 SPF SUNSCREEN, even though it may claim to provide UVA protection, may still allow UVA rays to penetrate the skin. Solumbra blocks more than 97 percent of both UVA and UVB rays, far better than a typical 30 SPF sunscreen or typical summer shirt.

See also CLOTHES AND SUN PROTECTION.

sore The common term for a skin lesion.

SPF See SKIN PROTECTION FACTOR.

spider angioma See NEVUS ARANEUS.

spider bite Although most of the 50,000 species of spiders in the United States have poison glands connected to their fangs, only a few are capable of piercing human skin, and only two—the black widow and the brown recluse—are harmful to humans. In general, most spider attacks occur when someone disturbs the nest while working outside.

Black Widow Spider

One of only two truly poisonous spiders found in the United States, all six species of black widow spider are venomous, although none are usually fatal. Reluctant to bite humans, these spiders are responsible for only about three deaths in the United States every year. The venom of the black widow spider is 15 times as deadly as the venom of the prairie rattlesnake, but because they inject only a small amount they are not usually very dangerous.

The bite of the black widow is not especially painful, and may produce just a bit of swelling with two tiny puncture marks, followed by a dull numbing pain that gets worse as time passes. The pain peaks within three hours, but continues for another two days. Within 40 minutes after the bite, the venom begins to attack the nerves, causing abdominal or chest muscles to get tight. At the same time, there may be stomach pain and muscle spasms in the arms and legs, along with breathing problems, chills, urinary retention, sweating, convulsions, paralysis, delirium, nausea and vomiting, drooping eyelids, headache, and fever. In rare cases, cardiac failure leads to death, but most patients recover without complication.

The wound should be kept clean and cool, with the affected limb elevated to heart level. Aspirin or Tylenol may used to relieve minor symptoms. A doctor or Poison Control (800-222-1222) should be called right away. Antivenin is available, but most people can be managed without it. Healthy people should recover rapidly in two to five days, but people under age 16 or older than 60, especially those with a heart condition, may require a hospital stay. A tetanus shot may be needed.

Brown Recluse Spider

The brown recluse is by far the most dangerous of the U.S. species, with a range from Texas and Arkansas to as far north as Massachusetts. This brown, half-inch-long spider gets its name from a shy habit of hiding in dresser drawers, closets, folds of clothing, garages, attics, and sheds, where they will not try to bite unless they are trapped. The venom of females is more deadly than males.

The physical reaction to a BROWN RECLUSE SPIDER BITE depends on how much venom was injected and the person's sensitivity to it. Some people are unaffected by a bite, whereas others experience immediate or delayed effects as the venom kills the tissues at the site. Typically, most people do not feel much pain at first, but within eight hours the pain becomes severe and the area begins to turn red. Any area on the skin that the spider has bitten will begin to die and slough off, because the venom contains a substance that is very destructive to skin. This leads to a large, spreading sore that will eventually become a dark, hard BLISTER within a few days. In some cases, this blister turns deep purple, and within two weeks becomes an open ulcer. As this ulcer develops, it often becomes infected, and in a small number of people the ulcer takes a very long time to heal.

The bite also may cause a number of body-wide reactions, including fever, chills, weakness, nausea and vomiting, joint pain, and RASH. Fatal bites usually kill within two days, as a result of kidney failure.

There is no specific antivenin, but ANTIHISTAMINES, muscle relaxants, and steroids may help. The surgical removal of affected skin was once standard procedure, but now experts believe this slows down wound healing. Some physicians administer high doses of systemic steroids, or oral DAPSONE to reduce the degree of tissue damage, but an effective treatment has not yet been found.

Risk Factors and Preventive Measures

Homeowners should be careful when working around areas where spiders may live, and should wear gloves and pay attention. To eradicate these spiders, homeowners should remove all materials where these spiders might hide, knocking down the webs and their round egg sacs with a stick and crushing them underfoot. Removing or destroying the egg sacs helps control the population.

spongiform pustule An accumulation of white blood cells between epidermal cells that may lead to a spongy appearance and the appearance of fluid between the cells. It is characteristic of PSORIASIS.

spongiosis Swelling between the epidermal cells. It is a hallmark of ECZEMA.

sporotrichosis A chronic fungal infection of the skin that often follows trauma caused by the fungus *Sporothrix schenckii,* characterized by the formation of painful ABSCESSES and ulcers. The fungus affects both men and women around the world who come in contact with the fungus through soil, vegetation, untreated plants, or decaying vegetables.

Symptoms and Diagnostic Path

There are several forms of the disorder; 80 percent of patients develop the acute chancriform or lympho-cutaneous type of sporotrichosis. In this form, numerous scaly papules that erode and form chronic ulcers usually form in a line starting at the initial site of injury, spreading up the limb.

A disseminated systemic form invades the eye, nervous system, or other organs in a true systemic fungal infection. The skin lesions that may accompany this type of musculoskeletal sporotrichosis are more chronic, and the outlook may not be so positive.

Treatment Options and Outlook

Specific treatment depends on the form of sporotrichosis. In the skin form, iodides (given as an oral solution of potassium iodide) are the preferred method of treatment for up to six weeks. Amphotericin B and flucytosine have also been used to treat the chancriform sporotrichosis. Itraconazole has also been found to be effective.

Systemic sporotrichosis does not respond well to iodide treatment. In this case, amphotericin B is usually necessary. Systemic sporotrichosis in particular may be fatal.

spun-glass hair See UNCOMBABLE HAIR SYNDROME.

squamous cell KERATIN-producing cells that make up most of the EPIDERMIS, lying above the BASAL CELL layer.

See also SQUAMOUS CELL CARCINOMA.

squamous cell carcinoma The second most common SKIN CANCER (after BASAL CELL CARCINOMA) that affects more than 200,000 Americans each year. This type of cancer begins in the SQUAMOUS CELLS that compose most of the upper layer of skin. Squamous cell cancers may be found on all areas of the body, including the mucous membranes, but they are most often found on areas exposed to the sun.

While squamous cell carcinomas start in the top layer of skin, they can eventually spread to underlying tissues if untreated. Rarely, they spread to distant tissues and organs; this can be fatal. Squamous cell carcinomas that metastasize most often begin from chronic inflammatory skin conditions or on the mucous membranes, lips, or ears.

Chronic exposure to sunlight causes most cases of squamous cell cancer, which is why tumors are usually found on areas of the body that are exposed to sunlight. The rim of the ear and the lower lip are particularly prone to this type of cancer.

Squamous cell cancers also may appear on skin that has been injured by burns, scars, long-standing sores, sites previously exposed to X-rays, or chemicals (such as arsenic and petroleum byproducts). In addition, chronic skin inflammation or medical conditions that suppress the immune system for long periods of time may encourage squamous cell carcinoma.

Sometimes squamous cell carcinoma begins spontaneously on what seems to be normal, healthy skin. Some researchers believe this type of cancer may be hereditary.

Anyone with a long history of sun exposure can develop squamous cell cancer, but those with fair skin, light hair, and blue, green, or gray eyes are at highest risk. Dark-skinned individuals are far less likely to develop any form of skin cancer, but more than two-thirds of all skin cancers in African Americans are squamous cell carcinomas found most often on sites of preexisting inflammatory skin conditions or burn injuries.

There are some skin conditions that are associated with eventual development of squamous cell carcinoma. These conditions include ACTINIC KERATOSIS, actinic cheilitis, LEUKOPLAKIA, and BOWEN'S DISEASE. These "precursor" conditions, if properly treated, can be prevented from developing into a squamous cell carcinoma.

Symptoms and Diagnostic Path

Symptoms include a persistent, scaly red patch with irregular borders that sometimes crust or bleed; an elevated growth with a central depression that sometimes bleeds; a wartlike crusting growth that may bleed; an open persistent sore that bleeds and crusts. The lesions usually look like rough, thick, scaly patches that bleed if bumped. They often look like warts, and sometimes an open sore will develop with a raised border and a crusty surface. A diagnosis is made after physical exam and biopsy (removal and examination of a piece of tissue). If tumor cells are found, the physician will outline possible treatment based on type, size, and location of the tumor and on the patient's age and health.

Treatment Options and Outlook

The most frequently used treatment is excision of the entire growth and an additional border of normal skin as a safety margin (excisional surgery). The site is then stitched closed and the tissue is sent to the lab to determine if all malignant cells have been removed.

A physician may use electrosurgery (curettage and electrodesiccation) in which cancerous tissue is scraped from the skin with a curette while an electric needle burns a safety margin of normal skin around the tumor at the base of the scraped area.

This technique is repeated several times to make sure the tumor has been completely removed.

With CRYOSURGERY, the physician does not cut the growth but instead freezes the lesion by applying LIQUID NITROGEN with a special spray or a cotton-tipped applicator; this method doesn't require anesthesia and produces no bleeding. It is easy to administer and is the treatment of choice for those who have bleeding disorders or are intolerant to anesthesia. Patients experience redness, swelling, or blistering, and crusting after this treatment.

LASER SURGERY is used to focus a beam of light onto the lesion either to excise it or destroy it by vaporization. The major advantage of this technique is that it seals blood vessels as it cuts.

In radiation therapy, X-rays are directed at the malignant cells. It usually takes several treatments several times a week for a few weeks to totally destroy a tumor. Radiation therapy is most often used with older patients or with those in poor health. Radiation may be less traumatic for the elderly.

Mohs' surgery (microscopically controlled surgery) involves the removal of very thin layers of the malignant tumor, checking each layer thoroughly under a microscope. This is repeated as often as necessary until the tissue is free of tumor. This method saves the most healthy tissue and has the highest cure rate. It is often used for tumors that recur, for large tumors, or for areas where recurrences are most common (nose, ears, and around the eyes).

When removed early, squamous cell carcinomas are easily treated, but the larger the growth the more extensive the treatment. While squamous cell carcinoma does not spread to vital organs very often, if it does it can be fatal. Since removal of a tumor scars the skin, large tumors may require reconstructive surgery and skin grafts.

If a patient is diagnosed with one squamous cell carcinoma, there is a greater chance of developing other squamous cell carcinomas in the future. Having had a BASAL CELL CARCINOMA also makes it more likely that a squamous cell cancer will develop. No matter how carefully a tumor is removed, another can develop in the same place (or nearby), usually within the first two years after surgery. If the cancer recurs, the physician may recommend a different type of treatment the second time. It is therefore important to examine the surgical site periodically.

See also MELANOMA, MALIGNANT.

staphylococcal infections A group of infections caused by staphylococci bacteria that are a common source of skin conditions. Staphylococcal bacteria are normally found on the skin of most people, but if the bacteria accumulate within the skin, they can cause a wide variety of skin infections (PUSTULES, BOILS, IMPETIGO, FOLLICULITIS, ABSCESS, STY, or CARBUNCLE).

One strain of the bacteria produces a toxin that can cause a severe blistering rash in newborn babies called staphylococcal SCALDED SKIN SYNDROME. Another produces the toxin responsible for TOXIC SHOCK SYNDROME.

staphylococcal scalded skin syndrome See also SCALDED SKIN SYNDROME.

Stein-Leventhal syndrome An endocrine disorder causing excess hairiness also known as polycystic ovary syndrome. In this disorder, the ovaries increase testosterone production, increasing blood levels of the male hormone. About 20 percent of women with this problem have ACNE.

Symptoms and Diagnostic Path

This disorder is characterized by incomplete development of follicles in the ovary due to inadequate secretion of luteinizing hormone; the follicles fail to ovulate and remain as multiple cysts, distending the ovary. Hormone imbalance results in obesity and hairiness (HIRSUTISM), and the sufferer becomes infertile due to the lack of ovulation.

Treatment Options and Outlook

Administration of antiandrogens such as spironolactone, cimetidine, or cyproterone acetate and the oral contraceptive pill to suppress gonadotropic hormones. A wedge resection of the ovaries may help some women.

Stevens-Johnson syndrome A rare condition involving the skin and mucous membranes (erythema multiforme major) characterized by fever and a variety of skin lesions, including red PAPULES, erosions, and BLISTERS. When the condition affects only the skin, it is called erythema multiforme minor, or simply erythema multiforme. The condition is most often caused by drug reactions, and while it may occur at any age, it is most common in children and young adults.

Symptoms and Diagnostic Path

A fever and malaise may precede by several days the appearance of skin lesions, and there may be extensive involvement of the skin, lips, oral areas, and mucous membranes.

Treatment Options and Outlook

Painkillers and sedatives may relieve the pain; while Stevens-Johnson patients usually respond to treatment, they may become seriously ill if shock or infection set in. Patients usually survive with some scarring, eye problems, and nail dystrophy. Controversy exists over whether systemic steroids are indicated in this condition.

See also ERYTHEMA MULTIFORME.

Stewart-Treves tumor A type of tumor that is closely related to angiosarcoma, which often appears in the upper extremities after radical mastectomy for breast cancer. The tumor, which is unrelated to the breast cancer, usually appears about 10 years after the original surgery and after long-standing swelling in the lymph nodes in the upper extremity.

Symptoms and Diagnostic Path

Onset of this tumor is usually fairly quick, with the appearance of a blue-purple patch on the upper arm followed by red-blue or purple NODULES or BLISTERS. Larger lesions may spread quickly, through the lymph system and blood vessels, to the lungs, pleura, and thoracic wall.

Treatment Options and Outlook

There is no truly effective treatment; the tumors and lesions usually recur even after radical surgery.

sting An injury caused by a plant or animal toxin introduced into the skin.

stork bite nevus A type of vascular malformation, this is a harmless small, flat, pink skin blemish found around the nape of the neck in up to 50 percent of newborn babies. It may persist indefinitely.

Salmon patches are similar blemishes found around the eyes in a similar percentage of newborns. These blemishes usually disappear within the first year.

stratum corneum Latin for the "horny layer," the top layer of EPIDERMIS that consists of dead cells. Because the surface of this layer is acidic, it is sometimes also referred to as the acid mantle. The *stratum corneum* gets its name from the fact that when tightly compacted, its cells toughen, like an animal's horn (and mammal horns are made of the same protein material that makes up the stratum corneum).

The cells of this SKIN layer are constantly sloughed from the skin's surface and are completely replaced about every two weeks by cells migrating upward from below. If for some reason horny cells accumulate on the skin surface, the result will be flaky skin. This is a particular problem for those with dark skin because of the sharp contrast between the gray flakes and the surrounding skin.

This layer of the skin provides the major physical barrier of the body, and also serves as a shield to the sun's harmful ultraviolet rays. It also blocks the penetration of most substances that touch the skin. Normally only substances smaller than a water molecule can easily penetrate the horny layer, which means that the skin cannot "drink up" vitamins, nutrients, COLLAGEN, or ELASTIN because their molecular structure is larger than water.

stratum germinativum The base of the EPIDERMIS also known as the basal layer where SKIN cells are constantly germinated anew. New cells are constantly produced in the basal layer, eventually migrating upward through the epidermis to the surface of the skin. The basal layer is composed not only of basal cells, but also of MELANOCYTES,

the pigment-forming cells of the skin that produce MELANIN, responsible for giving skin its color.

stratum granulosum A part of the EPIDERMIS, the stratum granulosum consists of two or three rows of cells lying directly below the STRATUM LUCIDUM, which lies below the STRATUM CORNEUM.

stratum lucidum The epidermal cell layer between the STRATUM CORNEUM and the STRATUM GRANULOSUM.

stratum malpighii The major layer of the EPIDERMIS, consisting of six to 10 layers of keratinocytes.

stratum spinosum The middle layer of the EPIDERMIS, also known as the SKIN's "prickle cell layer" because of its spiny, hairlike prickly projections linking the cells in this area. The cells within this thickest part of the epidermis are called SQUAMOUS CELLS (basal cells that have matured and migrated upward through the epidermis).

strawberry birthmark A bright red, raised, lumpy BIRTHMARK, also called strawberry nevus, strawberry HEMANGIOMA, or, the correct term, superficial HEMANGIOMA. About 2 percent of all infants develop this type of birthmark.

Symptoms and Diagnostic Path
They typically appear at about one to four weeks of age and may quickly grow over the new few months; they stop growing between six and 12 months and gradually disappear over the next few years. Experts cannot predict what will happen to a strawberry birthmark; some will disappear by age two and about 60 percent will be gone by age five. Between 90 and 95 percent will have disappeared by age nine.

Treatment Options and Outlook
Because these birthmarks eventually disappear on their own, treatment is not always recommended.

Data show a good response to the pulsed dye laser. The PULSED DYE LASER is effective at slowing growth during the proliferative phase, and may help to speed resolution of an already-regressing hemangioma.

DERMATOLOGISTS recommend that most superficial hemangiomas be left untreated. However, treatment should be started early if the hemangioma is on the face, or near the eyes, nose, or mouth, or if it grows rapidly or interferes with function of vital organs. Treatment of rapidly growing hemangiomas is performed every two weeks. Once growth has stabilized, treatment is given every four weeks.

streptocerciasis A type of infection caused by a roundworm (*Dipetalonema streptocerca*) found only in the tropical rain forests of western and central Africa that causes a chronic DERMATITIS similar to onchocerciasis (a tropical skin disease caused by a parasitic worm).

streptococcal infections A group of infections caused by bacteria of the streptococcus family, among the most common bacteria that affect humans.

Group A streptococcus is a bacterium responsible for a variety of health problems ranging from mild skin infection or "strep throat" to severe, life-threatening conditions such as TOXIC SHOCK SYNDROME and NECROTIZING FASCIITIS (flesh-eating disease). Experts estimate that more than 10 million mild throat and skin infections occur every year. Other strep infections responsible for a wide range of skin problems include ERIPSIPELAS, CELLULITIS, ECHTHYMA, and SCARLET FEVER. In addition to strep throat and superficial skin infections, group A strep bacteria can cause infections in tissues at specific body sites, including lungs, bones, spinal cord, and abdomen.

Strep infections can be spread by direct contact with saliva or nasal discharge from an infected person, usually not as a result of casual contact but from a crowded environment such as a dormitory or institutional setting. There also have been reports of contaminated food causing infection.

Symptoms and Diagnostic Path

Once exposed, a person can get sick within three days and can pass the infection to others for up to two or three weeks, even if there are no symptoms. After 24 hours of antibiotic treatment, the patient is no longer able to spread the germs.

Some types of group A strep bacteria cause severe infections, including BACTEREMIA, toxic shock syndrome, and necrotizing fasciitis. According to the Centers for Disease Control and Prevention, 4,844 cases of severe group A streptococcal disease were reported in 2003. All severe group A strep infections can cause shock, organ failure, and death.

These infections can be diagnosed with blood counts, urine tests, or cultures of blood or fluid from a wound site.

Treatment Options and Outlook

Antibiotics used to treat these severe infections include PENICILLIN, ERYTHROMYCIN, and CLINDAMYCIN. In severe cases of strep infection, a health care provider may need to remove the tissue surgically or amputate the limb.

stress and the skin The SKIN is the "window to the mind," and to an astonishing degree, it can reveal a person's emotional state. Humans blush when they are embarrassed; blanch when they are afraid, and turn red when angry.

It is not surprising that stress, which can have a profound impact on the emotions and the physical health of the body, also can cause profound effects – on the skin. In fact, experts believe a wide range of skin problems (ACNE, ECZEMA, ROSACEA, HERPES, PSORIASIS, and HIVES) can be worsened or even triggered by stress.

Stress can make new skin lesions appear, or make already existing skin problems worse. In fact, people who are most at risk for developing stress-related skin problems are those who have problem skin to start with. This is most likely due to the fact that when people are under stress, they may work long hours, eat unhealthy meals, neglect their exercise or sleep needs.

Abusing ALCOHOL also can damage the skin, since alcohol increases the flow of blood to the skin. Alcohol use is particularly troubling to skin conditions such as rosacea, hives, flushing, and psoriasis. Nicotine, on the other hand, constricts blood vessels, which reduces the supply of blood to the skin. This is one reason why the skin of chronic smokers looks pale and deeply lined, leading to the "smoker's mask."

Treatment Options and Outlook

If stress is worsening the condition of the skin, individuals should:

- avoid picking or scratching skin
- use a noncomedogenic moisturizer that clog pores, but will combat dryness
- avoid exotic ingredients that could cause an allergic reaction
- drink lots of water to improve the skin's tone and texture
- try relaxation techniques, biofeedback, and so on to lessen stress

stretch marks Also known medically as "striae," these lines on the skin are caused by thinning and loss of elasticity in the underlying skin area.

Symptoms and Diagnostic Path

Stretch marks first appear as red, raised lines that turn purple, flatten, and fade to form shiny streaks between a quarter-inch and a half-inch wide. These marks may strike during adolescence, appearing on thighs and hips of young girls during their growth spurt. They are also common in pregnancy; about 75 percent of pregnant women experience the marks on breasts, thighs, and lower abdomen. In addition, purple stretch marks may occur in patients with Cushing's syndrome and in those using excess CORTICOSTEROID hormones, which suppress the formation of collagen (skin fiber), causing COLLAGEN to waste away.

Treatment Options and Outlook

TRETINOIN (Retin-A) has been found to help fade red early stretch marks significantly, and in some cases even make them disappear, as long as the

marks are new and still pink. Retin-A dose not work on stretch marks that have turned white.

Caution: Pregnant women and nursing mothers should not use Retin-A, because it crosses the placenta and is also found in breast milk. For both red (early) and white (late) stretch marks, lasers are the treatment of choice. The pulsed-dye laser and the intense pulsed light source are two of several laser and light sources that improve stretch marks.

striae See STRETCH MARKS.

strongyloidiasis An intestinal infestation of tiny parasitic roundworms that cause itching and raised red patches on the skin where the worms enter. The disease, caused by *Strongyloides stercoralis*, is found throughout the tropics, especially in the Far East.

The worms are picked up by walking barefoot on soil contaminated with feces. The larvae enter the skin of the feet and migrate to the small intestines where they develop into adulthood, burrowing into the intestinal walls and producing larvae.

Symptoms and Diagnostic Path

After infestation, the worms cause redness, swelling, itching, or HIVES, fading within two days. If the larvae penetrate the perianal area, skin lesions begin to radiate from the anus down the thigh or across the buttocks or abdomen as itchy bands. While the individual lesion may fade away within a few days, an infestation may continue in the host for many years and cause recurrent problems.

Treatment Options and Outlook

Thiabendazole administered for two days is the treatment of choice. Rarely, death may occur from blood poisoning or meningitis many years after the infestation occurs.

Sturge-Weber syndrome (SW) A rare congenital condition (also called trigeminal angiomatosis) that affects the skin and brain. Sturge-Weber syndrome is caused by a spontaneous genetic mutation; it is not transmitted by parents who carry the gene. How often the condition occurs in babies is not known, and because it is not often diagnosed it is difficult to estimate how many people currently have the disease.

Symptoms and Diagnostic Path

The most obvious symptom is a facial PORT-WINE STAIN birthmark present at birth, usually over one side of the face, including at least one upper eyelid and the forehead. However, each case of Sturge-Weber is unique and symptoms vary.

Neurological problems include unusual blood vessel growths on the brain (angiomas) that usually cause seizures beginning before age one, and worsening with age. Convulsions usually appear on the side of the body opposite the port wine stain and vary in severity.

About 30 percent of patients with Sturge-Weber also develop glaucoma in the eye affected by the port-wine stain. Enlarging of the eye also can occur in the eye that is involved with the stain. In some cases, strokes can occur.

Treatment Options and Outlook

Visible light lasers (argon, dye, and heavy metal lasers) are the treatments of choice for children as young as 12 months, although lesions respond variably according to their color, thickness, size, and site. The birthmark can be hidden with specially designed masking makeup. Seizures can be controlled with anticonvulsant drugs, and in severe cases, surgery may be performed on the affected part of the brain to treat glaucoma and other eye problems.

See also CAMOUFLAGE COSMETICS.

sty   A small PUS-filled ABSCESS (also called a hordeolum) near the eyelashes caused by an infection with *Staphylococcus aureus.*

Treatment Options and Outlook

Warm compresses administered for 20 minutes, four times daily, may help eliminate the pus, reduce swelling, and decrease pain. An antibiotic ointment designed for the eyes can help prevent a recurrence.

subcutaneous   A medical term referring to the area beneath the SKIN.

subcutaneous fat, atrophy of   See FAT ATROPHY.

subcutaneous fatty tissue   Also known as subcutis, this is the bottommost layer of skin, found under the DERMIS. This layer serves as a cushion for internal organs and also as a storage site for reserve energy. The amount and distribution of this fatty tissue throughout the body is believed to be governed largely by heredity and by how much a person eats.

subcutis   See SUBCUTANEOUS FATTY TISSUE.

subungual hematoma   A blood-filled bruise under the fingernail caused by direct trauma, such as slamming the finger in a door. The pain can be eased by puncturing the nail plate with a drill or fine scalpel blade; otherwise, the nail may be shed. If the injury affects the matrix of the nail, it may form permanent deformity of the nail, with ridging or a split.

sulfapyridine   A long-acting sulfa drug used to treat blistering diseases such as DERMATITIS HERPETIFORMIS.

Side Effects

This drug can cause severe allergic reactions, anemia, and a decrease in the number of white cells in the body. To prevent kidney problems, patients should drink plenty of liquids.

sulfonamide drugs   The first available anti-bacterial drugs. These medications are used to treat skin infections, among other things. Before the development of PENICILLIN drugs, the sulfonamides were widely used to treat other infections.

The sulfa drugs are usually given by mouth, and most are quickly absorbed from the stomach and small intestines.

Side Effects

A variety of side effects may occur, including nausea, vomiting, headache, and appetite loss. More severe side effects include blood disorders, skin rashes, and fever. Patients taking sulfa drugs should avoid sun exposure.

sulfones One of a group of drugs closely related to the sulfa drugs in their structure and the way they act. Sulfones are powerful agents in the fight against bacteria that cause LEPROSY. The two sulfones most often used in dermatologic practices are DAPSONE and SULFAPYRIDINE. Other skin diseases in which sulfones are used include subcorneal pustular dermatosis, acne conglobata, PYODERMA GANGRENOSUM, BULLOUS PEMPHIGOID, cicatricial pemphigoid, chronic bullous dermatosis of childhood, erythema elevatum diutinum, relapsing POLYCHONDRITIS, GRANULOMA ANNULARE, granuloma faciale, bullous eruption of systemic lupus erythematosus, leukocytoclastic vasculitis, actinomycotic mycetoma, alopecia mucinosa, pustular psoriasis, HERPES GESTATIONNIS, PEMPHIGUS, Weber-Christian PANNICULITIS, BROWN RECLUSE SPIDER BITES, and HAILEY-HAILEY DISEASE.

Patients who take these drugs require frequent evaluation, including complete blood counts with differential white counts, a chemistry profile (including liver and kidney tests), urine tests, and methemoglobin level.

sulfur An important mineral component of vitamin B_1 and of several essential amino acids. Sulfur is particularly necessary for the body's production of COLLAGEN, which helps to form connective tissue. Sulfur is also a component of KERATIN, the chief ingredient in hair, skin and nails.

In addition, sulfur is one of the oldest of the modern drugs and a popular ACNE treatment, although its action is still not well understood. Researchers believe that it is effective by controlling bacteria and exfoliating the skin.

Many studies suggest that a combination of BENZOYL PEROXIDE and sulfur is more effective than sulfur used alone. Sulfur is thought to dissolve the top layer of dry dead cells and slow down oil-gland activity, which is why it is used in acne soaps, lotions and dandruff SHAMPOOS.

The highest concentration of sulfur in over-the-counter medication is 10 percent. Sulfur may cause a mild sensitivity and allergic reactions, and can irritate the eyes. Discontinue use if skin sensitivity occurs.

While most experts consider benzoyl peroxide and sulfur safe when used as single ingredients, products that combine the two increase the possibility of sensitivity to benzoyl peroxide. Therefore, combination products are not available without prescription.

In addition, sulfur is sometimes added to RESORCINOL (a drug that causes skin to peel) as an acne treatment, although experts aren't sure why this combination works. Resorcinol by itself is not considered to be effective against acne, but it appears to enhance the action of sulfur. Because resorcinol in concentrations above 3 percent appear to be toxic, products with this ingredient are only available over-the-counter in concentrations of 2 percent and less. Products containing resorcinol should not be applied to broken skin or to large areas of the body. In addition, resorcinol may discolor dark or black skin.

Sulfur is not the same as *sulfa,* an abbreviation for a group of antibacterial agents including sulfadiazole and sulfathiazole.

sun blocks See SUNSCREENS.

sunburn Inflammation of the skin as a result of overexposure to the sun. Sunburn occurs when the ultraviolet rays of the sun destroy skin cells in the outer layer of the skin, damaging tiny blood vessels underneath. Sunburn is a particular problem in light-skinned individuals whose skin does not produce much MELANIN, the protective pigment that can guard against damage from the sun.

Symptoms and Diagnostic Path

Sun-exposed skin turns red, becomes very painful and may develop BLISTERS; if the BURN is severe, the individual may also experience symptoms of sunstroke, including vomiting, fever, and collapse. Several days after the skin has burned, the skin may shed its dead cells by peeling. Repeated exposure to sunlight over the years may result in prematurely aged skin and SKIN CANCER; blistering sunburns before age 20 increase the risk of melanoma.

Treatment Options and Outlook

The best idea is to avoid getting sunburned in the first place, because once the skin is burned it has become damaged. While there are many so-called sunburn remedies, none are highly effective. Compresses may help, using a variety of ingredients such as skim milk and water, aluminum acetate baths (as contained in Buro-Sol antiseptic powder or Domeboro's powder), oatmeal, or witch hazel.

Cool (not cold) baths may also be soothing, especially if enhanced with one cup of white vinegar, Aveeno powder (made from oatmeal), or baking soda. Soap or bubble baths should not be used on sunburned skin (they can irritate tender flesh). After a compress or a soaking bath, moisturizer should be applied immediately afterward.

Other home remedies include application of a cornstarch paste, raw cucumber or potato slices, yogurt, or tea bags soaked in cool water. The oil from the aloe plant may be applied directly to the skin for sunburn relief, but the skin should first be tested for allergies.

Risk Factors and Preventive Measures

Exposure to strong sunlight should be limited to 15 minutes on the first day, especially for those with fair skin, increasing exposure slowly each day. Until the skin has tanned, it should be protected with a high-protection SUNSCREEN of at least 15 SPF. Fair-skinned individuals and those who are photosensitive should use a sunscreen with an SPF of 29 or higher. The sun should be avoided between the hours of 10 A.M. and 3 P.M.

Aspirin and nonsteroidal anti-inflammatory drugs (NSAIDs) can prevent sunburn only if taken before exposure to the sun. New types of protective clothing are now available that are equivalent to an SPF of 30; typical clothing is only about as effective as SPF 6.

See also SUN PROTECTION FACTOR; CLOTHES AND SUN PROTECTION; MELANOMA, MALIGNANT.

sun poisoning A common term for a temporary condition of red, itchy bumps caused by sun sensitivity. Some of the causes include POLYMORPHIC LIGHT ERUPTION, photocontact DERMATITIS involving an agent applied to the skin (such as PABA or oxybenzone in SUNSCREENS), and photosensitivity to a systemic drug (such as TETRACYCLINE). The bumps should disappear within a week. Patients should see a doctor if weeping, oozing blisters develop, since this may indicate a possible infection.

Treatment Options and Outlook

Cool compresses and over-the-counter hydrocortisone cream or oral antihistamines.

See also SOLAR WARNING INDEX; SUNBURN; SUNSCREEN; SKIN CANCER.

sun protection factor (SPF) A rating system for SUNSCREEN products that measures how effectively it works; the higher the SPF, the greater the amount of protection from the sun. For example, an SPF of 15 means that an individual using the sunscreen could spend up to 15 times longer in the sun without burning. An SPF value is assigned by manufacturers of sun protecting cosmetics for items such as sunscreens, creams, lipsticks, cosmetic milks, and lotions. Most SPF rating only apply to UVB rays. A burn is caused by ultraviolet-B (UVB) rays, which are strongest between the hours of 10 A.M. and 4 P.M. However, it is the ultraviolet-A (UVA) rays that age the skin, causing WRINKLES, sagging skin, and brown spots. Standardized ratings for blocking UVA rays are being developed, which is why there are few SPF ratings for UVA numbers on sunscreen bottles.

Experts suggest that sunscreen should have a minimum SPF of 15 to avoid the burning, drying, and wrinkling that results from overexposure to the harmful rays, which are the single most damaging element to the skin. On the other hand, experts at the U.S. Food and Drug Administration criticize sunscreens with SPFs up to 50, charging that consumers may have a false sense of security by using products with very high SPF values.

An SPF of 50 implies that a person can tolerate 50 times the amount of sun that it would normally take to burn, which is not necessarily true. And even a sunscreen with an SPF of 50 lets *some* UVB rays through, so using it does not allow a person to bake for hours in the sun without any risk of cancer or wrinkling, according to some DERMATOLOGISTs.

In addition, the higher the SPF number, the faster the proportional increase in protection diminishes. For example, the difference between an SPF of 45 and one of 30 is only a few percentage points. Most SUNBURNS can be prevented by using a product with an SPF of 30.

There are still some physicians and sunscreen manufacturers who believe that higher SPFs should be available for those who choose to use them. Sweating heavily, swimming, or participating in other water activities reduces the SPF because sweat or water on the skin will lessen the amount of protection the sunscreen provides. Sunscreen needs to be reapplied more frequently during these activities.

For overseas travelers, it is important to realize that not all SPFs are the same. In Europe, the SPF is called DIN (Deutsches Institut fur Normung, the company that developed the system). The DIN uses lower numbers than the American SPF system for equivalent sun protection. For example, an SPF 12 is equal to DIN 9; SPF 19 is DIN 15.

sunscreens   Products that protect the skin from the harmful effects of sunlight's harmful radiation; all sunscreen products protect against ultraviolet-B (UVB); some products protect against both ultraviolet-A (UVA) and UVB. Sunscreens are used primarily to avoid SUNBURN and suntanning, although they can also be used to prevent the rash in patients' PHOTOSENSITIVITY. They also prevent skin cancer and the aging effects of the sun on the skin.

While some skin exposure to sunlight is necessary for the body to produce VITAMIN D, overexposure can have a range of harmful effects, especially in fair-skinned people. Most sunscreens, including those preparations containing para-aminobenzoic acid (PABA) or benzophenone, work by absorbing ultraviolet rays of the sun. Products containing other substances (such as TITANIUM DIOXIDE, an uncolored relative of ZINC OXIDE) *reflect* the sun's rays.

Sunscreens are designed to protect against UVB light, the type of radiation that causes sunburn. No sunscreens screen out all UVA rays, another kind of ultraviolet light produced by the sun that can damage the skin and may play a role in malignant melanoma simply because sunlight contains so much of it. (Think UVA-*aging*, UVB-*burn* plus *aging*).

Some sunscreens may advertise protection from UVA rays; there is no standardized rating for UVA protection.

The best sunscreens offer a broad spectrum of protection, and include such ingredients as oxybenzone, titanium dioxide, zinc oxide, or Parsol 1789. But while sunscreens are not perfect, they do prevent sunburn, future freckling and brown spots, ACTINIC KERATOSES (precancerous lesions), and SKIN CANCER.

A French blocker called Mexoryl SX, made by the French skin care giant L'Oreal, and shown to be effective in several studies, is contained in some European and Canadian sunscreens, but is not yet approved in the United States. However, some con-

SAFE EXPOSURE TIMES USING SUNSCREENS			
PROTECTION FACTOR	**4**	**8**	**15**
SKIN TYPE	SAFE EXPOSURE TIME		
Fair	10 minutes	40–80 minutes	1.5–2 hours
Medium	50–80 minutes	2–2.5 hours	5–5.5 hours
Dark	1.5–2 hours	3.5–4 hours	all day
Black	4 hours	all day	all day

sumers are ordering the product online from out of the country and buying it on auction sites because it blocks both UVA and UVB light and provides better and longer UVA protection than other products available in the United States.

Sunscreens containing this blocker are available in Europe, Asia, and Latin and South America.

Consumers can still develop sun-induced aging and skin cancer even if they do not get a sunburn. The only way to completely protect against aging and skin cancer is to avoid the sun.

SPF

Sunscreen products are labeled with a SUN PROTECTION FACTOR (SPF), which is a measure of how effectively the sunscreen works; the highest factor indicates the greatest amount of protection. Sunscreen with a minimum SPF of 15 should be used to avoid burning, drying, and wrinkling that results from chronic overexposure. An SPF of 15 means that individuals using the sunscreen could spend up to 15 times longer in the sun without burning than if they weren't wearing it. However, the SPF applies only to UVB; no effective rating for UVA currently exists.

An SPF 15 blocks 94 percent of UVB rays and an SPF 30 blocks 98 percent. However, since many people skimp when applying sunscreen or apply it unevenly, experts rationalize that skimping when applying SPF 15 might mean the consumer ends up with the equivalent of an SPF 6, whereas skimping when using an SPF of 30 or higher still provides adequate protection. A full ounce should be applied each time.

The U.S. Food and Drug Administration (FDA) revised sunscreen labeling to include a maximum SPF 30 on all sunscreens, the use of the terms "water-resistant" and "very water resistant" instead of "waterproof," charts to match skin types with the appropriate SPF numbers, and stricter guidelines on anti-aging claims.

How to Apply

Experts suggest that adults should use an ounce of sunscreen (about a shot glass full) to properly protect an average-sized person. Sunscreens should be reapplied every two hours, and again after swimming; waterproof or water-resistant sunscreens can be applied less often, but experts recommend an extra application after swimming if there is any uncertainty about the need for more.

Sunscreen should be applied before going outside (even in cloudy weather, since 80 percent of the Sun's rays break through the clouds).

Sunscreen Allergies

Some people are allergic to the chemicals contained in sunscreens and can develop a skin rash. The most common ingredients to cause an allergic reaction are PABA and oxybenzone.

Fortunately, new chemical-free sunscreens are now being developed that contain physical sunblocks (such as titanium dioxide and talc) broken down into tiny particles that can be formulated into clear, invisible lotions instead of the white zinc-oxide creams. The nonchemical sunscreens block both UVA and UVB rays far better than most chemical sunscreens.

Other Protective Factors

A more controversial approach to sunscreen developments is the addition of other protective factors, such as VITAMINS E and C (antioxidants that neutralize free radicals, which are unstable oxygen molecules that damage skin). The goal is to prevent or delay damage to skin cells by screening out some of the premature-aging effects of sunlight while allowing the triggering of vitamin D, but many dermatologists are skeptical.

Because the wavelength of light that stimulates vitamin D production in the skin is UVB, some have voiced concern regarding the overuse of UVB sunscreens. However, since it takes only 15 minutes two or three times a week to spur vitamin D synthesis in the skin, very few people have to worry about not getting enough sun exposure.

Rating Sunscreens

The Skin Cancer Foundation rates sunscreens; consumers should look for their seal of approval on all sunscreen products. Sunscreens that have the foundation's "seal" on the label have met stringent criteria that exceed those of the FDA; in order to rate the foundation's approval, the product must prove that it helps prevent sun-induced damage to the skin. The product must have an SPF of 15 or higher and include substantiation for any claims that a sunscreen is waterproof, water-, or sweat-resistant. The seal is also granted to SELF-TANNING PRODUCTS that include a sunscreen; this sunscreen must meet the same requirements as regular sunscreen. Clothing is still considered to be the best protection against sun-induced skin aging and skin cancer of all types.

Protective Clothing

It is a good idea to wear some type of sun-protective clothing specially designed to block the harmful rays of the sun, such as SOLUMBRA.

See also PABA; SUN POISONING; SOLAR WARNING INDEX.

sunstroke Also called heatstroke, this condition is caused by excess exposure to heat and the sun, and is characterized by feelings of dizziness and nausea. However, in some people (especially the elderly) it can involve a very high body temperature and lack of sweating followed by loss of consciousness. For these individuals, this condition is potentially fatal unless treated quickly.

Treatment Options and Outlook

Quick cooling is the most important aspect of treatment for sunstroke. An ice bag or crushed ice should be applied; alternatively, the patient should be wrapped in a wet sheet and hosed down with cold water until emergency medical help arrives.

See also SUNBURN.

suntan The result of the body's attempt at protecting itself from the damage of the Sun's ultraviolet rays. During exposure to the Sun, the skin begins to produce more of the dark pigment called MELANIN to absorb the damaging rays. The result is a darkened skin tone.

While a suntan is widely considered to be desirable, it is in fact a sign that the skin has been damaged. Melanin provides some protection from skin damage and is the reason why dark-skinned individuals usually get fewer WRINKLES than fair-skinned individuals given the same amount of sun exposure.

Even with frequent applications of SUNSCREEN, sunbathers may be at risk for developing skin cancer, including melanoma (the most serious form of skin cancer). Newest findings have found that not only ultraviolet-B (UVB) light (rays that cause sunburn, between 280 and 320 nanometers) but also light with longer wavelengths—including ultraviolet-A (UVA) light—can fuel a series of changes in skin cells.

In the past several years, scientists began to agree that UVA light does indeed play a greater role in causing some skin disorders. Although experts still believe that UVB is responsible for much of the sun-related skin damage (especially SUNBURN) UVA is important in making the skin look aged (with wrinkles, brown spots) and to a lesser extent, SKIN CANCERS.

About 65 percent of melanomas and 90 percent of basal and squamous cell skin cancers are attributed to UV exposure. Although the exact wavelengths of UV light that contribute to the development of skin cancer is unknown, it is most likely a UVB wavelength. Most sunscreens do a good job blocking UVB, but fewer sunscreens filter out most of the UVA.

Controversy about how well sunscreen protects against cancer occurs because experts do not know whether melanoma and other skin cancers are caused by exposure to UVB, UVA, or both. Since most sunscreens protect only against UVB, using a sunscreen may be of no value if cancer is caused by UVA. Moreover, people using a UVB-only sunscreen may stay out longer than they would have in the sun, thus potentially increasing their risk.

The Sun's rays do not just stay on the surface of the skin; they also penetrate deep beneath the skin, where they can damage the COLLAGEN network, the springy web of fibers that support and strengthen skin. This damage actually can be reversed in part by staying out of the sun and by long-term use of Retin-A.

See also CLOTHES AND SUN PROTECTION; MELANOMA, MALIGNANT; SUNBURN; SUN PROTECTION FACTOR; TANNING BEDS.

suppuration The formation of pus at the site of bacterial infection. The pus may also accumulate, forming an ABSCESS (in solid tissue) or a BOIL or PUSTULE on the skin. Open sores often weep pus like this, especially when they do not heal well, because the exposed tissue gets reinfected with bacteria again and again.

surfer's nodules Lesions caused by repeated friction of the tops of the feet and the knees against a surfboard. This condition will disappear if the patient stops surfing; otherwise, local injections of a low-dose cortisone will help.

sweat Sweating is the body's way of keeping its internal temperature at a constant 98.6°. When the body's temperature rises, the body's SWEAT GLANDS are stimulated to start producing water to cool off the body. When this happens, sweating is heaviest on the forehead, upper lips, neck, and chest.

Sweat is made primarily of water and some tiny amounts of other substances (such as salt). Perspiration itself, regardless of the type of sweat gland from which it originates, is odorless—the smell occurs when sweat mixes with bacteria (especially in the armpits).

Sweating is an involuntary process, a response to the environment or to psychological factors such as embarrassment or stress. People who experience excess sweating (HYPERHIDROSIS) need to be

referred to a physician, since such sweating may be a sign of hormonal imbalance.

sweat glands Sweat glands are spread out all across the body in varying concentrations that are designed to produce perspiration. Each gland has a tube for secreting sweat and a narrow passage that carries sweat to the skin's surface. Most people have about 3 million sweat glands in two types—apocrine and eccrine glands.

Apocrine glands lie heavily coiled in mostly hairy areas (the armpits, the nipples, genital, and anal areas, and around the navel), located deep within the fatty tissue. This is the gland that secrets the type of sweat associated with body odor, mostly under the armpits. Apocrine glands secrete a milky sweat into the upper portion of the HAIR FOLLICLE, and from there to the skin surface. This sweat is broken down by bacteria on the skin, causing body odor. While it is believed that the apocrine glands in other mammals serve as a sexual stimulant, their function in humans is not known. Like SEBACEOUS GLANDS, the apocrine glands do not mature and begin secreting until puberty.

Eccrine glands are the most common (especially on hands and feet), and like apocrine glands they are heavily coiled in the fatty tissue layer. Eccrine glands secrete clear, watery sweat through their own pores, not along hair follicles. Exercise, hot weather, fever, and emotional stress can stimulate eccrine sweating over the entire surface of the body (but concentrated on the soles of the feet, forehead, palms, and armpits). They appear to be more strongly linked to stimulation by emotional stress than by heat. Eccrine glands are mostly water and do not cause body odor; they serve to regulate body temperature and to help eliminate waste salts.

See also HYPERHIDROSIS; SWEAT GLANDS, DISORDERS OF.

Cross Section of Skin Showing Sweat Glands

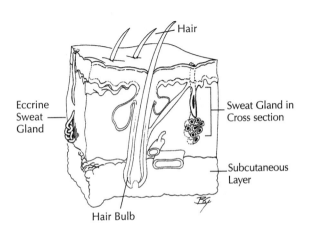

Eccrine Sweat Gland

Hair

Sweat Gland in Cross section

Subcutaneous Layer

Hair Bulb

sweat glands, disorders of There are a number of disorders that can affect the sweat glands. The most common is PRICKLY HEAT, an intense, irritating skin rash caused by blocked sweat glands. Less commonly, the sweat glands may be affected by HYPERHIDROSIS, a type of profuse sweating that often requires medical treatment and can cause highly embarrassing social problems. HYPOHIDROSIS (reduced sweating), a less common problem, occurs in ectodermal dysplasia syndrome.

swimmer's ear   See OTITIS EXTERNA.

swimmer's itch   The common name for cutaneous SCHISTOSOMIASIS, or cercarial dermatitis, this is an itchy skin inflammation caused by bites from flatworms. This disorder features a distinctive papular eruption after swimming in or having contact with freshwater populated by ducks and snails.

This type of dermatitis is a potential risk whenever people use an aquatic area with animals and mollusks who harbor the schistosomes. In the United States, the worst outbreaks occur in the lake regions of Michigan, Wisconsin, and Minnesota. A more serious tropical disease is visceral schistosomiasis.

Symptoms and Diagnostic Path

After exposure to water containing schistosomes, a prickling or itchy feeling begins that can last up to an hour while the flukes enter the skin. Small red MACULES form, but there may be swelling or wheals among sensitive people. Also these lesions begin to disappear, they are replaced after 10 or 15 hours by discrete, very itchy PAPULES surrounded by a red area. VESICLES and pustules form one or two days later; the lesions fade away within a week, leaving small pigmented spots. Different symptoms depend on how sensitive the patient is to the schistosome. Each reexposure causes a more severe reaction.

Treatment Options and Outlook

CALAMINE lotion or oral ANTIHISTAMINES may help control the itch until the lesions begin to disappear on their own.

Risk Factors and Preventive Measures

The best way to alleviate the problem is to destroy the snails by treating the water with copper sulfate and carbonate, or with sodium pentachloro-

phenate. A thick coating of grease or tightly woven clothes can protect against infestation. Bathing with a hexachlorophene soap before swimming may help to some degree. Briskly rubbing the skin with a towel after swimming may help remove some organisms.

swimming pool granuloma   A disorder of the skin caused by a mycobacterium in swimming pool water characterized by ABSCESSES on the hands, over the fingers, or on the knees. The problem is also found in those who own tropical fish tanks; if a person cleans the tank and scratches a hand against objects in the tank, the organism can penetrate the abrasion; weeks later, a lesion may form.

A swimming pool granuloma results when water contains an infectious organism, *Mycobacterium marinum*, enters a traumatized area of skin and produces a localized infection called a granuloma.

Symptoms and Diagnostic Path

Swimming pool granulomas appear approximately six to eight weeks after exposure to the organism, appearing as reddish bumps that slowly enlarge into purplish NODULES. The nodules may break down and ulcerate, leaving an open sore.

The lesions generally disappear over a period of months to more than a year. There is no evidence of systemic disease associated with *M. marinum*, but this organism may pose a threat to immunocompromised people.

The condition is diagnosed with a biopsy of the lesion, and a culture of lesion demonstrating *M. marinum*. A PPD tuberculin skin test will usually be positive.

Treatment Options and Outlook

Treatment includes local heat therapy and minocycline.

sycosis vulgaris   See BARBER'S ITCH.

syphilis   A sexually transmitted infection found around the world that causes (among other symptoms) a skin sore and rash. Also present as an infection at birth, syphilis was first recorded as a major epidemic in Europe during the 15th century.

Today, the infection is transmitted almost exclusively by sexual contact. Since the 1970s and early 1980s, the incidence of syphilis in the United States has been on the rise.

Syphilis is caused by a spirochete *Treponema pallidum* that enters broken skin or mucous membranes during sexual intercourse, by kissing, or by intimate bodily contact with an infected person. The rate of infection during a single contact with an infected person is about 30 percent.

Symptoms and Diagnostic Path

During the first (or primary) stage, a sore appears between three to four weeks after contact; the sore has a hard, wet painless base that heals in about a month. In men, the sore appears on the shaft of the penis. In women it can be found on the labia, although it is often hidden so well that the diagnosis is missed. In both sexes, the sore also may be seen on the lips or tongue.

Six to 12 weeks after infection, the patient enters the *secondary stage,* which features a skin rash that may last for months. The rash has crops of pink or pale red round spots, but in black patients the rash is pigmented and appears darker than normal skin. The eruption can be mistaken for PITYRIASIS ROSEA. In addition, the lymph nodes may be enlarged, and there may be backache, headache, bone pain, appetite loss, fever, fatigue, and sometimes meningitis. The hair may fall out and the skin may exhibit gray or pink patches (condylomata) that are highly infectious. The secondary stage may last up to a year.

The *latent stage* may last for a few years or until the end of a person's life. During this time, the infected person appears normal; about 30 percent of these patients will develop tertiary syphilis.

Tertiary syphilis (end stage) usually begins about 10 years after the initial infection, although it may appear after only about three years or as late as 25 years later. The person's tissues may begin to deteriorate (a process called "gumma formation"), involving the bones, palate, nasal septum, tongue, skin, or any organ of the body. The most serious complications in this stage include heart problems,

and brain damage (neurosyphilis) leading to insanity and paralysis.

Treatment Options and Outlook

PENICILLIN is the drug of choice for all forms of the disease; early syphilis can often be cured by a single large injection; later forms of the disease may require a longer course of the drug. More than half of syphilis patients treated with penicillin develop a severe reaction within six to 12 hours caused by the body's response to the sudden killing of large numbers of spirochete.

Risk Factors and Preventive Measures

Infection can be avoided by maintaining monogamous relationships; condoms offer some protection, but they are not absolutely safe. People with syphilis are infectious during the primary and secondary stages, but not in the late latent and tertiary stages.

syringomas Benign growths of the sweat ducts that look like small skin-colored lumps on the eyelids, trunk, and cheeks; they may occur among several family members.

Symptoms and Diagnostic Path

These harmless painless lumps, which are really enlarged, underdevelop SWEAT GLANDS, typically appear during adolescence and adulthood.

Treatment Options and Outlook

They can be removed by minor surgery for cosmetic reasons, but many individuals choose to ignore these skin growths.

systemic disease, skin symptoms of In many ways, the skin can be a window into the health of the body, mirroring internal disease. Changes can appear in thickness, color, texture, or sensation. Problems with immune function or with blood flow can trigger the appearance of HIVES, PURPURA (purple skin patches), BLISTERS, or deadened areas of skin.

Skin findings may be important in diagnosing cancer and a host of systemic diseases affecting any of the body's organ systems, such as the gastrointestinal tract, eye, kidneys, lungs, heart, blood vessels, cardiovascular system, musculoskeletal, or endocrine system.

Generalized itching is one skin symptom that may be associated with systemic disease. If there are no other skin diseases to explain it, itching of unknown origin (or "idiopathic" itching) may be associated with Hodgkin's disease, polycythemia rubra vera, liver or kidney disease, thyroid disease, hypoparathyroidism, infections, or drug reactions.

systemic lupus erythematosus (SLE) The more serious and potentially fatal form of the chronic circulatory disease LUPUS ERYTHEMATOSUS that affects many systems of the body, including the skin. (The milder form is DISCOID LUPUS ERYTHEMATOSUS, or DLE.)

SLE is probably not one, but several, conditions; although typically a disease of young women, it can affect either sex and all age groups without regard to race. The disease commonly waxes and wanes, and its etiology is affected by heredity, autoimmunity, certain drugs, sex hormones, ultraviolet light, and viruses.

The relationship between DLE and SLE is controversial. Between 2 and 20 percent of patients who are first diagnosed with DLE go on to develop SLE. It is not uncommon for typical SLE to go into remission, leaving lesions of chronic DLE. On the other hand, DLE may spontaneously subside, remain constant, worsen, or progress to active SLE after some stress.

Symptoms and Diagnostic Path

Typically there is a red scaly rash on the face, affecting the nose and cheeks, arthritis, and progressive kidney damage; the heart, lungs, and brain may also be affected by progressive attacks of inflammation followed by the formation of scar tissue. In the milder form (DLE) only the skin is affected.

Treatment Options and Outlook

Treatment depends on how active the disease is, and can range from nonprescription pain relievers and anti-inflammatories to prescription medica-

tion, therapy, dietary changes, and lifestyle changes (such as avoiding the sun, wearing sunblock, and avoiding stress).

Nonsteroidal anti-inflammatory drugs (NSAIDS) are used to relieve achy joints and arthritis in mild lupus when pain is limited and organs are not affected. Antimalarial drugs such as hydroxycholorquine are often prescribed for arthritis or skin problems. CORTICOSTERIODS such as prednisone are used for major organ involvement. The dosage prescribed will depend on the type of organ involvement, symptoms, and blood test results. Immunosuppressive agents such as AZATHIPRINE (Imuran), METHOTREXATE, CYCLOPHOSPHAMIDE, CYCLOSPORINE, and mycophenolate mofetil (CellCept), are strong drugs that help control the overactive immune system, helping to limit damage to major organs. However, these powerful drugs carry potentially serious side effects and complications.

The prognosis for patients with SLE depends on which organs are involved; kidney or central nervous system involvement implies a poor prognosis. In most patients the disease is chronic; more than 90 percent of patients survive for at least 10 years.

systemic necrotizing vasculitides A group of inflammatory diseases of the small and medium-size arteries causing palpable NODULES, ulcers, purple patches (PURPURA), or plaques. This group of diseases includes polyarteritis nodosa and WEGENER'S GRANULOMATOSIS.

The survival rate for untreated polyarteritis nodosa is 13 percent; CORTICOSTEROID treatment improves the survival rate to 48 percent and a combination approach using corticosteroids and immunosuppressive agents hikes the rate to 80 percent.

In a variety of polyarteritis nodosa, cutaneous polyarteritis nodosa, patients do not usually develop systemic signs and their prognosis is quite good.

Symptoms and Diagnostic Path

Skin symptoms include palpable purpura (see LEUCOCYTOELASTIC VASCULITIS), tender nodules, purple patches, LIVEDO RETICULARIS, and ulceration. There are a wide variety of nonskin symptoms, including fever, malaise, weight loss, joint or muscle problems, kidney problems, nausea and vomiting, abdominal pain, congestive heart failure, high blood pressure, strokes, and neuropathy.

Symptoms of Wegener's granulomatosis include ulcers, papules and plaques on legs, with ulcers in the mouth. "Saddle nose" may appear as a result of destruction of the cartilage in the nose.

Treatment Options and Outlook

A combination of corticosteroids (prednisone) and cyclophosphamide is the treatment of choice for both diseases, together with a careful control of high blood pressure. In addition, additional treatment with aspirin, sulfapyridine, and DAPSONE may be considered.

systemic sclerosis See SCLERODERMA.

tachyphylaxis The rapid decrease of response to topical steroids. Patients treated with topical COR-TICOSTEROIDS after only one or two weeks but usually after several weeks may find that the product seems to have stopped working. After a week-long rest of that specific corticosteroid, however, the drug usually begins working again.

Substituting one corticosteroid for another type with a slightly different chemical structure may eliminate this problem.

tacrolimus (Protopic) A nonsteroidal topical ointment for the treatment of ECZEMA (atopic dermatitis) that represents an advance in the development of topical steroids. It acts at the site of the immune imbalance to help stop the redness and itching of eczema inflammation. The 0.1 percent concentration of tacrolimus ointment was approved for the treatment of adults, while the lower 0.03 percent concentration was approved for the treatment of both children (ages two and above) and adults for short-term and intermittent long-term therapy.

Protopic's safety and effectiveness was evaluated in 28 worldwide trials with more than 4,000 adults and children, including those as young as 24 months. Research indicates that both concentrations of Protopic significantly improved or cleared the signs and symptoms of the condition in more than two-thirds of the subjects. Many subjects exhibited marked improvement after one week.

Side Effects

About 70 percent of patients experience burning and ITCHING with the application of Protopic; however, the incidence of these events decreased as the disease improved. The results of treatment are so dramatic, even in the worst cases, that the initial burning experienced at the beginning of treatment is worth the discomfort.

tan See SUNTAN.

tanning booths/beds A special booth or bed that emits ultraviolet (UVA) rays that cause the skin to tan. While an estimated 2 million Americans still aim for a rich golden tan from a bed or booth, experts have concluded that the practice is neither safe nor foolproof. In fact, researchers have found that people who use tanning devices have 2.5 times the risk of SQUAMOUS CELL cancer and 1.5 times the risk of BASAL CELL cancer.

These devices were once billed as a way to get a "safe" tan because the artificial ultraviolet light they emit is made up of primarily UVA rays, not UVB rays (the main component of sunlight). However, research suggests that in fact, both types of ultraviolet light are dangerous.

Research suggests that tanning beds may promote aging of the skin and SKIN CANCER. Many consumers do not realize that just 30 minutes in a tanning bed is equal to six to eight hours of nonstop sunning on the beach.

Experts also caution that there is no such thing as a "safe" tan, and a tan from a bed is just as damaging as a tan acquired at the beach.

Only 21 states have laws regulating indoor tanning, and there are no government standards for how much exposure time is safe for different skin types. Furthermore, many salons are staffed by part-time attendants who are poorly trained in safe tanning-bed procedures.

The World Health Organization in 2005 called for a ban on tanning beds and warned that the increasing popularity of tanning beds could result in an "epidemic" of skin cancer within a decade. For that reason, the United Nations health agency is urging governments around the world to pass laws regulating their use and banning them for all people under age 18. Still, the use of tanning beds and sun lamps is largely unregulated around the world, with France, Belgium, and Sweden among the few countries that have legislation on their use. In the United States, some states (including California, Texas, Tennessee, Illinois, and Wisconsin) have passed laws to keep children from using tanning beds.

Finally, many prescription drugs are photosensitizing, including some antibiotics (such as TETRACYCLINE) and thiazides (blood pressure pills). Anyone taking photosensitizing medication can experience severe consequences as a result of using a tanning bed.

tanning pills   Sometimes called "French bronzing pills," these are drugs designed to provide an artificial tan. They are sold outside the United States (and occasionally by mail order or through health food stores in this country). The drugs contain beta-carotene and/or canthaxanthin, chemicals that color the skin but also can damage the eyes and possibly the liver. They are not recommended by DERMATOLOGISTS.

Although canthaxanthin is approved by the U.S. Food and Drug Administration (FDA) for use as a color addictive in foods in small amount, its use in tanning pills is not approved. Imported tanning pills containing canthaxanthin may be automatically seized as products containing unsafe color additives.

Although at least one company applied for approval of canthaxanthin-containing pills as a tanning agent, it withdrew the application when side effects (such as crystals in the eye) were discovered. This is a common adverse effect associated with canthaxanthin use. Other side effects reportedly included nausea, cramping, diarrhea, severe ITCHING, and welts associated with the use of tanning pills.

Some tanning pills are advertised as a safe method of tanning, while others are designed to bolster resistance to sun damage. Regardless of the reason they are used, they should only be used with close medical supervision.

The U.S. FDA does not approve the sale of pills that contain beta-carotene and/or canthaxanthin, both relatives of VITAMIN A (although beta-carotene is available by prescription). According to both the FDA and the Skin Cancer Foundation, some of the ingredients in these pills can have toxic side effects.

Beta-carotene is a natural component of many fruits and vegetables (such as oranges, carrots, and tomatoes) and is sometimes used as a food additive in butter or cheese to add color. However, the pills may do the same thing to human skin, turning it yellow or orange instead of a handsome tan. In combination with the canthaxanthin, beta-carotene accumulates in the skin and colors it. At the same time, it forms deposits in the blood, fatty tissue, liver, and other organs, sometimes becoming toxic.

Another kind of tanning pill contains 5- or 8-methoxypsoralen, a form of PSORALEN that is used to treat PSORIASIS, ALOPECIA AREATA, and VITILIGO. Physicians have sometimes prescribed this chemical for those with sensitive skin as a way to resist sun damage on the theory that the chemical may thicken the skin and accelerate MELANIN production. It has been prescribed for those who are allergic to sunblocks, but can not avoid the sun.

It is recommended that it be used only under close medical supervision. It is available in other countries, and it does produce a deep, protective tan—but the risk of bleeding is significant.

tar compounds   Crude and refined tars are an effective treatment for psoriasis, and are used either alone or in combination with ultraviolet light therapy. Tar decreases the turnover of the top-most layer of skin, and helps to reduce scaling and flakiness. However, the color and smell of these products do not make them popular choices. Tar is usually applied to the skin a few hours before light therapy.

Tar is a mixture of hundreds of compounds; a more cosmetically acceptable tar compound is liquor carbonis detergens (LCD) usually mixed with COLD CREAM in a 5 percent to 10 percent concentration.

LCD is a distillate of crude coal tar not dissimilar to road tar. Other tar preparations are available as SOAPS, GELS, or SHAMPOOS. There are lots of newer cosmetically acceptable preparations, such as LCD tar-gel or fragrant clear shampoo.

Tar shampoos are one of the treatments of choice for scaly scalp conditions such as seborrheic dermatitis DANDRUFF, or PSORIASIS.

See also DERMATITIS, SEBORRHEIC

tattooing The process of instilling permanent colors into the skin, usually to create words or a design. Practiced for thousands of years as a form of identification or tribal marking, today tattoos are almost always used just for decoration. Even when performed by professionals, however, tattooing can be dangerous, leading to AIDS or hepatitis if the tattoo artist does not follow strict sterile procedures to clean needles that inject the dyes.

A "professional" tattoo is applied by an artist who may or may not be licensed, using non–FDA-approved pigments at a studio. A tattoo may be applied with or without consent from a parent or guardian, depending on state or local regulations.

Tattoo artists use an electrically powered, vertical vibrating instrument to inject the tattoo pigment 50 to 3,000 times per minutes into the second layer of the skin (DERMIS), at a depth of 1/64 to 1/16 of an inch. A single needle outlines the tattoo and the design is then filled in with five to seven needles in a needle bar.

State regulations of tattooing range from prohibiting tattooing to no regulations at all; in some states with no regulation, local cities have established their own standards. The law for any specific state may be obtained from state, country, or local health departments.

Because tattooing carries the risk of transmitting a blood-borne disease or infection, needles must be sterilized before use and should not be reused. Tattooists should use an autoclave to heat sterilize equipment between customers. Packaged, sterilized tattoo needles should be used only once and then thrown away in a special biohazard container. Leftover tattoo ink should be thrown away after each procedure; ink should never be poured into the bottle, and needles should never be inserted into the bottle. The tattooist should wear latex gloves and should change gloves if the tattooing procedure is interrupted for other activities such as answering the phone or leaving the room.

Tattoos can be removed using short pulsed lasers including the Q-switched ruby, Ng:YAG, alexandrite, and 510 nanometer pulsed dye laser. Amateur tattoos can usually be entirely removed, as can black professional tattoos. Multicolored professional tattoos are more difficult to remove and require several different wavelengths for the different colors.

Tegison The trade name for ETRETINATE.

telangiectasia An abnormal dilation of capillary blood vessels that often forms into an ANGIOMA (a tumor made of mostly of blood vessels). Telangiectasias may occur in ROSACEA, certain diseases such as SCLERODERMA, or in long-term therapy with topical fluorinated CORTICOSTEROIDS. Most causes are unknown. Telangiectasia also may occur as a result of an inherited disorders, such as hereditary hemorrhagic telangiectasia or LOUIS-BAR SYNDROME.

telogen The resting stage of the hair growth cycle.

telogen effluvium Generalized hair shedding, often after an acute illness or pregnancy. Normally, healthy adults lose between 75 and 100 hairs daily, but certain events can prompt an increase in hair loss by inducing the hair follicles to enter the telogen (resting) phase of hair growth.

About 95 percent of women develop some degree of hair loss after giving birth or after stopping birth control pills. Other causes may include high fever, surgery and psychiatric stress, bulimia, dieting, malnutrition, blood loss, and shock.

Treatment Options and Outlook
No treatment is needed, since new hairs replace those falling out. If hair loss persists for longer than three months, patients should see a dermatologist.

See also ALOPECIA AREATA.

tetracycline A group of antibiotic drugs used to treat a range of conditions with skin symptoms, including ACNE, SYPHILIS, and ROCKY MOUNTAIN SPOTTED FEVER.

Side Effects
Possible problems include nausea and vomiting, diarrhea, photosensitivity rash, and ITCHING. Tetracyclines may increase the overgrowth of yeasts in the vagina and interfere with the absorption of over-the-counter drugs taken concurrently. They may also discolor developing bones and teeth, and are not prescribed for youngsters under age 12 or for pregnant women. Tetracyclines also may worsen kidney disease in patients with kidney problems.

thalidomide The infamous antinausea drug never approved for use in the United States that caused widespread birth defects in other parts of the world when given to pregnant women.

In 1998 the U.S. Food and Drug Administration (FDA) approved thalidomide for use in treating LEPROSY symptoms. Studies are also being conducted to determine the effectiveness of thalidomide in treating symptoms associated with AIDS, Behcet disease, lupus, Sjogren syndrome, rheumatoid arthritis, inflammatory bowel disease, macular degeneration, and some cancers.

theque An island of MELANIN-producing cells situated at the junction of the DERMIS and EPIDERMIS, or within the dermis.

thrush The common name for candidiasis, a superficial fungal infection of the mucous membranes of the mouth.

See also CANDIDA INFECTION.

thymol An antiseptic derived from PHENOL that used to be used to treat ECZEMA, PSORIASIS, and ACNE. It is an effective drying agent for the treatment of PARONYCHIA.

thyroid disorders, skin symptoms of A range of skin symptoms accompany thyroid disorders.

Hyperthyroidism is characterized by fine, thin hair, red palms, increased sweating, onycholysis, diffuse darkening of skin, and ITCHING.

Hypothyroidism includes dry, lax skin; thick lips and tongue; cool skin; thinning hair; carotenemia; itching; xerosis; brittle nails.

Hashimoto's thyroiditis is associated with several other auto-immune conditions such as VITILIGO, ALOPECIA AREATA, DERMATITIS HERPETIFORMIS, PEMPHIGOID, LUPUS ERYTHEMATOSUS, and SCLERODERMA.

ticks and disease Ticks are not so much a primary cause of skin disease as carriers of infectious agents that produce diseases with skin symptoms, such as ROCKY MOUNTAIN SPOTTED FEVER, LYME DISEASE, and TULAREMIA.

Ticks bury their heads into the skin to feed, become engorged with their host's blood, and swell to many times their size.

Symptoms and Diagnostic Path
Sometimes generalized HIVES may develop. While a tick bite itself does not usually cause problems, it may result in persistent NODULES or PAPULES after forced removal of the tick. Other skin reactions to tick bites include papular HIVE-like lesions, patchy scalp hair loss, painful local swelling, ulceration, and erythema chronicum migrans in Lyme disease.

Treatment Options and Outlook
Gently pulling the tick parallel to the skin can often remove it completely.

Inflammatory papules and nodules caused by a tick bite can be treated with a topical CORTICOSTEROID cream. Excision of nodules may be necessary, although persistent reactions have occurred in spite of excision.

Risk Factors and Preventive Measures
Low concentrations of bug repellents such as Deet do not work very well at repelling ticks.

Tinactin See TOLNAFTATE.

tinea The medical term for RINGWORM, a group of common fungus infections of the skin, hair, or nails caused by various species of the fungi *Microsporum*, *Trichophyton*, and *Epidermophyton* that affect humans and animals. Ringworm is highly contagious and can be spread either by direct contact or via infected material. Infections can be contracted from other people, and from animals, soil, or an object (such as a shower stall).

The term *tinea* is often followed by the part of the body affected by the fungus, such as tinea pedis (ATHLETE'S FOOT).

Symptoms and Diagnostic Path

Symptoms vary according to the part of the body affected by the infection. The most common affected area is the foot (ATHLETE'S FOOT), with cracking, itchy skin between the toes. Tinea cruris (JOCK ITCH) is more common in males, and produces a red, itchy area from the genitals outward over the inside of the thighs. TINEA CORPORIS (ringworm of the body) is characterized by itchy circular skin patches with a raised edge. TINEA CAPITIS (ringworm of the scalp) causes round, itchy circles of hair loss found most commonly in children living in large cities or in overcrowded conditions. Tinea unguium (ringworm of the nails, or ONYCHOMYCOSIS) is characterized by thick white or yellow nails. Ringworm can also affect the skin under a beard (TINEA BARBAE) or the facial skin.

Treatment Options and Outlook

Antifungal drugs as creams, lotions, or ointments can successfully treat most types of tinea. For widespread infection (or those affecting hair or nails), systemic treatment is usually required. Treatment should continue after symptoms have faded to ensure the fungi have been destroyed. Mild infections on the surface of the skin may be treated for four to six weeks.

Toenail infections may require treatment with terfenebrin or itraconazole for months, but with the new drugs three-month treatment may be sufficient. Until recently, the standard treatment was GRISEOFULVIN. It is relatively effective for skin and hair fungal infections but of limited use in the treatment of nail infections.

tinea barbae RINGWORM infection of the skin under the beard, caused primarily by *Tinea mentagrophytes* or *T. verrucosum*.

See also TINEA.

tinea capitis The medical term for RINGWORM of the scalp, this fungal infection causes several round, itchy patches of hair loss on the scalp. It is most commonly found in children who are subject to crowded conditions where the fungi spread more easily.

Treatment Options and Outlook

Antifungal drugs, usually taken by mouth for four to six weeks, will cure the infection.

tinea corporis The medical term for RINGWORM of the body, this fungal infection is characterized by itchy round patches with raised edges. Tinea corporis is found throughout the world, occurring more often in hot, humid climates. *Tinea rubrum* is the most common infectious agent. In HIV-positive or other immunocompromised patients, significant symptoms of ITCHING or pain may develop, and, rarely, deep ABSCESSes or dissemination may occur.

Tinea corporis occurs in both men and women; women of childbearing age may be more frequently infected because they are more likely to come into contact with infected children.

Infection may occur through contact with infected humans, animals, or inanimate objects. The person may have had on-the-job exposure or environmental and recreational exposure during gardening, contact sports, or use of sports facilities.

The most common cause of tinea corporis is *T. rubrum*, although *M. canis*, *T. mentagrophytes*, and *T. tonsurans* are also known to cause infection.

Treatment Options and Outlook

Topical treatment is recommended for localized cases, applied to an area at least 2 cm beyond the edge of the identified lesion once or twice a day for at least two weeks, depending on which agent is used. ECONAZOLE, KETOCONAZOLE, clotrimazole,

MICONAZOLE, oxiconazole, sulconazole, and systemic azoles (fluconazole, itraconazole, ketoconazole) can be effective. Allylamines (naftifine, terbinafine) and the related benzylamine butenafine also may be prescribed.

Oral therapy may be indicated for tinea corporis cases that are extensive, involve immunocompromised patients, or are not responsive to topical therapy. Other drugs may include oral doses of micronized GRISEOFULVIN, ketoconazole, fluconazole, itraconazole, or terbinafine.

tinea cruris   See JOCK ITCH.

tinea manuum   RINGWORM infection most often caused by *Tinea rubrum*, often found together with a foot infection.

Symptoms and Diagnostic Path
The condition is characterized by thickened scaly skin of palms and fingers, especially in the creases of the skin.

Treatment Options and Outlook
Topical antifungal preparations such as imidazole or allylamine antifungals are preferred. Topical agents may not be enough to cure this problem; therefore, an oral antifungal drug (such as GRISEOFULVIN or KETOCONAZOLE) is usually required and should be taken for two to three months.

tinea nigra palmaris   A superficial RINGWORM infection of the palms, although the soles of the feet may also be affected. While the condition is found throughout the world in both men and women of all ages, it is uncommon in North America. Compared to other types of fungal infections, the incidence of tinea nigra palmaris is low, even in South America where it is most often found.

Symptoms and Diagnostic Path
The condition is characterized by the appearance on the palm or sole of a single brown-black MACULE with sharply defined margins that tends to spread in a circular pattern. It may mimic malignant melanoma

Treatment Options and Outlook
Most infections respond to topical antifungals such as Whitfield's ointment, topical imidazoles or allylamines, Keralyt gel, or 40 percent urea. Removal by scraping with an emery board may be helpful. Recurrence is rare.

See also MELANOMA, MALIGNANT.

tinea pedis   See ATHLETE'S FOOT.

tinea unguium   See ONYCHOMYCOSIS.

tinea versicolor   A common skin condition (also known as pityriasis versicolor) characterized by patches of white, brown, or salmon-colored flaky skin on the trunk and neck. It primarily affects young and middle-aged adult men, and is not contagious.

A yeast living on the skin causes the condition, when it colonizes the dead outer layer of skin.

Treatment Options and Outlook
Thorough application of antifungal cream or lotion from ears to knees for several consecutive nights after shampooing with an anti-yeast SHAMPOO, such as one containing selenium sulfide or KETOCONAZOLE, will eradicate the fungus, provided not one spot is missed. It is also important to wash underwear and night clothes and sheets thoroughly. The treatment will cure the condition, but it may take many months for the skin patches to return to a normal color. Relapses are frequent. A simpler approach requires taking an anti-yeast pill, ketoconazole, for just two doses.

tissue expansion   A technique of plastic surgery that uses neighboring skin to cover birth defects, injuries, or cosmetically displeasing areas by slowly stretching the skin.

This procedure began to gain popularity in the early 1980s and was first used to reconstruct breasts after mastectomy. Today it is also used to cover birth defects, areas of skin after tumor removal, skin damaged by trauma, as well as for breast enlargement and creation of new, hair-bearing scalp for bald men.

In the past, the only way to replace skin marred by defects or injuries was to cut a flap of healthy flesh from elsewhere on the body and transplant it over the problem area. Unfortunately, this caused scarring in both the donor and recipient area of the skin, as well as a mismatch between skin type. For example, the skin from the abdomen or back looks very different from the flesh on the breast or face in the color, thickness, texture, and ability to grow hair.

With the tissue expansion technique, a small expander is implanted beneath the skin. After the incisions have healed, the balloon is gradually filled by injection with saline solution until the skin has expanded enough to cover the desired area. This expansion process takes from six weeks to four months depending on the location and size. When the skin has been expanded enough, the balloon is withdrawn, any deformed tissue is removed, and the newly stretched skin is positioned and sutured into place. A permanent saline-filled implant may be inserted during a breast reconstruction procedure. Studies have shown that during expansion, the outer layer of skin (the EPIDERMIS) actually thickens as the cells multiply in reaction to the pressure.

In contrast, the underlying connective tissue, which is squeezed between the epidermis and the expanding balloon, becomes thinner. The body also forms a membrane of scar tissue around the expander, adding to the look of fullness.

toad skin   See PHRYNODERMA.

tobramycin (trade names: Nebcin, Tobrex)   An antibiotic drug used to treat severe skin infections, usually given by injection in combination with PENICILLIN.

Side Effects
Possible side effects when giving tobramycin in high doses may include kidney damage, nausea and vomiting, inner ear deafness, headache, and itchy rash.

toe web infection   Disorders of the spaces between the toes are usually called ATHLETE'S FOOT, and most are caused by fungal infections. Although the fungus is the primary cause of tissue destruction, subsequent bacterial infiltration can contribute to the problem and interfere with treatment success. Independent bacterial infection also produces toe web infection.

Symptoms and Diagnostic Path
Maceration, cracking, discomfort, foul smell, and oozing in the spaces between toes.

Treatment Options and Outlook
Because so many different types of organisms are involved in toe web infections, several different types of treatment must be used in order to be effective. If the lesions are dry and scaly, topical antifungal agents (such as imidazoles or allylamines) are effective. For soft, wet lesions, treatment must include removal of excess moisture, daily compresses with saline or albumin subacetate (BUROW'S SOLUTION), broad-spectrum topical antimicrobial agents, long-term use of antifungals, and oral GRISEOFULVIN.

tolnaftate (trade names: Aftate, Tinactin)   An antifungal treatment for some types of TINEA (including ATHLETE'S FOOT). It is available without a prescription as a cream, powder, or aerosol.

Side Effects
In rare cases, it may cause skin irritation or rash.

topical medications   Drugs that are applied to the skin surface (instead of being injected or swallowed). Topical drugs also include suppositories inserted into the vagina or rectum, and drugs administered to the ear canal or surface of the eye.

toxic epidermal necrolysis   See NECROLYSIS, TOXIC EPIDERMAL.

toxic shock syndrome An uncommon condition characterized by a distinctive skin rash resembling SUNBURN on the palms and soles of the feet that peels within one or two weeks.

The condition, first recognized in the 1970s, is associated with the use of certain brands of highly absorbent tampons (no longer available). About 70 percent of cases occur in women who are using tampons when symptoms begin. Most recent cases have been related to staphylococcal infections unrelated to tampon use.

The condition is caused by a toxin produced by *Staphylococcus aureus*.

Symptoms and Diagnostic Path

In addition to the skin rash, symptoms include sudden high fever, vomiting and diarrhea, headache, muscular aches and pains, dizziness, and disorientation. Blood pressure may drop rapidly and shock may develop. Death occurs in about 3 percent of cases, usually due to a prolonged drop in blood pressure or lung problems.

Treatment Options and Outlook

Antibiotic drugs and IV infusion (to prevent shock), plus treatment for any complications as they occur. Recurrence is common.

Risk Factors and Preventive Measures

Women who have had toxic shock syndrome should not use tampons, cervical caps, diaphragms, or vaginal contraceptive sponges.

transforming growth factor (TGF) beta A biological compound produced by the body that is essential for the normal production of COLLAGEN and ELASTIN. It lies beneath the skin and makes it supple. One of the newest compounds currently being studied, TGF may one day be available as a daily beauty treatment to slow down the physical signs of aging and keep skin young.

tretinoin (Retin-A, Renova) A synthetic form of VITAMIN A (RETINOIC ACID) used as a prescription ACNE medication and wrinkle cream; it also may prevent skin and cervix cancer. It is used to treat photoaging (the long-term effects of sun on the skin that cause wrinkling and blotchy pigmentation). Retinoin in the United States has been approved formally for the treatment of acne, but it is also widely used to treat sun-damaged, wrinkled skin. Renova (a 5 percent emollient cream) has been approved to treat photoaging.

Although tretinoin is in the same family as vitamin A, the two are not the same. For many years, different compounds of vitamin A have been included in cosmetics (as retinol, retinyl, retinyl-acetate, or retinyl palmitate) because these ingredients are not considered to be drugs by the U.S. Food and Drug Administration. Tretinoin, the acid of vitamin A, has unique properties and because it is available by prescription only in this country, it is not included in any cosmetic skin-care product. It is available without a prescription in Mexico.

The first reports of tretinoin's ability to smooth out wrinkles appeared in the *Journal of the American Medical Association* in 1988, when researchers at the University of Michigan reported that subjects with sun-damaged skin showed significant improvement in number of WRINKLES after applying it. Up to that time, dermatologists used tretinoin mostly for acne patients until Albert Kligman, M.D., a prominent dermatologist at the University of Pennsylvania, noted his acne patients' reports and began using tretinoin on sun-damaged skin.

Many studies have now shown that tretinoin is effective in removing facial wrinkles, smoothing coarse skin, and improving LENTIGINES. It is not effective for improving coarse wrinkles.

It is also extremely effective in the treatment of acne, although—as with the case of wrinkles—there is a lag time before it becomes effective. Some individuals even notice their skin becomes worse after the first two or three weeks. At the beginning, tretinoin can cause dryness and irritation.

Two types of SKIN CANCER, SQUAMOUS CELL cancer and BASAL CELL cancer, are caused by sun exposure and an individual's own risk factors. Cancer in the skin develops when cellular development goes awry; retinoids improve cellular differentiation, so experts think these medications may help prevent cancer. In fact, tretinoin does slow down the development of precancerous skin lesions such as ACTINIC KERATOSES. Individuals might choose to use tretinoin as a cancer preventive if they have a history of heavy sun exposure and previous sun-related lesions that were removed from their skin.

How to Apply

The higher the concentration of tretinoin, the faster and more significant the results. It is often irritating, however, and for this reason many doctors start patients with the milder forms available: 0.025 percent to 0.05 percent cream every other night, slowly increasing the strength and frequency of application.

Consumers should first wash the skin thoroughly with a gentle cleanser, pat dry, and then wait 15 minute. Then a tiny amount of cream is spread over the entire face. Tretinoin may be applied under the eyes. At first the skin may be pink and flaky; it takes three to six months before benefits are apparent. On less sensitive areas (such as the backs of the hands) it can be started more quickly and used every night.

Renova is a similar product containing retinoic acid in a moisturizing base. It is considered less irritating but as effective as tretinoin and is used in the same way.

Side Effects

Tretinoin is a powerful drug, and side effects can include burning eyes and peeling or reddening of the skin that lasts for weeks; this reaction is most common in women who sunburn easily and who normally have very sensitive skin. Benefits often do not appear until between six and 12 months. In study groups, some users experience results so distressing that they drop out, but these people were using a 0.1 percent cream twice a day.

Ironically, tretinoin makes the skin more vulnerable to ultraviolet light, causing users to sunburn more easily. Users should always layer a high SPF block under makeup (even during winter) to protect from harmful exposure, wear protective hats and avoid the sun.

The drug should be used under the supervision of a physician. Incorrect use of tretinoin can lead to extreme irritation so consumers should see a dermatologist to obtain a prescription.

Tretinoin is a class "C" drug, which means that pregnant women should use this medication only if the potential benefit outweighs the potential risk to the baby. Women who want to use tretinoin during pregnancy should consult with their doctors.

See also ACTINIC CONDITIONS; AGING AND SKIN; ALPHA HYDROXY ACIDS; EXFOLIANTS; ISOTRETINOIN; PHOTOSENSITIVITY; STRETCH MARKS.

triamcinolone (Trade names: Aristocort, Aristospan, Kenalog, Triacet, Triamolone) A CORTICO-STEROID hormone used to treat skin inflammations, with uses similar to cortisone. It reduces inflammation but does not cause water retention.

Side Effects

Dizziness, headache, muscle weakness, and low blood pressure may be evident.

trichauxis An increase in the size and number of hairs.

trichiasis Eyelashes that grow toward the eyeball instead of outward as they normally would. If the lashes grow to the point where they touch the eyeball, they can cause severe pain and may damage the cornea.

Treatment Options and Outlook

Temporary treatment consists of removing the eyelashes that are growing the wrong way, but the lashes will regrow. Permanent treatment requires the destruction of the growth follicles of the wayward eyelashes via ELECTROLYSIS.

trichosporosis Also known as piedra, this is a fungal condition in which the hair shafts are coated with hard masses of white (*Trichosporon cutaneum* or *T. beigelii*) or black (*Piedraia hortai*) fungus. The black fungus appears as small dark nodules along the hair shaft, visible to the naked eye and under the microscope. It occurs primarily in the Tropics. The white variety is found around the world, and is characterized by soft NODULES on primarily facial and pubic hair.

Treatment Options and Outlook

Removal of the affected hairs by clipping or shaving.

trichotillomania The habit of pulling out one's hair, often associated with psychological stress and sometimes mental illness or psychotic illness (such as schizophrenia). Hair-pulling also may take place among children who are anxious and frustrated. Typically, the patient pulls, twists, or breaks off chunks of hair, leaving bald spots. Children sometimes eat the removed hair, which may lead to a hairball in the stomach.

Treatment Options and Outlook

Psychotherapy and/or antipsychotic drugs are sometimes used.

tuberculin test A skin test used to determine whether or not a person has been infected with tuberculosis. The test is used to diagnose suspected cases of tuberculosis prior to vaccination against the disease.

During the test, the skin is first disinfected, usually with an alcohol swab, and a small dose of tuberculin (a protein extract of the tuberculosis bacilli) is introduced into the skin in one of a variety of ways. In the Mantoux test, the extract is injected into the skin with a needle—in the Sterneedle test, the extract is dropped on the forearm as a spring-loaded instrument circled with a sharp prong forces the tuberculin into the skin.

After two days, the skin is inspected at the site; if the skin is unchanged, the reaction is negative, indicating the person has never been exposed to tuberculosis and has no immunity. Skin that becomes red, firm, and raised after the injection indicates that the person has been exposed to tuberculosis, either through vaccination or infection.

See also TUBERCULOSIS, SKIN.

tuberculosis, skin Tuberculosis of the skin is characterized by breakdown of the skin over PUS-filled tuberculous glands, forming irregular-shaped ulcers tinged with blue. TB was uncommon and decreasing in prevalence in developed countries until the past few years. Recently, there has been a resurgence in TB cases, especially in urban areas.

Symptoms and Diagnostic Path

There are two basic forms of this type of TB: localized and disseminated.

The *localized* form may develop after the introduction of the tubercle bacilli into a wound in patients who have never been exposed to TB. It begins as an inflammatory nodule (called the "tuberculous chancre") and is followed by swelling of the lymph nodes. In those who are immune or partially immune, two types of lesions may appear: tuberculosis verrucosa and lupus vulgaris. In tuberculosis verrucosa, the bacilli leads to localized solid elevated lesions. Lupus vulgaris begins in early life, with patchy lesions studded with what look like soft yellowish brown "apple jelly" nodules, when compressed with a glass slide. This is followed by swelling, ulcers, and hypertrophy. In temperate climates, most lupus lesions are on the face, while those of tuberculosis verrucosa are on the hands; the distribution may be different in tropical areas.

Scrofuloderma is another form of localized skin TB, in which tuberculosis of the lymph nodes extends into the skin, causing the development of ulcers and fistulas beneath ridges of bluish skin.

In the *disseminated* form, bacteria spread by patients with fulminating TB result in miliary tuberculosis of the skin. Lesions that resemble ACNE appear on the face and arms and legs; these lesions end in CHICKEN POX–like scars.

Treatment Options and Outlook

Treatment usually combines three or four antibiotics in combination over six to nine months.

See also TUBERCULIN TEST.

tuberous sclerosis A genetic disorder that causes benign tumors (tubers) to form in many different organs, especially the skin, brain, eyes, heart, kidney, and lungs. It is called both tuberous sclerosis (TS) and tuberous sclerosis complex (TSC); the term *TSC* is used in scientific literature to distinguish tuberous sclerosis from Tourette syndrome.

The true prevalence of TS is unknown, but scientists estimate it occurs once in every 6,000 live births; this means approximately 25,000 to 40,000 individuals in the United States have TS. It occurs in both sexes and in all races and ethnic groups. It is often first recognized in children who have seizures and developmental disabilities, but the symptoms of TS vary greatly and may often not appear until later in life. There are presently no cures and there is no way to predict how severely or mildly an individual may be affected by TS.

Mutations in one of two genes, TSC1 and TSC2, have been identified as the cause of tuberous sclerosis. In some genetic conditions such as TS, a mutation in one copy of the gene is enough to cause the condition. About a third of people with TS inherit it from a parent who also has TS. If a parent has TS and passes on the copy of the gene with the mutation, then the child will also have TS. If the parent passes on the copy of the gene without the mutation, the child will not have TS. Thus, there is a 50 percent chance with each pregnancy for a parent with TS to have a child with TS. This is true regardless of the sex of the parent or the sex of the child. In the remaining two-thirds of people with TS, neither parent shows any symptoms or signs of TS. Instead, one of the normal genes from one parent changes to the abnormal form, leading to a new occurrence of TS in the child. Normally, these parents do not have another child with TS because the mutation was sporadic, not inherited. However, some families have more than one child with TS, even though neither parent showed symptoms or findings of TS.

Scientists have determined that a small number of physically unaffected parents of a child with TS actually have TS mutations in some of their cells. Because the mutation is limited to a small portion of all of the body's cells, these individuals show no signs of TS, but if a portion of the egg or sperm cells of a parent carries the TS mutation, that parent can have more than one affected child, possibly at the same 50/50 chance that people with TS have. A person who carries cells with TS mutations in egg or sperm supply has germline mosaicism. The occurrence of germline mosaicism has led geneticists to estimate a recurrence risk ranging from 1 percent to 3 percent. At this time, there is no simple way to determine whether an unaffected parent of a child with TS has germline mosaicism.

Although some individuals may inherit the disorder from a parent with TSC, most cases occur as spontaneous mutations. In these situations, neither parent has the disorder or the faulty gene. Instead, a faulty gene first occurs in the affected individuals.

First described in the 1880s, TS affects only some organs in most individuals.

Symptoms and Diagnostic Path

The skin, face, body, and nails are places where many people with TS experience symptoms. In some cases, skin growths can become obtrusive, but in most cases, the growths themselves are harmless. Skin lesions may include patches of skin lighter than the surrounding skin that can be any size or shape (or may be the classic "ash-leaf" shape), a shagreen patch (a patch of skin that is tough and dimpled like an orange peel), fibrous growths that appear around the fingernails and toenails, and benign tumors of the face. Fibrous plaques sometimes appear on the forehead of individuals with TS. There may also be fibrous, hairless scalp plaques surrounded by thin white tufts of hair.

Occasionally an individual with TS will have CAFÉ-AU-LAIT MACULES (areas of skin darker than the surrounding skin, but lighter and usually larger than a mole), but these skin lesions are not related to TS. A child with three or more or an adult with five or more café-au-lait spots may be diagnosed with NEUROFIBROMATOSIS, another genetic condition.

In most cases the first clue to recognizing TSC is the presence of seizures or delayed development. In other cases, the first sign may be white patches on the skin (hypomelanotic MACULES).

A physician will use a Wood's lamp (an ultraviolet light) to better visualize the white patches on the skin that often are difficult to see, especially on infants and people with very pale skin. The entire body should be examined, including the skin (for the wide variety of skin symptoms), the teeth for dental pits, and the eyes for dilated pupils. Some of the skin signs may not be present at birth; the facial tumors do not usually appear until between the ages of three and five at the earliest, and the fibrous growths do not usually occur until much later in life.

Other diagnostic tests include computed tomography (CT) or magnetic resonance imaging (MRI) of the brain and an ultrasound of the heart, liver, and kidneys.

Treatment Options and Outlook

Facial tumors can be removed using dermabrasion or laser treatment when they are small, before they enlarge and become fibrous. They most likely will recur and need further treatment, but they will be milder than if left untreated. Some cosmetic companies also manufacture makeup to cover lightened skin patches if they are large or in exposed areas of the skin.

Most people who are mildly affected by TS lead active and productive lives, but it is important to realize that TS is a life-long condition.

tularemia An infectious disease of wild animals occasionally transmitted to humans, characterized by a red spot at the site of infection that eventually forms an ulcer.

Humans may contract the disease through direct contact with an infected animal (most commonly a rabbit, squirrel, or muskrat). The bacteria enter the body through a cut or scratch in the skin, or may be acquired following a bite from a tick, flea, fly, or louse or (rarely) by eating infected meat.

A few hundred cases occur in North America, some parts of Europe, and Asia each year.

Symptoms and Diagnostic Path

In addition to the skin lesion, symptoms include enlarged lymph nodes, fever, headache, muscle pains, and malaise. Sometimes the eyes, throat, digestive tract, and lungs are affected.

Treatment Options and Outlook

Antibiotics (such as streptomycin, TETRACYCLINE, or intravenous gentamicin) treat the disease, with a less than 1 percent fatality rate. Untreated, tulare-

mia can be fatal in 5 percent of cases. The disease confers permanent immunity.

Risk Factors and Preventive Measures

A vaccine is available for those at high risk, such as hunters, trappers, game wardens, or lab workers.

tumbu fly bites A fly bite that causes myiasis (skin infestation with fly larvae). It most commonly occurs in South Africa.

tumefaction A swelling.

tunable dye laser Dye lasers use colored solids dissolved in organic solvents to produce laser light. The color of the laser light emitted depends on the color of solid material chosen. By changing the dye, the wavelength (or color) can be altered. Dye lasers are used for the treatment of blood vessel abnormalities (yellow light), and pigmented disorders (green light).

See also PULSED DYE LASER.

Tunga penetrans A species of fleas found in tropical and subtropical America, commonly referred to as jiggers, sand flies, or chigoes.

turban tumor Multiple benign growths called cylindromas that cover the scalp, giving the patient the appearance of a person wearing a turban.

Although the tumors are usually benign, they can become very large, ulcerated, or infected, requiring surgery to replace the affected areas with skin grafts. Turban tumors are more common in women; the male to female ratio ranges between 6 to 1 to 9 to 1.

Researchers have discovered the gene that causes multiple turban tumors on chromosome 16q12-q13. The gene codes for proteins that coordinate the attachment of structures inside the cell.

Solitary cylindromas This type of turban tumor usually occurs in middle and old age, affecting the face and scalp. This type of tumor does not seem to be inherited. The solitary form usually begins as a slow-growing, rubbery nodule with pink, red, or sometimes blue coloring, ranging in size from a few millimeters to several centimeters.

Multiple cylindromas   This type of turban tumor may cover almost the entire scalp, causing the disfiguring turban appearance and requiring extensive plastic surgery. The multiple form has numerous masses of pink, red, or blue NODULES, sometimes resembling bunches of grapes or small tomatoes (sometimes called "tomato tumor").

Multiple tumors, which are not as common as single tumors, are inherited in an autosomal dominant mode and may occur on the body, arms, and legs, as well as the head and neck. They usually begin in early adulthood and may progress over time. The inherited condition is known as familial cylindromatosis, and the cause appears to be due to a defect in a gene that is a tumor suppressor.

Malignant cylindromas   These tumors are very rare and appear to arise out of solitary cylindromas or—more often—as a complication of the multiple type. While the vast majority of cylindromas remain benign, at least 14 reports exist of malignant transformation.

The prognosis is not good with malignancy, since this type of cancer often spreads. A cylindroma occasionally will erode through the skull, causing hemorrhage and meningitis.

Treatment Options and Outlook

For solitary lesions, treatment is by excision or electrosurgery. For small cylindromas, a CARBON DIOXIDE LASER may be used. Multiple cylindromas usually require extensive plastic surgery, progressively removing a group of nodules in multiple procedures.

Because of the tendency for new lesions to develop and because of the risk of cancer, follow-up of patients with multiple cylindromas is recommended.

turtle oil   One of the oldest products used in skin care, whose effectiveness was discredited as early as 1934. Extracted from the genitals and muscles of the giant sea turtle, the oil does have some vita-

mins and—as all oils—it forms a film on the skin that helps retain moisture. It has no other value in skin-care products.

tylosis   Callus formation.

Tyndall light phenomenon   The reflection of light by particles suspended in a gas or liquid that imparts a blue tinge to objects. In skin, MELANIN particles found at levels of the dermis give the skin varying degrees of a bluish tinge. This is the same process as the scattering of particles in the atmosphere that makes the sky appear blue.

typhus   Any of a group of infectious diseases with similar symptoms, characterized by a measleslike rash, severe headache, back and limb pain, high fever, confusion, prostration, weak heartbeat, and delirium.

In the past, epidemic typhus spread by body lice was the most serious type of this disease. Epidemics swept across the world, killing hundreds of thousands of people during war, famine, and natural disaster. It is rare today, except in some areas of Africa and South America.

Typhus is caused by rickettsiae (microorganisms much like bacteria); in epidemic typhus, they are ingested by LICE from the blood of infected patients. The lice deposit feces containing the rickettsiae on another person's skin. When a person scratches the skin, the microorganisms enter the bloodstream.

Endemic (or murine) typhus is found in rats; it is spread to humans through flea bites. Scrub typhus is spread by mites in India and Southeast Asia.

Treatment Options and Outlook

Antibiotic drugs (TETRACYCLINES) treat typhus fever; other treatment is aimed at relieving symptoms. It may take a long time to recover from the disease. In the past, epidemic typhus was prevalent in crowded, unsanitary places and had a mortality rate close to 100 percent.

Untreated, a patient may die from blood poisoning, heart or kidney failure, or pneumonia.

Risk Factors and Preventive Measures

Epidemic typhus may be prevented by vaccination and control of lice via insecticides. Other types of typhus may be prevented by wearing protective clothes to prevent tick, mite, and flea bites.

tyrosine An amino acid that is used to produce MELANIN (skin pigment). Tyrosine is also used in some tan accelerators.

tyrosinemia type II See RICHNER-HANHART SYNDROME.

Tzanck smear Examination of cells from the floor of a BLISTER. It is used to diagnose HERPES VIRUS infections and some blistering disorders such as PEMPHIGUS. A DERMATOLOGIST removes the top of the blister and scrapes the jellylike material from the base of the blister onto a microscope slide. The results from this type of smear is better than in a culture of the virus in VARICELLA-ZOSTER virus infections, but less clear than that of a culture in herpes simplex. However, the test is inexpensive and very reliable.

ulcer An open sore on the skin caused by the destruction of surface tissue. Skin ulcers, typically caused by inadequate blood flow, may be found anywhere on the body; the site is often helpful in a diagnosis. Leg ulcers are mainly caused by inadequate blood flow or poor blood return to the heart. Skin cancer can ulcerate, as can trauma or burns. More rarely, ulcers may be caused by BASAL CELL CARCINOMA. Genital ulcers may be caused by sexually transmitted diseases, including SYPHILIS, gonorrhea, chancroid, and HERPES simplex.

ulerythema A rare, harmless skin disease causing atrophy and scarring, usually of the face, and hair loss. Typically, a portion of the eyebrow is affected and is lost. This disorder mainly affects children and young adults, affecting boys and girls equally. It is usually sporadic, although a few cases may be inherited in an autosomal dominant pattern. This means a defective gene inherited from just one parent causes the disease. Each child has a 50 percent chance of inheriting the affected gene and developing the disease.

Symptoms and Diagnostic Path

Symptoms include a red color on the central part of the face, especially the cheeks and on eyebrows, and occasionally with the loss of eyebrow hair later in life. The affected areas may feel rough, like fine sandpaper, and there may be scattered open and closed comedones and MILIA. Less often, similar lesions may be seen on the arms and legs.

Treatment Options and Outlook

Successful treatment with the PULSED DYE LASER has been reported. SUNSCREENS and sunblocks are recommended, because sun exposure and heat increase the flushing and may promote the redness.

ultraviolet light warning badge A self-adhesive waterproof badge that can be worn on clothing or on the skin that changes color with accumulated UV exposure. Watching the color changes on the badge helps even a child understand when excess exposure has occurred.

See also ULTRAVIOLET RADIATION.

ultraviolet radiation The energy that comes to the Earth from the Sun is emitted as radiation of various wavelengths, called the electromagnetic spectrum. Included in this spectrum are radio waves, X-rays, infrared rays, visible light, and ultraviolet radiation.

Infrared radiation is experienced as heat, representing 45 percent of the Sun's total energy. Another 49 percent of the total energy reaching the Earth makes up the *visible light* spectrum, which is perceived as color.

Ultraviolet radiation makes up the rest of the total energy from the Sun reaching the Earth—radiation strong enough to cause photochemical reactions and penetrate the skin.

There are three types of ultraviolet radiation emitted from sunlight: UVA, UVB, and UVC. UVC is toxic to human, plant, and animal life but it is absorbed by the Earth's atmosphere before it reaches the Earth. UVB (0.5 percent of the total energy reaching Earth) is responsible for inducing skin redness and burning by penetrating the top two layers of the skin. UVB has been considered to be more dangerous than UVA, and is believed to be the direct cause of a range of major skin and eye problems.

Until recently, UVA radiation was believed to be fairly harmless because it has a much lower intensity than UVB. But this type of ultraviolet radiation can penetrate the DERMIS (the third layer of the skin), and since UVA represents 5.5 percent of the total energy reaching the Earth, it has grave potential for damage.

Ultraviolet radiation stimulates melanocytes to produce brown pigment called MELANIN, which acts as a natural defense mechanism against ultraviolet radiation and gives skin a tanned look.

It is ultraviolet radiation that is responsible for both immediate and long-term damage to the skin from the sun. This radiation can cause anything from a tan to a painful SUNBURN. It causes skin to sag and wrinkle, brings out "sun spots," and ultimately can lead to SKIN CANCER.

The amount of ultraviolet radiation people receive depends on how close they are to the equator, what time of day it is, what season it is, their elevation, and the type of surrounding terrain. The potential for damage is greater at high altitudes because less atmospheric filtration occurs.

The closer to midday and the equator, the more damage from the Sun because of the position of the Sun in the sky: When the Sun is directly overhead, its rays reach the Earth vertically instead of at an angle, lessening the distance they must travel through Earth's protective atmosphere.

Seasonal changes also affect the ozone layer; the ozone layer is thinner and more dangerous, allowing more of the Sun's rays to penetrate the atmosphere. Snow can be very hazardous because it reflects the Sun more effectively even than sand and water. While clouds and pollution obstruct some ultraviolet radiation, they do not entirely eliminate it.

The ozone layer in Earth's stratosphere filters out most of this harmful radiation, but scientists warn that UV levels will climb as chemicals break down the ozone layer. Because the ozone layer is being depleted, higher concentrations of both UVA an UVB radiation are now reaching Earth, which has significantly increased the risk of skin cancer among all people.

In the last several years, instruments have detected significant thinning of stratospheric ozone over much of the world, but it is not clear how UV levels at the Earth's surface have changed, because no worldwide measurement network exists.

Interestingly, polluted air has been found to protect citizens from the ultraviolet radiation streaming through the Earth's damaged ozone layer. Studies found that levels of UV light were nearly twice as high in the relatively clean air of New Zealand as they were in the more polluted area of Germany. Similarly, measurements in the Alps show a strengthening of UV intensity; those in the United States show a weakening.

uncombable hair syndrome A rare hereditary hair-shaft defect characterized by coarse, curly, tangled hair. Also known as spun-glass hair, it mostly affects children aged three to 12. In some cases, the inheritance is autosomal dominant, whereas in others, the genetics are not clear.

Symptoms and Diagnostic Path

The hair of the head has a shaggy aspect, will not lie flat against the scalp, and cannot be combed or brushed. Dry and rough to the touch, the color is characteristically silver-blond. The eyebrows or eyelashes can be normal or thin. Slow hair growth and increased fragility are uncommon but have been reported. Uncombable hair syndrome is quite rare, with only about 60 cases reported between 1973 and 1998.

Onset may be in infancy or delayed until puberty, after which spontaneous improvement may occur.

Hair loss is possible because the hair is not always anchored in the hair follicle properly; also, the brittle nature of the hair means the hair is easy to break off. Problems with nails have been reported in association with uncombable hair syndrome. The nails can be short, brittle, and easy to split. Teeth may have problems, such as enamel defects. This is not surprising, since both nails and teeth have many similarities in basic structure with hair follicles.

The examination of the shaft under light microscopy may be normal, but under a scanning electron microscope, the cross section appears triangular in shape (pili trianguli) but may be kidney-shaped or oval. One or more depressions running along the length of the hair shaft resembling canals (pill canaliculi) may be seen. The cuticle is normal.

Treatment Options and Outlook

Spontaneous improvement occurs without treatment as the child enters adolescence.

ungual　Relating to the nail.

Unna's boot　A dressing of gelatin and ZINC OXIDE paste applied to the foot and leg to help to heal leg ulcers and other inflammatory skin conditions.

Urbach-Wiethe disease　A rare hereditary metabolic disease involving the skin as well as other tissues and organs. The condition is an autosomal recessive trait, which means that a defective gene must be inherited from both parents in order to cause the abnormality. Generally, both parents of an affected person are unaffected carriers of the defective gene. Each of their children has a one-in-four chance of being affected, and a two-in-four chance of being a carrier.

Symptoms and Diagnostic Path

In the first two years of life, skin symptoms include PUSTULES or BLISTERS on the face and exposed areas of the arms and legs that heal, leaving behind white scars. Subsequent skin lesions include NODULES and waxy yellow PAPULES on the face, back of the neck, hands, and fingers. Another characteristic sign is a line of lesions along the eyelids resembling a string of beads. In addition, there may be red warty plaques on elbows, knees, fingers, buttocks, and face. Some patients develop a general yellow thickened skin and lose hair on the scalp, beard area, eyebrows, and eyelashes.

Treatment Options and Outlook

There is no known treatment. Tracheostomy may be required for patients whose trachea becomes blocked with cartilage.

urticaria　See HIVES.

urticaria, contact　An acute localized allergic reaction characterized by HIVES after direct contact with an allergen, usually occurring within minutes after contact. It can be triggered by contact with a variety of antigens in food (especially fish or meat), drugs, cosmetics, and textiles. It also can be set off by other mechanisms, such as jellyfish, nettles, and chemicals.

Symptoms and Diagnostic Path

A red swollen area will appear at the point of contact with a substance to which a person is sensitized. It usually fades away within an hour or two. It can be confirmed by performing a skin prick test.

Treatment Options and Outlook

Antihistamines and anticholinergic drugs may sometimes provide relief.

Risk Factors and Preventive Measures

Avoiding a known irritant is the only prevention.
　See also URTICARIA, SOLAR.

urticaria, solar　A rare allergic response to sunlight characterized by the appearance of HIVES within minutes of exposure. The lesions last from a few minutes to an hour, depending on the intensity of the exposure as well as the sensitivity of the individual. This condition may be chronic. Solar urticaria sometimes develops in patients who are taking a drug (aspirin and morphine-like medicines) or are exposed to a particular chemical. When exposed to sunlight, the skin cells of someone with solar urticaria release HISTAMINE, and other inflammatory substances which widens the blood vessels and allows fluid to leak out, collecting within the skin.

Symptoms and Diagnostic Path

Symptoms include itchy skin covered with swollen red patches resembling weals or a rash that can take only a few minutes to longer than an hour to appear after exposure to light. Within an hour or so, they disappear, typical of hives. However, if a large area of the body is affected, the loss of fluid into the skin could cause light-headedness, pallor, and nausea.

A dermatologist who specializes in sun-sensitive conditions can diagnose the condition with blood tests or an instrument that studies the effects of light on the skin. In this test, different doses of ultraviolet and visible wavelengths are shone on the skin of the back to measure a person's sensitivity to each part of the light spectrum, with the response compared to that seen in normal subjects.

Risk Factors and Preventive Measures

Susceptible patients should avoid exposure to the sun by wearing protective clothes and opaque sunblocks. SUNSCREENS are not of much help. Gradual daily exposure to more and more sun will control the disease in many people, but this type of therapy is very difficult to carry out because of recurrent hives or even anaphylaxis; PUVA therapy is helpful in some patients.

urushiol oil The active ingredient in POISON IVY that is one of the most potent external toxins known. The amount necessary to cause a rash in a sensitive person is measured in nanograms (a nanogram is one billionth of a gram). This means that the amount of urushiol oil equal to the size of the period at the end of this sentence is enough to affect 500 people. Urushiol oil is also long-lasting; specimens of poison ivy several centuries old have been known to trigger a reaction in sensitive individuals.

UV light See ULTRAVIOLET LIGHT.

vaccinia   A viral cattle disease (cowpox) inoculated in humans to produce an antibody against SMALLPOX.

vaginal warts   See WARTS.

valacyclovir (Valtrex)   An antiviral drug used to treat HERPES infections. Easily absorbed and converted in the body to ACYCLOVIR, it is available in concentrations three to five times greater than that of acyclovir. The drug works by interfering with viral reproduction. Several large studies have shown that it is safe and well tolerated.

In treating SHINGLES, Valtrex reduces the lesions, shortens the duration of the infection, and shortens the pain. However, it is not clear whether it can reduce pain that lingers once the shingles clear.

Although valacyclovir will not cure shingles or genital herpes, it does help relieve the pain and discomfort and helps the sores heal faster. Valacyclovir works best if it is used within 48 hours after the first symptoms of shingles or genital herpes (for example, pain, burning, or BLISTERS) begin to appear. For recurrent outbreaks of genital herpes, valacyclovir works best if it is used within 24 hours after the symptoms begin to appear.

Side Effects

Side effects are rare. Valacyclovir can cause nausea and headache; the drug may damage the kidneys if patients are severely dehydrated. Because of potential kidney problems, people with existing kidney damage should use valacyclovir only under the close supervision of a physician.

varicella virus vaccine live (VariVax)   The CHICKEN POX vaccine approved in 1995 for all infants, children, teens, and young adults who have not had the disease.

One dose is needed for children up to age 12 (ideally given between 12 and 18 months of age); teenagers and adults need two shots, four to eight weeks apart. High-risk, susceptible patients may also obtain passive immunization with VZV immune globulin, which can abort or modify infection if administered within three days of exposure.

The vaccine is about 70 percent to 90 percent effective in preventing chicken pox, and 95 percent effective at preventing a moderate or severe case.

The vaccine is made from a live, weakened virus that works by creating a mild infection similar to natural chicken pox, but without related problems. The mild infection spurs the body to develop an immune response to the disease. These defenses are then ready when the body encounters the natural virus.

The vaccine is considered to be safe, but it is not yet known how long immunity will last in children who have received the chicken pox vaccine. Current studies suggest immunity lasts at least 20 years, since children who have received the vaccine 20 years ago are still immune. Although there has been no evidence of impaired immunity, if the vaccine should wear off later in life adults could then be vulnerable to infection at an age when chicken pox can be more serious. It is not currently believed that children will need a booster dose of the chicken pox vaccine.

If given within 72 hours after an exposure to someone with chicken pox, the vaccine may help to prevent the disease in a child who has not been vaccinated. People should not get chicken pox vaccine if they have ever had a life-threatening allergic reaction to gelatin, the antibiotic neomycin, or a previous dose of chicken pox vaccine. People who are sick at the time the shot is scheduled should usually wait until they recover before getting the vaccine. Pregnant women should wait to get the vaccine until after they have given birth, and they should not get pregnant for one month after getting chicken pox vaccine.

Some people should check with their doctor about whether they should get chicken pox vaccine, including anyone who has HIV/AIDS or another disease that affects the immune system, is being treated with drugs that affect the immune system (such as steroids) for two weeks or longer, or who has any kind of cancer or is undergoing cancer treatment with X-rays or drugs. People who recently had a transfusion or were given other blood products should ask their doctor when they may get chicken pox vaccine.

Side Effects

Mild problems or side effects that can occur after receiving the chicken pox vaccine include soreness or swelling where the shot was given, fever, and mild rash, which can occur for up to a month later. Rarely, it is possible for other people to catch a mild chicken pox infection from being in contact with this rash.

Moderate problems can include fever-related seizures. It is very rare for someone to have a serious problem after receiving the chicken pox vaccine, but side effects can also include acute cerebellar ataxia, pneumonia, and possibly (but unproven) severe brain reactions or a low blood and/or platelet count.

varicella-zoster virus A member of the family of HERPES viruses named after the two illnesses it causes—varicella (CHICKEN POX) and zoster (SHINGLES). The virus first enters the upper respiratory tract of a nonimmune host in childhood, and produces the skin lesions of chicken pox. The virus then becomes dormant in the nerve cells that transmit messages from the central nervous system to the skin.

A person's immune system usually can successfully keep the virus from reactivating until later in life, when the patient's immunity to VZV may deteriorate. At that time, the virus replicates within the ganglia, and causes shingles. Why and how the virus replicates is not well understood. In younger people shingles often may appear during periods of stress. It is much more likely, however, to affect people over age 50.

varicose veins Twisted, swollen veins just below the skin's surface, most often found in the legs. When valves in the leg veins become defective, they cause blood to pool in the superficial veins of the legs, which become swollen and distorted. Obesity, hormones during pregnancy or menopause, deep vein thrombosis, phlebitis, or pelvic vein pressure can all accelerate the formation of varicose veins. About 15 percent of adults suffer from varicose veins, which are more common among women and run in some families.

Symptoms and Diagnostic Path

If backflow of blood from varicose veins is severe enough to cut off oxygen and nourishment to tissue, the skin over the veins may become thin, tight, dry, scaly, and discolored, which can lead to ulcers. Bumping a large varicose vein may cause severe bleeding, which can be stopped by tying a clean handkerchief around the leg to apply moderate pressure and raising the affected leg.

Treatment Options and Outlook

In many cases, wearing elastic support stockings, exercising regularly, elevating the legs, and standing still as little as possible will alleviate the problem. SCLEROTHERAPY (injecting an irritant solution into the veins to scar and block them, forcing other healthy veins to take over) also is effective.

If they are very painful or if the overlying skin ulcerates, the veins may be removed using a surgical technique known as stripping. The patient must then keep the affected area bandaged for several weeks to help heal the wound.

Two techniques are replacing surgical stripping. Either a laser or a radiofrequency probe can be placed into the vessel. As it is slowly withdrawn, energy is applied to the vessel, causing it to collapse. These techniques, described as endovascular laser, are very promising.

variola Another name for SMALLPOX.

VariVax See VARICELLA VIRUS VACCINE LIVE.

vascular tumors Tumors related to or supplied with blood from blood vessels. They include HEMANGIOMAS (including superficial strawberry hemangioma, deep [cavernous] hemangioma, cherry angioma, pyogenic granuloma); ANGIOKERATOMAS, spider nevi, lymphangiomas, GLOMUS TUMORS, ANGIOSARCOMAS, STEWART-TREVES TUMORS, and PORT-WINE STAINS.

vasculitis Inflammation of blood vessels that usually leads to narrowed, blocked blood vessels, which eventually destroy the surrounding tissues supplied by those damaged vessels. This is the underlying basic disease process in a number of diseases such as SCLERODERMA, LUPUS, PERIARTERITIS NODOSA, ERYTHEMA NODOSUM, HENOCH-SCHONLEIN PURPURA, SERUM SICKNESS, temporal arthritis, and Buerger's disease. Symptoms depend on the size of vessel involved and their body location.

Vasculitis is caused in some cases by immune complexes in circulating blood. While these immune complexes would normally be destroyed by white blood cells, in certain disease states they settle in the blood vessel walls where they cause severe inflammation.

Symptoms and Diagnostic Path
Skin symptoms include red or purple dots on the legs; larger sports that may look like bruises are called PURPURA. These are the most common vasculitis skin lesions, but HIVES, itchy lumpy rash, and painful or tender lumps may appear. Areas of dead skin can look like ULCERS, and there may be small black spots at the end of the fingers or around the fingernails and toes, or GANGRENE of fingers or toes.

The diagnosis is based on a patient's medical history, symptoms, a complete physical examination, and the results of special lab tests.

Treatment Options and Outlook
Treatment depends on the disease severity and the patient's general health; many cases do not require treatment. For example, an occasional few spots on the skin may not require any treatment.

If treatment is chosen, physicians typically administer steroids such as prednisone, prednisolone, or methylprednisolone (Medrol). Some people with severe conditions that do not respond well will need to be treated with cytotoxic ("cell-killing") drugs to destroy the cells that are causing the inflamed blood vessels. The two most common are AZATHIOPRINE (Imuran) and cyclophosphamide (Cytoxan). These are often used together with prednisone and are often effective.

Other, experimental procedures that may help include: plasmapheresis, intravenous gammaglobulin, and CYCLOSPORIN, a medication used to prevent organ rejection in transplant patients.

Many patients whose vasculitis is confined to the skin may live a normal life, albeit with an annoying skin condition. Most people will find that treatment is at least partially successful.

venereal warts See WARTS.

vernix The pale cheesy substance covering newborn skin consisting of fatty secretions and dead cells. It protects and insulates the baby's skin before birth.

verruca The medical term for WART.

vesicle A small skin BLISTER (usually filled with clear fluid).

viral diseases with skin symptoms Viral diseases are a common cause of skin symptoms. Some of these skin symptoms (such as WARTS) are infections of the skin, whereas others (such as MEASLES and CHICKEN POX) are the symptoms of systemic disease.

Other viral diseases with skin symptoms include dengue, erythema infectiosum (HHV-6), EXANTHEM SUBITUM, HERPES simplex (HSV-1 and HSV-2), SHINGLES, MILKER'S NODULE, ORF, PAPULAR ACRODERMATITIS, RUBELLA, and COXSACKIE (hand, foot, and mouth disease).

Other viral infections that cause only mild skin symptoms include Epstein-Barr virus (infectious mononucleosis), hepatitis, and retroviruses (such as HIV).

vitamin A   The vitamin necessary to maintain healthy skin. Many foods contain this vitamin, but particularly good sources include liver, fish liver oils, egg yolk, milk and other dairy products, margarine, and a wide range of fruits and vegetables.

Deficiency of this vitamin is rare in developed countries, but a serious lack or excess intake can both cause dry, rough skin, among other problems.

Contrary to popular belief, ingesting too much carotene (by eating huge amounts of carrots) does *not* cause excess levels of vitamin A; however, it can produce carotenemia (high blood levels of carotene), which colors the skin deep yellow.

Synthetic vitamin A-like compounds called RETINOIDS, such as TRETINOIN, applied directly to the skin have been used to treat ACNE and skin WRINKLING and mottled pigmentation caused by chronic sun exposure. Used systemically, retinoids such as ISOTRETINOIN (Accutane) and ETRETINATE treat acne and help to prevent SKIN CANCER in those at very high risk.

vitamin A acid   See RETINOIC ACID.

vitamin A deficiency   The earliest signs of vitamin A deficiency appear in the eyes, causing night blindness, dry eyes, and corneal ulcers. Skin symptoms of vitamin A deficiency include dryness, fine scaling, and FOLLICULAR HYPERKERATOSIS.

vitamin B$_2$ (riboflavin) deficiency   Deficiency of this vitamin may cause chapped lips and a sore tongue, or sores in the mouth corners. While a balanced diet usually provides adequate amounts of riboflavin, some people are susceptible to a deficiency. This includes those taking phenothiazine antipsychotic drugs, tricyclic antidepressants, oral contraceptives, and those with malabsorption disorders or severe alcohol dependence. Deficiency also may result from serious illness or injury, or surgery.

vitamin B$_6$ (pyridoxine) deficiency   Deficiency of this vitamin causes a variety of skin conditions, inflammation of mouth and tongue and cracked lips. This vitamin plays a vital role in the activities of various enzymes and hormones involved in keeping skin healthy. Good dietary sources of vitamin B$_6$ are found in liver, chicken, pork, fish, whole grains, wheat germ, bananas, potatoes, and dried beans. A balanced diet will provide sufficient amounts of this vitamin, which is also produced in small amounts by intestinal bacteria.

People who are at risk for developing a vitamin B$_6$ deficiency include breast-fed infants, people with poor diets and those with malabsorption disorders, severe alcoholics, and patients taking certain drugs (including penicillamine, hydralazine, or birth control pills).

vitamin C   Also known by its chemical name (ascorbic acid), this vitamin plays an important role in healing wounds in the skin and in preventing SCURVY. The primary dietary source includes fresh fruits and vegetables, especially citrus fruits, tomatoes, green leafy vegetables, potatoes, green peppers, strawberries, and cantaloupe.

A balanced diet usually provides enough vitamin C, but slight deficiencies may occur after surgery, fever, constant inhalation of carbon monoxide in tobacco smoke and traffic fumes, serious injury, or use of oral contraceptives.

vitamin D   A naturally-occurring substance produced by the interaction of sunlight with chemicals in the skin that helps the body absorb calcium from the intestinal tract and provides for the healthy development and growth of bones. About 15 minutes outdoors a day is enough to meet the body's requirements for the vitamin, although it is also found in many foods. A deficiency of vitamin D, either through a poor diet or lack of sunlight, can lead to rickets. Vitamin D has been added to milk since the 1930s as a way to reduce the incidence of rickets.

Many other foods are fortified with vitamin D, and supplements are also available. Other good dietary sources of vitamin D include oily fish, liver, dairy products, and egg yolks. However, sunlight's interaction with the skin can provide enough vitamin D unless children drink no milk at all. Elderly people who do not drink milk and don't get out into the sunshine do have a potential risk for vitamin D deficiency.

Vitamin D is considered to be an antioxidant (see ANTIOXIDANT BEAUTY PRODUCTS) and anticarcinogen, and may play a role in skin pigmentation. Since it can be absorbed by the skin, applying this vitamin topically can have an effect on the skin's health.

Vitamin D is toxic in very large amounts (between 5,000 and 10,000 IU daily for several months for D3 or D4), and megadoses should be avoided. Sunbathing, however, will not result in an overdose.

vitamin E (tocopherol) This vitamin has a long history of usefulness in skin problems such as bruises, cuts, skin irritations, and to help heal WRINKLES. Scientifically, it has never been shown to be effective when used topically as anything other than a MOISTURIZER, since vitamin E cannot penetrate the outer skin's layers. Some studies have found that this vitamin can actually irritate the skin of the face, especially when it is used with an ACNE product that has a peeling effect. When spray-on vitamin E is forced through the layers of the skin it can lead to severe allergic reactions.

Vitamin E *is* an antioxidant that can help prevent FREE RADICAL damage. Based on the observation that skin damage caused by sunlight and by other environmental agents are induced by free radicals, there is the possibility that vitamin E may be effective in preventing skin damage. It is being used more and more in skin preparations as a way to fend off this damage.

Although topical use of vitamin E has few negative consequences other than the potential for allergic reaction, oral vitamin E overdoses can block the absorption of other fat-soluble vitamins such as A and D.

Vitamin E deficiency is extremely rare, and when it occurs it is usually caused by a disease that blocks its absorption from the gastrointestinal tract. This vitamin is found naturally in vegetable oils, including wheat germ oil; most people get an adequate supply by eating a typical American diet.

vitamins and the skin Experts have known for some time that vitamins affect the skin. Lack of vitamins can make skin lifeless, blotchy, dry, or oily. Healthy skin requires a variety of vitamins to keep it resilient; specifically, VITAMIN A (found in carrots, broccoli, leafy green vegetables, asparagus, cantaloupe, apricots, peaches, and sweet potatoes) and VITAMIN E (in whole grain breads, wheat germ, oatmeal, and eggs).

Furthermore, vitamins E and C (found in citrus fruits and vegetables) are the simplest forms of ANTIOXIDANT. Antioxidants may help prevent skin damage from free radicals, a dangerously mutant form of oxygen that in large doses (from pollution, sunlight, and so on) can break through the membrane that protects the skin's cells and cause inflammation, visible lines, and WRINKLES, among other damage.

Vitamin A may help prevent sun damage, and VITAMIN C may accelerate skin healing. There is also some evidence that vitamin C may pass through the layers of skin and help heal tissue damaged by burn or injury, although some experts dispute this. Vitamin D, absorbed through the skin's outer layers, may help heal the skin when applied topically, especially when combined with vitamin A.

vitiligo A common disease in which the skin loses pigment due to the destruction of pigment cells (melanocytes). In this condition, areas of the skin become white, especially in areas such as the groin or armpits, around body openings, and exposed areas like the face or hands. The unpigmented areas are extremely sensitive to ultraviolet radiation, and are especially obvious in dark-skinned people.

Between 2 to 5 million Americans have this condition, which occurs more often in people with thyroid conditions and some other metabolic diseases. However, most people who have vitiligo are in good health and suffer no symptoms other than areas of pigment loss.

About half of the people who develop this skin disorder experience some pigment loss before the age of 20, and about one-third of all vitiligo patients say that other family members also have this condition.

Medical researchers are not sure what causes vitiligo. Some researchers think the body may develop an allergy to its pigment cells; others believe that the cells may destroy themselves during the process of pigment production. MELANIN is the substance that normally determines the color of skin, hair, and eyes. This pigment is produced in cells called melanocytes. If melanocytes cannot form melanin or if their number decreases, skin color will become lighter or completely white—as in vitiligo.

A combination of genetic and immunologic factors is of major importance in most cases. In more than half the cases, there is a family history of vitiligo or early graying of hair. Many patients do not realize that anyone in the family has had vitiligo, either because they don't know that premature gray hair is a sign of vitiligo or because the affected area is hidden by clothing. In many cases of vitiligo, there is no family history of the disorder, and many vitiligo patients don't have either children or grandchildren with symptoms of pigment loss.

Many people report pigment loss shortly after a severe SUNBURN. Others relate the onset of vitiligo to emotional trauma associated with an accident, death in the family, or divorce. Patients with vitiligo appear to have normal pigment cells. An increase in something such as nitric oxide may be toxic for pigment cells or there may be a lack of growth factors that are required for normal pigment cells to be viable.

Vitiligo and Cancer

Vitiligo is neither a cancerous nor a precancerous condition. People with skin cancer sometimes develop vitiligo; in many of these cases, vitiligo seems to stop the cancer from spreading.

Symptoms and Diagnostic Path

Vitiligo often starts with a rapid loss of pigment, which may be followed by several months when the skin color does not change. The number and size of the light areas become stable and may remain so for a long time. Later, the pigment loss may resume, especially if the patient has suffered physical trauma or stress. Many vitiligo patients report that initial or later episodes of pigment loss are followed by periods of physical or emotional stress, which seem to trigger depigmentation in those who are predisposed. Sometimes, depigmented areas may spontaneously repigment. The loss of color may continue until for unknown reasons it suddenly stops. Cycles of pigment loss, followed by periods of stability, may continue indefinitely. However, it is rare for a patient with vitiligo to regain skin color. Most patients who say that they no longer have vitiligo may actually have become totally depigmented and are no longer bothered by contrasting skin color. While such patients appear to be "cured," they really are not. People who have vitiligo all over their bodies do not look like albinos because the color of their hair and eyes may not change.

In severe cases, the pigment loss extends over the entire body surface. The degree of pigment loss can also vary within each vitiligo patch, and a border of abnormally dark skin may encircle a patch of depigmented skin.

Treatment Options and Outlook

There is no cure for this disease, but the symptoms can be treated, although treatment may not be completely satisfactory. There are two basic methods: Try to restore the normal pigment (repigmentation), or try to destroy the remaining pigment cells (depigmentation). Current treatment options for vitiligo include medical and surgical options, along with camouflage cosmetics. Medical therapies include topical and oral PSORALEN photochemotherapy, topical steroid therapy, and DEPIGMENTATION. Surgical therapies include skin grafts from a person's own tissues, SKIN GRAFTS using BLISTERS, micropigmentation (TATTOOING), and laser therapy.

Repigmentation The most common method of repigmenting is a combination of a drug called PSORALEN (applied to the skin or taken orally) and regulated doses of sunlight. Some clinics use psoralen and indoor ultraviolet light treatments. When psoralen drugs are activated by ultraviolet (UVA) light called PUVA, they stimulate repigmentation by increasing the availability of color-producing cells at the skin's surface. The response varies among patients and body sites. The psoralen treatment is not always successful, but many patients find that it can help restore some degree of pigmentation to areas of the skin. About 75 percent of the patients who undergo psoralen–UVA light therapy respond to some extent, but complete repigmentation rarely occurs.

The psoralen drugs used for repigmentation therapy are trimethylpsoralen and 8-methyoxy-psoralen. A patient takes the prescribed dose by mouth two hours before lying in the sun or under artificial UVA light. The ideal time for natural sunlight is between 11 A.M. and 1 P.M. when the sun is highest. Treatment every other day is recommended. Too much ultraviolet light can be harmful. Treatment schedules can be adjusted for each patient. If the day is cloudy or if sun exposure is not possible on a scheduled treatment day, then the patient does not take any medication because the drug does not work without appropriate sunlight.

In northern United States, patients usually begin therapy in May and continue until September. Moderate repigmentation should take place during this time. Treatment is usually discontinued during the winter. Although artificial sources of UVA light can be used throughout the year, patients should consult their DERMATOLOGIST to determine whether such treatments are desirable. UVA light systems for home use are expensive and treatment can be time consuming. Ordinary sunlamps are not effective with the psoralen medications, since only UVA light produces the desired interaction.

After the initial two to three weeks of exposure to sunlight, patients will look worse since the contrast between light and tanned skin increases. With time, repigmentation will begin, and the appearance of the skin improves. If patients stop the therapy in winter, most will retain at least half of the color they achieved during the summer months.

A dermatologist's supervision is required during all aspects of repigmentation therapy. Patients with vitiligo should always protect their skin against excessive sun exposure by wearing protective clothing, staying out of the sun at peak periods except during treatment time, and applying SUNSCREEN lotions and creams. Patients with vitiligo should use a sunscreen with an SPF of 15 or higher, except during the hours of treatment. During treatment, an SPF of 8 to 10 protects against SUNBURN but does not block the UVA needed for treatment. Sunscreens should be reapplied after swimming or perspiring. To prevent potential damage to the eyes, special sunglasses with protective lenses should be worn during sunlight exposure and for the remainder of the day on which the psoralen drug is taken.

Another method of psoralen treatment, used occasionally for patients with small, scattered vitiligo patches, involves the application of a solution of the drug directly to the affected skin. The health expert applies a thin coat of psoralen to the patient's depigmented patches about 30 minutes before direct sun exposure, which then turns the affected area pink. The dose of UVA light is slowly increased over many weeks. Eventually, the pink areas fade and a more normal skin color appears. After each treatment, the skin is cleansed with soap and water and a sunscreen applied.

There are two main problems with topical psoralen-UVA (PUVA) therapy—severe sunburn and blistering and excess darkening of the treated patches, or of the normal skin surrounding the vitiligo (HYPERPIGMENTATION). Patients can lessen the chances of sunburn if they avoid exposure to direct sunlight after each treatment. Hyperpigmentation is usually a temporary problem and eventually disappears when treatment is stopped.

However, such topical treatment makes a person very susceptible to severe burn and blisters with too much sun exposure.

Hydrocortisone-type compounds when applied to the skin slow the process of depigmentation and sometimes even enhance repigmentation. However, the weak cortisones that are sold without a prescription (such as 1.0 percent hydrocortisone) are too weak to help. On the other hand, very potent cortisones when used daily for a long time produce side effects, such as thinning of the skin. Under the care of a dermatologist it is usually possible to adjust the treatment with topical hydrocortisones so that side effects are at a minimum.

Not everyone is a good candidate for repigmentation. The ideal person should have lost pigment no more than five years ago. In general, children and young adults respond better than older people. Patients should be at least 10 years old. While treatment is safe for younger children, the method is tedious, and better results are achieved when the child is interested in treatment. In addition, patients should be healthy, and no one with a sensitivity or allergy to sunlight can be treated. Pregnant women should not be treated because of the potential harmful effects of the drug on the developing baby.

Depigmentation People with vitiligo over more than half of the exposed areas of the body are not candidates for repigmentation. Instead, these people may want to try removing the pigmentation of the remaining skin so the patient is an even color. However, total depigmentation is tried only in very severe cases of vitiligo.

The drug for depigmentation is monobenzylether of hydroquinone. Many patients with vitiligo are at first apprehensive about the idea of depigmentation and reluctant to go ahead, but those who achieve complete depigmentation are usually satisfied with the end results. Unfortunately, some people become allergic to the medication and must discontinue therapy.

The major side effect of depigmentation therapy is skin inflammation, with ITCHING or dry skin. Depigmentation is permanent and cannot be reversed. Further, a person who undergoes depigmentation will always be abnormally sensitive to sunlight.

Skin grafts using blisters In this procedure, the doctor creates blisters on the patient's pigmented skin with heat, suction, or cold. The tops of the blisters are then cut out and transplanted to a depigmented skin area. Blister grafting can cause a cobblestone appearance, scars, or a lack of repigmentation, but there is less risk of scarring with this procedure than with other kinds of grafting.

Skin grafts In patients with small patches of vitiligo, the doctor may take a skin graft from a person's own tissues, removing skin from one part of a patient's body and attaching it to the depigmented section. Possible complications include infections, scarring, a cobblestone appearance, or spotty pigmentation. Sometimes the graft fails to repigment at all. Grafting is expensive and time-consuming, so most people find it unacceptable.

Tattooing (micropigmentation) Tattooing places pigment into the skin with a special surgical instrument, which works best for the lip area, particularly in people with dark skin; however, it is difficult for the doctor to match perfectly the color of the skin of the surrounding area. Tattooing tends to fade over time, while tattooing the lips may trigger episodes of herpes simplex blister outbreaks.

Experimental procedures In an autologous melanocyte transplant procedure, the doctor tries to grow pigment cells (melanocytes) from a sample of the patient's normal pigmented skin. When the melanocytes in the culture solution have multiplied, the doctor transplants them to the patient's depigmented skin patches. This procedure is still experimental.

Laser treatment The newly developed 308 nanometer excimer laser (XTrac) is a high-frequency source of UVB light that shows promise in repigmenting patches of vitiligo. Treatments are required two to three times a week for several months.

Cosmetics Most patients, even if they are responding well to treatment, would like to make the vitiligo less obvious. Many find that a combination of cosmetics can deemphasize the skin disorder. Cosmetics are not just for women, nor are they only for the face. Anyone can wear them anywhere on their body. Over-the-counter cosmetics exist in a wide range of skin tones; many are waterproof and do not rub off.

There are also special dermatological cosmetics that patients even with severe vitiligo find useful. Dermablend, Lydia O'Leary, Clinique, Fashion Flair, Vitadye, and Chromelin offer makeup or dyes that can help cover depigmented patches.

Vitiligo may spread to other areas, but there is no way of predicting whether or where it will spread. When vitiligo begins and how severe the pigment loss will be, differs with each patient, but illness and stress can result in more pigment loss. Light-skinned people usually notice the pigment loss during the summer, as the contrast between the vitiliginous skin and the suntanned skin becomes distinct. People with dark skin may observe the onset of vitiligo at any time.

Voigt's line(s) Also known as Futcher's lines, these normal color patterns are seen in dark-skinned people (especially African Americans and dark Japanese) in which the border between the darker segment of skin (usually on the upper arms) and the lighter area of skin is marked by a line.

voiles A type of spray-on fragrance that is non-drying because of a lack of alcohol. The voiles (French for "veils") are based on a water-in-oil emulsion and are helpful for consumers with dry skin who find alcohol-based fragrance to be too drying. The oil in the formulation helps skin retain moisture.

volar melanotic macules A condition primarily affecting the skin of African Americans, characterized by darker MACULES on palms and soles resulting from local accumulation of MELANIN. The discoloration lasts throughout life and requires no treatment.

Waardenburg's syndrome A hereditary disorder of pigmentation and hearing loss that was first described in 1951.

The disorder is genetically transmitted to offspring in a dominant manner, and carries a 50 percent risk that siblings may be born with a variation of the syndrome. Still, only a few people who have the abnormal form of the gene show all the features of the syndrome. Researchers believe there may be a connection between the development of pigmentation and hearing during pregnancy.

Symptoms and Diagnostic Path

Symptoms include a white forelock of hair with a triangular white area of skin on the forehead (60 percent); piebald spots on extremities or trunk (5 percent to 10 percent); medial folds of the eyes associated with flattening of the root of the nose (66 percent), and possibly two different colored eyes. About 50 percent of patients may have a nonprogressive sensorineural hearing loss ranging from mild to severe in one or both ears.

Treatment Options and Outlook

Therapy for the depigmentation of the skin is the same as for PIEBALDISM. Attempts to repigment the white areas of the skin with conventional methods (such as ultraviolet light and PSORALENS) have generally been unsuccessful. It is possible to surgically correct the problem with punch autografts, epidermal suction grafts, and thin split-thickness grafts. Repigmentation does occur, and the appearance is often satisfactory. Opaque cosmetics can be used to conceal the more obvious depigmented areas.

wart removal preparations Substances that remove WARTS from the skin. LIQUID NITROGEN is used to freeze a wart and form a blister that lifts off the growth. Sometimes a blister-producing liquid (cantharidin) or a corroding acid liquid or plaster is used. The last two product groups usually contain SALICYLIC ACID, lactic acid, or trichloracetic acid.

warts Harmless, contagious growths on the skin or mucous membranes caused by any of more than 50 varieties of PAPILLOMAVIRUS. Warts appear only on the very top layer of skin, without roots or branches. Occasionally, warts contain small black spots, which are capillaries that have become clotted due to the rapid skin growth caused by the virus. While all warts are basically the same type of growth, they may look different depending on where on the body they appear.

Symptoms and Diagnostic Path

Common warts are firm, well-defined growths up to a quarter-inch wide, often with a rough surface. They usually appear in areas that are frequently injured, such as the hands, fingers, feet, toes, knees, and face, especially in young children. They often appear in crops, and can disappear spontaneously.

Flat warts are flat-topped, sometimes itchy PAPULES found mainly on the wrists, backs of hands, legs and face.

Digitate warts are dark-colored growths with finger-like projections.

Filiform warts are long, slender growths found in the armpits, on eyelids, or the neck in middle-aged or overweight people.

Plantar warts are found on the soles of the feet, flattened by the pressure of the body on the bottom of the feet, forcing them to grow inward.

Genital warts are transmitted through sexual contact, and are characterized by pink or brown, flat, or raised cauliflowerlike groups of growths on the genitals. This type of wart needs prompt diagnosis and treatment, since there is evidence that some of these warts infecting a woman's cervix may predispose her to cervical cancer. *It is important that both partners be checked and rechecked, since the infection can be passed back and forth between them.* Condoms can prevent the transfer of warts. Warts present around the genitals of young children may be a sign of sexual abuse.

Treatment Options and Outlook

About half of all warts disappear on their own between six months to a year after they appear. In many cases they can be left untreated to spontaneously resolve.

Common, flat and plantar warts may be removed with liquid nitrogen or a blister-producing agent, corroding acids, or plasters. Surgical removal with a scalpel, electric needle, or laser also may be used.

Genital warts may be removed by surgery or by the application of podophyllin. Recurrence rates with this type wart are very high and there is no specific treatment available. All treatments are destructive and not that effective.

See also WART REMOVAL PREPARATIONS.

waxing A technique used to remove unwanted hairs (usually from the legs, bikini area, and upper lip) by stripping them from their root. In the procedure, solid wax and resin mixtures are heated until they melt, and are applied to the hairy areas. As the wax cools, it traps the hair; when the wax is pulled off, the hair comes off with it.

Alternatively, tacky material on strips of cloth or paper may be used to remove hair on the body or face.

Waxing is most often performed in beauty salons. When performed on the upper lip or legs around the hair follicle it may cause FOLLICULITIS, an inflammatory reaction.

webbing A flap of skin present at birth, located between toes or fingers that may affect two or more digits. Although mild webbing is harmless, surgery may be performed for cosmetic reasons. In severe cases, adjacent digits may be completely fused (called syndactyly). Webbing may have a genetic origin.

weeping Oozing of clear fluid from a superficial inflammation of the EPIDERMIS. When the ooze dries, it forms a crust.

Wegener's granulomatosis See GRANULOMA, LETHAL MIDLINE; SYSTEMIC NECROTIZING VASCULITIDES (VASCULITIS).

Weil's disease See LEPTOSPIROSIS.

Werner's syndrome A rare connective tissue disorder in men and women associated with premature aging and hardening of the skin, mottled skin color, and spidery veins in the skin. Other symptoms include a distinctive appearance with short stature, beaked nose, premature gray hair, diabetes mellitus, hypogonadism, and leg ulcers.

The disease usually starts in the 20s and 30s and is transmitted as an autosomal recessive trait, which means that a defective gene must be inherited from both parents to cause the abnormality. Generally, both parents of an affected person are unaffected carriers of the defective gene. Each of their children has a one in four chance of being affected, and a two in four chance of being a carrier.

This syndrome usually is associated with an increased risk of cancer, for which there is no known treatment. Death usually occurs as a result of accelerated hardening of the arteries (atherosclerosis), generally when the patient is in the 40s.

wheal A HIVE—a smooth, raised area of skin that is usually itchy.

Whipple's disease A rare disorder found most often among middle-aged men that causes (among other things) abnormal skin pigmentation.

The cause in unknown, but is probably due to an unidentified bacterial infection.

Symptoms and Diagnostic Path

Symptoms include abnormal skin color, malabsorption, diarrhea, abdominal pain, progressive weight loss, joint pain, swollen lymph nodes, anemia, and fever.

Treatment Options and Outlook

Antibiotics for at least one year is the typical treatment.

whitehead   Also known as an open comedone, this is a very common superficial dilated closed pore filled with debris and some white cells seen typically in patients with ACNE. Left untreated, some whiteheads progress to inflammatory pustules, which may then clear spontaneously.

See also MILIA.

Whitmore's disease   The common name for melioidosis, a bacterial infection of rodents caused by *Pseudomonas pseudomallei,* which is endemic in Southeast Asia and Australia. The disease, which is also found in pigs, cattle, sheep, and horses, can be acquired by humans who breathe the bacteria or come into contact with the bacteria via broken skin. The bacteria are also found in soil and water (especially rice paddies).

Symptoms and Diagnostic Path

In humans, the disease takes three forms—an acute septicemic (blood poisoning) with diarrhea; a typhoidal form with local abscess formation and severe HIVES; and a chronic variety. The disease may be milder and more common than had been thought.

Treatment Options and Outlook

ABSCESSES must be surgically drained; antibiotics (TETRACYCLINE with chloramphenicol, piperacillin, gentamicin, or doxycycline) are administered.

Wickham's striae   Pale network of whitish lines on the surface of the PAPULES of LICHEN PLANUS. The lines are also highly visible in the mouth.

Wilson's disease   An inborn defect of copper metabolism characterized by excess amounts of copper deposits in the liver (causing JAUNDICE and cirrhosis) or the brain (causing mental retardation and parkinsonism).

Symptoms and Diagnostic Path

Known medically as hepatolenticular degeneration, skin symptoms include skin darkening (hyperpigmentation) along the front portion of the legs; blue-colored nails, spider ANGIOMAS, and jaundice. Other symptoms include tremor, psychiatric problems, hepatitis or cirrhosis, discolored corneal membrane, bony abnormalities, and so on.

The gene that causes the disease prevents the liver from removing the excess copper ingested in food; eventually, the copper accumulates in the body, damages the liver, and leaks into the brain.

Treatment Options and Outlook

Administration of D-penicillamine for life. For those who cannot tolerate this drug, trientine is a safe alternative. If treated early, patients can expect to live a normal lifespan. Untreated patients eventually develop a fatal failure of many organs.

winter itch   Itchy, dry skin related to the cold winter season.

Wiskott-Aldrich syndrome   This rare hereditary disease is characterized by skin irritation that resembles atopic DERMATITIS, recurrent infections, and a reduced number of platelets in the blood.

The disease is an X-linked recessive trait, which means that it is caused by a defect on the X chromosome, usually leading to problems in males only. Women can be carriers of the defect, and half of their sons may be affected.

Symptoms and Diagnostic Path

The first sign of this disease is usually a bleeding irritation or infection; eventually, other infections appear, often followed by cancers.

Treatment Options and Outlook

Infections are treated by replacement of immuno-globulins and blood platelets; bone marrow transplants have helped some patients. This condition is often fatal.

See also DERMATITIS, ATOPIC.

witch hazel An extract of the leaves and bark of the *Hamamelis virginniana* plant used as an effective astringent. It can dry out spots, reduce oil on the skin, and soothe bruises and sprains. Puffy eyes can be refreshed with refrigerated witch hazel–soaked pads.

Woronoff ring A skin symptom of PSORIASIS in which a white halo forms at the periphery of skin lesions. It is thought to be related to vasoconstriction of vessels surrounding psoriatic plaques caused by the elaboration of prostaglandins.

wound Damage to the skin and/or underlying tissue resulting from an accident or surgery. Wounds in which the skin is broken are called *open* wounds; wounds associated with unbroken skin are called *closed* wounds.

Symptoms and Diagnostic Path

Incised wounds involve skin that is cleanly cut or surgically incised; an *abrasion* is a graze in which the surface skin is scraped away; a *laceration* involves torn skin. A *penetrating wound*, which penetrates all skin layers, would include a stab or gunshot wound, and a *contusion* is a bruise caused by a blunt instrument that damages underlying tissue.

Treatment Options and Outlook

Many minor wounds may be treated with first aid, but deeper wounds require professional care. Any foreign material or dead tissue must be removed. The wound should be cleaned with an antiseptic solution to decrease the chance of infection.

Clean, freshly incised wounds may be stitched closed, and usually heal with little scarring. Contaminated wounds are not usually stitched shut. Instead, they are usually filled with layers of sterile gauze and covered with a bandage. After four or five days, if there is no sign of infection, the wound can then be closed. Otherwise, the wound will be left open to heal on its own.

Cuts and scrapes heal best when treated with a broad-spectrum antibacterial ointment and a proper bandage.

It is best to keep cuts and scrapes clean and moist and not exposed to the air, which forms scabs that cut down on cell growth. Bandages that keep the wound moist (such as those impregnated with petroleum jelly) enable cells to regenerate rapidly.

wrinkles A crease or furrow in the skin caused by the natural process of aging or by excessive exposure to the Sun's damaging rays. Wrinkles are caused by reduced COLLAGEN production and subsequent loss of elasticity in the skin.

Symptoms and Diagnostic Path

While wrinkles are most obvious on exposed areas, they occur all over the body. "Expression lines" may be caused by the contraction of facial muscles during smiling or frowning; when these muscles contract, they pull the skin in, causing a line. The muscles controlling frown lines between the brows may contract even when the muscle is resting, causing deep lines.

Treatment Options and Outlook

Treatments aimed at reducing wrinkles do not permanently restore skin elasticity. These treatments include adding things to the skin to fill the wrinkles (such as collagen, silicone, fat, or Gortex) and removing tissue to smooth the surface (DERM-ABRASION, chemical peels, LASER RESURFACING, and FACE-LIFTS). Newer methods involve injections of BOTOX to paralyze facial muscles and ease frown lines. While all of these treatments are considered permanent solutions, they work best on fine, shallow wrinkles.

Laser resurfacing with a pulsed CO_2 laser or erbium YAG (Er:YAG) is a good technique for the treatment of medium-to-fine wrinkles, emitting a very brief pulse of high-intensity light that is fast enough to limit heat damage in the skin, yet strong enough to vaporize tissue cleanly. Since the heat penetrates the skin no deeper than half the thickness of a human hair, it can remove the wrinkled skin layer by layer without scarring. The procedure can be done on an outpatient basis, and takes on average about one to two hours.

Less expensive than a face-lift, laser resurfacing does not cause bleeding and does not require general anesthesia. While face-lifts are good for sagging skin, they are not ideal for too much sagging skin. While laser resurfacing cannot *replace* a face-lift, it can improve the appearance after a face-lift has been performed by removing the fine lines that may remain.

Unlike other cosmetic techniques, most patients report little or no pain during the pulsed CO_2 or Er:YAG laser treatment. Areas of the skin that can be completely anesthetized, such as the skin around the mouth, are usually pain free. After the technique, the skin may ooze and become puffy, crusting, and red. The skin remains reddened for about six weeks, but can be covered completely by makeup after the first few days. Full healing takes place within about three months.

Many dermatologists today believe the pulsed CO_2 or Er:YAG lasers are a better way to treat wrinkles than either dermabrasion and chemical peels because it allows for better control and safety.

Dermabrasion is the surgical removal of the top layer of skin by high-speed sanding; it can leave the skin smooth and soft, but it also carries a risk of scarring and pigment changes. In an age of blood-borne infections such as AIDS, dermabrasion can be risky to health care workers since the technique tends to spray a great deal of blood.

Deep *chemical peels* also are more risky than laser treatment since the extent of the burn can be difficult to control and the final appearance of the skin may appear artificial. A chemical peel causes a deep, controlled second-degree burn using caustic chemicals; at least one of the chemicals (phenol) may adversely affect someone with poor liver, heart, or kidney function.

Collagen injections, although temporary, is one of the less painful and more conservative methods to temporarily reduce the appearance of facial wrinkles. The procedure involves the injection of tiny drops of human collagen into the skin to minimize lines, filling in deep vertical wrinkles between the eyebrows, deep wrinkles running from mouth to nose, and forehead wrinkles. Results last only between three and 18 months. The entire treatment may take up to only about 10 minutes, and patients recover in two to three hours. Afterward, there may be some redness lasting up to 10 days. A few patients experience bruising, temporary stinging or burning, faint redness, swelling, or excessive fullness. Others may have no reaction. Risks include contour irregularities, infection, or local ABSCESSES. Like all cosmetic procedures, its success depends on the skill of the physician: Ill-placed collagen can leave a bumpy surface.

A face-lift can smooth out wrinkles by stretching the skin, but the effects only last for five to 10 years. In face-lifts and brow lifts, excess skin is removed at the edge of the face, leaving stretched, tighter skin behind.

BOTOX (*Botulinum* toxin), a purified form of the toxin that causes botulism, also can lessen wrinkles. Injected into the face, the substance temporarily and partially paralyzes the muscles underneath frown lines, giving the face a smoother, less furrowed look. While experts report up to a 90 percent reduction in wrinkling, the cost is high.

Risk Factors and Preventive Measures
Anything that protects the skin from sun exposure can help prevent wrinkles.

SOLUMBRA, a type of 30+ SPF sun-protective clothing, can provide medically accepted sun protection.

A typical 30 SPF SUNSCREEN, even though it may claim to provide UVA protection, may still allow UVA rays to penetrate the skin. Solumbra blocks more than 97 percent of both UVA and UVB rays, far better than a typical 30 SPF sunscreen or typical summer shirt.

Wrinkles in Men
Wrinkle-reducing products are also marketed to male consumers, because a man's skin tends to be thicker and oilier than a woman's and therefore needs unique skin-care products. Men's products tend to be more oil-free and concentrated.

xanthelasma   See XANTHOMA.

xanthogranuloma, juvenile   A benign disorder of infancy characterized by red-yellow NODULES that gradually grow larger and then fade away. They first appear in the first six months of life, but they also can occur in older children and adults.

Treatment Options and Outlook

These lesions usually require no treatment.

xanthoma   A yellow deposit of fatty material in the skin that may indicate a disorder of triglycerides or cholesterol.

Symptoms and Diagnostic Path

There are several types of xanthomas, depending on the lipid abnormality. Xanthelasmas are yellowish plaques on the eyelids that are related to lipid abnormality in 50 percent of patients.

Xanthomas may appear over joints such as elbows or knees (tuberous xanthomas) or scattered in showers over the trunk (eruptive xanthomas).

Symptoms and Diagnostic Path

These soft, yellowish bumps are located under the skin with a flat surface and sharply defined margins. The diagnosis is primarily on how the skin growth looks, especially if there is a history of an underlying disorder. A biopsy of the growth will show a fatty deposit.

Treatment Options and Outlook

Dietary changes and agents that lower blood lipid levels can be effective for tuberous and especially eruptive xanthomas. Eruptive xanthomas usually disappear as triglyceride levels return to normal.

xenograft   See HETEROGRAFT.

xeroderma pigmentosum   This rare inherited skin disease causes an extreme sensitivity to light, so that the skin (normal at birth) becomes dry, wrinkled, freckled, and prematurely old by age five, with various types of benign and malignant skin tumors. It is often accompanied by eye disorders such as photophobia and conjunctivitis.

The condition is caused by the lack of an enzyme present in normal individuals that corrects light-induced DNA damage. In affected patients, the lack of this enzyme causes cells to reproduce abnormally, leading to vast numbers of SKIN CANCERS.

Symptoms and Diagnostic Path

Infants or young children exposed to sunlight develop a prolonged skin redness, FRECKLES, and telangiectasia. Skin hardening causes distortions of eyes, nose, and mouth, and eye problems from damage caused by the sun. In some forms of the disease, there also may be microcephaly, mental retardation, and testicular hypoplasia.

Treatment Options and Outlook

Patients must avoid exposure to sunlight by wearing protective clothing and using SUNSCREENS with an SPF of at least 15. Skin cancer is treated by surgical removal or with anticancer drugs.

BASAL CELL CARCINOMA, SQUAMOUS CELL CARCINOMA, KERATOACANTHOMAS, and malignant melanoma are common at an early age and may be fatal.

See also MELANOMA, MALIGNANT.

xerosis   Abnormal dryness of the skin.

yaws One of the world's most prevalent infections, this is a childhood skin disease found throughout the poorer subtropical and tropical areas of the world, caused by a spirochete similar to the one responsible for SYPHILIS. Yaws, also known as frambesia, pian, or bouba, is found between the tropics of Cancer and Capricorn, where more than 50 million people have been treated with PENICILLIN in an effort to eradicate the disease. As a result, its incidence has been reduced in many areas, although it still occurs in many communities. It is transmitted by direct contact with infected persons, their clothing, and possibly by a fly. The spirochetes enter through skin abrasions.

Symptoms and Diagnostic Path

About a month after infection, a highly contagious, itchy tumor with yellow crusts appears on hands, face, legs, and feet. Scratching spreads the infection, leading to development of more growths on other parts of the skin that may deteriorate into deep ulcers.

Treatment Options and Outlook

A single dose of penicillin will cure this disease. Without treatment, growths heal slowly over about six months, but recurrence is common. About 10 percent of untreated patients experience widespread tissue loss leading to destruction of skin, bones, and joints of the legs, nose, palate, and upper jaw.

yeast infections Skin infections caused by types of yeast, the most important of which is *Candida albicans*. *Candida* can normally be found in the mouth, vagina, and large intestine, but for unknown reasons it can cause infection in its host—most commonly in those who take antibiotics, oral steroids, or birth control pills, or in diabetics and the overweight. Age or sex has no effect on these infections.

Symptoms and Diagnostic Path

This type of yeast causes THRUSH (white patches on the inside of the cheeks), cheesy vaginal discharge, monilial intertrigo (damp red eruptions under the breasts, the foreskin, and under-body folds in the obese). It also causes CANDIDA PARONYCHIA (redness and swelling around the nails).

Treatment Options and Outlook

Yeast infections respond to specific systemic agents designed to fight yeasts (such as Nystatin or KETOCONAZOLE).

yellow fever A short-acting infectious disease that gets its name from the jaundiced yellow skin that is its most striking symptom.

The yellow fever virus is transmitted by mosquitoes that spread the disease from monkeys to humans. Today it can be contracted only in Central America or Africa. In urban areas, the disease is transmitted between humans by *Aëdes aegypti* mosquitoes.

Symptoms and Diagnostic Path

Between three and six days after infection there is a sudden fever and headache accompanied by nausea and nosebleeds. Sometimes the patient recovers within three days, but often in more serious cases there is severe headache and neck, back, and leg pain, followed by liver and kidney damage, jaundice, and kidney failure. This may be followed by agitation, delirium, coma, and, in 10 percent of cases, death.

Treatment Options and Outlook

No drug is effective against the yellow fever virus, so treatment is aimed at maintaining blood volume via transfusion of fluids. In mild or moderate cases the prognosis is excellent. Relapses do not occur and one attack confers lifelong immunity.

Risk Factors and Preventive Measures

Vaccination confers long-lasting immunity and should always be obtained before traveling through affected areas. A vaccination certificate is required for entry to many countries.

A single injection of the vaccine gives protection for up to 10 years, but children under age one should not be vaccinated. In addition, eradication of the mosquito from populated areas has greatly reduced the incidence of the disease.

Yersinia (Pasteurella) pestis A small gram-negative bacterium that causes PLAGUE and is transmitted from rodents to humans. Streptomycin is the antibiotic of choice in combatting the bacterium.

zinc For many years, zinc has been used as an astringent, an antiseptic, and a skin protectant. However, a recent advisory panel of the U.S. Food and Drug Administration has determined that zinc salts (ZINC OXIDE, zinc stearate, and zinc sulfide) have no established effectiveness in the treatment of ACNE. Some dermatologists, however, recommend zinc to their patients for its anti-inflammatory effect, theorizing that zinc releases VITAMIN A, which may normalize cells, and suggesting patients add zinc-rich food to their diet (lean beef, cheese, and chicken). ZINC OXIDE also is an effective sunblock.

Deficiency of this element may cause skin inflammation and hair loss, diarrhea, and low zinc blood levels. Skin symptoms are very similar to those of ACRODERMATITIS ENTEROPATHICA. Zinc is a trace element essential for normal wound healing. Small amounts are found in a wide variety of foods, including lean meat, wholegrain breads and cereals, dried beans, and seafood.

A common cause of zinc deficiency is tube feeding without adequate zinc replacement, usually after the second or third month of tube feeding.

Zinc supplements rapidly reverse the deficiency.

zinc oxide An ingredient in many skin preparations that has a mild astringent action and soothing effect. It can be used to treat painful, itchy, or moist skin conditions (such as ECZEMA, DIAPER RASH, and BEDSORES) and is an ingredient in diaper rash ointment. It also can ease the pain and itch of INSECT BITES and stings and hemorrhoids, and will block the ultraviolet rays of the Sun. An inert ingredient, it is often used to thicken lotions and creams.

Zostrix An ointment whose active ingredient is CAPSAICIN, a red pepper derivative used to make chili powder, used to ease the pain of SHINGLES.

Z-plasty A plastic surgical technique used to change the direction of a scar so it can be hidden in natural skin creases or to relieve skin tension caused by a skin CONTRACTURE. It is especially helpful in reducing unsightly scars on the face, and for releasing scarring across joints (such as on the fingers or armpits) that restrict movement.

In the operation, a Z-shaped incision is made with the central arm of the Z along the scar; two V-shaped flaps are created by cutting the skin away from underlying tissue. The flaps are then transposed and stitched.

Zyderm See COLLAGEN.

APPENDIXES

I. Cosmetic Ingredients

II. Color Additive Terms

III. Cosmetic Ingredients to Avoid

IV. Types of Lesions

V. Organizations

VI. Professional Organizations

APPENDIX I
COSMETIC INGREDIENTS

ABRASIVE AGENT
pumice

ACNE TREATMENT
benzoyl peroxide
biotin
birch
ergocalciferol

ANTIBACTERIAL
methylbenzethonium chloride

ANTI-INFLAMMATORY AGENT
coltsfoot
elder
hypericum
juniper
restharrow

ANTIOXIDANT
ascorbyl palmitate
BHA
BHT
hydrogen peroxide
propyl gallate
salicyclic
sodium ascorbate
sodium bisulfate
tricosan

ANTIPERSPIRANT
aluminum chlorohydrate
sage

ANTISEPTIC
balsam
benzalkonium chloride
benzoin
boric acid
chamomile
colloidal sulfur
eucalyptus
geranium
horsetail
juniper
lemon
menthol
myrrh
phenol (carbolic acid)
pine needle
propylene glycol
resorcinol
thyme
zinc phenolsulfonate

ANTIWRINKLE
orange
rose
royal jelly
tocopherol
turtle oil

ASTRINGENT
ammonium alum
apricot
bentonite
birch
boric acid
coltsfoot
hectorite
horse chestnut

kaolin
lemon
nettle
potassium alum
quercus
rose
sage
salicylic acid
thyme
zinc sulfate

BLEACHING AGENT
ascorbic acid
fennel
hayflower
hydrogen peroxide
hydroquinone
lemon
linden
orange
parsley
phosphoric acid
wild lettuce

CLEANSER
acetone
ether
isoprophyl alcohol
mineral oil
petrolatum
SD alcohol
sodium laureth sulfate
yarrow

CONDITIONING AGENTS
alanine
amino acid

amniotic liquid
aspartic acid
benzoin
carrageenan
chondroitin sulfate
collagen
cysteine
cystine
elastine
glutamic acidglutathione
hydrolized animal proteins
lysine
menthionine
P.E.G. 2 stearyl quaternium 4
proteins
tyrosine

DEPILATORY

glyceryl thioglycolate

DETERGENT

benzalkonium chloride
sodium laureth sulfate

DISINFECTANT

benzoyl peroxide

DRAWS SKIN IMPURITIES TO THE SURFACE

almond bitter oil
bentonite
hectorite
kaolin
magnesium aluminum silicate
titanium dioxide
silica
zinc oxide

DRYING AGENT

benzoyl peroxide
kelp

EMOLLIENTS

acetamide
almond sweet oil
althea

apricot kernel oil
avocado oil
beeswax
benzoin
butyl stearate
caprylic/capric triglyceride
carnauba
carrot
castor oil
ceresin
cetearyl alcohol
cetearyl octanoate
cetyl alcohol
cocoa butter
cocoanut acid
cocoanut oil
coltsfoot
diisopropyl adipate
glycerin
glyceryl monostearate
hexyl alcohol
hexylene glycol
isocetyl stearate
isopropyl isostearate
isopropyl myristate
isopropyl palmitate
isostearic acid
laneth
lanolin
lanolin alcohol
lanolin hydrogenate
lard
lauryl alcohol
lauryl lactate
lecithin
magnesium lanolate
microcrystalline wax
mineral oil
mink oil
myristyl alcohol
myristyl lactate
oleic acid
oleyl alcohol
olive oil
palm oil
petrolatum
polyethylene
polyethylene glycols
polyoxethylene lauryl ether

poilyoxypropylene 15 stearyl
   ether
P.P.G. (followed by a number)
propylene glycol stearate
purceline
sesame oil
silicone
spermaceti
squalane
stearic acid
steryl alcohol
vegetable oils
wheat germ

EMULSIFIER

acetamide M.E.A.
ammonium laureth sulfate
ceteareth
ceteth
choleth
disodium monolauryl
   sulfosuccinate
disodium phosphate
glyceryl stearate
isopropyl (lanolate, linoleate,
   myristate, oleate, palmitate
   or stearate)
isosteareth 20
lanolinamide DEA
lauramide DEA
laureth
lauroyl sarcosine
linoleamide
magnesium lauryl sulfate
nonoxynol
octoxy glyceryl palmitate
octoxynol
oleamide DEA
oleth
pareth
poloxamer
polysorbate
quaternium
sodium borate
sodium cocoyl isethionate
sodium isostearoyl 2 lactylate
sorbeth (followed by a number)
sorbitan
steareth

stearic acid
stearoyl sarcosine
sucrose

HEALING, SOOTHING AGENT

allantoin
allantoin acetyl methionine
aloe
apricot
arnica
azulene
balm mint
biotin
birch
boric acid
calendula
coltsfoot
cucumber
elder
honey
hops
horsetail
hypericum
mallow
menthol
peach
peppermint
restharrow
riboflavin
spearmint
thyme
tocopherol
witch hazel

HUMECTANTS

amniotic liquid
butylene glycol
cholesterol
diethylene glycol
glycerin
glycol (usually followed by
    another name)
lactic acid
laneth
lavender
lecithin
lime
P.P.G. (followed by a number)
propylene glycol

royal jelly
sorbitol solution
stearic acid
urea

MISCELLANEOUS

chlorhexidine (skin activity
    booster)
dimethicone (silicone)
folic acid (essential for cell
    growth)
ginseng (promotes cell growth)
papaya (natural exfoliant)
pyridine (helps synthesize
    vitamins)
pyridoxine (helps metabolize fat)
resorcinol (peels dead cells)
retinol (improves dry skin)
rosemary (tonic, antispasmodic)
salicylic acid (peels dead skin
    cells)
sodium bicarbonate (increases
    pH of a cosmetic)
sodium xexameta phosphate
    (water softener)
titanium dioxide (whitens
    powders)
tocopherol (slows
    formation of dark spots)

PIGMENTS

bismuth oxycholoride
chromium oxide green
D&C and FD&C
erric ammonium ferrocyanide
ferric ferrocyanide
iron oxides
manganese violet
mica
titanium dioxide (white
    pigment)
ultramarine blue

PRESERVATIVES, ANTIOXIDANTS, AND CHEMICAL STABILIZERS

benzylparaben
benzoin

boric acid
butylparaben
disodium EDTA
ethylparaben
fructose
imidazolidinyl
lactic acid
methylparaben
parabens (ethyl-, methyl- and
    butyl-)
potassium sorbate
propylparaben
quaternium-15
sodium chloride
sodium dehydroacetate
sorbic acid

SEBACEOUS GLAND REGULATOR

camphor
eucalyptus
hops
lime
linoleic acid
menthol
methionine
myrrh
rosemary
royal jelly
thyme

SOLVENTS

acetone
alcohol
ascetic acid
ether
ethoxydiglycol
isopropyl alcohol
toluene

STABILIZERS/VISCOSITY BUILDERS

amphoteric
cholesterol
glycol
lecithin
phosphoric acid (stabilizer)
sodium laureth sulfate

STIMULANT

anise
apricot kernel oil
chamomile
dandelion
gentian
juniper
matricaria
myrrh
parsley
thyme
sunscreen
cetyl dimethyl paba (escalol)
cucumber
dihydroxyacetone
homosalate
matricaria
myrrh
para-aminobenzoic acid (PABA)

THICKENING/STIFFENING/ SUSPENDING AGENTS

acacia
acrylate/acrylamide copolymer
agaraluminum stearate
carbomer
cellulose
dextrin
gelatin
glutam gum
hydrated silica
potassium alginate
potassium carrageenan
rosin
xanthan

TONER

althea
balsam
hops
horse chestnut
hydrolized animal proteins
lavender
matricaria
mint
pine needle
quercus
rose
spearmint
thiamine H.C.I.
turtle oil
witch hazel

VASO-CONSTRICTOR

camphor
elder
geranium
horsetail
lime
menthol
mint
pine needle
witch hazel

APPENDIX II
COLOR ADDITIVE TERMS

A variety of color additives may be included in cosmetics. The following describe some of the most common:

allura Red AC The common name for uncertified FD&C Red No. 40

certifiable color additives Colors manufactured from petroleum and coal sources listed in the Code of Federal Regulations for use in foods, drugs, cosmetics, and medical devices

coal-tar dyes Coloring agents originally derived from coal sources

D&C A prefix designating that a certifiable color has been approved for use in drugs and cosmetics

erythrosine The common name of FD&C Red No. 3

exempt color additives Colors derived primarily from plant, animal, and mineral (other than coal and petroleum) sources that are exempt from Food and Drug Administration certification

Ext. D&C A prefix designating that a certifiable color may be used only in externally applied drugs and cosmetics

FD&C A prefix designating that a certified color can be used in foods, drugs, or cosmetics

indigotine The common name for uncertified FD&C Blue No. 2

lakes Water-insoluble forms of certifiable colors that are more stable than straight dyes and ideal for product in which leaching of the color is undesirable (coated tablets and hard candies, for example)

permanent listing A list of allowable colors determined by tests to be safe for human consumption under regulatory provisions

provisional listing A list of colors, originally numbering about 200, that the Food and Drug Administration allows to continue to be used pending acceptable safety data

straight dye Certifiable colors that dissolve in water and are manufactured as powders, granules, liquids, or other special forms (used in beverages, baked goods, and confections, for example)

tartrazine A common name for uncertified FD&C Yellow No. 5

APPENDIX III
COSMETIC INGREDIENTS TO AVOID

CONDITIONERS

Irritants: Quaternium 15, Benzalkonium chloride, stearalkonium chloride
Carcinogens: DEA

DEODORANTS

Irritants: Fragrance, lanolin, parabens, propylene glycol, triclosan
Carcinogens: Cocamide DEA

LIPSTICKS

Allergens/irritants: Synthetic colors
Carcinogens: Some synthetic colors, octyl dimethyl PABA

LOTIONS

Irritants: Lanolin, beeswax, propylene glycol, parabens, some preservatives
Carcinogens: TEA

MOISTURIZERS

Irritants: Beeswax, cocoa butter, PABA, propylene glycol, parabens, preservatives
Carcinogens: Polyethylene glycol, TEA, octyle dimethyl PABA

SHAMPOO

Allergens/irritants: Sodium lauryl sulfate, preservatives
Carcinogens: Cocamide DEA

SHAVING CREAMS

Allergens/irritants: Lanolin
Carcinogens: Cocamide DEA, TEA

SOAPS

Allergens/irritants: Almond, coconut, lavender, oak moss, potassium hydroxide
Carcinogens: DEA

SUNSCREENS

Irritants: PABA, octyl methoxycinnamate, lanolin, cocoa butter, coconut oil
Carcinogens: TEA; padimate-0 or octyl-dimethyl PABA *may* be carcinogenic

APPENDIX IV
TYPES OF LESIONS

ABNORMAL KERATIN FORMATION
Acanthosis nigricans
Actinic keratosis
Ichthyosis
Keratosis of soles and palms
Keratosis follicularis
Warts

BLISTERS
Burns
Chemical warfare
Dermatitis herpetiformis
Drug eruption
Epidermolysis bullosa
Erythema multiforme
Frostbite
Herpes gestationis
Impetigo
Pemphigoid
Pemphigus
Phototoxicity
Plant allergies
Porphyria
Toxic epidermal necrolysis
Toxic dermatitis

DEPOSITS
Amyloid: systemic amyloidosis
Calcinosis: scleroderma,
　dermatomyositis
Cholesterol: xanthoma and
　xanthelasma
Mucus: mucinosis, diffuse
　myxedema, pretibial
　myxedema

ERYTHRODERMA
Allergic contact dermatitis
Atopic dermatitis
Congenital ichthyosiform
　erythroderma
Dermatoleukemia
Lymphoma
Psoriasis

HIVES
Cold, warmth, or irradiation
Food or drug allergies
Insect bites

MACULES
Drug eruptions
Infectious exanthemas

NODULES
Erythema nodosum
Granuloma annulare
Leishmaniasis
Leprosy
Lymphomas
Nodular vasculitis
Sarcoidosis
Tumors

PAPULES
Atopic dermatitis
Leishmaniasis
Leprosy
Lichen planus
Localized neurodermatitis
Lymphocytoma

Metabolic disorders
Molluscum contagiosum
Rosacea
Sarcoidosis
Secondary syphilis
Tuberculosis
Warts

PUSTULES
Acne
Folliculitis barbae
Fungal infections
Mercury dermatitis
Pustular psoriasis
Pyodermas
Reiter's disease

VESICLES
Allergies
Contact dermatitis
Dermatitis herpetiformis
Duhring's disease
Fungal infections
Herpes simplex
Miliaria
Mycosis
Nummular eczema
Shingles

APPENDIX V
ORGANIZATIONS

ALLERGIES

Asthma and Allergy Foundation of America
1233 20th Street, NW, Suite 402
Washington, DC 20036
(202) 466-7643
info@aafa.org
http://www.aafa.org/

A nonprofit organization founded in 1953 for people with asthma and allergies. AAFA provides practical information, community-based services, and a national network of chapters and support groups. AAFA organizes state and national advocacy efforts and funds research.

American Latex Allergy Association
3791 Sherman Road
Slinger, WI 53086
888-972-5378 (tollfree)
alert@latexallergyresources.org
http://www.latexallergyresources.org

A national nonprofit organization that provides information about latex allergy and supports latex-allergic individuals. The association offers education and provides support to individuals with latex allergy.

ALOPECIA

American Hair Loss Council
125 Seventh St.
Suite 625
Pittsburgh, PA 15222
http://www.ahlc.org

A group of dermatologists, plastic surgeons, cosmetologists, barbers, and interested lay members that provides information regarding treatments for hair loss in both men and women. The group facilitates communication and information exchange between specialists in different areas, maintains a library, conducts educational programs, offers children's services and a placement service, and compiles statistics.

National Alopecia Areata Foundation
P.O. Box 150760
San Rafael, CA 94915-0760
710 C Street
Suite 11
San Rafael, CA 94901
(415) 472-3780
http://www.alopeciaareata.com

A support group for individuals with alopecia areata, that develops public awareness, provides a support network, raises funds for research, maintains a medical advisory board, and offers research grants. Founded in 1981, the group publishes a bimonthly newsletter covering treatment, research, and development (including wig and cosmetic tips). The foundation also sponsors an annual conference.

BEHCET'S SYNDROME

American Behcet's Association
P.O. Box 19952
Amarillo, TX 79114
(800) 7 BEHCETS
http://www.behcets.com

A support group for Behcet's syndrome. The association conducts educational programs, maintains a speakers' bureau, and publishes a quarterly newsletter, brochures, and pamphlets.

BIRTHMARKS

Klippel-Trenaunay Support Group
5404 Dundee Road
Edina, MN 55436
(612) 925-2596
http://www.k-t.org

The Klippel-Trenaunay Support Group was founded in 1986; its Web site has been established to provide information about the group and about Klippel-Trenaunay syndrome.

BURNS

Burns United Support Groups
P.O. Box 36416
Detroit, MI 48236
(313) 881-5577

A support group for burn survivors and their families that provides support services and information on burn care and prevention. The group conducts educational programs and children's services and operates a speakers' bureau.

International Society for Burn Injuries
http://www.worldburn.org

The ISBI was founded in the city of Edinburgh, Scotland, in 1965 to establish a permanent organization to reduce the incidence of burns and improve patient care, especially in developing countries, and to stimulate prevention in the field of burns.

National Burn Victim Foundation
32-34 Scotland Road
Orange, NJ 07050
(973) 676-7700
(973) 267-8660

A professional group for anyone interested in burns, fire prevention, and burn care that maintains a 24-hour emergency burn referral service and crisis intervention team to provide counseling to burn victims and their families. The group provides free blood services to burn victims, sponsors a self-help group, and conducts burn care seminars and workshops for health-care experts.

The group also provides private helicopters to transport medical teams to disaster sites. It offers consultation and evaluation services regarding suspected child abuse or neglect to the Division of Youth and Family Services and to law enforcement agencies, and presents burn awareness and prevention programs to schools, civic organizations, and day-care centers. It also maintains speakers' bureaus, compiles statistics, and conducts specialized education, children's services, and research programs.

The foundation offers videos and publishes the quarterly newsletter Update.

Phoenix Society for Burn Survivors
1835 R. W. Behrends Drive, SW
East Grand Rapids, MI 49519
(800) 888-BURN (2876)
(616) 458-2773
info@phoenix-society.org
http://www.phoenix-society.org

A self-help service organization for burn survivors and their families that works to ease the psychosocial adjustment of severely burned and disfigured persons during and after hospitalization. The group offers a training program for volunteers, educates the public about disfigurement, discourages concealment of disfigurement, conducts research on psycho-logical ramifications of burn disfigurement, and disseminates information on burns and trauma and their treatment. The society conducts school programs for burned children returning to class and presents the Heroism Award to burn rescuers. It maintains a speakers' bureau and contains books on burn recovery, films, and videocassettes.

CANCER

American Cancer Society
1599 Clifton Road, NE
Atlanta, GA 30329
(404) 320-3333; (800) 227-2345
http://www.cancer.org

The American Cancer Society is a nonprofit organization dedicated to eliminating cancer. This nationwide, community-based voluntary health organization has state divisions and more than 3,400 local offices.

Cancer Care Inc. National Office
275 7th Avenue
New York, NY 10001
(212) 302 2400
(800) 813-HOPE (4673)
http://www.cancercare.org/

Cancer Care is a national nonprofit organization that provides free professional support services to anyone affected by cancer.

Look Good . . . Feel Better
(800) 395-LOOK
http://www.lookgoodfeelbetter.org

A free public service program of classes taught by makeup, hair, and nail aestheticians to help cancer patients cope with the cosmetic crises that may accompany chemotherapy or other treatments, such as loss of hair, eyelashes and eyebrows; uneven skin tone and texture or fragile fingernails. The program was founded by the Cosmetics, Toiletry and Fragrance Association Foundation in partnership with the American Cancer Society.

Skin Cancer Foundation
245 Fifth Avenue
Suite 1403
New York, NY 10016
1-800-SKIN-490
info@skincancer.org
http://www.skincancer.org

The only international organization concerned solely with skin cancer. The nonprofit foundation conducts education programs and provides support for medical training and research.

The major goals of the foundation are to increase public awareness of the importance of preventive sun overexposure and to publicize the warning signs of skin cancer.

It distributes brochures, posters, books, newsletters, and audiovisual materials.

The foundation publishes an annual journal (the Skin Cancer Foundation Journal) and a quarterly newsletter (Sun & Skin News). It also grants its Seal of Recommendation to sunscreens of SPF15 or higher that meet its stringent criteria.

DYSTROPHIC EPIDERMOLYSIS BULLOSA

Dystrophic Epidermolysis Bullosa Research
   Association of America
An association for people with epidermolysis bullosa and their families that raises funds to support research into the cause, nature, and treatment and to provide practical advice, guidance, and support.

ECTODERMAL DYSPLASIA

National Foundation for Ectodermal Dysplasias
401 East Main Street
Box 114
Mascoutah, IL 62258
(618) 566-2020
http://www.nfed.org
A support group for families of ectodermal dysplasia patients and the medical community. The group helps physicians acquire information, locates treatment facilities and makes referrals, provides funds to qualified applicants for care, conducts educational meetings, helps with research projects, and establishes regional centers for diagnosis and treatment. The group also provides children's services, compiles statistics and publishes a number of brochures and newsletters.

EPIDERMOLYSIS BULLOSA

Dystrophic Epidermolysis Bullosa Research
   Association of America
5 West 36th Street
Suite 404
New York, NY 10018
(212) 868-1573
http://www.debra.org
The only national nonprofit organization dedicated to both promoting research to find new treatments and a cure for epidermolysis bullosa and providing information and support for people with EB and their families.

HEREDITARY HEMORRHAGIC TELANGIECTASIA

Hereditary Hemorrhagic Telangiectasia (HHT)
   Foundation International
P.O. Box 329
Monkton, MD 21111

(800) 448-6389; (410) 357-9932
http://www.hht.org
A support group that promotes research into the treatment, causes, and cure of hereditary hemorrhagic telangiectasia (HHT), also known as Osler-Weber-Rendu disease. Founded in 1991, the foundation publishes the quarterly HHT Newsletter.

HERMANSKY-PUDLAK SYNDROME

Hermansky-Pudlak Syndrome
One South Road
Oyster Bay, NY 11771
(516) 922-3440 or (800) 789-9HPS
appell@worldnet.att.net
http://www.medhelp.org/web/hpsn.htm
A volunteer nonprofit support group for those dealing with Hermansky-Pudlak syndrome. Founded in 1992, the network provides education and research, publishes a newsletter and a pamphlet, and maintains a bibliography of materials. The group promotes research activities and is involved in research.

ICHTHYOSIS

Foundation for Ichthyosis and Related Skin Types
   (F.I.R.S.T.)
1601 Valley Forge Road
Lansdale, PA 19446
(215) 631-1411
http://www.scalyskin.org
An educational foundation for persons suffering from ichthyosis, a group of rare hereditary diseases that cause the skin to be thick, dry, taut, and scaly.

The group provides information about the technical, social, and psychological aspects of the disease. Its publications include booklets and a quarterly, Ichthyosis Focus.

KLIPPEL-TRENAUNAY SYNDROME

Klippel-Trenaunay Syndrome Support Group
5404 Dundee Road
Edina, MN 55436
(616) 925-2596
http://www.k-t.org
A support group for individuals affected by Klippel-Trenaunay syndrome and for their families. The support group acts as a clearinghouse of information and correspondence between members. Founded in 1986, the group publishes a quarterly K-T newsletter and holds a biennial conference.

LEPROSY

American Leprosy Foundation
11600 Nebel Street
Suite 210
Rockville, MD 20852
(301) 984-1336
http://www.userserols.com/lwm-alf

A health and research foundation concerned with microbiological research of leprosy, conducting research programs in the United States and the Philippines. The foundation supports clinical and basic lab research and epidemiological surveys and sponsors an exchange program.

American Leprosy Missions
1 ALM Way
Greenville, SC 29601
(800) 543-3135; (864) 271-7040
http://www.leprosy.org

An international medical Christian mission for those with leprosy supporting more than 100 programs in 30 countries with antileprosy drugs, surgical intervention, training, research, public information, and physical and vocational rehabilitation assistance. The group collaborates with member agencies of the International Federation of Anti-Leprosy Associations. As leprosy treatment becomes integrated with community health care, ALM includes those who are disabled from causes other than leprosy in its rehabilitation programs. Founded in 1906 by Protestant missionaries, the group works closely with committees of the World Health Organization and with the U.S. Public Health Service Hospital in Carville, Louisiana. ALM also supports training and research centers in India, Ethiopia, and Brazil. The group also publishes a quarterly newsletter (Word & Deed), pamphlets, reports, and brochures.

Damien Dutton Society for Leprosy Aid
616 Bedford Avenue
Bellmore, NY 11710
(516) 221-5829

A group of religious leaders and laypeople interested in helping sufferers of leprosy that provides relief, research, and recreation to patients all over the world. Founded in 1944, the society has 30,000 members and publishes the quarterly newsletter Damien-Dutton Call.

LICE

National Pediculosis Association
50 Kearney Road
Needham, MA 02484
(781) 449-NITS
http://www.headlice.org

A nonprofit organization established to build awareness about head lice and to standardize head lice control policies nationwide. The NPA seeks to dispel myths about pediculosis while encouraging research and development for safer and more effective management procedures. Its program of education, prevention, and early detection work is an effort to raise pediculosis as a public health priority for the protection of American children and their families.

LUPUS ERYTHEMATOSUS

The American Lupus Society
260 Maple Court
Suite 123
Ventura, CA 93003
(800) 331-1802

A support group for those interested in information on lupus erythematosus, a noncontagious disease that may affect the skin, alone or in addition to other symptoms. The society offers patients support, funds research, holds patient seminars, and publishes the quarterly newsletter The American Lupus Society—Lupus Today.

L.E. Support Club
8039 Nova Court
North Charleston, SC 29420
(803) 764-1769

A patient support group designed to aid people with lupus erythematosus and other autoimmune diseases that offers support and self-help education via newsletters and personal interchange and also provides information on nutrition and medication. Founded in 1984, the club contributes to lupus research and publishes the bimonthly newsletter LE Beacon.

Lupus Foundation of America
2000 L Street
Suite 710
Washington DC 20036
(202) 349-1155
http://www.lupus.org

A nonprofit voluntary health foundation serving patients with lupus erythematosus by providing patient education, services, and support and education to the medical community and the public. The foundation offers a fellowship grant for lupus research and publishes the Lupus News *three times a year, together with other publications.*

Lupus Network
230 Ranch Drive
Bridgeport, CT 06606
(203) 372-5795

An informational group for educators, medical professionals, and individuals suffering from systemic lupus erythema-

tosus. Established in 1985, the group publishes the quarterly newsletter Heliogram, *pamphlets, and reprints.*

MAFFUCCI'S SYNDROME

Ollier/Maffucci Self-Help Group
1824 Millwood Road
Sumter, SC 29150
(803) 775-1757

A nonprofit group established in 1998 for individuals with Olliers/Maffucci's syndrome, their families, and physicians. The group supports research, helps families cope, provides information, and offers a geographic database of physicians and hospitals with expertise in Maffucci's. The group also offers a newsletter, videos, and brochures.

NECROTIZING FASCIITIS FOUNDATION

National Necrotizing Fasciitis Foundation
180 Lafayette Avenue
Suite 10-D
Passaic, NJ 07055
http://www.nnff.org

The foundation tries to educate the public about recognition of symptoms and preventive measures, offers resources, and offers support for those affected by necrotizing fasciitis.

NEUROFIBROMATOSIS

Children's Tumor Foundation
95 Pine Street
16th Floor
New York, NY 10005
(800) 323-7938
http://www.nf.org

A foundation that helps provide surgical and rehabilitation service programs for patients suffering facial disfigurements who are unable to afford private care. The group also trains health professionals, encourages research, and educates the public. The group maintains a patient referral service; founded in 1951, the group publishes an annual newsletter and offers brochures.

PEMPHIGUS

International Pemphigus Foundation
1540 River Park Drive
Suite 208
Sacramento, CA 95815
(916) 922-1298
http://www.pemphigus.org/

Foundation dedicated to providing information and support to people living with pemphigus and pemphigoid.

PEUTZ-JEGHERS SYNDROME

Network for Peutz Jeghers an Juvenile Polyposis
    Syndrome
http://www.epigenetic.org~pjs/homepage.html

Online information site dedicated to Peutz-Jeghers and juvenile polyposis syndrome, with information, related Web sites, a support group, and genetic information.

PLASTIC/RECONSTRUCTIVE SURGERY

Children's Craniofacial Association
13140 Coit Road
Suite 307
Dallas, TX 75251
(214) 570-8811; (800) 535-3643
http://www.ccakids.com

A national nonprofit organization dedicated to improving the quality of life for people with facial differences and their families. CCA addresses the medical, financial, psychosocial, emotional, and educational concerns relating to craniofacial conditions. CCA's mission is to empower facially disfigured children and their families.

National Foundation for Facial Reconstruction
317 East 34th Street
Room 901
New York, NY 10016
(212) 263-6656
http://www.nffr.org/

The mission of the National Foundation for Facial Reconstruction (NFFR) is to enable people (primarily children) with craniofacial conditions to lead productive, fulfilling lives. The NFFR supports the Institute of Reconstructive Plastic Surgery at the New York University Medical Center. Its programs include comprehensive surgical rehabilitation; medical research and professional training; help with social, psychological, and financial needs; and programs to change attitudes.

PORPHYRIA

American Porphyria Foundation
P.O. Box 22712
Houston, TX 77227
(713) 266-9617
http://www.porphyriafoundation.com

A support group for anyone interested in the treatment of porphyria, a class of seven rare (usually inherited) metabolic disorders that affect either the skin or the nervous system. The foundation provides financial support for research, offers educational programs, and maintains a lending library of videotapes, papers, and pamphlets. Founded in 1981, the group sponsors an annual meeting and physician lecture series.

PSEUDOXANTHOMA ELASTICUM

PXE International, Inc.
4301 Connecticut Avenue, NW
Suite 404
Washington, DC 20008
(202) 362-9599
http://www.pxe.org

A nonprofit organization offering services for individuals with pseudoxanthoma elasticum and their families, including a quarterly newsletter and support group meetings. PXE International, Inc. was founded in 1995 to initiate, fund and conduct research; support affected individuals and their families; and provide resources to clinicians.

PSORIASIS

National Psoriasis Foundation
6600 S.W. 92nd Avenue
Suite 300
Portland, OR 97223
(503) 244-7404; (800) 723-9166
http://www.psoriasis.org

A professional organization for people suffering from psoriasis, their families and friends, and health-care workers. The foundation supports research, makes physician referrals, offers a pen-pal program, and sponsors group sessions. The group provides information to schools, libraries, and the media and supplies members with samples of new nonprescription products. Established in 1968, the foundation maintains a library of major medical journals and personal histories of psoriasis patients. Publications include an annual report, a bimonthly newsletter, pamphlets, brochures, and flyers.

ROSACEA/ACNE

National Rosacea Society
800 South Northwest Highway
Suite 200
Barrington, IL 60010
(888)-No-Blush
http://www.rosacea.org

An educational organization that provides information on rosacea to physicians, patients, and the public.

SCLERODERMA

Scleroderma Foundation
12 Kent Way
Suite 101
Byfield, MA 01922
(800) 722-4673; (978) 463-5843
http://www.scleroderma.org

A professional organization that promotes medical research to find a cure for scleroderma. It provides information and referrals to local organizations and medical specialists, offers encouragement and consultation services, a speakers' bureau, and publishes a range of brochures and the quarterly Scleroderma Voice.

Scleroderma International Foundation
704 Gardner Center Road
New Castle, PA 16101
(724) 652-3109

International organization for individuals with scleroderma, family and friends of patients, and health-care workers. It sponsors research into the cause, cure, and control of the disease, and provides information and a quarterly newsletter, pamphlets, and other brochures.

Scleroderma Research Foundation
2320 Bath Street
Suite 315
Santa Barbara, CA 93105
(805) 563-9133
http://www.srfcure.org

A support and research group for interested individuals with firsthand experience of scleroderma that supplements medical research on the cause, treatment, and cure of the disease. The foundation also seeks to develop a national network of support centers for patients and their families; informs the medical community and public about symptoms; and encourages donations, bequests, and memorials. It publishes a quarterly newsletter, the Advance, *and the quarterly* Advance Research and Treatment.

International Scleroderma Network
7455 France Avenue South
Suite 266
Edina, MN 55435 USA
(800) 564-7099
(952) 831-3091
http://www.sclero.org

A nonprofit organization operating a Web site, publishing a book series, and supporting research. It also manages the Scleroderma Webmaster's Association, which provides links to many scleroderma resources.

SHINGLES

Varicella Zoster Virus Research Foundation
24 East 64th Street
5th Floor
New York, NY 10021
(212) 371-7280
vzv@vzvfoundation.org
http://www.vzvfoundation.org
  Nonprofit organization dedicated to funding research into shingles and the VZV virus.

SJOGREN'S SYNDROME

National Sjogren's Syndrome Association
P.O. Box 22066
Beachwood, OH 44122
(800) 395-NSSA; (216) 292-3866
http://www.sjogrenssyndrome.org
  The association promotes public awareness of Sjogren's syndrome and encourages research into the cause and cure of the disorder, sponsors support groups, offers information to the medical community, conducts educational and research programs, and maintains a speakers' bureau. Its publications include the quarterly Patient Education Series, *the quarterly* Sjogren's Digest, *and the guide* Learning to Live with Sjogren's Syndrome.

Sjogren's Syndrome Foundation
8120 Woodmont Avenue
Bethesda, MD 20814
(516) 933-6365; (800) 4 sjogren
http://www.sjogrens.com

SKIN DISORDERS

National Institute of Arthritis and Musculoskeletal
  and Skin Diseases
9000 Rockville Pike
Building 31, Room 4C02
31 Center Drive MSC 2350
Bethesda, MD 20892
(301) 496-8190
http://www.nih.gov/niams
  The mission of the institute is to support research into the causes, treatment, and prevention of arthritis and musculoskeletal and skin diseases; the training of basic and clinical scientists to carry out this research; and the dissemination of information on research progress in these diseases.

STURGE-WEBER SYNDROME

Sturge-Weber Foundation
P.O. Box 418
Mt. Freedom, NJ 07970
(973) 895-4445; (800) 627-5482
http://www.sturge.weber.com
  A support group for patients with Sturge-Weber syndrome and their families that serves as an information clearinghouse on the syndrome, port-wine stains, and Klippel-Trenaunay Weber syndrome. The group, founded in 1986, provides information, offers support, maintains a speakers' bureau, compiles statistics, and funds research. The foundation publishes Branching Out.

TUBEROUS SCLEROSIS

Tuberous Sclerosis Alliance
801 Roeder Road
Suite 750
Silver Spring, MD 20910
(301) 562-9890; (800) 225-6872
http://www.tsalliance.org
  A nonprofit organization founded in 1974 to provide fellowship, generate awareness, and provide hope to those who shared the common bond of tuberous sclerosis. The group also supports research and offers a range of brochures and books.

VITILIGO

National Vitiligo Foundation
700 Olympic Plaza Circle
Suite 404
Tyler, TX 75701
(903) 595-3713
http://www.vitiligofoundation.org
  A professional group for physicians, patients, and supporters that provides information and counseling to vitiligo patients and their families. Founded in 1985, the group raises funds for scientific and clinical research on the cause, treatment, and care of vitiligo.

APPENDIX VI
PROFESSIONAL ORGANIZATIONS

American Academy of Allergy, Asthma and
Immunology
555 East Wells Street
Milwaukee, WI 53202
(414) 272-6071; (800) 822-2762
http://www.aaaai.org

A professional society of specialists in allergy and allergic diseases. The group conducts research and educational programs, maintains a speakers' bureau, bestows annual grants and research awards, operates a placement service, and compiles statistics. Founded in 1943, the academy publishes the annual journal, a quarterly newsletter, and a monthly journal.

American Academy of Cosmetic Surgery
737 North Michigan Avenue
Suite 2100
Chicago, IL 60611
(312) 981-6760; (800) 221-9808
http://www.cosmeticsurgery.org

A professional group that represents practitioners of dermatology, ophthalmology, otorhinolaryngology, plastic and reconstructive surgery, oral surgery, general surgery, and cosmetic dentistry. The group seeks to encourage high-quality cosmetic medical and dental care, provides continuing education for cosmetic surgeons, and promotes research. The academy also compiles statistics, operates the American Board of Cosmetic Surgery, and is the nation's largest organization representing cosmetic surgeons.

American Academy of Dermatology
P.O. Box 4014
930 North Meacham Road
Schaumburg, IL 60168
(847) 330-0230
http://www.aad.org

The world's largest society representing dermatologists, which conducts educational programs, provides placement services, bestows awards, and compiles statistics. Its publications include the bimonthly Bulletin, *the biennial* Directory of the American Academy of Dermatology, *and the monthly* Journal of the American Academy of Dermatology.

American Academy of Facial Plastic and
Reconstructive Surgery
310 South Henry Street
Alexandria, VA 22314
(703) 299-9291
http://www.facemd.org

A professional association for physicians specializing in facial plastic surgery that promotes research and study in the field, maintains a speakers' bureau, conducts education and charitable programs, and compiles statistics. Founded in 1964, the academy is the world's largest specialty association whose members are board-certified surgeons with a focus on surgery of the face, head, and neck.

American Association of Plastic Surgeons
900 Cummings Center
Suite 221-U
Beverly, MA 01915
(978) 927-8330
http://www.aaps1921.org

A professional group of plastic surgeons founded in 1921. Formerly the American Association of Oral and Plastic Surgeons, the group sponsors an annual scientific program each spring.

American Board of Dermatology
Henry Ford Health System
1 Ford Place
Detroit, MI 48202
(313) 874-1088
http://www.abderm.org

The examining and certifying body for U.S. dermatologists offers board certification to those who meet its requirements and pass its examination. The board establishes requirements of postdoctoral training and creates and conducts an annual comprehensive examination to determine the competence of physicians who meet the requirements.

American Board of Plastic Surgery
7 Penn Center
Suite 400
1635 Market Street
Philadelphia, PA 19103
(215) 587-9322
http://www.abplsurg.org

A group established in 1937 and officially recognized in 1941 as the only specialty board responsible for certifying plastic surgeons, the board has 20 directors who meet twice a year to judge the education, training, and knowledge of plastic surgeons. Certification by the board is not required to practice plastic surgery, but it is a status that plastic surgeons voluntarily obtain as an indication of competence. Requirements for certification include graduation from an accredited medical school; at least three years of clinical training in general surgery, completion of an approved residency in orthopedic surgery, or certification by the American Board of Otolaryngology; at least two years of approved residency training in plastic surgery in the United States or Canada; and successful completion of the certification examination.

American Burn Association
625 North Michigan Avenue
Suite 2550
Chicago, IL 60611
(312) 642-9260
http://www.ameriburn.org

A professional organization for anyone interested in the care of burn injuries dedicated to improving the care and treatment of burns. Founded in 1967, the association publishes an annual book of abstracts, a directory of burn care services in North America, and a bimonthly Journal of Burn Care and Rehabilitation.

American Dermatological Association
P.O. Box 554
Millwood, NY 10546
(914) 923-8540
http://www.amer-derm-assn.org

Founded in 1876, this professional society of physicians specializing in dermatology promotes teaching, practice, and research in dermatology.

American Electrology Association
106 Oakridge Road
Trumbull, CT 06611
http://www.electrology.com

A professional group for electrologists interested in education, professional advancement, and uniform legislative standards. The association sponsors the International Board of Electrologist Certification and maintains referral, refer-ence, advisory, and consulting services. Founded in 1958, the association publishes brochures, the quarterly newsletter Electrolysis World *and the semiannual* Journal of the American Electrology Association, *and the semiannual* Medical/Professional News.

American Osteopathic College of Dermatology
1501 East Illinois Street
P.O. Box 7525
Kirksville, MO 63501
(660) 665-2184; (800) 449-2623
http://www.aocd.org

A professional association for osteopaths or those involved in dermatology that conducts specialized education programs and improves the standards of dermatology practice.

American Society for Aesthetic Plastic Surgery
11081 Winners Circle
Suite 200
Los Almitos, CA 90720
(800) 364-2147; (562) 799-2356
http://www.surgery.org

The leading organization of board-certified plastic surgeons specializing in cosmetic plastic surgery. Active member plastic surgeons are certified by the American Board of Plastic Surgery or the Royal College of Physicians and Surgeons of Canada. The Web site offers information on tummy tuck, breast augmentation, breast lift, breast reduction, brow lift, eyelid surgery, face-lift, liposuction and rhinoplasty; non-surgical cosmetic procedures, including laser hair removal, skin resurfacing; and injectable treatments such as Botox and collagen.

American Society for Dermatologic Surgery
930 North Meacham Road
Schaumburg, IL 60204
(847) 330-9830
http://www.asds-net.org

A professional organization for physicians specializing in dermatologic surgery that seeks to maintain the highest possible standards in medical education, clinical practice, and patient care. The group promotes high standards in allied health professions and maintains an audiovisual library. Founded in 1970, its publications include the monthly Journal of Dermatologic Surgery. *The group can provide consumers with a list of local physicians qualified to perform dermatologic laser surgery.*

American Society for Laser Medicine and Surgery
2404 Stewart Square
Wausau, WI 54401
(715) 845-9283
http://www.aslms.org

A professional group for physicians, physicists, and other scientists, nurses, dentists, podiatrists, veterinarians, paramedical personnel, technicians, and commercial representatives concerned with the medical application of lasers. The society exchanges information about lasers and publishes the bimonthly journal Lasers in Surgery and Medicine.

American Society of Dermatopathology
930 North Meacham Road
Schaumburg, IL 60173
(847) 330-9830
http://www.asdp.org

A professional association that seeks to improve the quality of dermatopathology. The group provides information, supports continuing education and research, conducts seminars and courses, and bestows awards. Founded in 1962, it hosts an annual scientific conference and an annual meeting in conjunction with the International Academy of Pathology. Its publications include the bimonthly Journal of Cutaneous Pathology *and its annual membership directory.*

American Society of Plastic and Reconstructive Surgeons
444 East Algonquin Road
Arlington Heights, IL 60005
(708) 228-9900; (800) 635-0635
http://www.plasticsurgery.org

A professional organization founded in 1931 to promote quality care for plastic surgery patients, provide educational programs, and support the activities of its members. To become a member, each plastic surgeon must be certified by the American Board of Plastic Surgery. In addition to its professional activities, the society maintains a patient referral service to help patients choose a plastic surgeon and a speakers bureau.

Cosmetic, Toiletry and Fragrance Association
1101 17th Street, NW
Suite 300
Washington, DC 20036
(202) 331-1770
http://www.ctfa.org

The leading U.S. trade association for the personal-care products industry, with about 600 member companies. Founded in 1894, the CTFA works to protect the freedom of the industry to compete in a fair and responsible marketplace. CTFA also supports the cosmetic ingredient review, a program it helped establish in 1976 that assesses the safety of ingredients used in cosmetics in an unbiased, independent forum with an expert panel composed of world-renowned physicians and scientists.

Dermatology Foundation
1560 Sherman Avenue
Suite 870
Evanston, IL 60201
(847) 328-2256
http://www.dermfnd.org

A foundation for members of national and regional dermatological societies and board-certified dermatologists that raises funds to help control skin cancer and disease through research, improved education, and better patient care. Established in 1964, the foundation's publications include the quarterly Dermatology Focus, *the quarterly* Progress in Dermatology, *and an annual report,* Stewardship Report.

International Guild of Professional Electrologists
803 North Main Street
Suite A
High Point, NC 27262
(800) 830-3247
http://www.igpe.org

A professional organization for electrologists, electrology schools, and manufacturers and suppliers of electrolysis equipment that works to improve the image of electrolysis and promote it as an acceptable allied health profession. It establishes standards for practice, promotes licensing, compiles statistics, provides a referral service, and conducts seminars and research programs. The organization publishes brochures, a quarterly newsletter, and biennial conference reports.

International Society for Burn Injuries
http://www.worldburn.org

A professional society for those who treat or research burns that seeks to disseminate knowledge and stimulate prevention in the field. The society promotes scientific, clinical, and social research in burns; promotes first aid, nursing, and other types of education in all phases of burn care; and offers awards for research. Affiliated with the World Health Organization, the society was founded in 1965 and publishes the monthly journal Burns.

International Society of Dermatology
930 North Meacham Road
Schaumburg, IL 60173
(847) 330-9830
http://www.intsocdermatol.org

An international organization of dermatologists and general physicians that promotes interest, education, and research in dermatology. The group was founded in 1960 and publishes a biennial directory and a monthly, International Journal of Dermatology.

Interplast
300-B Pioneer Way
Mountain View, CA 94041
(650) 962-0123
http://www.interplast.org
   A professional group of medical professionals that sends volunteer teams into developing countries to perform free reconstructive surgery on patients with burns, birth defects, or other deformities. An estimated 37,000 free surgeries have been performed in Ecuador, Peru, Peru, Honduras, Nepal, Mexico, Brazil, China, Thailand, Vietnam, and the Philippines. The group also conducts teaching programs during visits to these countries.

National Foundation for Facial Reconstruction
317 East 34th Street
Suite 901
New York, NY 10016
(212) 263-6656; (800) 422-FACE
http://www.nffr.org

North American Clinical Dermatologic Society
Mayo Clinic
4500 San Pablo Road
Jacksonville, FL 32082
(908) 223-2000
http://www.nacds.com

Plastic Surgery Educational Foundation
444 E. Algonquin Road
Arlington Heights, IL 60005
(708) 228-9900; (888) 475-2784
http://www.plasticsurgery.org
   A professional group for plastic and reconstructive surgeons that sponsors demonstrations, lectures, educational seminars, symposia, and workshops focusing on plastic surgery techniques and procedures. Founded in 1948, the group publishes the Plastic and Reconstructive Surgery *journal, booklets, and* Plastic Surgery News.

Plastic Surgery Research Council
45 Lyme Road
Suite 304
Hanover, NH 03755
(603) 643-2325
http://www.ps-rc.org
   A professional group designed to foster fundamental research in the fields of plastic and reconstructive surgery.

Society for Clinical and Medical Hair Removal, Inc.
2810 Crossroads Drive
Suite 3800
Madison, WI 53718
(608) 443-2470
homeoffice@scmhr.org
http://scmhr.org
   An international nonprofit organization with members in the United States, Canada, Australia, Japan, and beyond. SCMHR supports all methods of hair removal and is dedicated to the research of new technology that will keep its members at the pinnacle of their profession, offering safe, effective hair removal to clients. The society also provides information on the newest technology in hair removal and offers the only national certification for physicians, nurses, and medical estheticians.

Society for Investigative Dermatology
820 West Superior Avenue
Suite 340
Cleveland, OH 44113
(216) 579-9300
http://www.sidnet.org
   A professional society promoting research in dermatology and allied subjects. Founded in 1937, the society publishes the monthly Journal of Investigative Dermatology.

Society for Pediatric Dermatology
5422 North Bernard
Chicago, IL 60625
(773) 583-9780
http://www.spdnet.org
   A professional organization of pediatricians, dermatologists, pediatric or dermatologic house officers, manufacturers of children's skin products, and researchers in pediatric biomedicine. Founded in 1975, the group conducts research programs and bestows awards. Publications include the quarterly Society for Pediatric Dermatology.

GLOSSARY

abdominoplasty A tummy tuck.

abrasion A slight loss of epithelium (usually caused by a scrape) that causes oozing and crusting.

abscess A clearly defined walled-off inflammatory area (usually caused by infection) that contains pus.

actininc Relating to sunshine.

actinic keratosis Rough slightly raised, pink, or red papules that appear singly or in groups on sun-damaged skin.

acute condition A condition that appears suddenly.

adnexa Term that refers to hair, nails, sweat, and oil glands.

allergen Substance that causes allergic reactions.

alopecia Hair loss.

anagen Growth phase of hair.

anaphylactic shock A severe life-threatening reaction that occurs in people with an extreme sensitivity to a particular substance that causes the release of massive amounts of histamines and other inflammatory chemicals that affect body tissues. The dilation of blood vessels cause a drop in blood pressure; other symptoms include hives, constriction of the airway, leading to breathing problems, abdominal pain, and swelling of the tongue.

androgen Male hormone.

angioedema A soft tissue swelling of skin caused by excess fluid.

angioma A tumor comprising blood or lymph vessels.

anhidrosis Absence of the ability to sweat.

annular Ring-shaped.

antifungal A substance that destroys or suppresses the growth/reproduction of fungi.

antigen Any substance foreign to the body's system that causes an immune response.

antihistamine A drug that counteracts the action of histamine.

aplasia Lack of development of a tissue or organ.

apocrine A gland that releases cellular material and fluid. It usually applies to the type of sweat gland found only in hairy areas of the body and that develop after puberty.

atrophy Wasting away.

Auspitz's sign Pinpoint bleeding when the scale of a psoriatic lesion is removed.

axillary Referring to the armpit area of the body.

basal cells Cells found along the bottom layer of the top layer of the skin.

benign Not malignant.

blackhead A darkened plug of sebum and keratin blocking the outlet of a sebaceous (oil-forming) gland in the skin. (Another name for open comedo.)

blanch To make white or pale.

bromhidrosis Foul-smelling sweat produced by the apocrine sweat glands, caused by bacterial decomposition.

bubo Enlarged, inflamed lymph node (especially under the arm or in the groin) caused by infections (such as plague, tuberculosis, or syphilis).

bulla A fluid-filled blister.

café-au-lait macules Medium brown-colored patches that may appear without an underlying disorder or in patients with neurofibromatosis.

callus Area of skin that is thickened in certain areas (especially on the hands and feet), in response to friction or pressure.

canker sore A small painful ulcer usually found in the mouth or on the lips.

carbuncle A deep-seated infection involving clustered hair follicles.

carcinoma A malignant growth of cells.

carcinoma in situ Limitation of cancer to its place of origin.

carotenemia Yellowed skin (similar to jaundice) caused by too much carotene in the skin. It is most often caused by eating too many carrots.

cavernous hemangioma A vascular tumor of large blood vessels found in the deep dermis (middle layer of the skin), extending into the subcutaneous fat.

cellulitis Inflammation of tissues of the skin usually caused by bacterial infection.

chancre A papule or ulcer at the site of infection in the skin caused by diseases such as syphilis or tuberculosis.

cold sore The common term for a herpes simplex infection (usually on the lips).

collagen The primary supportive protein of the skin.

comedo Thick secretion of dead skin cells and oily substances that plug a pore or follicle. When open, it is called a blackhead; when closed, a whitehead.

corn A tender, horny, thickened growth produced by friction or pressure, resulting in a cone-shaped mass pointing into the middle layer of skin (dermis).

corticosteroids A group of anti-inflammatory drugs similar to hormones produced by the adrenal glands.

crust Outer layer of solid material caused by drying of a secretion by the body.

curettage The removal of skin tissue with a curette.

curette An instrument with a tip shaped like a spoon or loop used to remove abnormal tissue or growths.

cutis The skin.

cyst A sac containing either a liquid or semisolid.

depigmentation Loss of pigment (usually melanin).

dermabrasion Surgical removal by mechanical methods of the epidermis (outermost layer of skin) and as much of the dermis (middle skin layer) as necessary.

dermatitis Skin inflammation.

dermatofibroma A benign skin nodule found most often on the arms and legs.

dermis Part of the skin lying directly under the epidermis, made up primarily of connective tissue.

diaphoretic A substance that produces or increases perspiration.

ecchymosis Bruise.

eccrine The name for the common sweat gland and its related structures.

edema Collection of excess fluid in the skin leading to swelling.

elastosis Degeneration of elastic tissue.

electrodesiccation Dehydration and destruction of skin tissue using a high-frequency electric current.

emollient A substance used to moisten, soften, or smooth the skin.

emulsifier A substance that binds two dissimilar substances together (such as the mixture of an egg, oil, and vinegar to make mayonnaise).

emulsion One liquid broken down into globules and distributed throughout a second liquid.

ephelis Freckle (plural: ephelides).

epidermis The very thin outer layer of the skin that covers the dermis; it contains the stratum basal, stratum spinosum, stratum granulosum, stratum lucidum, and stratum corneum.

erosion A superficial ulcer, resulting in loss of epidermis (outer skin layer) that heals without scars.

eruption Visible rash or production of lesions.

erythema Red, warm skin usually caused by inflammation due to infection or injury.

erythroderma Generalized redness of the skin.

eschar Crusted dead skin produced by burns, corrosive agents, or gangrene.

exfoliative Diffuse scaling.

factitial Produced artificially.

fibroma A tumor of fibrous or mature connective tissue.

fissure Crack or split in the skin.

flush Redness and warmth (usually of the face and neck).

follicle A sac, cavity, or depression.

fungus Simple parasitic life forms that make up a plant phylum (including yeasts, rusts, molds, smuts, mushrooms, mildews, and so on).

granular The presence of granules or grains.

granuloma A chronic, proliferative lesion of cells often associated with chronic inflammation anywhere in the body.

hemangioma A benign tumor composed of blood vessels.

hematoma A localized accumulation of blood (usually clotted) in skin caused by a rupture of a blood vessel wall.

hidradenitis Inflammation of a sweat gland (usually an apocrine gland).

histamine A chemical found in cells all over the body that is released during an allergic reaction; it is one of the substances responsible for inflammation.

hives An eruption of itchy wheals (raised white lumps surrounded by red areas) on the skin (also called urticaria).

hyperhidrosis Excessive sweating.

hyperpigmentation An abnormal excess of pigmentation (or darkening) of the skin.

hyperplasia An increase in the number of keratocytes that cause a thickened epidermis (topmost layer of the skin).

hypersensitivity A condition of heightened reactivity in that the body responds with an exaggerated reaction to a foreign substance.

hypertrichosis Excess hair growth.

hypertrophic scar Enlarged or thickened scar.

hypertrophy Thickened epidermis (topmost skin layer) caused by the increase in keratinocyte size.

hypopigmentation A reduction of pigment resulting in a lightening of skin.

integument The skin.

keloid A sometimes tender scar that is sharply elevated and larger than the original wound.

keratin   The principal protein constituent of epidermis, hair, and nails.

keratinization   The process by which the epidermal cells (outer layer of the skin) turn into keratin.

kerion   A deep fungal infection of hair-bearing skin that produces a nodular swelling covered with pustules.

laceration   Torn, ragged skin wound.

lanugo   The fine hair covering the fetus.

lentigo   Pigmented macule on the skin (liver spot).

lichenification   Thickened epidermis with exaggerated normal markings.

liniment   Oily liquid preparation.

lipoma   A benign tumor composed of mature fat cells.

lotion   A liquid preparation in suspension or dispersion for external application to the body.

macerate   Soften by wetting or soaking.

macule   Nonpalpable area of skin that has a different color or texture from surrounding skin, but flush with surrounding skin.

malignant   Cancerous.

melanin   Dark pigment contained in special cells in the hair and skin.

melanocyte   Melanin-producing cells found in the bottom layer of the top skin layer (epidermis).

mesoderm   The middle layer of the three primary germ layers of the embryo.

milia   Small white cysts.

mole   A nevocellular nevus.

morbilliform   Eruption resembling measles.

mycosis   Any disease caused by a fungus.

necrosis   Death of cells.

ointment   A greasy semisolid preparation applied to the skin.

papule   Raised pimple that is smaller than a pea.

petechia   A tiny non-blanchable red spot caused by a capillary hemorrhage.

pH   A measure of acidity or alkalinity using a scale from 0 to 14 (the lower the number, the more acidic; the higher the number, the more alkaline). Vinegar has a pH of 2.3; the skin has a slightly acid pH (between 5.5 and 6.8). Most soaps are pH 8 to 10.

pilar   Pertaining to the hair.

poikiloderma   Dappled, mottled with areas of hypo- and hyperpigmentation and atrophy.

porphyria   A group of diseases caused by dysfunction in porphyrin metabolism, characterized by increased production and excretion of porphyrins.

poultice   A moist hot pack applied to the skin.

prurigo   An itchy area of skin.

pruritus   Itching.

purpura   The generic term for hemorrhage into tissue. It may appear as pinpoint bleeding (petechiae) or larger areas (bruise).

pus   A liquid caused by inflammation consisting of leukocytes, dead tissue, and fluid.

pustule   A raised skin lesion (papule), usually less than 1 cm, containing pus.

pyoderma   A condition of the skin involving pus-filled lesions.

rash   Skin eruption.

scale   The thin cells that build up on the outer layer of the skin due to abnormal formation and shedding of the top layers.

schlerosis   Hardening.

seborrhea   Excess secretion of sebum.

sebum   The oily secretion produced by the oil (sebaceous) glands, consisting of fats and waxes designed to lubricate the skin and keep it supple.

shake lotion   A suspension of a powder in a lotion.

squamous cell   Flat cell that makes up most of the top skin layer (epidermis).

systemic   Affecting many or all of the organs or systems of the body.

telangiectasia   Dilation of small group of blood vessels that look like small red lines.

tinea   Superficial fungal skin infection of skin, hair, or nails.

topical medication   Drugs that are applied directly to the surface of the skin.

tumefaction   Swelling.

ulcer   An erosion or loss of skin layers from the surface of the skin downward.

urticaria   The medical term for hives or wheals.

vascular   Related to blood vessels.

verruca   A wart.

vesicle   A small blister less than .5 cm in diameter.

wheal   Solid, distinct raised lesion formed by swelling welt that may be white to dark pink.

xerosis   Skin dryness.

BIBLIOGRAPHY

Abel, Elizabeth, Lionel Bercovitch, and Howard L. Stoll Jr. "When actinic keratoses are a problem," *Patient Care* 26 (July 15, 1992): 115–128.

Adler, Tina. "Sunscreen can't give blanket protection," *Science News* 145 (January 22, 1994): 54–55.

Alam, M., and Jeffrey S. Dover. "On beauty: Evolution, psychosocial considerations, and surgical enhancement," *Archives of Dermatology.* 147, no. 6 (June 2001): 795–807.

Alora, M. B., Jeffrey S. Dover, and K. A. Arndt. "Lasers for vascular lesions," *Dermatologic Nursing* 11, no. 2 (April 1999): 97–102, 105–107.

Alam, M., J. S. Dover, and K. A. Arndt. "Pain associated with injection of botulinum A exotoxin reconstituted using isotonic sodium chloride with and without preservative: A double-blind, randomized controlled trial," *Archives of Dermatology* 138, no. 4 (March 2002): 510–514.

———. "Treatment of facial telangiectasia with variable-pulse high-fluence pulsed-dye laser: Comparison of efficacy with fluences immediately above and below the purpura threshold," *Dermatologic Surgery* 29, no. 7 (July 2003): 681–684.

———. "Energy delivery devices for cutaneous remodeling: lasers, lights, and radio waves," *Archives of Dermatology* 139, no. 10 (October 2003): 1,351–1,360.

Alam, M., K. A. Arndt, and J. S. Dover. "Severe, intractable headache after injection with botulinum a exotoxin: Report of 5 cases," *Journal of the American Academy of Dermatology* 46, no. 1 (January 2002): 62–65.

Alam, M., N. E. Omura, J. S. Dover, and K. A. Arndt. "Glycolic acid peels compared to microdermabrasion: A right-left controlled trial of efficacy and patient satisfaction," *Dermatologic Surgery* 28, no. 6 (June 2002): 475–479.

———. "Clinically significant facial edema after extensive treatment with purpura-free pulsed-dye laser," *Dermatologic Surgery* 29, no. 9 (September 2003): 920–924.

Alam, M., T. S. Hsu, J. S. Dover, D. A. Wrone, et al. "Nonablative laser and light treatments: Histology and tissue effects—a review," *Lasers in Surgery and Medicine* 33, no. 1 (2003): 30–39.

Alam, M., J. S. Dover, A. W. Klein and K. A. Arndt. "Botulinum A exotoxin for hyperfunctional facial lines: Where not to inject," *Archives of Dermatology* 138, no. 9 (August 2002): 1,180–1,185.

Alam, M., L. Pantanowitz, A. M. Harton, K. A. Arndt, et al. "A prospective trial of fungal colonization after laser resurfacing of the face: Correlation between culture positivity and symptoms of pruritus," *Dermatologic Surgery* 29, no. 3 (March 2003): 255–260.

Anastasi, Joyce, and Julie Rivera. "Identifying the skin manifestations of HIV," *Nursing* 22 (November 1992): 58–61.

Armstrong, B. K., and A. Kricker. "How much melanoma is caused by sun exposure?" *Melanoma Research* 3, no. 6 (December 1993): 395–401.

Armstrong, Robert. "Clinical panel assessment of photodamaged skin treated with isotretinoin using photographs," *Journal of the American Medical Association* 268 (August 12, 1992): 720.

Arndt, K. A., M. S. Kaminer, and J. S. Dover. "What is cosmetic surgery?" *Seminars in Cutaneous Medicine and Surgery* 21, no. 1 (March 2002): 1–2.

Arnott, Nancy. "Your baby head to toe," *American Baby* 54 (June 1992): 48–51.

"Artificial fat aids skin replacement," *USA Today*, June 1993, 53.

Ash, L. R., and T. C. Orihel. *Atlas of Human Parasitology.* Chicago: American Society of Clinical Pathologists, 1997.

Atlas, E., and A. Yee. "Bites of the brown recluse spider," *New England Journal of Medicine* 352, no. 19 (May 2005): 2,029–2,030.

Batra, R. S., J. S. Dover, L. Hobbs, and T. J. Phillips. "Evaluation of the role of exogenous estrogen in postoperative progress after laser skin resurfacing," *Dermatologic Surgery* 29, no. 1 (January 2003): 43–48.

Batra, R. S., C. I. Jacob, L. Hobbs, K. A. Arndt, et al. "A prospective survey of patient experiences after laser skin resurfacing: Results from 2 ½ years of follow-up," *Archives of Dermatology* 139, no. 10 (October 2003): 1,295–1,299.

Belcove, Julie, Cara Kagan, and Soren Larson. "Beauty companies ride acid wave," *Women's Wear Daily,* March 18, 1994, S4–5.

Beljaards, R. C., K. P. de Roos, and F. G. Bruins. "NewFill for skin augmentation: A new filler or failure?" *Dermatological Surgery* 31, no. 7 (July 2005): 772–776.

Bernstein, E. F. "Hair growth induced by diode laser treatment," *Dermatological Surgery* 31, no. 5 (May 2005): 584–586.

Biesman, B. S., J. S. Dover, K. A. Arndt, and R. G. Geronemus. "Lasers in facial plastic surgery," *Archives of Facial and Plastic Surgery* 4, no. 4 (October to December 2002): 270–127.

Bleicher, P. A., Jeffrey S. Dover, and Kenneth A. Arndt. "Lichenoid dermatoses and related diseases, Part I" *Journal of American Academy of Dermatology* 22 (February 1990): 288–292.

———. "Lichenoid dermatoses and related diseases, Part II" *Journal of American Academy of Dermatology* 22 (April 1990): 671–675.

Bondeson, J., and A. Rausing. "Reversible scleroderma, fasciitis and perimyositis," *Clinical and Experimental Rheumatology* 12, no. 1 (January/February 1994): 71–73.

Bonifas, J. M., A. L. Rothman, and E. H. Epstein, Jr. "Epidermolysis bullosa simplex: Evidence in two families for keratin gene abnormalities," *Science* 254 (November 22, 1991): 1,202–1,206.

Bourguignon, Jean-Pierre, Gerald Pierard, Christian Ernould, Claudine Heinrichs, Margarita Graen, Pierre Rochiccioli, Jorge Arrese, and Claudine Franchimont. "Effects of human growth hormone therapy on melanocytic naevi," *Lancet* 341 (June 12, 1993): 1,505–1,507.

Bouzari, N., K. Nouri, H. Tabatabai, Z. Abbasi, et al. "The role of number of treatments in laser-assisted hair removal using a 755-nm alexandrite laser," *Journal of Drugs and Dermatology* 4, no. 5 (September–October 2005): 573–578.

Boyer, Pamela. "The perfect tan: Save-your-skin tans without the dangers of sun exposure," *Prevention,* (May 1993): 116–121.

———. "Moisturizers for the 21st century," *Prevention,* (December 1992): 81–85.

Brazzelli, V., et al. "Effects of fluid volume changes during hemodialysis on the biophysical parameters of skin," *Dermatology* 188 (2) 1994: 113–116.

Brincat, M. P., Y. M. Baron, and R. Galea. "Estrogens and the skin," *Climacteric* 8, no. 2 (June 2005): 110–123.

Bronaugh, R. L. "Dose response relationship in skin sensitization," *Food and Chemical Toxics* 32 (February 1994): 113–117.

Brumberg, Elaine. "What Price Beauty?" *Modern Maturity,* August/September 1993, 74.

Bulengo-Ransby, Stella, Christopher Griffiths, Candace Kimbrough-Green, et al. "Topical tretinoin therapy for hyperpigmented lesions caused by inflammation of the skin in black patients," *The New England Journal of Medicine* 328 (May 20, 1993): 1,438–1,443.

Burnham, Gilbert. "Ivermectin where Loa loa is endemic," *Lancet* (July 5, 1997): 2–3.

Cahill, J., and R. Sinclair. "Cutaneous manifestations of systemic disease," *Australian Family Physician* 34, no. 5 (May 2005): 335–340.

Caldwell-Brown, Dorothea, Robert S. Stern, et al. "Lack of efficacy of phenytoin in recessive dystrophic epidermolysis bullosa," *Journal of the American Medical Association* 327 (July 16, 1992): 163–168.

Campbell, Laurel. "Assessing pediatric rashes," *RN* 56 (April 1993): 58–65.

Cantor, J. "Cosmetic dermatology and physicians' ethical obligations: More than just hope in a jar," *Seminars in Cutaneous Medicine and Surgery* 24, no. 3 (September 2005): 155–160.

Cassano, N., N. Arpaia, and G. A. Vena. "Diode laser hair removal and isotretinoin therapy," *Dermatologic Surgery* 31, no. 3 (March 2005): 380–381.

Champsi, Jamila, and Stanley Deresinski. "Cutaneous tuberculosis," *Journal of the American Medical Association* 268 (September 9, 1992): 1,339.

Colwell, Shelley. "Treatment cosmetics: more than just a pretty face," *Soap-Cosmetics-Chemical Specialties* 70 (March 1994): 22–26.

Committee to Advise on Tropical Medicine and Travel (CATMAT). "Statement on personal protective measures to prevent arthropod bites," *Canada Communicable Disease Report* 15, no. 31 (May 2005): 1–18.

Consumer Reports editors. "Indoor tanning: unexpected dangers," *Consumer Reports* 70, no. 2 February 2005): 30–33.

Consumer Reports editors. "It won't kill you to dye," *Consumer Reports On Health,* June 1994, 69.

Coopman, Serge, et al. "Cutaneous disease and drug reactions in HIV infection," *The New England Journal of Medicine* 328 (June 10, 1993): 1,670–1,675.

Cowen, Ron. "Dermatophagy: Waste Not, Want Not?" *Science News* (June 19, 1993): 397.

Current Health editors. "Birthmarks: lifelong companions," *Current Health* 18 (April 1992): 30–32.

Darmstadt, G. I., and M. H. Karizler. "Subcutaneous fat necrosis of newborn," *Archives of Pediatrics and Adolescent Medicine* 148 (January 1994): 61–62.

Davis, Donald. "Boggy ground," *Drug & Cosmetic Industry* 154 (March 1994): 22.

Dawber, R. P. "Guidance for the management of hirsutism," *Current Medical Research and Opinion* 21, no. 8 (August 2005): 1,227–1,234.

DeCoste, Susan, and Robert Stern. "Diagnosis and treatment of nevomelanocytic lesions of the skin: A community-based study," *Journal of the American Medical Association* 269 (March 24, 1993): 1,554.

van Deuren, Marcel. "Rapid diagnosis of acute meningococcal infections by needle aspiration or biopsy of skin lesions," *Journal of the American Medical Association* 270 (July 21, 1993): 326.

Dellavalle, R. P., L. M. Schilling, A. K. Chen, and E. J. Hester. "Teenagers in the UV tanning booth? Tax the tan," *Archives of Pediatric and Adolescent Medicine* 157, no. 9 (September 2003): 845–846.

Demko, C. A., E. A. Borawski, S. M. Debanne, K. D. Cooper, and K. C. Stange. "Use of indoor tanning facilities by white adolescents in the United States," *Archives of Pediatric and Adolescent Medicine* 157, no. 9 (September 2003): 854–60.

DermNet NZ. "Seaweed Dermatitis," DermNet NZ. Available online. URL: http://www.dermnetnz.org/dermatitis/plants/seaweed.html. Downloaded May 29, 2005.

Diaz, J. H. "The epidemiology, syndromic diagnosis, management, and prevention of spider bites in the South," *Journal of the Louisiana State Medical Society* 157, no. 1 (January–February 2005): 32–38.

DiBernardo, B. E., and A. Cacciarelli. "Cutaneous lasers," *Clinical Plastic Surgery* 32, no. 2 (April 2005): 141–150.

Discover. "Skin deep," *Discover,* August 1991, 16.

Dover, J. S. "My skin has become drier and more fragile as I've aged. Why is that, and what can I do about it?" *Health News* 8, no. 8 (August 2002): 12.

Dover, J. S. "Roundtable discussion on laser skin resurfacing," *Dermatologic Surgery* 25, no. 8 (August 1999): 639–653.

Dover, Jeffrey S., and Kenneth Arndt. "Dermatology," *Journal of the American Medical Association* 265 (June 19, 1991): 3,111–3,114.

———. "New approaches to the treatment of vascular lesions," *Lasers Surgical Medicine* 26, no. 2 (2000): 158–163.

Dover, Jeffrey S., and R. A. Johnson. "Basal cell carcinoma," *New England Journal of Medicine* 329 (August 1993): 545.

———. "Cutaneous manifestation of HIV-infected patients, Part I" *Archives of Dermatology* 127 (September 1991): 1,383–1,391.

———. "Cutaneous manifestation of HIV-infected patients, Part II" *Archives of Dermatology* 127 (October 1991): 1,549–1,558.

Dover, Jeffrey S., S. I. Kilmer, and R. R. Anderson. "What's new in cutaneous laser surgery," *Journal of Dermatologic Surgery and Oncology* 19 (April 1993): 295–298.

Dover, J. S., N. S. Sadick, and M. P. Goldman. "The role of lasers and light sources in the treatment of leg veins," *Dermatologic Surgery* 25, no. 4 (April 25, 1999): 328–335.

Dover, J. S., et al. "Guidelines of care for laser surgery, American Academy of Dermatology. Guidelines/Outcomes Committee," *Journal of the American Academy of Dermatology* 41, no. 3; pt. 1 (September 1999): 484–495.

Dworkin, R. H., and R. K. Portenoy. "Pain and its persistence in herpes zoster," *Pain* 67 (1996): 241–251.

Eden, Alvin. "A sensitive subject—diaper rash," *American Baby* 54 (December 1992): 10–11.

———. "Getting to the bottom of diaper rash," *American Baby* 54 (November 1991): 16–17.

Edlich, R. F., K. L. Winters, L. D. Britt, W. B. Long, K. D. et al. "Difficult wounds: an update," *Journal of Long-Term Effects of Medical Implants* 15, no. 3 (2005): 289–302.

Edwards, Libby. "Treatment of cutaneous squamous cell carcinomas by intralesional interferon alfa-2b therapy," *Journal of the American Medical Association* 269 (February 3, 1993): 578.

Eikje, N. S., K. Aizawa, and Y. Ozaki. "Vibrational spectroscopy for molecular characterisation and diagnosis of benign, premalignant and malignant skin tumours," *Biotechnological Annual Review* 11 (2005): 191–225.

Elias, S., D. S. Emerson, et al. "Ultrasound-guided fetal skin sampling for prenatal diagnosis of genodermatoses," *Obstetrics and Gynecology* 83 (March 1994): 337–341.

Eller, Daryn. "Danger: Rays. How safe are we from UVAs?" *Health* 23 (May 1991): 74–80.

Elston, D. M., S. D. Miller, R. J. Young, J. Eggers, et al. "Comparison of colchicine, dapsone, triamcinolone, and diphenhydramine therapy for the treatment of brown recluse spider envenomation: A double-blind, controlled study in a rabbit model," *Archives of Dermatology* 141, no. 5 (May 2005): 595–597.

Elston, Dirk, and Wilma Bergfeld. "Skin diseases of the hands and feet," *The Physician and Sportsmedicine* 22 (March 1994): 40–48.

Epstein, Ervin. "Molecular genetics of epidermolysis bullosa," *Science* 256 (May 8, 1992): 799–805.

Esgleyes-Ribot, T., R. A. Chandraratna, et al. "Response of psoriasis to a new topical retinoid," *Journal of the American Academy of Dermatology* 30 (April 1994): 581–590.

Ezzell, Carol. "Skin genes underlie blistering disorder," *Science News* 140 (September 28, 1991): 197.

Fackelmann, Kathy A. "Vitamin A-like drug may ward off cancers," *Science News* 141 (May 30, 1992): 358.

Fairley, Janet. "Tretinoin revisited," *The New England Journal of Medicine* 328 (May 20, 1993): 1,436–1,437.

Farndon, P. A., R. G. Del Mastro, D. Evans, and M. Kilpatrick. "Location of gene for Gorlin syndrome," *Lancet* 339 (March 7, 1992): 581–582.

Feldman, S. R., A. Liguori, M. Kucenic, S. R. Rapp, et al. "Ultraviolet exposure is a reinforcing stimulus in frequent indoor tanners," *Journal of the American Academy of Dermatology* 51, no. l (July 2004): 45–51.

Fernandez, D. F., A. H. Wolff, and M. P. Bagley. "Acute cutaneous toxoplasmosis presenting as erythroderma," *International Journal of Dermatology* 33 (February 1994): 129–130.

Fincher, E. F., and R. L. Moy. "Cosmetic blepharoplasty," *Dermatologic Clinics* 23, no. 3 (July 2005): 431–42, vi.

Fitzpatrick, T. B., et al., eds. *Dermatology in General Medicine*. 4th ed. New York: McGraw-Hill, 1993.

Fobi, G., et al. "Ocular findings after ivermectin treatment of patients with high Loa loa microfilaremia," *Ophthalmic Epidemiology* (March 2000): 27–39.

Freeman, L. E., L. K. Dennis, C. F. Lynch, J. B. Lowe, et al. "Test-retest of self-reported exposure to artificial tanning devices, self-tanning creams, and sun sensitivity showed consistency," *Journal of Clinical Epidemiology* 58, no. 4 (April 2005): 430–432.

Freundlich, Naomi. "Homing in on the genetic flaw that causes skin cancer," *Business Week*, November 23, 1992, 87.

Frey, Nadine. "Skin outlook," *Harper's Bazaar*, January 1991, 15–16.

Gage, Diane. "Fighting back: the side effects of Retin-A," *American Health* 9 (June 1990): 18–19.

Galer, B. S., et al. "Topical lidocaine patch relieves postherpetic neuralgia more effectively than a vehicle topical patch: Results of an enriched enrollment study," *Pain* 80 (1999): 533–538.

Gallagher, R. P., J. J. Spinelli, and T. K. Lee. "Tanning beds, sunlamps, and risk of cutaneous malignant melanoma," *Cancer Epidemiology, Biomarkers, and Prevention* 14, no. 3 (March 2005): 562–566.

Gannon, Kathi. "Glycolic acid found helpful in treating problems of the skin," *Drug Topics* 135 (May 6, 1991): 43–44.

Ganske, Mary Garner. "Nine skin signals that can save your life," *Family Circle*, November 3, 1992, 52–54.

Garcia, Lynne. *Diagnostic Medical Parasitology*. Washington, D.C.: ASM Press, 2001.

Garrett, Anne Wolven. "Dermal irritation continued," *Drug & Cosmetic Industry* 152 (June 1993): 16–17.

———. "IPD—immediate pigment darkening," *Drug & Cosmetic Industry* 149 (August 1991): 12.

Gavenas, Mary Lisa. "New cure for wrinkles?" *Glamour*, February 1993, 54.

Geller, A. C., G. Colditz, S. Oliveria, K. Emmons. "Use of sunscreen, sunburning rates, and tanning bed use among more than 10,000 US children and adolescents," *Pediatrics* 109, no. 6 (June 2002): 1,009–1,014.

Gentile, R. D. "Multimodality aesthetic skin rejuvenation," *Facial and Plastic Surgery* 21, no. 2 (May 2005): 120–130.

Gibran, N. S., F. F. Isik, et al. "Basic fibroblast growth factor in the early human burn wound," *Journal of Surgical Research* 56 (March 1994): 226–234.

Gillespie, Sheila, Matthew Carter, Steven Asch, James Rokos, William Gary, Cecelia Tsou, David Hall, Larry Anderson, and Eugene Hurwitz. "Occupational risk of human parvovirus B19 infection for school and daycare personnel during an outbreak of erythema infectiosum," *Journal of the American Medical Association* 263 (April 18, 1990): 2,061–2,064.

Glaser-Sommer, Marjorie. "Taking a shot at wrinkles," *American Health* 11 (May 1992): 28.

Gleason, Suzanne Gleckman. "Facing the bar," *Vogue*, January 1994, 80.

Gorden, P. and O. Gavrilova. "The clinical uses of leptin," *Current Opinion in Pharmacology* 3, no. 6 (December 2003): 655–659.

Gorman, Christine. "Does sunscreen save your skin?" *Time*, May 24, 1993, 69.

Green, Howard. "Cultured cells for the treatment of disease," *Scientific American* 265, November 1991, 96–102.

Greene, Eva-Lynne. "Old wine in new bottles," *American Health* 11 (September 1992): 45.

Gregory, Richard, Randall Roenig, and Ronald Wheeland. "When and when not to use cutaneous laser therapy," *Patient Care* 25 (November 30, 1991): 67–84.

Griffiths, Christopher, Andrew Russman, et al. "Restoration of collagen formation in photodamaged human skin by tretinoin," *The New England Journal of Medicine* 329 (August 19, 1993): 530–536.

Grimes, P. E. "Microdermabrasion," *Dermatological Surgery* 31 (September 2005): 1,160–1,165.

Grossbart, Ted, and Carl Sherman. *Skin Deep: A Mind/Body Program for Healthy Skin*. New York: William Morrow, 1986.

Grosse, G. "Cutaneous histoplasmosis as opportunistic initial infection in AIDS," *Journal of the American Medical Association* 271 (January 19, 1994): 186H.

Gupta, M. A., and B. A. Gilchrest. "Psychosocial aspects of aging skin," *Dermatologic Clinics* 23, no. 4 (October 2005): 643–648.

Habif, T. *Clinical Dermatology: A Color Guide to Diagnosis and Therapy. 3rd ed.* St. Louis, Mo.: Mosby, 1996.

Hall, E. G., et al. "Acyclovir-resistant varicellazoster and HIV infection," *Archives of Diseases in Childhood* 70 (February 1994): 133–135.

Hoffman, Michelle. "A layer by layer look at the skin blister diseases," *Science* 254 (November 22, 1991): 1,111–1,112.

Hom, D. B. "The wound healing response to grafted tissue," *Otolaryngologic Clinics of North America* 27 (February 1994): 13–24.

Hornung, R. L., K. H. Magee, W. J. Lee, L. A. Hansen, and Y. C. Hsieh. "Tanning facility use: Are we exceeding Food and Drug Administration limits?" *Journal of the American Academy of Dermatology* 49, no. 4 (October 2003): 655–661.

Horowitz, H. W., K. Sanghera, et al. "Dermatomyositis associated with Lyme disease: case report and review of Lyme myositis," *Clinical Infectious Diseases* 18 (February 1994): 166–171.

Hruza, G. J., R. G. Geronemus, and J. S. Dover. "Lasers in dermatology," *Archives of Dermatology* 129 (August 1993): 1,026–1,035.

Hruza, G. J., J. S. Dover, et al. "Q-switched ruby laser irradiation of normal human skin," *Archives of Dermatology* 127 (December 1991): 1,799–1,805.

Hsu, T. S., J. S. Dover, M. S. Kaminer, K. A. Arndt, et al. "Why make patients exercise facial muscles for 4 hours after botulinum toxin treatment?" *Archives of Dermatology* 139, no. 7 (July 2003): 948.

Hsu, T. S., B. Zelickson, J. S. Dover, S. Kilmer, et al. "Multicenter study of the safety and efficacy of a 585 nm pulsed-dye laser for the nonablative treatment of facial rhytides," *Dermatologic Surgery* 31, no. 1 (January 2005): 1–9.

Hsu, T. S., J. S. Dover, and K. A. Arndt. "Effect of volume and concentration on the diffusion of botulinum exotoxin A," *Archives of Dermatology* 140, no. 11 (November 2004): 1,351–1,354.

Hughes, B. R., and W. J. Cunliffe. "A prospective study of the effects of isotretinoin on the follicular reservoir and sustainable sebum excretion in patients with acne," *Archives of Dermatology* 130 (March 1994): 31–38.

Iglesias, M. E., A. Espana, et al. "Generalized skin reaction following *Tinea pedis*," *Journal of Dermatology* 211 (January 1994): 31–34.

Imai, S. "Reactions of uninvolved psoriatic skin and normal skin to ultraviolet radiation," *Journal of the American Academy of Dermatology* 30 (April 1994): 657–660.

Isbister, G. K., M. R. Gray, C. R. Balit, R. J. Raven, et al. "Funnel-web spider bite: A systematic review of recorded clinical cases," *Medical Journal of Australia.* 182, no. 8 (April 2005): 407–411.

Isbister, G. K., and R. S. Vetter. "Loxoscelism and necrotic arachnidism: More myths and minor corrections," *Annals of Emergency Medicine* 46, no. 2 (August 2005): 205–206.

Jacob, C. I., J. S. Dover, and M. S. Kaminer. "Acne scarring: a classification system and review of treatment options," *Journal of the American Academy of Dermatology* 45, no. 1 (July 2001): 109–117.

Jaroff, Leon. "Giant step for gene therapy: An experiment on a young girl opens a new era in the fight against hereditary diseases," *Time*, September 24, 1990, 74–77.

Jick, Susan, Barbara Terris, and Hershel Jick. "First trimester topical tretinoin and congenital disorders," *Lancet* 341 (May 8, 1993): 1,181–1,182.

Jimenez, Sherry. "Measles, mumps and pregnancy: here's how to protect yourself and your unborn baby from the effects of these childhood illnesses," *American Baby* 52 (November 1990): 64–66.

Journal of the American Medical Association. "Anogenital warts in children: Clinical and virologic evaluation for sexual abuse," *Journal of the American Medical Association* 265 (April 17, 1991): 1,934.

Kahn, Henry, Dorothy Nelson, Michael Klag, Paul Whelton, Josef Coresh, Clarence Grim, and Lewis Kuller. "Blood pressure and skin color," *Journal of the American Medical Association* 265 (June 12, 1991): 2,957–2,958.

Kalter, D. C. "Laboratory tests for diagnosing and evaluating of leishmaniasis," *Dermatologic Clinics* 12 (January 1994): 37–50.

Kang, S., and Jeffrey S. Dover. "Successful treatment of eruptive pyoderma gangrenosum with IV vancomycin and mezlocillin," *British Journal of Dermatology* 121, no. 3 (September 1990): 389–393.

Kanazi, G., R. W. Johnson, and R. H. Dworkin. "Treatment of postherpetic neuralgia. An update," *Drugs* 59, no. 5 (May 2000): 1,113–1,126.

Karagas, Margaret, Therese Stukel, E. Robert Greenberg, John Baron, et al. "Risk of subsequent basal cell carcinoma and squamous cell carcinoma of the skin among patients with prior skin cancer," *Journal of the American Medical Association* 267 (June 24, 1992): 3,305–3,310.

Karimipour, D. J., S. Kang, T. M. Johnson, J. S. Orringer, et al. "Microdermabrasion: A molecular analysis following a single treatment," *Journal of the American*

Academy of Dermatology 52, no. 2 (February 2005): 215–223.

Karlsrud, Katherine, and Dodi Schultz. "What to do about birthmarks," *Parents*, September 1993, 70–72.

Kauvar, A. N. and J. S. Dover. "Facial skin rejuvenation: laser resurfacing or chemical peel: Choose your weapon," *Dermatologic Surgery* 27, no. 2 (February 2001): 209–212.

Klein, Nancy. "Face off against wrinkles," *Muscle & Fitness*, May 1992, 36–37.

Klinger, Georgette, and Barbara Rowes. *Skincare*. New York: William Morrow, 1979.

Koh, Howard. "Cutaneous melanoma," *The New England Journal of Medicine* 325 (July 18, 1991): 171–183.

Koike, Tadashi, et al. "Severe symptoms of hyperhistaminemia after treatment of acute promyelocytic leukemia with tretinoin," *The New England Journal of Medicine* 327 (August 6, 1992): 385–387.

Kraemer, K. H., et al. "Risk of cutaneous melanoma in dysplastic nevus syndrome types A and B," *New England Journal of Medicine* 315 (1986): 1,615–1,616.

Kurimoto, Il, M. Arana, and J. W. Streilein. "Role of dermal cells from normal and ultraviolet B-damaged skin in induction of contact hypersensitivity and tolerance," *Journal of Immunology* 152, no. 7 (April 1, 1994): 3,317–3,323.

van Laborde, S., J. S. Dover, M. Moore, B. Stewart, et al. "Reduction in injection pain with botulinum toxin type B further diluted using saline with preservative: A double-blind, randomized controlled trial," *Journal of the American Academy of Dermatology* 48, no. 6 (June 2003): 875–877.

Laman, S. D., and T. T. Provost. "Cutaneous manifestations of lupus erythematosus," *Rheumatic Disease Clinics of North America* 20 (February 1994): 195–212.

Larson, Connie, and Dennis West. "Photoreactions and photoprotection," *Drug Topics* 135 (April 8, 1991): 77–83.

Laskin, J. D. "Cellular and molecular mechanisms in photochemical sensitization studies on the mechanism of action of psoralens," *Food and Chemicals Toxics* 32 (February 1994): 119–127.

Lazarus, G. S., D. M. Cooper, et al. "Definitions and guidelines for assessment of wounds and evaluation of healing," *Archives of Dermatology* 130 (April 1994): 489–493.

Lebowitz, Lisa. "Pollution solutions," *Harper's Bazaar*, October 1991, 147–148.

Lebowitz, Lisa, and Constance Cardozo. "Beauty blooms," *Harper's Bazaar*, January 1992, 84–89.

Lee, M. N., S. Gellis, and J. S. Dover. "Eczematous plaques in a patient with liver failure," *Archives of Dermatology* 128 (February 1992): 257, 260.

Lee, M. S. and H. H. Bernstein. "Immunizations, neonatal jaundice, and animal-induced injuries," *Current Opinion in Pediatrics* 17, no. 3 (June 2005): 418–429.

Leffell, David. "Aggressive-growth basal cell carcinoma in young adults," *Journal of the American Medical Association* 267 (March 18, 1992): 1,456.

Lesher, Jack, Norman Levine, and Patricia Treadwell. "Fungal skin infections: common but stubborn," *Patient Care* 28 (January 30, 1994): 16–31.

———. "Antifungals in office dermatology," *Patient Care* 28 (March 15, 1994): 59–69.

Levine, Norman, Scott Sheftel, Ted Eytan, Robert Dorr, et al. "Induction of skin tanning by subcutaneous administration of a potent synthetic melanotropin," *Journal of the American Medical Association* 266 (November 28, 1991): 2,730–2,737.

Lewin, A. H., et al. "Evaluation of retinoids as therapeutic agents in disease," *Pharmacology Research* 11 (February 1994): 192–200.

Lipper, G. M., K. A. Arndt, and J. S. Dover. "Recent therapeutic advances in dermatology," *Journal of the American Medical Association* 283, no. 2 (January 2000): 175–177.

Lister, Pamela. "Skin spots: not every blemish is cause for concern," *New Choices for the Best Years* 30 (August 1990): 34–36.

Littlefield, Robin Wiest. "Are they safe? (sunscreens)," *American Health* 9 (May 1990): 20.

———. "Long-distance dermatology; computer technology expert diagnosis," *American Health* 10 (January–February 1991): 20.

Longley, B., et al. "Altered metabolism of mast-cell growth factor in cutaneous mastocytosis," *The New England Journal of Medicine* 328 (May 6, 1993): 1,302–1,305.

Maheux, R. "A randomized, double-blind, placebo-controlled study of the effects of conjugated estrogens on skin thickness," *American Journal of Obstetrics and Gynecology* 170 (February 1994): 642–649.

Martin, Paul. "Skin cancer: scourge of the sun," *Safety & Health* 143 (May 1991): 82–85.

Marwick, Charles. "Additional steps proposed to ensure antiacne drug used only in appropriate patient population," *Journal of the American Medical Association* 263 (June 20, 1990): 3,125–3,126.

Mayo Clinic editors. "How do I know if laser hair removal is a good option for me?" *Mayo Clinic Women's Healthsource* 9, no. 8 (August 2005): 10.

———. "One on one. Are tanning beds really as bad for you as people say?" *Mayo Clinic Women's Healthsource* 6, no. 10 (October 2002): 8.

Mayo Clinic editors. "Melanoma: What's your risk of developing this type of skin cancer?" *Mayo Clinic Health Letter* 9 (August 1991): 1–3.

———. "Skin cancer: Tried-and-true ways for dealing with the diagnosis," *Mayo Clinic Health Letter* 12 (March 1994): 1–3.

Maytin, E. V., R. F. Horan, and J. S. Dover. "Tumorous nodules on the lower extremity in systemic mastocytosis," *Archives of Dermatology* 127 (March 1991): 406–410.

McCann, Jean. "FDA set to classify all sunscreen products as drugs," *Drug Topics* 137 (January 25, 1993): 67–68.

McCarthy, Laura Flynn. "Research shows hair loss occurs among women for many reasons," *Vogue* 181 (January 1991): 88.

———. "Today's skin-care products give increasingly scientific explanations of their various benefits," *Vogue*, July 1990, 86.

———. "Overdoing cleansing or using the wrong products can irritate skin, but the marriage of medicine and cosmetics is helping to better educate consumers," *Vogue*, April 1990, 216.

Megahed, H., and K. Scharffetter-Kochanek. "Epidermolysis bullosa acquisita: Successful treatment with colchicine," *Archives of Dermatological Research* 286 (1)1994: 35–46.

Men's Health editors. "Just a trim, please. Leave some character," *Men's Health*, 6 October 1991, 20.

Menter, Marcia. "Winning the wrinkle wars," *Redbook*, October 1991, 62–66.

Miles, R. H., T. P. Paxton, et al. "Systemic administration of interferon-gamma impairs wound healing," *Journal of Surgical Research* 56 (March 1994): 288–294.

Miller, C. C., et al. "Ultraviolet B injury increases prostaglandin synthesis through a tyrosine kinase-dependent pathway," *Journal of Biological Chemistry* 269, no. 5 (February 4, 1994): 3,529–3,533.

Miller, Laura. "Feeling the heat: sun protection for professionals," *Working Woman* 16 (July 1991): 74–77.

Mitchnick, Mark. "Microfine zinc oxide: A transparent total sunblock," *Drug & Cosmetic Industry* 153 (August 1993): 38–43.

Monheit, G. D. "Suspension for the aging face," *Dermatologic Clinics* 23, no. 3 (July 2005): 561–573.

Moran, S. A., N. Patten, J. R. Young, et al. "Changes in body composition in patients with severe lipodystrophy after leptin replacement therapy," *Metabolism* 53, no. 4 (April 2004): 513–519.

Morbidity and Mortality Weekly, "Recommendations of the Advisory Committee on Immunization Practices: Use of Anthrax Vaccine in the United States." *Morbidity and Mortality Weekly Report*, Vol. 49 (rr15) (December 15, 2000): 1–20.

Munavalli, G. S., R. A. Weiss, and R. M. Halder. "Photoaging and nonablative photorejuvenation in ethnic skin," *Dermatologic Surgery* 31 (September 2005): 1,250–1,261.

Niamtu, J. 3rd. "Anterior face-lift for correction of middle face aging utilizing a minimally invasive technique," *Dermatologic Surgery* 31, no. 8 (August 2005): 977

Nish, W. A. "The effects of immunotherapy on cutaneous late phase response to antigen," *Journal of Allergy and Clinical Immunology* 93 (February 1994): 484–493.

Nursing Times editors. "Emollient cream," *Nursing Times* 101, no. 31 (August 2005): 31.

Ohtake, N., et al. "Brown papules and leukoderma in Darier's Disease," *Dermatology* 188 (2) 1994: 157–159.

Olbricht, Suzanne, Michael Bigby, and Kenneth Arndt, eds. *Manual of Clinical Problems in Dermatology*. Boston: Little, Brown, 1992.

Omura, N. E., J. S. Dover, K. A. Arndt, and A. N. Kauvar. "Treatment of reticular leg veins with a 1064 nm long-pulsed Nd:YAG laser," *Journal of the American Academy of Dermatology* 48, no. 1 (January 2003): 76–81.

Orkin, Milton, Howard Maibach, and Mark Dahl. *Dermatology*. Norwalk, Conn.: Appleton & Lange, 1991.

Osborne, R., and M. A. Perkins. "An approach for development of alternative test method based on mechanics of skin irritations," *Food and Chemical Toxics* 32 (February 1994): 133–142.

Paller, A. S. "Laboratory tests for ichthyosis," *Dermatologic Clinics* 12 (January 1994): 99–107.

Patient Care editors. "Melanoma detection: a new, improved method," *Patient Care* 26 (May 30, 1992): 13–23.

Pavllichko, Joseph, and Phil Band. "The science of minimizing wrinkles," *Soap-Cosmetics-Chemical Specialties* 68 (February 1992): 33–37.

Pearce, D. J., A. Boles, H. M. Greist, and S. R. Feldman. "Biologic therapy for psoriasis: telephone triage," *Dermatological Nursing* 17, no. 4 (August 2005): 265–270, 295.

Peters, Sue. "A new light on birthmarks," *Health* 7 (January–February 1993): 26–27.

Phillips, Tania, and Jeffrey S. Dover. "Recent advances in dermatology," *The New England Journal of Medicine* 326 (January 16, 1992): 167–179.

Pope, Deborah. "Benign pigmented nevi in children: Prevalence and associated factor," *Journal of the American Medical Association* 268 (November 18, 1992): 2,641.

Posten, W., D. A. Wrone, J. S. Dover, K. A. Arndt, et al. "Low-level laser therapy for wound healing: Mechanism and efficacy," *Dermatologic Surgery* 31, no. 3 (March 2005): 334–340.

Preston, Diana, and Robert S. Stern. "Nonmelanoma cancers of the skin," *The New England Journal of Medicine* 327 (December 3, 1992): 1,649–1,662.

Prevention editors. "Fake and Bake: Indoor tanning is no day at the beach," *Prevention*, May 16, 1993.

———. "Warning spots: mole location may indicate melanoma risk," *Prevention*, July 1990, 11–12.

———. "Smoking's new wrinkle," *Prevention*, October 1991, 12.

———. "Skin cancer preventive: study shows potential for vitamin A derivative," *Prevention*, February 1990, 19–20.

Probert, Christina. *Vogue Beauty and Health Encyclopedia*. London: Octopus Books, 1986.

Rae, Stephen. "Retin-A: acne remedy or wrinkle reducer?" *Modern Maturity*, December–January 1991, 76.

Rafal, Elyse, et al. "Topical tretinoin treatment for liver spots associated with photodamage," *The New England Journal of Medicine* 326 (February 6, 1992): 368–374.

Ramirez, R., and J. Schneider. "Practical guide to sun protection," *The Surgical Clinics of North America* 83, no. 1 (Feb 2003): 97–107.

Ramirez, M. A., M. M. Warthan, T. Uchida, and R. F. Wagner. "Double exposure: Natural and artificial ultraviolet radiation exposure in beachgoers," *Southern Medical Journal* 96, no. 7 (July 2003): 652–655.

Ramon, Y., A. Fodor, and Y. Ullmann. "Deep phenol peeling and fat injection: Treatment option for perioral wrinkles in a scleroderma patient," *Dermatologic Surgery* 31, no. 7 (July 2005): 777–779.

Reali, V. M. "Sonographic evaluation of dermis and subcutaneous tissues during and after skin expansion," *Plastic and Reconstructive Surgery* 93, no. 5 (April 1994): 1,050–1,055.

Reid, Ken, and Luba Vikhanski. "The sun's ominous side: skin cancer," *Medical World News* 33 (February 1992): 18–25.

Roddi, R. "Progressive hemifacial atrophy in patient with lupus erythematosus," *Plastic and Reconstructive Surgery* 93, no. 5 (April 1994): 1,067–1,072.

Rose, Jeanne. *Kitchen Cosmetics*. Berkeley, Calif.: North Atlantic Books, 1990.

Rostan, E. F. "Laser treatment of photodamaged skin," *Facial and Plastic Surgery* 21, no. 2 (May 2005): 99–109.

Rowbotham, M. C., et al. "Gabapentin for the treatment of postherpetic neuralgia: A randomized controlled trial," *Journal of the American Medical Association* 280 (1998): 1,837–1,842.

Rowbotham, M. C., et al. "Lidocaine patch: Double-blind controlled study of a new treatment method for postherpetic neuralgia," *Pain* 65 (1996): 39–44.

Roy, D. "Ablative facial resurfacing," *Dermatologic Clinics* 23, no. 3 (July 2005): 549–559.

Rubenstein, Hal. "Dying of thirst: Reviving your skin," *The New York Times Magazine*, March 27, 1994, S18.

Rudolf, Patricia. "Is your back fit to bare?" *Redbook*, June 1990, 128–129.

Rundle, Rhonda. "Cells 'tricked' to make skin for burn cases," *The Wall Street Journal*, March 17, 1994, B1, E.

Rustad, O. J. "Outdoors and active: Relieving summer's siege on skin," *The Physician and Sportsmedicine* 20 (May 1992): 162–176.

Ryval, Michael. "The facts about fifth disease: How the virus affects children and pregnant women," *Chatelaine*, February 1993, 32.

Saladi, R. N., and A. N. Persaud. "The causes of skin cancer: a comprehensive review," *Drugs Today* 41, no. 1 (January 2005): 37–53.

Sams, W. M. *Principles and Practice of Dermatology*. New York: Churchill, 1990.

Sangiorgio, Maureen, Greg Gutfeld, and Linda Rao. "Helping bad cells age," *Prevention*, February 1992, 18–19.

Sangiorgio, Maureen, Melissa Meyers, and Greg Gutfeld. "So long stretch marks: Vitamin A offshoot may erase unwanted scars," *Prevention*, December 1990, 22.

Scarlett, W. L. "Ultraviolet radiation: sun exposure, tanning beds, and vitamin D levels. What you need to know and how to decrease the risk of skin cancer," *Journal of the American Osteopathic Association* 103, no. 8 (August 2003): 371–375.

Schempp, Christoph. "Further evidence of *Borrelia burgdorferi* infection in morphea and lichen schlerosus et atrophicus confirmed by DNA amplification," *Journal of the American Medical Association* 270 (October 20, 1993): 1801.

Schneider, Phyllis. "Skin caring," *Redbook*, 17 February 1990, 92–93.

Schneiderman, Henry. "What's your diagnosis: pearly penile papules," *Consultant* 31 (July 1991): 39–40.

Schorr, Lia. *Skin Care for Men*. Englewood Cliffs, N.J.: Prentice-Hall, 1985.

Science News editors. "Hot answers to some 'bad hair' problems," *Science News* 144 (December 11, 1993): 391.

———. "Mutation reveals skin's exposure to sun," *Science News* 145 (January 22, 1994): 60.

Schwartz, R. A. "Acanthosis nigricans," *Journal of the American Academy of Dermatology* 31, no. 1 (July 1994): 1–19.

Schwetz, Bernard A. "Artificial skin for grafts," *Journal of the American Medical Association* 285, no. 13 (April 4, 2001).

Scrivner, Charles R., et al., *The Metabolic and Molecular Bases of Inherited Disease*, 7th ed. New York: McGraw Hill, Health Professions Division, 1995.

Scuderi, N., and M. G. Onesti. "Anti-tumor agents," *Annals of Plastic Surgery* 32 (January 1994): 39–44.

Shorell, Irma. *A Lifetime of Skin Beauty.* New York: Simon and Schuster, 1982.

Shum, D. T. "Usefulness of the dissecting microscope in surgical management of skin cancers," *Journal of Dermatologic Surgery and Oncology* 20 (April 1994): 266–271.

Sioutos, N., et al. "Primary Cutaneous Hodgkin's Disease," *American Journal of Dermatopathology* 16, no. 1 (February 1994): 2–8.

Smith, Mark. "Saving your skin," *Saturday Evening Post,* April 1994, 32–33.

Smith, Walter P. "Hydroxy acids and skin aging," *Soap-Cosmetics-Chemical Specialties* 69 (September 1993): 54–58.

Sommi, Roger W. "Drugs that go on top," *Current Health II* 17 (April 1991): 14–15.

Spencer, J. M. "Microdermabrasion," *American Journal of Clinical Dermatology* 6, no. 2 (2005): 89–92.

Stambler, Irwin. "Tissue R&D produces skin replacements," *R&D* 35 (July 1993): 18.

Stehlin, Dori. "Beyond measles and chicken pox: Other childhood diseases cause rashes," *FDA Consumer* 26 (April 1992): 32–35.

Steigleder, Gerd Klaus, and Howard Maibach. *Pocket Atlas of Dermatology.* New York: Thieme Medical Publishers, 1993.

Stratigos, A. J., J. S. Dover, and K. A. Arndt. "Laser treatment of pigmented lesions—2000: How far have we gone?" *Archives of Dermatology* 136, no. 7 (July 2000): 915–921.

Stratigos, A. J., S. Tahan, and J. S. Dover. "Rapid development of nonmelanoma skin cancer after CO2 laser resurfacing," *Archives of Dermatology* 138, no. 5 (May 2002): 696–697.

Sugarman, J. L., T. H. McCalmont, J. Frieden, J. Dover, et al. "Gigantic metameric seborrheic keratosis," *Plastic and Reconstructive Surgery* 111, no. 5 (April 15, 2003): 1,775–1,776.

Sumitra, S., and P. Yesudian. "Friction amyloidosis: a variant or etiologic factor in amyloidosis cuta," *International Journal of Dermatology* 33 (January 1994): 74.

Szentgyorgyi, Tom. "Artificial skin goes on trial," *Popular Science,* April 1991, 24.

Tan, M. H., J. S. Dover, T. S. Hsu, K. A. Arndt, et al. "Clinical evaluation of enhanced nonablative skin rejuvenation using a combination of a 532 and a 1,064 nm laser," *Lasers in Surgery and Medicine* 34, no. 5 (2004): 439–445.

Tardio, Amy. "The black man's guide to skin care," *Gentleman's Quarterly,* March 1994, 174–175.

Taylor, H. S. "Judging a book by its cover: estrogen and skin aging," *Fertility and Sterility* 84, no. 2 (August 2005): 295.

Teot, L., and J. P. Bosse. "The use of scapular skin island flaps in the treatment of axillary postburn scar contractures," *British Journal of Plastic Surgery* 47, no. 2 (March 1994): 108–111.

Thami, G. P., S. Kaur, A. J. Kanwar. "Association of juvenile xanthogranuloma with café-au-lait macules," *International Journal of Dermatology* 40, no. 4 (April 2001): 283–285.

Toutexis, Anastasia. "Fountain of youth in a jar," *Time,* October 14, 1991, 83–84.

Tran, L. P., et al. "Familial multiple glomus tumors," *Annals of Plastic Surgery* 32 (January 1994): 89–91.

Trelles, M. A., X. Alvarez, and M. J. Martin-Vazquez, et al. "Assessment of the efficacy of nonablative long-pulsed 1064-nm Nd:YAG laser treatment of wrinkles compared at 2, 4, and 6 months," *Facial and Plastic Surgery* 21, no. 2 (May 2005): 145–153.

Trelles, M. A., P. Brychta, J. Stanek, and I. Allones, et al. "Laser techniques associated with facial aesthetic and reparative surgery," *Facial and Plastic Surgery* 21, no. 2 (May 2005): 83–98.

Tsao, S. S., J. S. Dover, K. A. Arndt, and M. S. Kaminer. "Scar management: keloid, hypertrophic, atrophic, and acne scars," *Seminars in Cutaneous Medicine and Surgery* 21, no. 1 (March 2002): 46–75.

Tucker, M. A., and A. M. Goldstein. "Melanoma etiology: where are we?" *Oncogene* 22, no. 20 (May 2003): 3,042–3,052.

Turchin, I., B. Barankin, K. W. Alanen, and L. Saxinger. "Dermacase. Dermatophyte infection (tinea)," *Canadian Family Physician* 51 (April 2005): 499–501.

Ujihara, M., S. Hamanaka, et al. "Pemphigus vulgaris associated with autoimmune hemolytic anemia and elevated TNF alpha," *Journal of Dermatology* 21, no. 1 (January 1994): 56–58.

U.S. Preventive Services Task Force. "Counseling to prevent skin cancer: Recommendations and rationale of the U.S. Preventive Services Task Force," *Morbidity and Mortality Weekly Reports: Recommendations and Reports* 52 (October 2003): 13–17.

Valmy, Christine. *Skin Care and Makeup Book.* New York: Crown, 1982.

Vetter, R. S. "Arachnids submitted as suspected brown recluse spiders (Araneae: Sicariidae): Loxosceles spiders are virtually restricted to their known distributions but are perceived to exist throughout the United States," *Journal of Medical Entomology* 42, no. 4 (July 2005): 512–521.

Walker, S. L., J. Morris, A. C. Chu, and A. R. Yong. "Relationship between the ability of sunscreens containing 2-ethylhexyl-4-methoxcinnamate to protect against UVA-induced inflammation, depletion of epidermal

Langerhans cells and suppression of alloactivating capacity of murine skin in vivo," *Journal of Photochemistry and Photobiology* 22 (January 1994): 29–36.

Walzer, Richard. *Healthy Skin: A Guide to Life-long Skin Care.* Mount Vernon, N.Y.: Consumers' Report Books, 1989.

Wang, L. L., et al. "Clinical manifestations in a cohort of 41 Rothmund-Thomson syndrome patients," *American Journal of Medical Genetics* 102, no. 1 (July 2001): 11–17.

Wasco, James. "What your hands say about your health," *Woman's Day,* February 6, 1990, 26.

Wasserman, G. S. "Bites of the brown recluse spider," *New England Journal of Medicine* 352, no. 19 (May 2005): 2,029–2,030.

Watson, C. B. N., and N. Babul. "Efficacy of oxycodone in neuropathic pain: A randomized trial in postherpetic neuralgia," *Neurology* 50 (1998): 1,837–1,841.

Watson, C. B. N. et al. "Nortriptyline versus amtriptyline in postherpetic neuralgia: a randomized trial," *Neurology* 51 (1998): 1,166–1,171.

Weis, Rick. "Melanoma shrinks from human monoclonals," *Science News* 137 (May 26, 1990); 324.

Weiss, R. A. and J. S. Dover. "Leg vein management: Sclerotherapy, ambulatory phlebectomy, and laser surgery," *Seminars in Cutaneous Medicine and Surgery* 21, no. 1 (March 2002): 76–103.

———. "Laser surgery of leg veins," *Dermatologic Clinics* 20, no. 1 (January 2002): 19–36.

Widmer, J., P. Elsner, and G. Burg. "Skin irritant reactivity following experimental cumulative irritant contact dermatitis," *Contact Dermatitis* 30 (January 1994): 35–39.

Wildenberg, S. C. et al. "The gene causing Hermansky-Pudlak Syndrome in a Puerto Rican population maps to Chromosome 10q2," *American Journal of Human Genetics* 57 (1995): 755–765.

Wilson, J. R., C. O. Hagood, and I. D. Prather. "Brown recluse spider bites: A complex problem wound. A brief review and case study," *Ostomy Wound Management* 51, no. 3 (March 2005): 59–66.

Wolff, Klauss, Richard A. Johnson, and Richard Surmond. *Fitzpatrick's Color Atlas & Synopsis of Clinical Dermatology.* New York: McGraw-Hill, 2005.

Woodley, David, Alvin Zelickson, Robert Briggaman, Ted Hamilton, et al. "Treatment of photoaged skin with topical tretinoin increases epidermal-dermal anchlring fibrils: A preliminary report," *Journal of the American Medical Association* 263 (June 13, 1990): 3,057–3,059.

Wooldridge, Wilfred. "Skin conditions that require further investigation," *Consultant* 32 (February 1992): 31–38.

Yaghmai, D., J. M. Garden, A. D. Bakus, E. A. Spenceri, et al. "Hair removal using a combination radio-frequency and intense pulsed light source," *Journal of Cosmetic Laser Therapy* 6, no. 4 (August 2004): 201–207.

Yee, S. "Laser hair removal in Fitzpatrick type IV to VI patients," *Facial Plastic Surgery* 21, no. 2 (May 2005): 139–144.

INDEX

AUG   2008

Northport-East Northport Public Library

To view your patron record from a computer, click on
the Library's homepage: **www.nenpl.org**

You may:
- request an item be placed on hold
- renew an item that is overdue
- view titles and due dates checked out on your card
- view your own outstanding fines

151 Laurel Avenue
Northport, NY 11768
631-261-6930